Dictionary of
Medicinal Drugs

Dictionary of
Medicinal Drugs

Grange
BOOKS

Grange Books
The Grange
Kingsnorth Industrial Estate
Hoo, Near Rochester
Kent ME3 9ND
www.Grangebooks.co.uk

This edition is published by Magpie Books,
an imprint of Constable & Robinson Ltd, for Grange Books 2005

The text of this book was originally published by Oxford University Press as
the *A Z of Medicinal Drugs*© Market House Books Ltd 2000, 2003 reprinted here
by arrangement with Oxford University Press.

A copy of the British Library Cataloguing in Publication Data
is available from the British Library

ISBN 1 84013 886 6

Printed and bound in the European Union

Chief contributor

Jan Hawthorn BSc, PhD

Editor

Elizabeth Martin MA

Production editor

Anne Stibbs BA

Keyboarding

Sandra McQueen

Advisers

J. K. Aronson MA, MBChC, DPhil, FRCP
Richard M. Crosby BSc, MRPharmS, DipPharmPrac
Sarah E. Crotty BPharm, MCPP, DipClinPharm, MRPharmS
Funmi Fajemisin BPharm, DipClinPharm, MRPharmS
Raj Gokami MSc, MRPharmS
Emma Green BPharm, DipClinPharm, MRPharmS
Jane Hough BPharm, MSc, ADCPT, MRPharmS
Y. K. Loke MBBS, MRCP
Jenny J. Mizen BPharm, DipClinPharm, MRPharmS
Jo Panniers BPharm, MRPharmS
Helen Ritchie BSc, DipClinPharm, MRPharmS
Sarah Stoll BSc, MSc, MRPharmS
Lesley Tilson BPharm, DipClinPharm, MRPharmS

AAA Spray (Manx) *See* BENZOCAINE.

abciximab A *monoclonal antibody that has *antiplatelet activity and is used in patients undergoing balloon angioplasty and other forms of heart surgery. It may also be used in the treatment of patients with unstable *angina. Abciximab is used only under specialist supervision, with careful monitoring of blood clotting; it is available as a solution for injection on *prescription only.
Side effects: include excessive bleeding, high blood pressure, nausea, vomiting, blood disorders, and a fast heart rate.
Precautions: abciximab should not be used in people who have had a stroke within the previous two years or recent major surgery, or who have other risk factors for spontaneous bleeding, or by women who are pregnant or breastfeeding. It is also not recommended for patients with certain blood platelet disorders or severe kidney or liver disease.
Proprietary preparation: ReoPro.

Abelcet (Liposome Company) *See* AMPHOTERICIN.

Abidec (Warner-Lambert Consumer Healthcare) A proprietary combination of *vitamin A, vitamins of the B group (*see* VITAMIN B COMPLEX), *vitamin C, and *vitamin D, used as a multivitamin supplement. It is freely available *over the counter in the form of drops.

acamprosate calcium A drug that is used in the treatment of alcohol dependence, for helping people who have achieved a state of abstinence to refrain from drinking again. It should be started as soon as possible after abstinence has been achieved and is usually taken for a period of one year (this is variable), even if the patient has occasional relapses. Acamprosate is available as tablets on *prescription only.
Side effects: include diarrhoea, nausea, vomiting, abdominal pain, and occasionally rash; there may be fluctuations in libido.
Precautions: acamprosate should not be taken by people with severe liver or kidney impairment or by women who are pregnant or breastfeeding.
Proprietary preparation: Campral EC.

acarbose An *oral hypoglycaemic drug that acts by temporarily inhibiting digestive enzymes in the intestine that break down starch and sucrose into glucose: it therefore delays the absorption of glucose and reduces the high blood-glucose concentrations that occur after a meal. Acarbose is used as an *adjunct to *metformin or *sulphonylureas when these have failed to control blood-glucose concentrations in people with noninsulin-dependent (type II) *diabetes mellitus. It is available as tablets on *prescription only.

Side effects: include flatulence, diarrhoea, and abdominal distension and pain; rarely, liver damage may occur.

Precautions: acarbose should be not be taken by people with impaired liver or severely impaired kidney function, inflammatory bowel disease, or a history of bowel surgery or by women who are pregnant or breastfeeding. It may increase the hypoglycaemic effects of *insulin and sulphonylureas.

Interactions with other drugs:

Neomycin: increases the hypoglycaemic effect of acarbose and the severity of gastrointestinal side effects.

Pancreatin: reduces the effect of acarbose.

Proprietary preparation: Glucobay.

Accolate (AstraZeneca) *See* ZAFIRLUKAST.

Accupro (Parke-Davis Medical) *See* QUINAPRIL.

Accuretic (Parke-Davis Medical) A proprietary combination of *quinapril (an ACE inhibitor) and *hydrochlorothiazide (a thiazide diuretic), used in the treatment of *hypertension. It is available as tablets on *prescription only.

Side effects, precautions, and interactions with other drugs: *see* ACE INHIBITORS; THIAZIDE DIURETICS.

See also ANTIHYPERTENSIVE DRUGS; DIURETICS.

acebutolol A cardioselective *beta blocker used for the treatment and prevention of heart *arrhythmias and the treatment of *angina. It is also used in the treatment of *hypertension. It is available as tablets or capsules on *prescription only.

Side effects, precautions, and interactions with other drugs: *see* BETA BLOCKERS.

Proprietary preparations: Sectral; SECADREX (combined with hydrochlorothiazide).

See also ANTI-ARRHYTHMIC DRUGS; ANTIHYPERTENSIVE DRUGS.

aceclofenac An *NSAID used for the treatment of pain and inflammation in rheumatoid arthritis, osteoarthritis, and ankylosing spondylitis (a type of arthritis affecting the spine). It is available as tablets on *prescription only.

Side effects, precautions, and interactions with other drugs: *see* NSAIDS.

Proprietary preparation: Preservex.

ACE inhibitors (angiotensin-converting-enzyme inhibitors) A class of drugs that dilate the arteries (*see* VASODILATORS). They act by suppressing the action of an enzyme that converts an inactive chemical, angiotensin, into angiotensin II, a substance in the bloodstream and tissues that normally narrows the arteries. ACE inhibitors are used for treating *hypertension (high blood pressure); the addition of a *thiazide diuretic can enhance the blood-pressure-lowering effects in those who are not well controlled. ACE inhibitors are also used in the treatment of *heart failure as they reduce the workload of the heart. In addition to reducing the blood pressure they also reduce blood volume by improving the blood supply to the kidneys and increasing the excretion of salt in urine. This latter effect reduces excess body fluids and prevents further accumulation of fluid. *See* CAPTOPRIL; CILAZAPRIL; ENALAPRIL HYDROCHLORIDE; FOSINOPRIL; LISINOPRIL; MOEXIPRIL HYDROCHLORIDE; PERINDOPRIL; QUINAPRIL; RAMIPRIL; TRANDOLAPRIL.

Side effects: ACE inhibitors can cause the blood pressure to fall too rapidly, especially when they are first used; the first dose is therefore usually taken when the patient is in bed and often under medical supervision. Other possible side effects include headache, skin rash, dry cough (which is treatable by *sodium cromoglycate <cromoglicate>) and, less commonly, nausea, muscle cramps, sore throat, and (especially in the elderly and those with kidney disease) impaired kidney function; tests for kidney function should be carried out regularly in the early stages of treatment.

Precautions: people taking ACE inhibitors should generally not take *potassium supplements or potassium-sparing diuretics.

Interactions with other drugs:

Anaesthetics: their effects in lowering blood pressure are increased.

Cyclosporin: increases the risk of high concentrations of potassium in the blood.

Diuretics: their effects in lowering blood pressure are increased; potassium-sparing diuretics can increase concentrations of potassium in the blood and cause toxic effects.

Lithium: levels of lithium in the blood may be increased and cause toxic effects.

NSAIDs: increase the risk of kidney damage.

acemetacin An *NSAID that is a derivative of *indomethacin <indometacin>. It is used for the treatment of pain and inflammation in rheumatoid arthritis and other disorders of the joints and muscles and for the relief of pain after an operation. Acemetacin is available as capsules on *prescription only.

Side effects and precautions: see INDOMETHACIN <INDOMETACIN>; NSAIDS.
Interactions with other drugs: see NSAIDS.
Proprietary preparation: Emflex.

acenocoumarol *See* NICOUMALONE.

Acepril (Ashbourne Pharmaceuticals) *See* CAPTOPRIL.

acetazolamide A *carbonic anhydrase inhibitor that is used for the treatment of *glaucoma: it reduces pressure inside the eye by reducing the formation of aqueous fluid in the eye. It may be used in the treatment of epilepsy (though rarely) and to prevent mountain sickness (although it does not have a *licence for this use). Acetazolamide produces a moderate loss of fluid as urine but is now little used as a *diuretic. It is available, on *prescription only, as tablets, *modified-release capsules, or a form for intravenous injection.

Side effects: the main side effect is *potassium loss, which can result in 'pins and needles', weakness, lethargy, and cramps; nausea, vomiting, flushing, headache, and thirst are among the other side effects. Less commonly drowsiness, rashes, and blood disorders have been reported.

Precautions: acetazolamide is not usually recommended for long-term treatment. It should not be taken by people with low blood concentrations of potassium or sodium, severe liver disease, or kidney disease. It should be used with caution in people with lung diseases, such as asthma or emphysema. Anyone taking acetazolamide should report unusual rashes to their doctor.

Interactions with other drugs:

Antiepileptic drugs: there is an increased risk of potassium loss if carbamazepine is taken with acetazolamide, and acetazolamide increases the plasma concentration of carbamazepine; the risk of osteomalacia may be increased if phenytoin is taken with acetazolamide.

Digoxin and digitoxin: their adverse effects are increased due to potassium depletion by acetazolamide.

Lithium: its excretion is increased (and therefore its effects may be reduced) by acetazolamide.

Quinidine: its excretion is reduced (and therefore its effects enhanced) by acetazolamide.

Proprietary preparations: Diamox; Diamox SR (modified-release capsules).

acetic acid An organic acid that has weak antimicrobial and antifungal activity. It is used in vaginal gels and douches to treat nonspecific vaginal infections by restoring the normal acidity of the vagina. Acetic acid is an ingredient of solutions and paints for application to the skin or nails and of ear drops to treat infections caused by bacteria, fungi, or protozoa. It is also used as a spermicide, an astringent lotion, and as a treatment for warts and calluses. Weak solutions are used to treat coughs in babies. A solution of 4% acetic acid is also known as **artificial vinegar**. Acetic acid is available without a prescription.

Proprietary preparations: Aci-Jel (vaginal jelly); Baby Meltus (cough linctus); GODDARD'S WHITE OIL EMBROCATION (combined with turpentine oil and dilute ammonia solution); OTOMIZE (combined with dexamethasone and neomycin sulphate); PHYTEX (combined with antifungal drugs).

acetylcholine A substance that conveys messages from nerve cells (i.e. it is a neurotransmitter) in the *parasympathetic nervous system. It acts on very small specialized areas of cells of the target tissues called receptors, of which there are two main types: **muscarinic** receptors, found, for example, in smooth muscle (e.g. of the gut and bladder), heart muscle, and endocrine glands; and **nicotinic** receptors, in (for example) skeletal muscle. Drugs whose action resembles that of acetylcholine are called *cholinergic drugs and include *anticholinesterases (or cholinesterase inhibitors). Drugs that prevent the action of acetylcholine include *antimuscarinic (or anticholinergic) drugs and *muscle relaxants used in general anaesthesia.

acetylcholine chloride A salt of *acetylcholine that is used to keep the pupil of the eye dilated during eye surgery. It is available, on *prescription only, as a solution for bathing the eye.
Proprietary preparation: Miochol.

acetylcholinesterase inhibitors A class of drugs that inhibit the action of acetylcholinesterase, an enzyme that breaks down the neurotransmitter *acetylcholine. They therefore increase the amount of acetylcholine that is available for the transmission of nerve impulses. The acetylcholinesterase inhibitors *donepezil hydrochloride and *rivastigmine exert their effects in the brain. They are used in the treatment of Alzheimer's disease, which is associated with a loss in the activity of acetylcholine-secreting nerve cells in the brain.

acetylcysteine A *mucolytic drug that breaks down the mucus that accumulates as filaments in the eye and causes dry eyes. It is also given intravenously as the antidote to *paracetamol overdosage. Acetylcysteine is available, on *prescription only, as eye drops or a solution for intravenous infusion.
Side effects: intravenous infusion of acetylcysteine may cause rashes or allergic reactions.
Precautions: eye drops should not be used with soft contact lenses; intravenous infusions of acetylcysteine should be used with caution in people with asthma.
Proprietary preparations: Parvolex (injection); ILUBE (combined with hypromellose).

acetylsalicylic acid *See* ASPIRIN.

Acezide (Ashbourne Pharmaceuticals) A proprietary combination of *captopril (an ACE inhibitor) and *hydrochlorothiazide (a thiazide diuretic), used in the treatment of mild to moderate *hypertension. It is available as tablets on *prescription only.
Side effects, precautions, and interactions with other drugs: see ACE INHIBITORS; THIAZIDE DIURETICS.
See also ANTIHYPERTENSIVE DRUGS; DIURETICS.

Achromycin

Achromycin (Wyeth Laboratories) *See* TETRACYCLINE HYDROCHLORIDE.

aciclovir (acyclovir) An *antiviral drug that is used specifically to treat herpesvirus infections, including chickenpox, shingles, cold sores, genital herpes, and herpes infections of the eyes or mouth. It works by inhibiting DNA polymerase, the enzyme within human cells that is used by the virus to make viral DNA, which is necessary if the virus is to replicate. Although it may not completely eradicate the virus, aciclovir is more effective if started early after the onset of infection and can be life-saving in patients whose immune systems are compromised. It is also used to prevent infection or recurrence of previous infection in immunocompromised patients. Aciclovir is available, on *prescription only, as dispersible tablets and a suspension for oral use, a solution for intravenous infusion, and as an eye ointment; creams for topical application are available without a prescription, but only from pharmacies.

Side effects: include rashes, nausea and vomiting, headache, dizziness, and fatigue; intravenous infusions may cause local inflammation and (rarely) confusion, hallucinations, and agitation. Local burning, stinging, irritation, or inflammation can occur with topical application; the cream may cause flaking of the skin.

Precautions: people taking aciclovir orally or as an infusion must maintain an adequate intake of fluids. The drug should be used with caution in those with impaired kidney function and in women who are pregnant or breastfeeding. The cream should not be used in the eyes or on mucous membranes (for example in the mouth or vagina) as it may be irritant.

Interactions with other drugs:

Mycophenolate mofetil: the plasma concentrations of both drugs may be increased.

Probenecid: increases the plasma concentration of aciclovir.

Proprietary preparations: Boots Avert (cream); Herpetad (cream); Soothelip (cream); Virasorb (cream); Virovir (tablets); Zovirax; Zovirax Cold Sore Cream.

Acid-Eze (Norton Healthcare) *See* CIMETIDINE.

acid-peptic diseases Conditions associated with the action of gastric (stomach) acid on the lining of the oesophagus (gullet), stomach, or upper sections of the small intestine causing **dyspepsia** (indigestion), marked by pain (**heartburn**) or discomfort. The normal stomach secretes hydrochloric acid as part of the digestive process; however, if the acid enters the lower part of the oesophagus (**gastro-oesophageal reflux**), it can cause pain or actual tissue damage, giving rise to **reflux oesophagitis** (inflammation of the oesophagus). Reflux oesophagitis is more common in people with a **hiatus hernia** (a condition in which a part of the stomach has been pushed upwards through the diaphragm). Pregnant women may suffer reflux and heartburn in the later stages of pregnancy due to the pressure of the fetus on the stomach. **Peptic ulcers**, which most commonly affect the stomach, the lower part of the oesophagus, or the duodenum, may occur when gastric acid is present in abnormally high concentrations but more usually result from other conditions that make the lining of the digestive tract more susceptible to attack by acid. These include the presence of the bacterium *Helicobacter pylori* and the use of *NSAIDs and certain other drugs (e.g. corticosteroids). Ulcers may also be caused or exacerbated by stress, smoking, and alcohol. A rare cause of peptic ulceration is the **Zollinger-Ellison syndrome**, a disorder in which excessive secretion of gastric acid is triggered by the hormone gastrin released by a pancreatic tumour.

Drug treatments for acid-peptic diseases include *antacids, *proton pump inhibitors, and *H_2-receptor antagonists; less commonly *cytoprotectant agents or *antimuscarinic drugs are used. *Helicobacter pylori* is eradicated by a combination of two of the following antibiotics – *clarithromycin, *amoxycillin <amoxicillin>, *metronidazole – and a proton pump inhibitor or *ranitidine bismuth citrate (an H_2-receptor antagonist).

Aci-Jel (Janssen-Cilag) *See* ACETIC ACID.

acipimox A *lipid-lowering drug that is a *nicotinic acid derivative. It lowers both *triglycerides and *cholesterol and is therefore used in the treatment of a variety of *hyperlipidaemias. It acts by inhibiting the breakdown of fats in fatty tissue, thereby typically causing a 20% fall in plasma LDL-cholesterol (*see* LIPOPROTEINS). It is available as capsules on *prescription only.

Side effects: vasodilatation, flushing, itching, and rashes may occur. Occasional side effects are heartburn, pain in the stomach region, nausea, headache, and diarrhoea.

Precautions: acipimox should not be taken by people with severely impaired kidney function or peptic ulcer or by women who are pregnant or breastfeeding because of a lack of data on its safety.

Proprietary preparation: Olbetam.

Acitak (Opus) *See* CIMETIDINE.

acitretin A *retinoid that is used for the treatment of severe extensive *psoriasis that is resistant to other treatments and of severe ichthyosis (abnormal scaling of the skin). It is available as capsules on *prescription only, and treatment must be under hospital supervision.

Side effects: include dryness and thinning of the mucous membranes (for example in the mouth), dryness, redness, and itching of the skin, and dryness of the eyes (which can affect the wearing of contact lenses). Other side effects that may occur include hair loss, muscle or joint aches, nausea, headache, drowsiness, and sweating.

Precautions: acitretin should not be taken by women who are pregnant or breastfeeding, and contraception must be used for one month before and during treatment and for at least two years after stopping treatment (*see* RETINOIDS). It should not be taken by people with impaired liver or kidney function and is not recommended for children. Patients should avoid exposure to ultraviolet light (including excessive sunlight). Tests to monitor liver function, blood sugar, and blood fats should be performed before and during treatment. Donation of blood should be avoided during treatment and for at least a year after stopping treatment.

Interactions with other drugs:

Keratolytics: should not be used with acitretin.

Methotrexate: its plasma concentration (and therefore side effects) are increased by acitretin.

Vitamin A: the risk of vitamin A poisoning is increased if supplements are taken with acitretin.

Warfarin: its anticoagulant effect may be reduced by acitretin.

Proprietary preparation: Neotigason.

Aclacin (Medac) *See* ACLARUBICIN.

aclarubicin A *cytotoxic antibiotic that is similar to *doxorubicin. It is given intravenously for the treatment of leukaemias (*see* CANCER) that are resistant to standard therapy. Aclarubicin is available as an injection on *prescription only.

Side effects: *see* DOXORUBICIN; CYTOTOXIC DRUGS.

Precautions: aclarubicin should not be given to pregnant women and should be used with caution in people with impaired liver or kidney function. *See also* DOXORUBICIN; CYTOTOXIC DRUGS.

Proprietary preparation: Aclacin.

acne (acne vulgaris) A common inflammatory disorder of the sebaceous glands. These grease-producing glands in the skin are under *androgen control, but the cause of acne is unknown. It involves the face, back, and chest and is characterized by the presence of blackheads with papules, pustules, and – in more severe cases – cysts and scars. Mild to moderate acne usually responds to topical therapy with *benzoyl peroxide, *azelaic acid, antibiotics (such as *clindamycin or *erythromycin), or retinoids; other topical treatments include *nicotinamide. More refractory conditions require treatment with long-term oral antibiotics (such as *oxytetracycline or *tetracycline hydrochloride) or (for treating women only) *Dianette (cyproterone and ethinyloestradiol <ethinylestradiol>). Severe acne may need treatment with oral *isotretinoin (a retinoid).

Acnecide (Galderma) *See* BENZOYL PEROXIDE.

Acnidazil (Janssen-Cilag) A proprietary combination of *miconazole nitrate (an antifungal drug) and *benzoyl peroxide (a keratolytic and antiseptic), used for the treatment of acne. It is available as a cream without a *prescription, but only from pharmacies.

Side effects: there may be transient irritation and peeling of the skin.

Precautions: the cream should not come into contact with the eyes, mouth, or mucous membranes, and contact with clothing should be avoided.

Acnisal (DermaPharm) *See* SALICYLIC ACID.

Acoflam, Acoflam 75 SR (Goldshield Pharmaceuticals) *See* DICLOFENAC SODIUM.

Acriflex Cream (Seton Scholl Healthcare) *See* CHLORHEXIDINE.

acrivastine One of the newer (non-sedating) *antihistamines, used to relieve the symptoms of such allergic conditions as hay fever and urticaria. It is available as capsules on *prescription, and packs containing no more than 10 days' supply can be obtained from pharmacies without a prescription.
Side effects, precautions, and interactions with other drugs: *see* ANTIHISTAMINES.
Proprietary preparations: Benadryl Allergy Relief; Semprex.

Actal (Seven Seas) *See* ALEXITOL SODIUM.

Actifed (Warner-Lambert Consumer Healthcare) A proprietary combination of *pseudoephedrine (a decongestant) and *triprolidine (an antihistamine), used to relieve the symptoms of coughs, colds, and hay fever. Actifed is available as a syrup without a prescription, but only from pharmacies. It cannot be prescribed on the NHS.
Side effects and interactions with other drugs: *see* ANTIHISTAMINES; DECONGESTANTS; EPHEDRINE HYDROCHLORIDE.
Precautions: Actifed should not normally be given to children under two years old. *See also* ANTIHISTAMINES; DECONGESTANTS; EPHEDRINE HYDROCHLORIDE.

Actifed Compound Linctus (Warner-Lambert Consumer Healthcare) A proprietary combination of *dextromethorphan (a cough suppressant), *pseudoephedrine (a decongestant), and *triprolidine (an antihistamine), used for the relief of dry coughs and congestion of the upper airways (including that due to hay fever and similar allergic conditions). It is available without a prescription, but only from pharmacies. It cannot be prescribed on the NHS.
Side effects and interactions with other drugs: *see* ANTIHISTAMINES; DECONGESTANTS; DEXTROMETHORPHAN; EPHEDRINE HYDROCHLORIDE; OPIOIDS.
Precautions: this medicine should not normally be given to children under two years old. *See also* ANTIHISTAMINES; DECONGESTANTS; EPHEDRINE HYDROCHLORIDE; OPIOIDS.

Actifed Expectorant (Warner-Lambert Consumer Healthcare) A proprietary combination of *guaiphenesin <guaifenesin> (an expectorant), *pseudoephedrine (a decongestant), and *triprolidine (an antihistamine), used for the relief of productive coughs associated with nasal congestion. It is available as a liquid without a prescription, but only from pharmacies. It cannot be prescribed on the NHS.

Side effects and interactions with other drugs: see ANTIHISTAMINES; DECONGESTANTS; EPHEDRINE HYDROCHLORIDE; GUAIPHENESIN <GUAIFENESIN>.

Precautions: this medicine should not normally be given to children under two years old. *See also* ANTIHISTAMINES; DECONGESTANTS; EPHEDRINE HYDROCHLORIDE; GUAIPHENESIN <GUAIFENESIN>.

Actifed Junior Cough Relief (Warner-Lambert Consumer Healthcare) A proprietary combination of *dextromethorphan (a cough suppressant) and *triprolidine (an antihistamine) used for the relief of dry coughs in children. It is available as a liquid without a prescription, but only from pharmacies. It cannot be prescribed on the NHS.

Side effects, precautions, and interactions with other drugs: see DEXTROMETHORPHAN; OPIOIDS; ANTIHISTAMINES.

Actilyse (Boehringer Ingelheim) *See* ALTEPLASE.

Actinac (Hoechst Marion Roussel) A proprietary combination of *chloramphenicol (an antibiotic), *hydrocortisone (a corticosteroid), the *keratolytics butoxyethyl nicotinate and *sulphur, and *allantoin (an abrasive agent and astringent), used for the treatment of acne. It is available as a lotion on *prescription only.

Side effects: include reddening of the skin.

Precautions: Actinac should not be used during pregnancy. *See also* TOPICAL STEROIDS.

actinomycin D *See* DACTINOMYCIN.

activated charcoal An agent that can adsorb (bind) many poisons in the stomach and therefore prevent them from being absorbed. It is used after swallowing poisons or taking an overdose of drugs and should be taken as soon as possible after the poisoning has occurred, although it may still be effective up to two hours after the poison has been consumed. Activated charcoal is also included in dressings to absorb the odour of infected wounds. Charcoal itself reduces flatulence and abdominal distension and is included as an ingredient in some preparations for the treatment of indigestion. Activated charcoal is available as a powder, effervescent granules, or a suspension and can be obtained without a prescription, but only from pharmacies.

Proprietary preparations: Carbomix (powder); Liqui-Char (suspension); Medicoal (granules); CARBELLON (combined with magnesium hydroxide and peppermint oil).

Actonorm Gel (Wallace Manufacturing) A proprietary combination of *aluminium hydroxide and *magnesium hydroxide (antacids), activated *dimethicone <dimeticone> (an antifoaming agent), and *peppermint oil (an antispasmodic), used for the treatment of flatulence, indigestion, and discomfort due to overeating. It is available as a suspension and can be obtained without a prescription, but only from pharmacies.

Side effects and interactions with other drugs: see ANTACIDS.

Precautions: Actonorm Gel is not recommended for children. *See also* ALUMINIUM HYDROXIDE; MAGNESIUM SALTS.

Actonorm Powder (Wallace Manufacturing) A proprietary combination of *atropine sulphate and *peppermint oil (antispasmodics), and *aluminium hydroxide, *calcium carbonate, *magnesium trisilicate, *magnesium carbonate, and *sodium bicarbonate (all antacids), used for the treatment of indigestion (except that caused by ulcers) and flatulence. It is available from pharmacies without a prescription and cannot be prescribed on the NHS.

Side effects and precautions: see ATROPINE SULPHATE; MAGNESIUM SALTS; ANTACIDS.

Interactions with other drugs: see ATROPINE SULPHATE; ANTACIDS.

Acular (Allergan) *See* KETOROLAC TROMETAMOL.

Acupan (3M Health Care) *See* NEFOPAM.

acyclovir *See* ACICLOVIR.

Adalat (Bayer) *See* NIFEDIPINE.

adapalene A drug that resembles the *retinoids and is used for the treatment of mild to moderate acne in which blackheads and pustules predominate. It is available as a gel on *prescription only.

Side effects: adapalene may irritate the skin. If irritation is severe, treatment should be stopped.

Precautions: adapalene should not be used on broken or sunburnt skin, by people with eczema or a personal or family history of skin cancer, or by pregnant women (effective contraception should be used during treatment). It should not be applied near the eyes, lips, nostrils, or mouth, and excessive exposure of treated skin to sunlight should be avoided. Adapalene should not be used with retinoids or *keratolytics.

Proprietary preparation: Differin.

Adcortyl (Bristol-Myers Squibb) *See* TRIAMCINOLONE ACETONIDE.

Adcortyl in Orabase (Bristol-Myers Squibb) A proprietary combination of *triamcinolone acetonide (a potent steroid) and *carmellose (a protective agent), used for the treatment of mouth ulcers, sores, and ulcers caused by ill-fitting dentures, trauma, or gingivitis. It is available as a paste on *prescription only, but a 5-gram tube for the treatment of mouth ulcers can be obtained from pharmacies without a prescription.

Side effects: see TOPICAL STEROIDS.

Precautions: see TOPICAL STEROIDS. In addition, this preparation should not be used in people with untreated infections of the mouth or throat or in those with tuberculosis.

Adcortyl with Graneodin (Bristol-Myers Squibb) A proprietary combination of *triamcinolone acetonide (a potent steroid) and the antibiotics *neomycin sulphate and *gramicidin, used for the treatment of skin conditions when bacterial infections may be present and infected insect bites. It is available as a cream on *prescription only.

Side effects and precautions: see TOPICAL STEROIDS.

addiction *See* DEPENDENCE.

Adenocor (Sanofi Winthrop) *See* ADENOSINE.

adenosine A drug that is used for rapid restoration of normal heart rhythm and to help diagnose different types of *arrhythmia. A *prescription only drug in the form of a sterile solution for injection, it is available only for use in hospitals.

Side effects: include transient flushing, chest pain, breathlessness, a choking sensation, nausea, and light-headedness.

Precautions: adenosine should not be given to people with asthma or heart block. *See also* ANTI-ARRHYTHMIC DRUGS.

Interactions with other drugs:

Dipyridamole: enhances the effects of adenosine, therefore a reduction in the dose of adenosine is recommended if it is prescribed with dipyridamole.

Theophylline: inhibits the action of adenosine.

Proprietary preparation: Adenocor.

See also ANTI-ARRHYTHMIC DRUGS.

Adipine MR (Trinity Pharmaceuticals) *See* NIFEDIPINE.

Adizem-XL, Adizem-SR (Napp Pharmaceuticals) *See* DILTIAZEM HYDROCHLORIDE.

adjunct A drug that is used in conjunction with another to provide additional beneficial effects in order to achieve the best treatment of a condition. The adjunct has the role of 'helping' or 'supporting' the main drug used in the treatment. The adjunct may have a mode of action that is different from that of the principal drug. For example, ranitidine bismuth citrate (an H_2-receptor antagonist) is used as an adjunct to antibiotics for the eradication of *Helicobacter pylori*, the bacterium associated with peptic ulcers.

adrenaline <epinephrine> A hormone that is secreted by the centre (medulla) of the adrenal glands into the bloodstream in conditions of stress. It acts on *adrenoceptors to cause constriction of some blood vessels and dilatation of others, increasing blood flow to the heart and skeletal muscles. The heart rate is increased, while the muscles of the intestine and airways relax. As a drug, adrenaline is available in various forms on *prescription only. It is given by intramuscular injection to relieve the effects of anaphylactic shock (an extreme and potentially fatal allergic reaction; *see* ANAPHYLAXIS) and by intravenous injection to treat cardiac arrest. It is given with *local anaesthetic preparations because it constricts blood vessels and thus confines the local anaesthetic to the area of application. It is also available as eye drops to treat *glaucoma, in which it reduces the production of aqueous fluid in the eye and increases its outflow.

Side effects: when adrenaline is given by injection side effects include dry mouth, palpitation, cold hands and feet, nervousness, tremor, and headache; there may be stomach pain after inhalation. Side effects with eye drops include smarting and redness of the eye and headache.

Interactions with other drugs:

Anaesthetics: irregular heartbeats (*arrhythmias) may occur if adrenaline is given with certain anaesthetics.

Antidepressants: hypertension (raised blood pressure) and arrhythmias may occur if adrenaline is given with tricyclic antidepressants.

Beta blockers: severe hypertension may occur if these drugs are given with adrenaline.

Dopexamine: may increase the effects of adrenaline.

Entacapone: may increase the effects of adrenaline.

Proprietary preparations: Epipen and Epipen Junior (disposable pens for self-injection); Eppy (eye drops); Min-I-Jet Adrenaline (injection); Simplene (eye drops); GANDA (combined with guanethidine monosulphate).

adrenoceptors Specialized areas in the membranes of cells on which noradrenaline <norepinephrine>, and to a lesser extent adrenaline <epinephrine>, act to convey messages from the nerves of the *sympathetic nervous system to their target tissues. There are two main types of adrenoceptors: **alpha receptors** and **beta receptors**. Stimulation of alpha receptors by noradrenaline <norepinephrine> causes (among other effects) constriction of arteries (*vasoconstriction); stimulation of beta receptors causes an increase in heart rate, widening of airways, relaxation of the muscle of the uterus, and dilatation of arteries (*vasodilatation).

Drugs that act on adrenoreceptors either stimulate them and increase their normal activity or block them and prevent their normal actions. Drugs that mimic the effects of noradrenaline <norepinephrine>are called *sympathomimetic drugs. There are two classes of drugs that block the effects of noradrenaline <norepinephrine>; they are known as *alpha blockers and *beta blockers (they used to be called sympatholytic drugs). Some drugs (*carvedilol and *labetalol) block both alpha and beta receptors and are used to treat *hypertension.

Adult Meltus Expectorant with Decongestant (Seton Scholl Healthcare) A proprietary combination of *guaiphenesin <guaifenesin> (an expectorant), *pseudoephedrine (a decongestant), and *menthol, used to relieve the symptoms of coughs and colds. This liquid is freely available *over the counter. It cannot be prescribed on the NHS.

Side effects and interactions with other drugs: see EPHEDRINE HYDROCHLORIDE; GUAIPHENESIN <GUAIFENESIN>.

Precautions: this medicine should not be taken by children under 12 years old. *See also* EPHEDRINE HYDROCHLORIDE.

Advil, Advil Extra Strength (Whitehall Laboratories) *See* IBUPROFEN.

AeroBec Autohaler, AeroBec Forte (3M Health Care) *See* BECLOMETHASONE <BECLOMETASONE> DIPROPIONATE.

Aerocrom (Castlemead Healthcare) A proprietary combination of *sodium cromoglycate <cromoglicate> (a chromone) and *salbutamol (a bronchodilator), used for the prevention of asthma in individuals who require both drugs. It is available in a metered-dose aerosol on *prescription only. **Aerocrom Syncroner** is fitted with a spacer device.

Side effects: include low potassium concentrations in blood, fine tremor, headache, coughing, throat irritation, and rarely wheezing and breathlessness.

Precautions: Aerocrom should be used with caution by people with an overactive thyroid gland, angina, high blood pressure, or *arrhythmias and by women who are pregnant or breastfeeding.

Interactions with other drugs:

Sympathomimetic drugs: increase the risk of adverse effects and should not to be used in conjunction with Aerocrom.

Aerolin Autoinhaler (3M Health Care) *See* SALBUTAMOL.

aerosol A suspension of extremely small liquid or solid particles (about 0.001 mm diameter) in a gas. Drugs in aerosol form may be administered by inhalation (*see* INHALER).

Afrazine (Schering-Plough) *See* OXYMETAZOLINE.

agonist A drug that acts at a cell-receptor site to produce an effect that is the same as, or similar to, that of the body's normal chemical messenger. *Cholinergic drugs, which have effects similar to the neurotransmitter acetylcholine, are examples.

AIDS (acquired immune deficiency syndrome) *See* HIV.

Ailax, Ailax Forte (Galen) *See* CO-DANTHRAMER.

Airomir (3M Health Care) *See* SALBUTAMOL.

Akineton (Knoll) *See* BIPERIDEN.

Aknemin (Merck Pharmaceuticals) *See* MINOCYCLINE.

albendazole An *anthelmintic used for the treatment of hydatid cysts (caused by the tapeworm *Echinococcus*); it may be used in conjunction with surgery. Albendazole is available as tablets on *prescription only.
Side effects: include stomach and bowel upsets, headache, and dizziness; rarely there may be reversible baldness, rash, fever, and blood disorders.
Precautions: albendazole should not be taken during pregnancy; contraception should be used during treatment and for up to one month after stopping treatment. The drug should be used with caution by women who are breastfeeding. Blood counts and liver tests should be carried out during treatment.
Proprietary preparation: Eskazol.

alclometasone dipropionate A moderately potent *topical steroid used for the treatment of a variety of skin disorders. It is available as a cream or ointment on *prescription only.
Side effects and precautions: see TOPICAL STEROIDS.
Proprietary preparation: Modrasone.

Alcobon (ICN Pharmaceuticals) *See* FLUCYTOSINE.

Alcoderm (Galderma) *See* LIQUID PARAFFIN.

Aldactide 25, Aldactide 50 (Searle) *See* CO-FLUMACTONE.

Aldactone (Searle) *See* SPIRONOLACTONE.

aldesleukin An *interleukin produced by genetic engineering techniques and used for the treatment of certain patients with cancer of the kidney that has produced secondary tumours. A *prescription only medicine, it is given by intravenous infusion, but only in specialist units.
Side effects: aldesleukin is highly toxic, causing *bone marrow suppression, damage to the liver, kidneys, thyroid gland, brain, and spinal cord, and pulmonary *oedema with low blood pressure.
Interactions with other drugs:
  Antihypertensive drugs: aldesleukin increases the blood-pressure-lowering effect of these drugs.
Proprietary preparation: Proleukin.

Aldomet (Merck Sharp & Dohme) *See* METHYLDOPA.

Alec (Britannia Pharmaceuticals) *See* PUMACTANT.

alendronic acid A *bisphosphonate used for the treatment of osteoporosis in postmenopausal women: it acts by preventing loss of calcium from bone and therefore increases bone density. It is available as tablets on *prescription only.

Side effects: include ulcers and inflammation of the oesophagus (gullet), abdominal pain and distension, diarrhoea or constipation, flatulence, muscle pain, and headache; rarely, nausea and vomiting, peptic ulcers, or a rash may occur.

Precautions: if there are any signs of irritation of the oesophagus (difficulty in swallowing, new or worsening heartburn), the drug should be discontinued immediately and a doctor contacted. Food and some drugs (see below) bind to alendronic acid in the stomach and intestine and prevent its absorption. Therefore the tablets should be swallowed whole, with a full glass of water, on an empty stomach at least 30 minutes before breakfast. The patient should then remain standing or sitting upright for at least 30 minutes and not lie down until after eating breakfast. The tablets should not be taken at bedtime or before rising. Alendronic acid should not be taken by anyone with disorders of the oesophagus or peptic ulcers. It should be used with caution by those with impaired kidney function and should not be taken by women who are pregnant or breastfeeding.

Interactions with other drugs:

Aminoglycosides: in combination with alendronic acid, they may cause abnormally low concentrations of calcium in the plasma.

Antacids: reduce the absorption of alendronic acid.

Calcium supplements: reduce the absorption of alendronic acid.

Iron supplements: reduce the absorption of alendronic acid.

NSAIDs: alendronic acid may increase the gastrointestinal effects of NSAIDs.

Proprietary preparation: Fosamax.

alexitol sodium An aluminium-containing drug that is used as an *antacid for the relief of indigestion and stomach upsets. It is freely available *over the counter in the form of tablets.

Side effects, precautions, and interactions with other drugs: see ALUMINIUM HYDROXIDE; ANTACIDS.

Proprietary preparation: Actal.

alfacalcidol A derivative of *vitamin D used to prevent and treat the bone disease that may occur in kidney dialysis patients and to treat low blood calcium levels due to lack of *parathyroid hormone in people with poorly functioning parathyroid glands. It is also used to treat rickets that does not respond to vitamin D and osteomalacia (softening of the bones). Alfacalcidol is available as capsules or a solution on *prescription only.

Side effects, precautions, and interactions with other drugs: *see* VITAMIN D.

Proprietary preparations: Alfa D (capsules); One Alpha (capsules or solution).

Alfa D (APS-Berk) *See* ALFACALCIDOL.

alfuzosin hydrochloride An *alpha blocker used to relieve urinary obstruction in men with an enlarged prostate gland. It is available as tablets or *modified-release tablets on *prescription only.
Side effects and interactions with other drugs: *see* ALPHA BLOCKERS.
Precautions: alfuzosin should not be taken by people with severely impaired liver function. *See also* ALPHA BLOCKERS.
Proprietary preparations: Xatral; Xatral SR (modified-release tablets).

Algesal (Solvay Healthcare) *See* DIETHYLAMINE SALICYLATE.

Algicon (Rhône-Poulenc Rorer) A proprietary combination of *aluminium hydroxide, magnesium alginate (*see* ALGINIC ACID), *magnesium carbonate, and *potassium bicarbonate, used as an *antacid for the relief of heartburn associated with gastric reflux, reflux oesophagitis, hiatus hernia, pregnancy, and increased secretion of stomach acid (*see* ACID-PEPTIC DISEASES). It is available as tablets or a suspension and can be obtained from pharmacies without a prescription.
Side effects and interactions with other drugs: *see* ANTACIDS.
Precautions: Algicon is not recommended for children under 12 years old and should not be taken by people with kidney failure. The tablets have a high sugar content and should therefore be used with caution by people with diabetes.

alginic acid A complex carbohydrate extracted from certain brown seaweeds (kelps). It absorbs water to form a slightly sticky gel. Alginic acid or its compounds, **magnesium alginate** and **sodium alginate**, are included in many *antacid preparations because they form a thick layer on the surface of the stomach contents, providing a mechanical barrier to protect the oesophagus from reflux (*see* ACID-PEPTIC DISEASES).
Proprietary preparations: Gaviscon Infant (sugar-free powder of sodium alginate and magnesium alginate); ALGICON (combined with aluminium hydroxide, magnesium carbonate, and potassium bicarbonate); ASILONE HEARTBURN (combined with aluminium hydroxide, magnesium trisilicate, and sodium bicarbonate); GAVISCON ADVANCE (combined with potassium bicarbonate); GAVISCON LIQUID (combined with sodium bicarbonate and calcium carbonate); GAVISCON TABLETS (combined with aluminium hydroxide, magnesium trisilicate, and sodium bicarbonate); PEPTAC (combined with sodium bicarbonate and calcium carbonate); PYROGASTRONE (combined with carbenoloxone sodium, magnesium trisilicate, sodium bicarbonate, and aluminium hydroxide).

Algipan Rub (Whitehall Laboratories) A proprietary combination of the rubefacients *capsicum oleoresin, *glycol salicylate, and *methyl nicotinate in the form of a cream, used for the relief of muscular and rheumatic aches, pains, and stiffness, including backache, sciatica, lumbago, and fibrositis. It is freely available *over the counter.
Side effects and precautions: see RUBEFACIENTS.

Algitec (SmithKline Beecham Pharmaceuticals) A proprietary combination of *cimetidine (an H$_2$-receptor antagonist) and *alginic acid, used for the treatment of gastro-oesophageal reflux disease (*see* ACID-PEPTIC DISEASES). It is available, on *prescription only, as chewable tablets (**Algitec Chewtab**), which should be thoroughly chewed, or as a sugar-free suspension.
Side effects, precautions, and interactions with other drugs: see CIMETIDINE.

alglucerase An enzyme preparation used to replace an enzyme deficiency that gives rise to Gaucher's disease, an inherited disorder in which lipids accumulate in the bone marrow, liver, spleen, lymph nodes, and other tissues. Alglucerase is available as a form for intravenous infusion on *prescription only; its use is restricted to specialists.
Side effects: include abdominal pain, diarrhoea, nausea, vomiting, pain and irritation at the injection site, and possibly allergic reactions.
Precautions: alglucerase should not be given to people with certain types of cancer and should be used with caution in women who are pregnant or breastfeeding.
Proprietary preparation: Ceredase.
See also IMIGLUCERASE.

alimemazine tartrate *See* TRIMEPRAZINE TARTRATE.

alkaloids A group of nitrogen-containing substances that are produced by plants and can have potent effects on body functions. Many alkaloids are medicinally important drugs, including *morphine, *quinine, and *atropine.

Alka-Seltzer (Bayer) *See* ASPIRIN.

Alka-Seltzer XS (Bayer) A proprietary combination of *aspirin and *paracetamol (analgesics) and *caffeine (a stimulant), used for the relief of headache and other symptoms caused by overindulgence in alcohol and food. It is freely available *over the counter as effervescent tablets.
Side effects and precautions: see ASPIRIN; PARACETAMOL; CAFFEINE.
Interactions with other drugs: see ASPIRIN.

Alkeran (GlaxoWellcome) *See* MELPHALAN.

alkylating drugs A class of *cytotoxic drugs that prevent cell replication by binding to DNA and preventing the separation of two DNA chains during cell division. They are widely used to treat a variety of cancers. These drugs cause the side effects common to all cytotoxic drugs but are particularly damaging to eggs and sperm and may therefore cause infertility. Their long-term use has also been associated with an increase in the incidence of non-lymphocytic leukaemia. The common alkylating drugs are *cyclophosphamide, *ifosfamide, *chlorambucil, *melphalan, *busulphan <busulfan>, *lomustine, *carmustine, *mustine <chlormethine>, *estramustine, *treosulfan, and *thiotepa.

allantoin An abrasive and *astringent agent that is included in preparations for the treatment of acne, *psoriasis, and other skin disorders and in preparations for the relief of *haemorrhoids and other irritating conditions of the anus or rectum.

Proprietary preparations: ACTINAC (combined with chloramphenicol, hydrocortisone acetate, butoxyethyl nicotinate, and sulphur); ALPHOSYL (combined with coal tar); ALPHOSYL HC (combined with coal tar and hydrocortisone); ANODESYN (combined with lignocaine <lidocaine>); DERMALEX (combined with hexachlorophane and squalane).

Allegron (Dista) *See* NORTRIPTYLINE.

Aller-eze (Novartis Consumer Health) *See* CLEMASTINE.

Aller-eze Cream (Novartis Consumer Health) *See* DIPHENHYDRAMINE.

Aller-eze Plus (Novartis Consumer Health) A proprietary combination of *phenylpropanolamine (a decongestant) and *clemastine (an antihistamine), used for the treatment of hay fever and other allergic conditions associated with nasal and sinus congestion. It is available as tablets without a prescription, but only from pharmacies.

Side effects, precautions, and interactions with other drugs: see ANTIHISTAMINES; DECONGESTANTS; EPHEDRINE HYDROCHLORIDE.

allopurinol A drug used for the prevention and long-term treatment of gout and for the treatment of kidney stones; it acts by reducing the formation of uric acid in the body. It is not used to control acute attacks of gout, and may in fact exacerbate symptoms if started during an attack. It may be used in conjunction with *probenecid or *sulphinpyrazone <sulfinpyrazone>. Allopurinol is available as tablets on *prescription only.

Side effects: rashes may indicate a serious allergic condition and should be reported to a doctor; other side effects include nausea and (rarely) malaise and headache.

Precautions: people taking allopurinol must maintain an adequate fluid intake (at least 2 litres a day) to prevent crystals of uric acid being passed in the urine (which can cause pain and bleeding). Alcohol should be avoided. Allopurinol should not be taken by people with liver or kidney disease.

Interactions with other drugs:

Anticoagulants: allopurinol enhances the anticoagulant effects of warfarin and nicoumalone <acenocoumarol>.

Captopril: allopurinol increases the risk of captopril causing adverse effects.

Cyclosporin: allopurinol increases plasma concentrations of cyclosporin and may cause adverse effects.

Cytotoxic drugs: allopurinol prevents the breakdown of azathioprine and mercaptopurine and markedly increases the risk of their adverse effects.

Proprietary preparations: Caplenal; Cosuric; Rimapurinol; Xanthomax; Zyloric.

Almodan (Cox Pharmaceuticals) *See* AMOXYCILLIN <AMOXICILLIN>.

almond oil An oil expressed from almond nuts. It is used as an *emollient in skin creams and is also used to soften earwax.

Proprietary preparations: EAREX EAR DROPS (combined with camphor and arachis oil); IMUDERM THERAPEUTIC OIL (combined with liquid paraffin); INFADERM THERAPEUTIC OIL (combined with liquid paraffin).

aloes *See* ALOIN.

aloin A compound derived from **aloes**, the juice of leaves of various species of *Aloe*. Both aloin and aloes are *stimulant laxatives used for the relief of constipation and its associated discomfort. Aloin is available as tablets that can be obtained without a prescription, but only from pharmacies. Aloes is an ingredient of a compound laxative.

Side effects: *see* STIMULANT LAXATIVES.

Precautions: this laxative is not recommended for children. *See also* STIMULANT LAXATIVES.

Proprietary preparations: Beechams Pills; Calsalettes; POTTER'S CLEANSING HERB (combined with cascara and senna).

Alomide (Galen) *See* LODOXAMIDE.

aloxiprin A compound of *aspirin and *aluminium oxide. It has the same actions as aspirin and is used as an *analgesic and antipyretic agent. Aloxiprin is available as an ingredient in *over the counter analgesics.

Side effects, precautions, and interactions with other drugs: *see* ASPIRIN.

Proprietary preparation: ASKIT (combined with aspirin and caffeine).

alpha blockers (α-blockers; in full **alpha-adrenoceptor blockers**) *Vasodilator drugs that act by blocking the effect of noradrenaline <norepinephrine> on peripheral blood vessels. Noradrenaline normally acts at alpha-*adrenoceptors to constrict blood vessels; therefore opposing these actions causes widening of small arteries (arterioles) and a drop in blood pressure. This arteriolar widening also improves blood flow to areas of poor blood flow and therefore improves oxygen supply. Alpha blockers act on blood vessels and the ring of muscle that controls the opening of the bladder; they are used to treat *hypertension and in the management of bladder problems due to an enlarged prostate. Alpha blockers have beneficial effects on plasma lipids and are suitable for people with diabetes or heart failure.

See ALFUZOSIN HYDROCHLORIDE; DOXAZOSIN; INDORAMIN HYDROCHLORIDE; PHENOXYBENZAMINE HYDROCHLORIDE; PHENTOLAMINE; PRAZOSIN; TAMSULOSIN HYDROCHLORIDE; TERAZOSIN; THYMOXAMINE <MOXISYLYTE>.

Side effects: sedation, dizziness (especially when standing up suddenly), and hypotension (low blood pressure) are quite common. Less common side effects are drowsiness, weakness and loss of energy, depression, headache, dry mouth, stuffy nose, nausea, urinary retention (difficulty in passing urine), and palpitation.

Precautions: the first dose may cause low blood pressure (especially in elderly people) and should be given when the patient is lying down or about to lie down. For this reason people may be started on low dosages and the dosage increased as necessary. Alpha blockers must be taken with caution, after appropriate dosage reduction, by people taking other antihypertensive medication. See also ANTIHYPERTENSIVE DRUGS.

Interactions with other drugs: a number of drugs enhance the action of alpha blockers in lowering blood pressure. These include antidepressants, beta blockers, calcium antagonists, and diuretics. Thymoxamine <moxisylyte> can interact with other alpha blockers to cause a severe fall in blood pressure on standing up.

Alphaderm (Procter & Gamble) A proprietary combination of *hydrocortisone (a corticosteroid) and *urea (a hydrating agent), used for the treatment of *eczema and dermatitis. It is available as a cream on *prescription only.
Side effects and precautions: see TOPICAL STEROIDS.

Alphagan (Allergan) See BRIMONIDINE TARTRATE.

Alphaglobin (Grifols) See IMMUNOGLOBULINS.

Alpha Keri Bath (Bristol-Myers Squibb) A proprietary combination of *liquid paraffin and *lanolin oil (both emollients), used for the treatment of dry skin conditions. It is available as a bath oil and can be obtained without a prescription, but only from pharmacies.

Alphanate (Grifols) See FACTOR VIII.

Alpha-Nine (Grifols) See FACTOR IX.

Alphaparin (Grifols) See CERTOPARIN.

alpha stimulants (alpha agonists) *See* SYMPATHOMIMETIC DRUGS.

alpha tocopheryl acetate *See* VITAMIN E.

Alphosyl (Stafford-Miller) A proprietary combination of *coal tar extract (a keratolytic) and *allantoin (an abrasive and astringent), used for the treatment of *psoriasis. It is available as a cream or lotion and can be obtained without a prescription, but only from pharmacies.
Precautions: see COAL TAR.

Alphosyl 2-in-1 Shampoo (Stafford-Miller) *See* COAL TAR.

Alphosyl HC (Stafford-Miller) A proprietary combination of *hydrocortisone (a corticosteroid), *coal tar extract (a keratolytic), and *allantoin (an abrasive and astringent), used for the treatment of *psoriasis. It is available as a cream on *prescription only.
Side effects and precautions: see TOPICAL STEROIDS; COAL TAR.

alprazolam A long-acting *benzodiazepine used for the short-term treatment of anxiety. It is available as tablets on *prescription only and cannot be prescribed on the NHS.
Side effects and precautions: see DIAZEPAM; BENZODIAZEPINES.
Interactions with other drugs:
  Antiviral drugs: indinavir and ritonavir increase the risk of profound sedation and should not be used with alprazolam.
  See also BENZODIAZEPINES.
Proprietary preparation: Xanax.

alprostadil A *prostaglandin that produces dilatation of blood vessels. It is used for the treatment of erectile impotence and to aid diagnosis, being administered by injection into the erectile tissue of the penis or by application into the urethra. Treatment is not started until the possibility of any underlying treatable cause of the condition has been excluded. Alprostadil is also available as a solution for infusion to treat newborn babies who are awaiting surgery for congenital heart disease. It acts by preventing the closure of the ductus arteriosus, a blood vessel that enables the circulation to bypass the lungs in the fetus but normally closes after birth to allow the lungs to be included in the circulation. Both forms of alprostadil are only available on *prescription.
Side effects: in men, these may include penile pain, prolonged erection, reactions at the injection site, testicular pain and/or swelling, blood in the urine, nausea, dry mouth, sweating, dizziness, and headache. Men who experience erections lasting four hours or longer should seek immediate medical help; treatment of prolonged erection should not be delayed more than six hours. Side effects in babies include breathlessness (particularly in infants under 2 kg), flushing, a slow heart rate, and low blood pressure; there may be oedema, diarrhoea, fever, and convulsions.
Precautions: alprostadil should not be taken by men with a

predisposition to prolonged erection (as seen in sickle-cell anaemia, multiple myeloma, or leukaemia) or anatomical deformity of the penis. It should not be used in conjunction with other drugs for the treatment of erectile dysfunction or when sexual activity is medically inadvisable. Alprostadil should not be given to babies with a history of haemorrhage.

Interactions with other drugs:

Antihypertensive drugs: their effect in lowering blood pressure may be enhanced by alprostadil.

Proprietary preparations: Caverject (intracavernosal injection); MUSE (pellet for direct urethral application); Prostin VR (infusion); Viridal (intracavernosal injection).

Altacite Plus (Hoechst Marion Roussel) A proprietary combination of *hydrotalcite (an antacid) and activated *dimethicone <dimeticone> (an antifoaming agent), used for the relief of flatulence and heartburn associated with *acid-peptic diseases; this combination is also known as **co-simalcite**. It is available as a suspension and can be obtained without a prescription.

Side effects, precautions, and interactions with other drugs: see ANTACIDS.

alteplase A *fibrinolytic drug used to dissolve blood clots in the coronary arteries (which supply the heart) in people who have had a heart attack; treatment should be started within 12 hours of the attack. Alteplase is also used to treat pulmonary embolism (*see* THROMBOSIS). It is available in a form for intravenous injection or infusion on *prescription only.

Side effects, precautions, and interactions with other drugs: see FIBRINOLYTIC DRUGS.

Proprietary preparation: Actilyse.

altretamine A *cytotoxic drug used for the treatment of advanced ovarian cancer when other treatments have failed. *Antiemetics are recommended to prevent the nausea and vomiting that are common side effects of treatment with this drug. Altretamine is available as capsules on *prescription only.

Side effects: include nausea and vomiting, nerve damage, rash, itching, and damage to the liver and kidneys. *See also* CYTOTOXIC DRUGS.

Precautions: altretamine should not be taken by women who are pregnant or breastfeeding and should be used with caution in people with liver or kidney disease. *See also* CYTOTOXIC DRUGS.

Interactions with other drugs:

Antidepressants: there is a risk of severe low blood pressure on standing if monoamine oxidase inhibitors or tricyclic antidepressants are taken with altretamine.

Pyridoxine: reduces the effect of altretamine.

Proprietary preparation: Hexalen.

Alu-Cap (3M Health Care) *See* ALUMINIUM HYDROXIDE.

Aludrox (Pfizer Consumer Healthcare) *See* ALUMINIUM HYDROXIDE.

aluminium acetate A salt of aluminium that has *astringent properties. It is used to cleanse weeping wounds and patches of eczema and to treat inflammation of the outer ear. Aluminium acetate is available as a lotion or ear drops that can be obtained without a prescription, but only from pharmacies.

aluminium chlorhydroxyallantoinate *See* DERMIDEX.

aluminium chloride A powerful antiperspirant that is used for the treatment of excessive sweating of the armpits, hands, or feet. At lower concentrations, it is included as an ingredient of many proprietary antiperspirant preparations. Aluminium chloride is available as a solution, usually in a roll-on applicator, and can be obtained without a prescription, but only from pharmacies.
Side effects: aluminium chloride may cause skin irritation.
Precautions: aluminium chloride should not be allowed to come in contact with the eyes, mouth, or other mucous membranes and should not be applied to broken or inflamed skin. The armpits should not be shaved or treated with depilatories for 12 hours before or after applying aluminium chloride.
Proprietary preparations: Anhydrol Forte; Driclor.

aluminium hydroxide An *antacid used in the treatment of indigestion (*see* ACID-PEPTIC DISEASES). It is also used as a *phosphate-binding agent to absorb phosphates from the diet. Aluminium hydroxide is available, without a prescription, in the form of tablets, a mixture (gel), capsules, or a suspension; some preparations that contain aluminium hydroxide as an ingredient can only be obtained from pharmacies. Some preparations cannot be prescribed on the NHS. *See also* CO-MAGALDROX.
Side effects: aluminium hydroxide may cause constipation. *See also* ANTACIDS.
Precautions: aluminium hydroxide should be used with caution in people undergoing kidney dialysis.
Interactions with other drugs: see ANTACIDS.
Proprietary preparations: Aludrox (mixture); Alu-Cap (capsules); ACTONORM GEL (combined with magnesium hydroxide, dimethicone <dimeticone>, and peppermint oil); ALGICON (combined with magnesium alginate, magnesium carbonate, and potassium bicarbonate); ASILONE HEARTBURN (combined with alginic acid, magnesium trisilicate, and sodium bicarbonate); ASILONE SUSPENSION (combined with magnesium oxide and dimethicone <dimeticone>); BIRLEYS (combined with magnesium trisilicate and magnesium carbonate); DIJEX SUSPENSION (combined with magnesium hydroxide); DIJEX TABLETS (combined with magnesium carbonate); DIOVOL (combined with magnesium hydroxide

and dimethicone <dimeticone>); GASTROCOTE (combined with alginic acid, magnesium trisilicate, and sodium bicarbonate); GAVISCON TABLETS (combined with alginic acid, magnesium trisilicate, and sodium bicarbonate); KOLANTICON GEL (combined with magnesium hydroxide, dimethicone <dimeticone>, and dicyclomine hydrochloride); Maalox (*see* CO-MAGALDROX); MAALOX PLUS (combined with magnesium hydroxide and dimethicone <dimeticone>); MOORLAND (combined with bismuth, magnesium trisilicate, magnesium carbonate, calcium carbonate, and kaolin); MUCAINE (combined with oxethazaine <oxetacaine> and magnesium oxide); Mucogel (*see* CO-MAGALDROX); PYROGASTRONE (combined with carbenoloxone sodium, magnesium trisilicate, sodium bicarbonate, and alginic acid); TOPAL (combined with magnesium carbonate and alginic acid).

aluminium oxide An abrasive agent used for the treatment of acne in the form of a paste containing fine or medium-sized particles in a cleansing base. It is freely available *over the counter.
Precautions: the paste should not be used by people with telangiectasia (in which spidery red spots of distended blood vessels can be seen beneath the skin). It should not come into contact with the eyes.
Proprietary preparation: Brasivol.

Alupent (Boehringer Ingelheim) *See* ORCIPRENALINE SULPHATE.

Alvedon (Novex Pharma) *See* PARACETAMOL.

Alvercol (Norgine) A proprietary combination of *sterculia (a bulking agent) and *alverine citrate (an antispasmodic), used for the treatment of irritable bowel syndrome. It is available as granules to be swallowed with plenty of water and can be obtained without a prescription, but only from pharmacies.
Side effects: Alvercol may cause abdominal distension.
Precautions: Alvercol should not be taken immediately before going to bed. It should not be taken by people with intestinal obstruction and should be used with caution during the first three months of pregnancy.

alverine citrate An *antispasmodic used in the treatment of irritable bowel syndrome, diverticular disease (which causes abdominal pain and altered bowel habit), and painful periods caused by spasms of the uterus. It is available as capsules and can be obtained without a prescription, but only from pharmacies.
Side effects: include nausea, headache, itching, rash, and dizziness.
Precautions: alverine citrate should not be taken by people with intestinal obstruction due to loss of intestinal movement or during the first three months of pregnancy.
Proprietary preparations: Relaxyl; Spasmonal; Spasmonal Forte (a stronger formulation); ALVERCOL (combined with sterculia).

amantadine hydrochloride An *antiparkinsonian drug that acts by increasing the activity of *dopamine in the brain. It provides moderate relief of symptoms but *tolerance to its effect may develop. Amantadine is also an *antiviral drug that acts by inhibiting viral replication; it is used particularly in the prevention and treatment of influenza type A$_2$ and rarely in the treatment of shingles. It is available, on *prescription only, as capsules or a syrup.

Side effects: include nervousness, inability to concentrate, insomnia, dizziness, and (rarely) convulsions and hallucinations; nausea and loss of appetite may also occur.

Precautions: amantadine should be used with caution in people who have liver or kidney disease, congestive heart disease, or states of confusion or hallucination. It should not be taken by people with epilepsy or a history of peptic ulcers or by women who are pregnant or breastfeeding. Withdrawal of the drug at the end of treatment should be gradual.

Interactions with other drugs:

Antimuscarinic drugs: the side effects of these drugs are increased.

Antipsychotics: *extrapyramidal reactions can occur.

Methyldopa and metirosine: extrapyramidal reactions can occur.

Proprietary preparation: Symmetrel.

Amaryl (Hoechst Marion Roussel) *See* GLIMEPIRIDE.

AmBisome (NeXstar Pharmaceuticals) *See* AMPHOTERICIN.

Ambre Solaire (Laboratoires Garnier) A proprietary *sunscreen preparation consisting of a cream containing avobenzone, 4-methylbenzylidene camphor, terephthalylidene dicamphor sulphonic acid, and *titanium dioxide. It protects against both UVA and UVB (SPF 60) and can be prescribed on the NHS or obtained without a prescription.

amethocaine <tetracaine> A potent *local anaesthetic used in the form of a cream to relieve the pain of bites and stings and as a gel to anaesthetize the skin before intravenous injections or the insertion of a cannula. It is also used in eye drops to induce anaesthesia for minor eye operations and is an ingredient of a spray for treating mouth and throat conditions. Most preparations of amethocaine can be obtained without a prescription but eye drops are available on *prescription only.

Side effects: amethocaine may cause redness, itching, or irritation of the skin.

Precautions: amethocaine should not be applied to inflamed or damaged skin. It should not be used for prolonged periods or over extensive areas.

Proprietary preparations: Ametop (gel); Anethaine (cream); Minims Amethocaine Hydrochloride (single-dose preservative-free eye drops); ELUDRIL SPRAY (combined with chlorhexidine).

Amias (AstraZeneca; Takeda) *See* CANDESARTAN CILEXETIL.

Amidox (APS-Berk) *See* AMIODARONE.

amifostine A drug that is used to reduce the risk of infection in
patients whose natural immunity has been compromised by the
administration of *cisplatin and *cyclophosphamide for the treatment of
advanced ovarian *cancer. These *cytotoxic drugs cause a reduction in
the numbers of neutrophils (a type of white blood cell; *see* BONE MARROW
SUPPRESSION), which have an important role in defending the body
against infection. Amifostine is also used to protect against kidney
damage caused by cisplatin. A *prescription only medicine for specialist
use, it is often given with antiemetics before chemotherapy and is
available as an injection.
Side effects: include a fall in blood pressure, nausea, vomiting, flushing,
chills, dizziness, sleepiness, hiccups, coughing, sneezing, and allergic
reactions.
Precautions: amifostine should not be given to people with low blood
pressure or liver or kidney disease, or to women who are pregnant or
breastfeeding. Patients should be given plenty of fluids before treatment
starts.
Interactions with other drugs:
  Antihypertensive drugs: their effects in lowering blood pressure are
    enhanced; antihypertensives should therefore be withheld for 24
    hours before a dose of amifostine, and blood pressure should be
    monitored carefully during treatment.
Proprietary preparation: Ethyol.

amikacin An *aminoglycoside antibiotic used for the treatment of
serious infections that are resistant to *gentamicin. It is given as an
*intramuscular or *intravenous injection and is available on
*prescription only.
Side effects, precautions, and interactions with other drugs: see
GENTAMICIN.
Proprietary preparation: Amikin.

Amikin (Bristol-Myers Squibb) *See* AMIKACIN.

Amilamont (Rosemont Pharmaceuticals) *See* AMILORIDE
HYDROCHLORIDE.

Amil-Co (Norton Healthcare) *See* CO-AMILOZIDE.

Amilmaxco 5/50 (Ashbourne Pharmaceuticals) *See* CO-AMILOZIDE.

amiloride hydrochloride A *potassium-sparing diuretic used in the
treatment of *hypertension and *oedema associated with heart failure,

liver disease, or kidney disease. It is available, on *prescription only, as tablets or a solution. *See also* CO-AMILOFRUSE; CO-AMILOZIDE.

Side effects, precautions, and interactions with other drugs: see POTASSIUM-SPARING DIURETICS.

Proprietary preparations: Amilamont (solution); Amilospare (tablets); Amil-Co (*see* CO-AMILOZIDE); Amilmaxco 5/50 (*see* CO-AMILOZIDE); Aridil (*see* CO-AMILOZIDE); BURINEX A (combined with bumetanide); Delvas (*see* CO-AMILOZIDE); Fru-Co (*see* CO-AMILOFRUSE); Froop-Co (*see* CO-AMILOFRUSE); FRUMIL (*see* CO-AMILOFRUSE); KALTEN (combined with atenolol and hydrochlorothiazide); LASORIDE (*see* CO-AMILOFRUSE); MODUCREN (combined with timolol maleate and hydrochlorothiazide); Moduret 25 (*see* CO-AMILOZIDE); Moduretic (*see* CO-AMILOZIDE); NAVISPARE (combined with cyclopenthiazide); Zida-Co (*see* CO-AMILOZIDE).

See also ANTIHYPERTENSIVE DRUGS; DIURETICS.

Amilospare (Ashbourne Pharmaceuticals) *See* AMILORIDE HYDROCHLORIDE.

aminacrine hydrochloride <aminoacridine hydrochloride> A disinfectant used in dilute solutions as an *antiseptic. It is included in preparations for treating minor sores and infections of the mouth.
Proprietary preparation: MEDIJEL (combined with lignocaine <lidocaine> hydrochloride).

aminoacridine hydrochloride *See* AMINACRINE HYDROCHLORIDE.

aminobenzoic acid A vitamin of the B group (*see* VITAMIN B COMPLEX). It is included as an ingredient of some *sunscreen preparations as it absorbs UVB, a range of ultraviolet light of medium wavelength that causes reddening and burning of the skin. Aminobenzoic acid is also included in some vitamin B supplements but there is no evidence of its value.
Side effects: sunscreens containing aminobenzoic acid may cause allergic rashes in the presence of sunlight.
Proprietary preparation: SPECTRABAN (combined with padimate-O).

aminoglutethimide A drug that inhibits the conversion of androgens to oestrogens (*see* AROMATASE INHIBITORS); it also acts on the adrenal glands to inhibit the productions of *corticosteroids. Aminoglutethimide is used for the treatment of advanced breast *cancer in postmenopausal women or women who have had their ovaries removed. It is also used to treat advanced cancer of the prostate gland and overproduction of corticosteroids (Cushing's syndrome) due to malignant disease. Aminoglutethimide is available as tablets on *prescription only.
Side effects: include drowsiness, lethargy, rash, and fever (which usually settle as treatment proceeds), dizziness, and nausea; other side effects include headache, depression, insomnia, confusion, blood disorders, and reduced activity of the thyroid gland.

Precautions: aminoglutethimide should not be taken by women who are pregnant or breastfeeding or by people with porphyria. Replacement corticosteroid therapy is usually given to people being treated for cancer and may also be required for those with Cushing's syndrome.

Interactions with other drugs:

Anticoagulants: the effects of warfarin and nicoumalone <acenocoumarol> are reduced.

Corticosteroids: their effects are reduced (see precautions above).

Diuretics: there is an increased risk of low plasma sodium concentrations.

Medroxyprogesterone: its effect is reduced.

Oral antidiabetics: their rate of metabolism may be increased and therefore their effects may be reduced.

Tamoxifen: its plasma concentration is reduced.

Theophylline: its effect may be reduced.

Proprietary preparation: Orimeten.

aminoglycosides A group of bactericidal antibiotics (i.e. they kill bacteria, rather than just inhibiting their growth). Because of their toxicity (possible side effects include ear damage, causing impaired hearing and balance, and kidney damage), they are used only when less toxic antibacterials are ineffective or inadvisable. As most of their side effects are dose-related, care must be taken with dosage. Aminoglycosides are excreted by the kidneys, therefore they must be used with caution in people with kidney disease as toxic concentrations of the aminoglycosides can accumulate. Most aminoglycosides are not continued for longer than seven days. Aminoglycosides are not absorbed from the gut unless this is damaged, so they must be administered by injection.

See AMIKACIN; GENTAMICIN; KANAMYCIN; NEOMYCIN SULPHATE; NETILMICIN; TOBRAMYCIN.

aminophylline A *xanthine that is a compound of *theophylline and ethylenediamine and is used for the treatment of *asthma and in some cases of emphysema and chronic bronchitis (*see* BRONCHODILATORS). It is available from pharmacies without a prescription in the form of tablets or *modified-release tablets; an injection is available on *prescription only.

Side effects, precautions, and interactions with other drugs: see THEOPHYLLINE; XANTHINES.

Proprietary preparations: Amnivent 225 SR (modified-release tablets); Norphyllin SR (modified-release tablets); Phyllocontin Continus (modified-release tablets).

aminosalicylates A class of drugs used for the treatment of ulcerative colitis (inflammation and ulceration of the large bowel) and to maintain patients in remission from it. They are also used to treat Crohn's disease (inflammation and ulceration of the gastrointestinal tract) that affects the large bowel. The aminosalicylates include *mesalazine (aminosalicylic acid), *balsalazide sodium, *olsalazine sodium, and *sulphasalazine <sulfasalazine>; they are taken by mouth or rectally and are available on *prescription only.

Side effects: include diarrhoea, nausea, headache, allergic reactions (including rashes), and exacerbation of the symptoms of colitis. Rare side effects include blood disorders (see precautions below).

Precautions: aminosalicylates should not be taken by people who are allergic to *salicylates or by those with severe kidney disease. They should be used with caution in women who are pregnant or breastfeeding. Bleeding, bruising, sore throat, or fever should be reported immediately to a doctor as this can indicate a blood disorder; in this case treatment should be discontinued.

amiodarone A class III *anti-arrhythmic drug, which works by slowing nerve impulses in the heart. It is given to control and prevent ventricular and supraventricular tachycardia and atrial fibrillation (*see* ARRHYTHMIA). This drug can have serious side effects and it should be initiated under hospital or specialist supervision, when it may be given as tablets or by injection. It is available on *prescription only.

Side effects: harmless deposits may form on the cornea of the eyes, which usually cause no symptoms and reverse when the medication is stopped. In the long term amiodarone can have a number of adverse effects on the liver, eyes, lungs, and thyroid gland. About one-third of people taking the drug become more sensitive to the sun, and everyone taking amidarone should take care in the sun until they have established whether or not they are affected; people who tan easily are no more or less likely to be affected than very fair-skinned people. Sensitivity may be overcome by the use of sunscreens.

Precautions: amiodarone should not be taken by people with thyroid disorders or by women who are pregnant or breastfeeding. *See also* ANTI-ARRHYTHMIC DRUGS.

Interactions with other drugs: amiodarone interacts with a number of other drugs to increase the risk of ventricular arrhythmias. These drugs should therefore not be taken with amiodarone (see below).

Other anti-arrhythmic drugs: amiodarone should not be taken with disopyramide, flecainide, procainamide, or quinidine.

Antibiotics: amiodarone should not be taken with erythromycin (given by injection) or co-trimoxazole.

Anticoagulants: amiodarone increases the anticoagulant effects of warfarin, nicoumalone <acenocoumarol>, and phenindione.

Antihistamines: amiodarone should not be taken with astemizole, terfenadine, or mizolastine.

Antimalarial drugs: amiodarone should not be taken with mefloquine, chloroquine, quinine, hydroxychloroquine, or halofantrine.

Antipsychotic drugs: amiodarone should not be taken with the phenothiazines, haloperidol, pimozide, or sertindole.

Antiviral drugs: amiodarone should not be taken with nelfinavir or ritonavir.

Beta blockers: amiodarone should not be taken with sotalol; the risk of bradycardia (slow heart rate) is increased if amiodarone is taken with other beta blockers.

Calcium antagonists: the risk of bradycardia is increased if amiodarone is taken with diltiazem or verapamil.

Cisapride: should not be taken with amiodarone.

Digoxin: amiodarone increases the plasma concentration of digoxin, whose dosage should therefore be reduced.

Pentamidine isethionate <isetionate>: should not be taken with amiodarone.

Phenytoin: its plasma concentration is increased by amiodarone.

Tricyclic antidepressants: should not be taken with amiodarone.

Proprietary preparations: Amidox (tablets); Cordarone X (tablets or injection).

amisulpride An atypical *antipsychotic drug that is used in the treatment of schizophrenia; it controls both the positive symptoms (e.g. delusions) and the negative symptoms (e.g. apathy) of the disease. Amisulpride is available as tablets on *prescription only.

Side effects: include weight gain, dizziness, low blood pressure on standing (which can cause fainting in some people), insomnia, anxiety, agitation, sleepiness, constipation, nausea, vomiting, dry mouth, raised concentrations of prolactin in the blood (causing breast pain and enlargement and menstrual problems), and (rarely) slowing of the heart rate.

Precautions: amisulpride should not be taken by women who are pregnant or breastfeeding or by people with phaeochromocytoma (a tumour of the adrenal gland) or tumours that are stimulated by prolactin. It should be used with caution in people with cardiovascular disease, a history of epilepsy, or Parkinson's disease.

Interactions with other drugs:

Anaesthetics: their effect in lowering blood pressure is increased.

Antidepressants: there is an increased risk of *antimuscarinic effects and *arrhythmias if amisulpride is taken with tricyclic antidepressants.

Antiepileptic drugs: amisulpride antagonizes the effects of these drugs in controlling seizures.

Antihistamines: there is an increased risk of arrhythmias if amisulpride is taken with astemizole or terfenadine.

Halofantrine: there is an increased risk of arrhythmias if this drug is taken with amisulpride.

Ritonavir: may increase the effects of amisulpride.

Sedatives: the sedative effects of amisulpride are increased if it is taken with anxiolytic or hypnotic drugs, or any other drug that causes sedation.

Proprietary preparation: Solian.

amitriptyline hydrochloride A *tricyclic antidepressant drug used for the treatment of depressive illness, especially when sedation is required, and to treat bedwetting in children. It is available, on *prescription only, as tablets, capsules, or a solution for oral use and as a solution for injection.

Side effects: include dry mouth, sedation, blurred vision, constipation, nausea, difficulty in urinating, palpitation and fast heart rate, sweating, tremor, rashes and allergic reactions, behavioural disturbances, confusion (especially in the elderly), and interference with sexual function. There may be increased appetite and weight gain, drowsiness, nervousness or insomnia, weakness and fatigue, and changes in blood sugar concentrations.

Precautions and interactions with other drugs: see TRICYCLIC ANTIDEPRESSANTS.

Proprietary preparations: Domical; Elavil; Lentizol; Tryptizol; TRIPTAFEN (combined with perphenazine).

Amix (Ashbourne Pharmaceuticals) *See* AMOXYCILLIN <AMOXICILLIN>.

amlodipine A class II *calcium antagonist used for the treatment of *angina and as a first-line treatment for *hypertension. It has a longer duration of action than *nifedipine or *nicardipine and is therefore usually given once daily. It is available as tablets on *prescription only.

Side effects and interactions with other drugs: see CALCIUM ANTAGONISTS.

Precautions: amlodipine should not be used to treat patients with unstable angina and should not be taken by women who are pregnant or breastfeeding.

Proprietary preparation: Istin.

See also ANTIHYPERTENSIVE DRUGS.

ammonia solution A solution that gives off a pungent vapour. Strong or weak ammonia solutions are used in *decongestant and *rubefacient preparations.

Precautions: ammonia can be caustic and irritating, depending on the concentration. It can irritate eyes and mucous membranes and should not be swallowed, as it can burn the lining of the gullet and stomach.

Proprietary preparations: BN LINIMENT (combined with ammonium chloride and turpentine oil); GODDARD'S WHITE OIL EMBROCATION (combined with dilute acetic acid and turpentine oil); MACKENZIES SMELLING SALTS (combined with eucalyptus oil).

ammonium acetate *See* EXPECTORANTS.

ammonium carbonate *See* EXPECTORANTS.

ammonium chloride A compound that is included as an *expectorant in some proprietary cough medicines. Ammonium chloride is also used to acidify the urine, which reduces the reabsorption of some drugs from the urine back into the body, and so enhances their excretion; it can therefore be used as an antidote to poisoning by these drugs.

Proprietary preparations: BENYLIN CHESTY COUGHS ORIGINAL (combined with diphenhydramine and menthol); BOOTS BRONCHIAL COUGH MIXTURE (combined with ammonium carbonate and guaifenesin <guaifenesin>); BRONALIN EXPECTORANT (combined with diphenhydramine); ECDYLIN (combined with diphenhydramine); GUANOR EXPECTORANT (combined with diphenhydramine and menthol); HISTALIX (combined with diphenhydramine and menthol).

Amnivent 225 SR (Ashbourne Pharmaceuticals) *See* AMINOPHYLLINE.

amobarbital *See* AMYLOBARBITONE.

Amoram (Eastern Pharmaceuticals) *See* AMOXYCILLIN <AMOXICILLIN>.

amorolfine An *antifungal drug applied topically as the hydrochloride for treating ringworm infections of the nails and skin and pityriasis versicolor (a chronic fungal infection of the skin). It is available as a cream or nail lacquer on *prescription only.

Side effects: amorolfine may rarely cause transient burning or reddening of the skin.

Precautions: amorolfine should not be used during pregnancy or breastfeeding. It should not be used in or around the eyes, ears, and mucous membranes.

Proprietary preparations: Loceryl; Loceryl Lacquer.

amoxapine A *tricyclic antidepressant drug used for the treatment of depression. It is available as tablets on *prescription only.

Side effects: see AMITRIPTYLINE HYDROCHLORIDE; TRICYCLIC ANTIDEPRESSANTS. In addition, involuntary facial and limb movements and (in women) menstrual irregularities, breast enlargement, and milk secretion may occur.

Precautions and interactions with other drugs: see TRICYCLIC ANTIDEPRESSANTS.

Proprietary preparation: Asendis.

amoxicillin *See* AMOXYCILLIN.

Amoxil (SmithKline Beecham Pharmaceuticals) *See* AMOXYCILLIN <AMOXICILLIN>.

amoxycillin <amoxicillin> A broad-spectrum *penicillin very similar to *ampicillin. It is used for the treatment of middle-ear and sinus infections, chest infections (including exacerbations of chronic bronchitis), *Salmonella* infections, urinary-tract infections, and gonorrhoea. It is available, on *prescription only, as capsules or a syrup for oral use and as an injection.

Side effects, precautions, and interactions with other drugs: see AMPICILLIN.

Proprietary preparations: Almodan; Amix; Amoram; Amoxil; Galenamox; Rimoxallin; Augmentin (*see* CO-AMOXICLAV).

amphetamines A group of *sympathomimetic drugs that have a marked *stimulant action on the central nervous system. They alleviate fatigue and produce a feeling of mental alertness and well-being. Amphetamines have limited uses in clinical medicine since they can cause *dependence and psychotic states; the most important member of the group is *dexamphetamine <dexamfetamine> sulphate, which is used in the treatment of narcolepsy in adults and attention deficit disorder in children. Amphetamines should not be used to treat depressive illness, obesity, senility, or tiredness.

Amphocil (AstraZeneca) *See* AMPHOTERICIN.

amphotericin (amphotericin B) An *antifungal drug that is active against a wide range of organisms and can be used to treat most fungal infections; it is especially effective in treating systemic (generalized) infections. When taken orally or applied topically, for treating superficial infections, side effects are rare. For systemic infections amphotericin is given by intravenous injection, which must be under medical supervision because side effects can be severe. A *prescription only medicine, amphotericin is available as tablets, lozenges to be dissolved in the mouth, and solutions or suspensions for injection.

Side effects: when injected, amphotericin can cause nausea, vomiting, loss of appetite, diarrhoea, stomach pains, fever, headache, muscle and joint pains, anaemia, allergic reactions, kidney damage, and (less frequently) changes in blood pressure, abnormal heart rhythms, blood disorders, liver damage, hearing loss, double vision, and convulsions.

Precautions (with injections): since severe allergic reactions can occur, a test dose of amphotericin should be given before the full dose. Tests for liver and kidney function during treatment are necessary. Amphotericin should be used with caution in people taking corticosteroids or anti-cancer drugs and in women who are pregnant or breastfeeding.

Interactions with other drugs:

Aminoglycoside antibiotics: increase the risk of toxic effects on the kidney.

Cyclosporin: increases the risk of toxic effects on the kidney.

Digoxin and digitoxin: the toxic effects of these drugs are increased if amphotericin causes potassium concentrations in the blood to fall.

Diuretics: amphotericin increases the risk of loop and thiazide diuretics causing low potassium concentrations in the blood.

Proprietary preparations: Abelcet; AmBisome; Amphocil; Fungilin; Fungizone.

ampicillin A broad-spectrum penicillin that is inactivated by penicillinase (*see* PENICILLINS). It is used for the treatment of middle ear and sinus infections, chest infections (including exacerbations of chronic bronchitis), *Salmonella* infections, urinary-tract infections, and gonorrhoea. It is available, on *prescription only, as capsules or a syrup for oral use and as an injection.

Side effects: may include diarrhoea, nausea, and rashes. Rashes, which should be reported to a doctor, are most common in patients suffering from glandular fever, chronic lymphatic leukaemia, and HIV infection and in patients who are also taking *allopurinol.

Precautions: ampicillin should not be taken by anyone with known allergy to penicillins, and it should be used with caution in people with severe kidney disease.

Interactions with other drugs:

Methotrexate: concentrations of methotrexate in the blood are increased, which may cause toxic effects.

Oral contraceptives: their contraceptive effect may be reduced. Additional contraceptive precautions should therefore be taken with short courses of ampicillin and for seven days after stopping; if these days run beyond the end of a packet of oral contraceptives, the next packet should be started immediately without a break.

Proprietary preparations: Penbritin; Rimacillin; Vidopen; Flu-Amp (see CO-FLUAMPICIL); Magnapen (see CO-FLUAMPICIL).

amsacrine A *cytotoxic drug used for the treatment of acute myeloid leukaemia (see CANCER). It is similar to *doxorubicin and is available as a solution for intravenous infusion on *prescription only.

Side effects and precautions: see DOXORUBICIN.

Proprietary preparation: Amsidine.

Amsidine (Goldshield Pharmaceuticals) *See* AMSACRINE.

amylmetacresol An *antiseptic used as an ingredient of lozenges for the treatment of minor infections of the mouth and throat.

Proprietary preparations: STREPSILS (combined with dichlorobenzyl alcohol); STREPSILS DUAL ACTION LOZENGES (combined with dichlorobenzyl alcohol and lignocaine <lidocaine>).

amylobarbitone <amobarbital> An intermediate-acting *barbiturate. Amylobarbitone and its sodium salt, **amylobarbitone sodium**, are used for the short-term treatment of severe insomnia in people who are already taking barbiturates; amylobarbitone sodium is also given by injection to treat status epilepticus (repeated epileptic seizures). Amylobarbitone is available as tablets, its sodium salt as capsules or an injection (only for use in specialist epilepsy centres); both are *controlled drugs.

Side effects, precautions, and interactions with other drugs: see BARBITURATES.

Proprietary preparations: Amytal (tablets); Sodium Amytal (capsules or injection); TUINAL (combined with quinalbarbitone <secobarbital>).

Amytal (Flynn Pharma) *See* AMYLOBARBITONE <AMOBARBITAL>.

Anabact (ASTA Medica) *See* METRONIDAZOLE.

anabolic steroids Steroids that promote the growth of tissues, especially muscles. Anabolic steroids are synthetic forms of male sex hormones (*androgens) that have fewer masculinizing effects in women than androgens. They have not proved to be effective for promoting weight gain in severely underweight patients, and their use as body builders by athletes is banned by athletic authorities. **Oxymetholone** is occasionally used to stimulate production of blood cells by the bone marrow in people with aplastic *anaemia; other anabolic steroids used clinically are *nandrolone and *stanozolol. Prolonged use of anabolic steroids can cause liver damage.
Interactions with other drugs:
   Anticoagulants: anabolic steroids increase the anticoagulant effects of warfarin, nicoumalone <acenocoumarol>, and phenindione.

Anacal (Sankyo Pharma) A proprietary combination of *heparinoid (an anticoagulant) and laureth '9' (a *lauromacrogol), used to relieve the discomfort and pain of *haemorrhoids, anal fissures, proctitis (inflammation of the rectum), or itching of the anal region. It is available as ointment or suppositories and can be obtained without a prescription, but only from pharmacies.

Anadin (Whitehall Laboratories) A proprietary combination of *aspirin (an analgesic and antipyretic) and *caffeine (a stimulant), used for the treatment of mild to moderate pain (including headache, neuralgia, toothache, and period pains) and fever and to relieve the symptoms of influenza and colds. It is available as tablets or capsules; **Anadin Maximum Strength** is a stronger formulation in the form of capsules. These preparations are available without a prescription, but larger packs can only be obtained from pharmacies.
Side effects and interactions with other drugs: see ASPIRIN.
Precautions: these medicines are not recommended for children, except on medical advice. *See also* ASPIRIN; CAFFEINE.

Anadin Extra, **Anadin Extra Soluble** (Whitehall Laboratories) Proprietary combinations of *aspirin and *paracetamol (analgesics and antipyretics) and *caffeine (a stimulant), used for the treatment of mild to moderate pain (including headache, neuralgia, toothache, and period pains) and fever and to relieve the symptoms of influenza and colds. They are available as tablets or soluble tablets without a prescription, but larger packs can only be obtained from pharmacies.
Side effects and interactions with other drugs: see ASPIRIN.
Precautions: these medicines should not be given to children, except on medical advice. *See also* ASPIRIN; PARACETAMOL; CAFFEINE.

Anadin Paracetamol (Whitehall Laboratories) *See* PARACETAMOL.

Anadin Ultra (Whitehall Laboratories) *See* IBUPROFEN.

anaemia A condition that arises when the amount of haemoglobin, the oxygen-carrying pigment of the red blood cells, is reduced. Those affected are pale, constantly feel tired, become breathless on exertion, and have poor resistance to infection. There are many causes. **Iron-deficiency anaemia** (*see* IRON) may be due to loss of blood or lack of dietary iron. **Haemolytic anaemias** result from the increased destruction of red blood cells; this occurs, for example, in haemolytic disease of the newborn, in which the red cells of the fetus are destroyed by antibodies in the mother's blood (*see* ANTI-D (RH$_0$) IMMUNOGLOBULIN). Anaemia can also occur when the production of red cells is impaired. This may be due to a deficiency of the factors necessary for red cell production, such as vitamin B$_{12}$ or intrinsic factor (causing **pernicious anaemia**; *see* VITAMIN B COMPLEX), *folic acid, or *erythropoietin, or by suppression of red cell production in the bone marrow, which occurs in leukaemia (*see* CANCER). Such anaemias are characterized by the presence of abnormal red blood cells; for example megaloblasts are present in the bone marrow in folic acid or vitamin B$_{12}$ deficiency (**megaloblastic anaemias**). In **aplastic anaemia** the numbers of red blood cells are very much reduced due to failure of the bone marrow to produce them.

anaesthetics *See* LOCAL ANAESTHETICS.

Anafranil, Anafranil SR (Novartis Consumer Health) *See* CLOMIPRAMINE HYDROCHLORIDE.

analeptic drugs (respiratory stimulants) *See* STIMULANTS.

analgesics Drugs used for controlling pain. **Non-opioid analgesics**, mainly *aspirin and *paracetamol, provide effective relief of such pains as headache, toothache, and mild rheumatic pain. **Opioid analgesics** (sometimes colloquially called narcotic analgesics) include *codeine and more potent drugs (such as *morphine and *pethidine) that are only used under medical supervision (*see* OPIOIDS). The non-steroidal anti-inflammatory drugs (*see* NSAIDS) are a large group of analgesics widely used for treating rheumatic conditions (including rheumatoid arthritis).

analogue A drug that differs structurally in minor ways from its parent compound. These minor differences in molecular structure can result in important changes in action. Examples are *calcipotriol (an analogue of vitamin D) and *betahistine (an analogue of histamine). Useful analogues of existing drugs are either more potent, cause fewer side effects, or are better absorbed after oral administration.

anaphylaxis A severe allergic reaction to a particular antigen (foreign protein), which interacts with antibody that is bound to certain cells (mast cells) to bring about the release of *histamine and other chemicals, causing local or widespread symptoms. These range from pain and itchy weals on the face (especially the lips, eyelids, and tongue) accompanied by swelling (**angioedema**) to widespread tissue swelling (which can involve the larynx), constriction of the airways, and a fall in blood pressure leading to circulatory collapse (**anaphylactic shock**). This is a medical emergency requiring prompt treatment (including the injection of *adrenaline <epinephrine>).

Substances that can provoke anaphylaxis include insect stings, certain foods (such as peanuts, fish, and eggs), and a variety of drugs (especially if injected), including antibiotics (such as *penicillins), aspirin and other *NSAIDs, vaccines, and blood products.

anastrozole An *aromatase inhibitor used for the treatment of advanced breast *cancer in postmenopausal women. It is usually given to women in whom treatment with *tamoxifen has failed. Anastrozole is available as tablets on *prescription only.

Side effects: include hot flushes, sweating, vaginal dryness and irritation, thinning of the hair, nausea, vomiting, diarrhoea, weakness, insomnia, headache, and rash.

Precautions: anastrozole should not be taken by women who are pregnant or breastfeeding, have moderate to severe liver or kidney disease, or who have not yet reached the menopause.

Proprietary preparation: Arimidex.

Anbesol (Whitehall Laboratories) A proprietary combination of *lignocaine <lidocaine> hydrochloride (a local anaesthetic), *cetylpyridinium chloride (an antiseptic), and *chlorocresol (a disinfectant), used for the treatment of mouth pain and minor irritations and infections of the mouth. It is available as a gel, a liquid, or a teething gel formula (in which the lignocaine concentration is lower) and can be obtained without a prescription, but only from pharmacies.

Andrews Antacid (SmithKline Beecham Consumer Healthcare) A proprietary combination of *magnesium carbonate and *calcium carbonate, used for the relief of upset stomach, heartburn, indigestion, and trapped wind. It is freely available *over the counter in the form of chewable tablets.

Side effects and precautions: Andrews Antacid is not recommended for children. *See also* MAGNESIUM SALTS.

Interactions with other drugs: see ANTACIDS.

Andrews Salts *See* ORIGINAL ANDREWS SALTS.

Andrews Seltzer Extra (SmithKline Beecham Consumer Healthcare) A proprietary combination of *caffeine (a stimulant), *paracetamol (an analgesic), and *sodium bicarbonate (an antacid), used for the relief of stomach upsets, particularly those caused by overindulgence in food or alcohol. It is freely available *over the counter as effervescent tablets.

Side effects: *see* CAFFEINE; PARACETAMOL; SODIUM BICARBONATE.

Precautions: this preparation is not recommended for children. *See also* CAFFEINE; PARACETAMOL; SODIUM BICARBONATE.

Androcur (Schering Health Care) *See* CYPROTERONE ACETATE.

androgens The male sex hormones, which stimulate the development of male sex organs and male secondary sexual characteristics (beard, deep voice, body hair). These *steroid hormones are produced primarily in the testes but also, in small amounts, in the ovaries and adrenal cortex. Production is stimulated by a *gonadotrophin secreted by the pituitary gland. The main androgen is *testosterone. Androgens are used mainly as replacement therapy in castrated adult men and to treat men whose testicular function is impaired because of disease of the pituitary gland or testes. When pituitary function is poor androgen therapy can lead to normal sexual development and potency but not fertility (if fertility is desired, treatment is with gonadotrophins). *See also* MESTEROLONE.

Andropatch (SmithKline Beecham Pharmaceuticals) *See* TESTOSTERONE.

Anethaine (Torbet Laboratories) *See* AMETHOCAINE <TETRACAINE>.

Anexate (Roche Products) *See* FLUMAZENIL.

Angettes 75 (Bristol-Myers Squibb) *See* ASPIRIN.

Angeze, Angeze SR (Opus) *See* ISOSORBIDE MONONITRATE.

Angilol (DDSA Pharmaceuticals) *See* PROPRANOLOL HYDROCHLORIDE.

angina Chest pain that results from lack of oxygen in the heart muscle. It is usually caused by narrowing of the coronary arteries, the vessels that supply blood (and therefore oxygen) to the heart muscle. In **classic** or **exertional angina**, the most common form, pain typically occurs during physical exertion or emotional stress or after a heavy meal; the underlying cause is likely to be *atherosclerosis. **Unstable angina** can occur at rest and results from spasm and constriction of the coronary arteries. Angina is most commonly treated with *nitrates, *beta blockers, or *calcium antagonists.

angioedema *See* ANAPHYLAXIS.

Angiopine, Angiopine MR (Ashbourne Pharmaceuticals) *See* NIFEDIPINE.

angiotensin II inhibitors (angiotensin II antagonists) Drugs that inhibit the action of angiotensin II, a hormone that constricts blood vessels. They have similar effects to *ACE inhibitors and are used in the treatment of *hypertension. Unlike ACE inhibitors they do not produce a dry cough. *See* CANDESARTAN CILEXETIL; IRBESARTAN; LOSARTAN POTASSIUM; VALSARTAN.

Side effects: these are usually mild; dizziness occassionally occurs, more rarely rash and oedema (swelling) of the face.

Precautions: angiotensin II inhibitors should be avoided in pregnancy.

Interactions with other drugs: see ACE INHIBITORS.

Angiozem (Ashbourne Pharmaceuticals) *See* DILTIAZEM HYDROCHLORIDE.

Angitil SR (Trinity Pharmaceuticals) *See* DILTIAZEM HYDROCHLORIDE.

Anhydrol Forte (Dermal Laboratories) *See* ALUMINIUM CHLORIDE.

anistreplase A *fibrinolytic drug used to dissolve blood clots in the coronary arteries (which supply the heart) in people who have had a heart attack; treatment should be started within 12 hours of the attack. Anistreplase is given by intravenous injection and is available on *prescription only. Because antibodies are formed against anistreplase, it may not be effective if used on more than one occasion within the space of a year.

Side effects: see FIBRINOLYTIC DRUGS. In addition, anistreplase may cause allergic reactions (such as rashes).

Precautions and interactions with other drugs: see FIBRINOLYTIC DRUGS.

Proprietary preparation: Eminase.

Anodesyn (Seton Scholl Healthcare) A proprietary combination of *lignocaine <lidocaine> (a local anaesthetic) and *allantoin (an astringent), used for the relief of pain and irritation associated with external haemorrhoids. It is freely available *over the counter in the form of an ointment or suppositories.

Anquil (Janssen-Cilag) *See* BENPERIDOL.

Antabuse (Cox Pharmaceuticals) *See* DISULFIRAM.

antacids Drugs that neutralize stomach acid. Antacids are used to treat any *acid-peptic disease. They produce rapid but brief relief of symptoms by making the stomach less acidic (raising the pH). They are best taken when symptoms are likely to occur, usually after meals or at bedtime, and are often taken four or more times daily. Antacids are alkaline salts of metals. The most commonly used ones are *aluminium hydroxide, magnesium salts (including *magnesium carbonate and *magnesium trisilicate), carbonates (especially *sodium bicarbonate), and *calcium carbonate. Aluminium and magnesium compounds are relatively insoluble in water and therefore long-acting in the stomach. Many antacid preparations contain salts of *alginic acid (e.g. magnesium alginate), which provide protection against reflux oesophagitis. Since bicarbonate salts liberate carbon dioxide, activated *dimethicone <dimeticone>, which allows gas bubbles to coalesce and be expelled, is often added to antacid salts. This may cause belching and/or flatulence.

Side effects: magnesium-containing antacids are laxative, whereas aluminium and calcium salts are constipating. The combination of different salts usually results in a preparation with few or no side effects on the bowel. Carbonates cause belching and/or flatulence.

Precautions and interactions with other drugs: antacids can alter the *electrolyte balance and can affect the absorption of some vitamins, minerals, and other drugs. Drugs whose absorption is reported to have been reduced in the presence of antacids, and should therefore not be taken at the same time, include the following: most tetracyclines (which should not be taken within two hours of antacids); fosinopril; diflunisal; azithromycin; cefpodoxime; ciprofloxacin; isoniazid; nitrofurantoin; norfloxacin; ofloxacin; rifampicin; gabapentin; phenytoin; itraconazole; ketoconazole; dipyridamole; chloroquine; hydroxychloroquine; phenothiazines; bisphosphonates; mycophenolate mofetil; penicillamine.

antagonist A drug that opposes the action of another drug or natural body chemical. Examples are the *oestrogen antagonists.

antazoline An *antihistamine used in topical preparations. **Antazoline sulphate** is an ingredient of eye drops for the treatment of allergic conjunctivitis, such as that associated with hay fever. **Antazoline hydrochloride** is used in an ointment for the relief of insect stings and bites. Preparations containing antazoline can be obtained without a prescription, but only from pharmacies.

Side effects: the ointment may cause allergic reactions.

Precautions: the ointment should not be used for longer than three days and should not be used for treating eczema.

Proprietary preparations: Wasp-Eze Ointment; OTRIVINE-ANTISTIN (combined with xylometazoline).

Antepsin (Wyeth Laboratories) *See* SUCRALFATE.

anthelmintics (antihelminthics) Drugs used to destroy parasitic worms (such as tapeworms, roundworms, and threadworms) and/or to expel them from the intestine. *See* ALBENDAZOLE; MEBENDAZOLE; NICLOSAMIDE; PIPERAZINE; THIABENDAZOLE <TIABENDAZOLE>.

Anthisan (Rhône-Poulenc Rorer) *See* MEPYRAMINE.

Anthisan Plus (Rhône-Poulenc Rorer) A proprietary combination of *mepyramine maleate (an antihistamine) and *benzocaine (a local anaesthetic), used to relieve pain and itching (for example, caused by

insect stings). It is available as a spray and can be obtained from
pharmacies without a prescription.

Side effects: the spray may occasionally cause allergic reactions.

Precautions: the spray should not be applied to the eyes, mouth, or other
mucous membranes or to broken skin.

anthracyclines *See* CYTOTOXIC ANTIBIOTICS.

anti-androgens Drugs that antagonize the action of *androgens. They
are used for the treatment of severe hypersexuality and sexual deviation
in men and can also be used as an *adjunct in the treatment of prostate
cancer and excessive body hair and acne in women. *See* BICALUTAMIDE;
CYPROTERONE ACETATE; FINASTERIDE; FLUTAMIDE.

anti-arrhythmic drugs (anti-arrhythmics) Drugs used for treating
disordered heart rhythms (*see* ARRHYTHMIA). Anti-arrhythmic drugs either
slow the flow of electrical impulses to the heart muscle or inhibit the
ability of heart muscles to contract; they are classified as class I, II, III, or
IV anti-arrhythmics, depending on their mode of action. Class I drugs
affect the response of the heart muscle to the signal received and may be
subdivided into classes Ia (e.g. *quinidine bisulphate and *disopyramide);
Ib (e.g. *lignocaine <lidocaine> and *mexiletine); and Ic (e.g.
*propafenone hydrochloride and *flecainide acetate). Class II anti-
arrhythmic drugs are *beta blockers, which reduce the ability of the
pacemaker to pass electrical signals to the heart muscle. Class III drugs
include *amiodarone and *bretylium tosylate <tosilate>. Class IV
comprise some, but not all, *calcium antagonists, which interfere with
the conduction of nerve impulses in the atria. Other drugs used are
*cardiac glycosides (digitalis drugs, such as *digoxin), which affect the
way signals are transmitted in the heart, and *adenosine.

Side effects: many of these drugs can depress normal heart function and
may produce dizziness on standing (postural hypotension) or
breathlessness on exertion. Mild nausea and visual disturbances are quite
common. Side effects specific to particular drugs are listed in their
entries.

Precautions and interactions with other drugs: the effects of anti-
arrhythmic drugs tend to be additive, therefore specialist care is
necessary if two or more are used. Most of the drugs that control
arrhythmias can also provoke them in some circumstances. Low
*potassium concentrations can enhance this effect; it is important,
therefore, that when people are taking diuretics with anti-arrhythmic
drugs, a potassium-sparing diuretic is used either alone or in combination
with a loop diuretic or a thiazide diuretic. Details of specific interactions
are given at entries for individual drugs.

antibacterial drugs *See* ANTIBIOTICS.

antibiotics Originally, natural products secreted by microorganisms
(microbes) that inhibit the growth of other microorganisms. The term is

now commonly used, however, to denote any drug, natural or synthetic, that has a selective toxic action on bacteria, protozoans, or other single-celled microorganisms. Antibiotics are not active against viruses (*see* ANTIVIRAL DRUGS). The more accurate term is therefore **antimicrobials**. While many are now produced synthetically, they are still based on the natural compounds. Antibiotics used to treat bacterial infections are called **antibacterial** drugs. Antibacterials may kill bacteria, in which case they are described as **bactericidal**, or they may prevent bacterial growth, when they are referred to as **bacteriostatic**. They are usually designed to exploit some aspect of bacterial structure that is not present in mammalian cells and therefore they do not harm human cells. For example, *penicillins and *cephalosporins (collectively known as **beta-lactam antibiotics**) attack bacterial cell walls; mammalian cells do not have cell walls. *Aminoglycosides and *tetracyclines attack bacterial ribosomes (the protein-synthesizing machinery of the cell), which are different from mammalian ribosomes. Antibiotics that are active against a wide variety of microorganisms are known as **broad-spectrum antibiotics**; those effective only against particular microbes are called **narrow-spectrum antibiotics**. Widespread use of antibiotics results in bacteria developing resistance to these agents. Antibiotics are therefore, in most Western countries, *prescription only medicines. The normal healthy human body contains several types of bacteria and other microbes, notably in the gut. Use of antibiotics can have a harmful effect on some of these microbes, which results in the overgrowth of others causing **superinfections**, which may present more problems than the original infection.

anticholinergic drugs *See* ANTIMUSCARINIC DRUGS.

anticholinesterases Drugs that inhibit the action of cholinesterases, the enzymes that break down *acetylcholine. They therefore prolong the activity of acetylcholine and cause an exaggerated response of the *parasympathetic nervous system, i.e. they are *cholinergic drugs. They have the opposite action to *antimuscarinic drugs. Anticholinesterases are used at the end of surgical operations to reverse the paralysis induced by skeletal *muscle relaxants. They are also used to treat myasthenia gravis, an autoimmune condition in which nerve impulses to the muscles are diminished, causing extreme weakness and fatigability of the muscles. By preventing the breakdown of acetylcholine, anticholinesterases enable the transmission of nerve impulses to the muscles to be prolonged. Anticholinesterases have a limited role in relieving urinary retention and paralysis of the bowel, especially after surgery. The commonly used anticholinesterases are *pyridostigmine, *distigmine bromide, and *neostigmine.

anticoagulants Drugs used to prevent the formation of blood clots, or the extension of an existing blood clot, in the veins. They are widely used for the prevention and treatment of deep-vein *thrombosis in the legs. Anticoagulants are less effective at preventing blood-clot formation in the arteries, but they are used to prevent clots forming in cardiac aneurysms (balloon-like swellings in the walls of the arteries in the heart) or on artificial heart valves. Anticoagulants may be given before open-heart surgery or kidney dialysis, and patients may be given them after surgery to prevent deep-vein thrombosis.

Oral anticoagulants (mainly *warfarin sodium; *nicoumalone <acenocoumarol> and *phenindione are now rarely used) act by antagonizing the effects of vitamin K, which is essential for the formation of clotting factors. It may take 72 hours before their full anticoagulant effect occurs. *Heparins, which are given by injection, directly interfere with the blood-clotting process. They are relatively fast acting. The two types of anticoagulants may be given in combination. Often patients are started on a combination of heparin and warfarin and the heparin is discontinued once the warfarin takes full effect.

Side effects and precautions: the most serious adverse effect of anticoagulants is the risk of excessive bleeding, usually from overdosage. People who are taking anticoagulant therapy therefore need to have the clotting times of their blood measured frequently. Clotting times are usually expressed in terms of the **INR** (International Normalized Ratio). Prolonged clotting times (indicating overdosage) may be shown by easy bruising. For other side effects and precautions, as well as interactions with other drugs, *see* HEPARIN; WARFARIN SODIUM.

anticonvulsant drugs Drugs used to prevent or reduce the severity and frequency of seizures (convulsions). Seizures occur when the electrical activity in the brain that controls the movement of the limbs becomes paroxysmal and chaotic. The most common form of seizures is **epilepsy**. Since not all seizures involve convulsions, and not all types of convulsion are epileptic seizures, the term **antiepileptic** is often preferred to describe medication for treating epilepsy. Most people with epilepsy need to take anticonvulsants on a regular basis until they have been free of seizures for two years. The type of drug used will depend on the type of epilepsy, although a patient's age and response to treatment may also affect the choice of drug.

Tonic-clonic (or major) seizures (formerly called 'grand mal'), in which a period of unconsciousness is followed by convulsions, usually last only a few minutes; prolonged attacks, in which repeated seizures occur with no intervening recovery of consciousness, are called **status epilepticus**. The main drugs used to treat major seizures are *carbamazepine, *phenytoin, and *sodium valproate; *phenobarbitone <phenobarbital> and *primidone may also be used but are more sedating. Drugs used in the treatment of status epilepticus include *diazepam, phenytoin, and *paraldehyde. Absence seizures (formerly called 'petit mal'), which usually affect children and consist of a momentary loss of consciousness during which posture and balance are maintained, are treated with *ethosuximide, sodium valproate, and (less commonly) *clonazepam. Partial seizures, in which the nature of the seizure depends on the part of the brain that is affected, are most commonly treated with phenytoin, sodium valproate, and carbamazepine; phenobarbitone and primidone may also be effective. *Lamotrigine, *vigabatrin, *gabapentin, *tiagabine, *topiramate, and *piracetam are newer anticonvulsants that may be used as *adjuncts to (or replacements for) older medicines.

anti-D (RH$_0$) immunoglobulin An *immunoglobulin that is given to a rhesus-negative woman who has recently given birth to a baby who is rhesus-positive (or who has miscarried or aborted a rhesus-positive fetus) in order to prevent her from forming antibodies to rhesus-positive fetal cells that may pass into her blood during subsequent pregnancies. The aim is to protect her subsequent children from haemolytic disease of the newborn (*see* ANAEMIA). Anti-D immunoglobulin is available as a solution for intramuscular injection on *prescription only.
Proprietary preparation: Partobulin.

antidepressant drugs Drugs that act to relieve the symptoms of moderate to severe depression. Antidepressant drugs usually need to be taken for 2 weeks before their effect is apparent, and full benefit may not be felt for 6–8 weeks. They are generally continued for 4–6 months after the depression has resolved, and if the condition is recurrent, medication may be continued for years. Most antidepressants are dangerous in overdose and should therefore be prescribed in small quantities (prescriptions for one month are common). If stopped suddenly after having been taken for eight weeks or more, withdrawal symptoms (including nausea, vomiting, and weakness) may occur. Depression is thought to be related to abnormal function of the transmitters *noradrenaline <norepinephrine> and/or *serotonin. After these transmitters have been released in the brain they will stimulate brain cells and then be taken up again by nerve endings, broken down, and hence inactivated. Some antidepressant drugs inhibit the reuptake mechanism, while others prevent breakdown of the transmitters; both actions result in a longer duration of action of these transmitters. The mechanism of action of other antidepressants is less clear.

Antidepressants elevate mood, increase the capacity for physical activity, improve the appetite, and restore activity in everyday life. Some antidepressants are sedative in nature and are especially useful when depression is accompanied by anxiety and insomnia. The main classes of antidepressants are the *tricyclic antidepressants, the *monoamine oxidase inhibitors (MAOIs), the selective serotonin reuptake inhibitors (*SSRIs), and *lithium salts. *See also* MIRTAZAPINE; REBOXETINE; TRYPTOPHAN.

antidiabetic drugs *See* INSULIN; ORAL HYPOGLYCAEMIC DRUGS.

antidiarrhoeal drugs Drugs used for the treatment of diarrhoea. *Electrolyte solutions are used to replace fluid and salts that are lost in acute diarrhoea (*see* ORAL REHYDRATION THERAPY). *Bulk-forming laxatives, such as *methylcellulose, are used for treating chronic diarrhoea associated with diverticular disease and irritable bowel syndrome, and to adjust consistency of the faeces in other diseases of the bowel. Adsorbents, such as *kaolin, adsorb irritant substances that cause diarrhoea, but they are not recommended for treating acute diarrhoea. Opioids, such as *codeine phosphate, *loperamide hydrochloride, *co-phenotrope, and *morphine, act by slowing down the movement of the gut and increasing transit time and are used as *adjuncts in the treatment of acute diarrhoea and some chronic diarrhoeas.

antidiuretic hormone *See* VASOPRESSIN.

antiemetics Drugs that stop or prevent vomiting and, to a lesser extent, nausea. They are used to prevent motion sickness and the nausea associated with Ménière's disease, to prevent or treat the nausea and vomiting caused by *cytotoxic drug therapy for cancer and some other drug treatments, and to treat nausea and vomiting associated with diseases of the stomach, duodenum, liver, and gall bladder or experienced after some types of surgery. Antiemetics should not be taken unless the reason for the vomiting and/or nausea is known. In some circumstances, for example after the ingestion of a poison or contaminated food, vomiting is beneficial and should not be stopped. On the other hand, severe or prolonged vomiting may be a sign of a more serious underlying condition and should be reported to a doctor. Antiemetics should not be given to people with obstruction of the gut, and they are not advised during the first three months of pregnancy unless the vomiting is so severe that a doctor considers them necessary.

Antiemetics include *hyoscine hydrobromide and certain *antihistamines (for motion sickness), *phenothiazines, *domperidone, *metoclopramide, *ondansetron, *granisetron, and *tropisetron.

antiepileptic drugs *See* ANTICONVULSANT DRUGS.

antifibrinolytic drugs *See* HAEMOSTATIC DRUGS.

antifungal drugs Drugs that are used to treat infections caused by fungi (including yeasts). The most common fungal infections are **tinea (ringworm)** and **candidiasis (thrush)**. Tinea is caused by fungi called dermatophytes, which feed on keratin (the principal protein of the skin, hair, and nails). Tinea most commonly affects the skin between the toes (athlete's foot), the scalp, the skin beneath a beard, the groin, and the nail bed (where it can be deep-seated). Thrush is caused by overgrowth of the yeast *Candida albicans*, normally a harmless inhabitant of the gastrointestinal tract and vagina. This can occur when the normal balance of the body's microorganisms is upset, for example in people taking drugs (e.g. antibiotics, oral contraceptives), or when the body's resistance to infection is lowered, for example in people with diabetes and pregnant women. The infection is usually confined to the mouth, vagina, or skin folds (it can infect napkin rash in babies), but in severely immunocompromised people (for example those whose immune systems are impaired by AIDS) candidiasis can spread throughout the body. Such people are also susceptible to other systemic fungal infections (e.g. *Cryptococcus neoformans*).

A variety of drugs is available for treating fungal infections; some of them are also active against bacteria (*see* ANTIBIOTICS). Many of them act on the cell walls of fungi to make them permeable so that the contents of the cell leak out and the fungus dies. The *imidazole antifungal drugs are used mainly to treat candidiasis (especially of the vagina) and various forms of tinea; they are usually applied locally (as pessaries, creams, powders, etc.), although some can also be taken orally for treating persistent infections (*see* CLOTRIMAZOLE; ECONAZOLE NITRATE; FENTICONAZOLE; ISOCONAZOLE NITRATE; KETOCONAZOLE; MICONAZOLE; SULCONAZOLE; TIOCONAZOLE). The triazoles (*see* FLUCONAZOLE; ITRACONAZOLE) are usually taken orally. Other antifungal drugs include *griseofulvin and *terbinafine (usually taken orally for treating tinea) and *nystatin. For treating deep-seated or systemic infections, such drugs as *amphotericin and fluconazole are administered by injection; *flucytosine is used specifically for treating systemic yeast infections. Antifungal drugs applied topically rarely cause side effects, but treatment by mouth or injection may produce severe adverse effects and must be monitored carefully. *See also* AMOROLFINE; TOLNAFTATE; UNDECENOIC ACID.

antihaemophilic factor *See* FACTOR VIII.

antihelminthics *See* ANTHELMINTICS.

antihistamines (H₁-receptor antagonists) A class of drugs that antagonize the effect of *histamine, a substance released by the body in large amounts during allergic reactions. Antihistamines act by blocking H_1 receptors in the skin, nose, and airways: these receptors – when stimulated by histamine – produce the symptoms of an allergic response. They relieve the sneezing, running nose, and itching associated with allergic rhinitis, including hay fever (seasonal allergic rhinitis). They are also used to treat urticaria (an itchy rash commonly occurring as an allergic reaction to eating such foods as shellfish and strawberries), other itching skin conditions, and the histamine-induced reaction to insect bites or stings. For allergic reactions antihistamines may be given as nasal sprays or inhaled; they are also taken by mouth to prevent or treat symptoms. Antihistamines may be injected intravenously as an *adjunct to *adrenaline <epinephrine> and/or corticosteroids to relieve life-threatening *anaphylaxis – an extreme allergic reaction. Some antihistamines (e.g. *cinnarizine, *cyclizine, *dimenhydrinate, and *promethazine) are used as *antiemetics or to treat vertigo or Ménière's disease. The older antihistamines (especially promethazine, *diphenhydramine, *trimeprazine <alimemazine>, dimenhydrinate, and – to a lesser extent – *chlorpheniramine <chlorphenamine>, cyclizine, and *mequitazine) cause drowsiness and some of them are used for their *hypnotic effect, for example in preparations used for treating coughs and colds and in non-prescription sleeping tablets. These antihistamines can impair the ability to drive or operate machinery; alcohol enhances this effect. The newer antihistamines (*acrivastine, *astemizole, *cetirizine, *fexofenadine, *loratadine, and *terfenadine) are less sedating.

See also AZATADINE MALEATE; AZELASTINE HYDROCHLORIDE; BROMPHENIRAMINE MALEATE; CLEMASTINE; CYPROHEPTADINE HYDROCHLORIDE; HYDROXYZINE HYDROCHLORIDE; LEVOCABASTINE; PHENIRAMINE MALEATE; TRIPROLIDINE HYDROCHLORIDE.

Side effects: the older antihistamines cause sedation or drowsiness and (less commonly) headache, antimuscarinic effects (e.g. difficulty in urinating, dry mouth, blurred vision), and stomach upsets. The newer antihistamines are less sedating and are less likely to cause antimuscarinic effects.

Precautions: alcohol enhances the sedating effects of the older antihistamines. Antihistamines should be used with caution by people with epilepsy, an enlarged prostate gland, glaucoma, or liver disease and by women who are pregnant or breastfeeding.

Interactions with other drugs:

Antidepressants: there is an increased risk of abnormal heart rhythms (*see* ARRHYTHMIA) if antihistamines are taken with monoamine oxidase inhibitors or tricyclic antidepressants. Astemizole and terfenadine also interact with a number of other drugs to increase the risk of arrhythmias; these drugs are listed in the entries for astemizole and terfenadine.

antihypertensive drugs (antihypertensives) Drugs used in the treatment of *hypertension (high blood pressure), either alone or in combination. They work in a variety of ways, some of which are not completely understood, and some antihypertensive drugs have more than one action. The main classes of antihypertensive drugs are *ACE inhibitors, *alpha blockers, *beta blockers, *calcium antagonists, *diuretics, and *vasodilators. Some drugs act centrally (on the brain) to reduce blood pressure (*see* CLONIDINE HYDROCHLORIDE; METHYLDOPA). The overall aim of treatment is to reduce the pressure in the arterial system.

Side effects: see entries for individual classes of drugs.

Precautions: some dosage adjustment may be needed at the start of treatment. It is important to continue taking antihypertensive medication even if the problem appears to be under control. Sudden withdrawal of some of these drugs may cause a potentially dangerous 'rebound' increase in blood pressure; dosage reduction needs to be gradual and under medical supervision.

anti-inflammatory drugs Drugs that act against the body's chemicals that initiate or maintain inflammation. The main class comprises the non-steroidal anti-inflammatory drugs (*see* NSAIDS). Other drugs with anti-inflammatory activity include the glucocorticoids (*see* CORTICOSTEROIDS).

antimetabolites A class of *cytotoxic drugs that act by combining with enzymes in cells to prevent the synthesis of nuclear material (DNA)

and cell division. They are used for the treatment of a wide variety of
*cancers. The most commonly used antimetabolites are *methotrexate,
*cytarabine, *fludarabine, *cladribine, *gemcitabine, *fluorouracil,
*raltitrexed, *mercaptopurine, and *thioguanine <tioguanine>.

antimicrobial drugs See ANTIBIOTICS.

antimuscarinic drugs (anticholinergic drugs) A class of drugs that
block the activity of *acetylcholine at **muscarinic** receptors (a
subdivision of acetylcholine receptors). They tend to relax smooth muscle
(including that of the airways and the gut), reduce the secretion of saliva,
digestive juices, and sweat, and dilate the pupil of the eye. They are used
as *antiparkinsonian drugs, as *antispasmodics in the treatment of
gastrointestinal pain, and as *bronchodilators; they are also used to dilate
the pupil of the eye in ophthalmic examinations, to antagonize the
effects of *anticholinesterases, and to increase the heart rate in certain
circumstances.

Side effects: characteristic side effects of antimuscarinic drugs include dry
mouth, thirst, blurred vision, dry skin, increased heart rate (following an
initial slowing of the heart rate), and difficulty in urinating. Side effects
occurring more rarely include confusion (especially in elderly people),
drowsiness, dizziness, nausea, and vomiting.

Precautions: antimuscarinics should not be taken by people with closed-
angle (acute) *glaucoma, myasthenia gravis, intestinal obstruction due to
loss of movement in the intestine, pyloric stenosis, and enlargement of
the prostate. They should be used with caution in children and the
elderly and in people with reflux oesophagitis, diarrhoea, ulcerative
colitis, hypertension (high blood pressure), and conditions causing a fast
heart rate.

Interactions with other drugs: taking two or more antimuscarinic drugs
together can increase their side effects. Drugs that can increase
antimuscarinic effects include amantadine, antihistamines,
disopyramide, nefopam, MAOIs, and tricyclic antidepressants.

anti-oestrogens See OESTROGEN ANTAGONISTS.

antiparkinsonian drugs Drugs used to treat Parkinson's disease or
parkinsonism. These conditions result from a disease process affecting
the basal ganglia, the part of the brain responsible for controlling
voluntary movement at a subconscious level, and are associated with a
deficiency of the neurotransmitter *dopamine. This gives rise to an
imbalance between the actions of dopamine and another
neurotransmitter, *acetylcholine, and results in disorders of movement,
notably tremor, rigidity, and slow movements. A distinction is sometimes
made between Parkinson's disease, a degenerative condition associated
with ageing, and parkinsonism, parkinsonian symptoms due to other
causes; for example, the long-term use of antipsychotic drugs (*see*
EXTRAPYRAMIDAL REACTIONS).

A variety of drugs are available for treating the condition. *Levodopa, which is converted to dopamine in the body, is used as replacement therapy. *Selegiline prevents the breakdown of dopamine in the body. Dopamine agonists (*see* BROMOCRIPTINE; CABERGOLINE; ENTACAPONE; LYSURIDE <LISURIDE> MALEATE; PERGOLIDE; QUINAGOLIDE; ROPINIROLE) increase the action of dopamine by stimulating dopamine receptors in the brain. *Antimuscarinic drugs block the activity of acetylcholine in the brain and thus act to correct the imbalance between dopamine and acetylcholine. They are less effective than levodopa, although they often supplement its action. Patients with mild symptoms may be treated initially with antimuscarinic drugs (alone or with selegiline), levodopa being added at a later stage as symptoms progress. They are also useful in reversing drug-induced extrapyramidal reactions. The common antimuscarinic drugs used in treating parkinsonism are *benzhexol <trihexyphenidyl> hydrochloride, *benztropine mesylate <benzatropine mesilate>, *biperiden, *orphenadrine, and *procyclidine. *See also* AMANTADINE HYDROCHLORIDE.

antiplatelet drugs A class of drugs that reduce the ability of platelets (specialized blood cells) to stick together, which occurs normally as part of the blood-clotting process. Antiplatelet drugs are used to prevent the formation of blood clots in arteries, when *anticoagulants are ineffective (*see* THROMBOSIS). The most commonly used antiplatelet drugs are *aspirin and *dipyridamole. They are used for the prevention of strokes or heart attacks in those at risk, especially in people who have had a previous stroke or heart attack. Aspirin is also given (in low daily doses) after heart bypass surgery to reduce the risk of clots obstructing the grafts. Other antiplatelet drugs include *clopidogrel, *abciximab, and *epoprostenol.

Antipressan (APS-Berk) *See* ATENOLOL.

antipruritics Agents that relieve itching (pruritus). Examples are *calamine, *crotamiton, *camphor, and *lauromacrogols, applied in creams or lotions. Some *antihistamines, in the form of creams or tablets, are used if the itching is due to an allergy.

antipsychotic drugs (neuroleptic drugs) A group of drugs formerly known as **major tranquillizers** (*compare* ANXIOLYTIC DRUGS). Antipsychotic drugs are used in the short term to calm or sedate patients who are severely disturbed, agitated, hostile, or aggressive. They control the acute symptoms of mania (such as extreme overactivity, incoherence, and extravagant behaviour) and relieve acute positive symptoms of schizophrenia (such as disordered thinking, delusions, and hallucinations); long-term treatment is usually required for patients with schizophrenia in order to prevent relapses. Most antipsychotic drugs are less effective in treating the negative symptoms of schizophrenia (e.g. apathy and withdrawal), although some have an alerting effect. Antipsychotic drugs are also used for the short-term treatment of severe anxiety and some also have an *antidepressant effect. Antipsychotic drugs produce their actions by reducing the activity of the neurotransmitter *dopamine in the brain; however, they also affect other body functions controlled by dopamine, which causes a group of troublesome side effects known as *extrapyramidal reactions. These drugs also interfere with the action of other neurotransmitters, including acetylcholine, which produces antimuscarinic effects (*see* ANTIMUSCARINIC DRUGS).

Antipsychotic drugs belong to various different chemical groups, including the *phenothiazines (e.g. *chlorpromazine), **butyrophenones** (e.g. *haloperidol, *droperidol, and *benperidol), and **thioxanthenes** (e.g. *flupenthixol <flupentixol>, *zuclopenthixol); other antipsychotics are *sulpiride, *oxypertine, and *loxapine. The **atypical antipsychotics** are a group of more recently developed drugs that have less effect on dopamine activity, producing their action by interfering with other neurotransmitters, especially *serotonin (5-hydroxytryptamine). They therefore have less pronounced extrapyramidal reactions than conventional antipsychotic drugs. Atypical antipsychotic drugs are used to treat patients who have not responded to, or cannot tolerate, conventional antipsychotic drugs; they include *amisulpride, *olanzapine, *risperidone, *quetiapine, *clozapine, and *zotepine.
Side effects, precautions, and interactions with other drugs: see entries for individual drugs.

antipyretics Drugs that reduce fever by lowering body temperature. The most commonly used antipyretics are *aspirin and *paracetamol.

antisecretory drug Any drug that reduces the normal rate of secretion of a body fluid, usually one that reduces acid secretion into the stomach. Such drugs include *antimuscarinic drugs, *H_2-receptor antagonists, and *proton pump inhibitors.

antiseptic A chemical that destroys or inhibits the growth of disease-causing bacteria and other microorganisms and is sufficiently nontoxic to be applied to the skin or mucous membranes to cleanse wounds and prevent infections or to be used internally to treat infections of the intestine and bladder. Examples are *cetrimide, *chlorhexidine, *hexamine <methenamine> hippurate, *triclosan, *cetylpyridinium chloride, and *dequalinium.

antispasmodics Drugs that relax the smooth muscle of the gut. They are used as an *adjunct in the treatment of indigestion not associated with peptic ulcers, of irritable bowel syndrome, and of diverticular disease (which causes abdominal pain and altered bowel habit). The main agents are *antimuscarinic drugs (such as *dicyclomine <dicycloverine> hydrochloride, *propantheline bromide, *atropine sulphate, and *hyoscine butylbromide), *alverine citrate, *mebeverine hydrochloride, and *peppermint oil.

antitussives *See* COUGH SUPPRESSANTS.

antiviral drugs Drugs used to treat infections caused by viruses. Because viruses can only function within the cells of their hosts, it has been difficult to produce drugs that act specifically against viruses without damaging their host cells. The effectiveness of antiviral drugs is therefore limited: frequently they will contain an outbreak of viral activity but are not capable of totally eradicating the infection, which can recur (as with cold sores). Fortunately, the majority of viral infections resolve spontaneously in most people and do not require specific medication. However, in immunocompromised individuals, whose ability to fight infection is impaired because of drug therapy (e.g. immunosuppressants) or disease (e.g. AIDS), antiviral treatment may be life-saving.

Many antiviral drugs act by interfering with DNA production and thus prevent the virus from replicating (*see* ACICLOVIR; CIDOFOVIR; FAMCICLOVIR; FOSCARNET; GANCICLOVIR; PENCICLOVIR; VALACICLOVIR). Some are **nucleoside analogues**: similar to the nucleosides (building blocks) of DNA, they become incorporated into the new DNA being made by the virus, but – since they are not the correct nucleoside – they will stop any further DNA synthesis (*see* IDOXURIDINE; TRIBAVIRIN). The mechanisms of action of other antiviral drugs are less well understood (*see* AMANTADINE HYDROCHLORIDE; INOSINE PRANOBEX).

The **reverse transcriptase inhibitors** are antiviral drugs that act specifically against a particular group of viruses, the retroviruses, the best known of which is the human immunodeficiency virus (*HIV), which causes AIDS. Retroviruses contain RNA (rather than DNA) as their genetic material; this is converted to DNA by the virus inside its host cell by means of the enzyme reverse transcriptase. The nucleoside analogue reverse transcriptase inhibitors prevent retroviral replication by becoming incorporated into the growing strand of viral DNA (*see* DIDANOSINE; LAMIVUDINE; STAVUDINE; ZALCITABINE; ZIDOVUDINE). Non-nucleoside reverse transcriptase inhibitors (*see* NEVIRAPINE) bind directly to the enzyme to prevent its action. The **protease inhibitors** act by preventing the action of a protease, a protein-cleaving enzyme that is needed by the virus to produce mature virus particles (*see* INDINAVIR; NELFINAVIR; RITONAVIR; SAQUINAVIR). These drugs are used in combination with other antiviral drugs in the treatment of HIV infection. However they also inhibit an enzyme system in the liver that is involved in metabolizing many drugs; there is therefore a potential for drug interactions in people taking protease inhibitors.

See also INTERFERONS.

Anturan (Novartis Consumer Health) *See* SULPHINPYRAZONE <SULFINPYRAZONE>.

Anugesic-HC (Parke-Davis Medical) A proprietary combination of *zinc oxide and *bismuth oxide (astringents), *pramoxine <pramocaine> hydrochloride (a local anaesthetic), *hydrocortisone (a corticosteroid), *Peru balsam, and benzyl benzoate (a *surfactant), used to relieve the discomfort of *haemorrhoids, anal itching, and other painful conditions of the anorectal region. It is available as a cream on *prescription only.

Side effects: see CORTICOSTEROIDS.

Precautions: Anugesic-HC should not be used when viral or fungal infection is present and should not be used for longer than seven days. It is not recommended for children.

Anugesic-HC Suppositories (Parke-Davis Medical) A proprietary combination of *zinc oxide, *bismuth subgallate, and *bismuth oxide (astringents), *pramoxine <pramocaine> hydrochloride (a local anaesthetic), *hydrocortisone (a corticosteroid), *Peru balsam, and benzyl benzoate (a *surfactant), used to relieve the discomfort of *haemorrhoids, anal itching, and other conditions of the anorectal region. It is available on *prescription only.

Side effects: see CORTICOSTEROIDS.

Precautions: these suppositories should not be used when viral or fungal infection is present and should not be used for longer than seven days. They are not recommended for children.

Anusol (Warner-Lambert Consumer Healthcare) A proprietary combination of *zinc oxide and *bismuth oxide (astringents) and *Peru balsam, used to relieve the discomfort of *haemorrhoids, anal itching, and other painful anorectal conditions. It is available as a cream; Anusol ointment and suppositories also contain *bismuth subgallate. All these preparations are freely available *over the counter.

Anusol-HC (Parke-Davis Medical) A proprietary combination of *zinc oxide, *bismuth subgallate, and *bismuth oxide (astringents), *hydrocortisone (a corticosteroid), *Peru balsam, and benzyl benzoate (a *surfactant), used for the relief of *haemorrhoids and other painful anorectal conditions. It is available as an ointment or suppositories on *prescription only; **Anusol Plus HC** ointment or suppositories can be obtained from pharmacies without a prescription.

Side effects: see CORTICOSTEROIDS.

Precautions: Anusol-HC should not be used when viral or fungal infection is present and should not be used for longer than seven days. It is not recommended for children.

anxiolytic drugs (sedatives) Drugs that reduce anxiety; they were formerly known as **minor tranquillizers** (*compare* ANTIPSYCHOTIC DRUGS). Anxiolytics should only be used to relieve anxiety that is severe or disabling. They will also induce sleep when taken at night (*see* HYPNOTIC DRUGS). Physical and psychological *dependence can develop with prolonged use, and these drugs should only be used for short periods and then withdrawn gradually. The lowest effective dosage should be used and discontinued as soon as possible. Anxiolytics may impair judgment and increase reaction time, affecting the ability to drive or operate machinery. They increase the effects of alcohol, and the hangover effects of a night-time dose may impair driving the following day. The most commonly used anxiolytics are the *benzodiazepines and *buspirone.

apomorphine hydrochloride An *antiparkinsonian drug used for the treatment of 'off' episodes in Parkinson's disease, when the condition is poorly controlled by *levodopa. It acts by stimulating *dopamine receptors in the brain. *Domperidone is given before, and during the first weeks of, treatment with apomorphine in order to minimize the nausea that this drug causes (see below). Apomorphine is available as a solution for injection on *prescription only.

Side effects: include instability of posture with a tendency to fall, nausea and vomiting, impairment of cognitive abilities, confusion, and personality changes.

Precautions: apomorphine should not be given to people who are hypersensitive to opioids or who have psychiatric problems. It should be used with caution in people who have a tendency to nausea and vomiting, in those with lung, liver, or heart disease, and in the elderly.

Interactions with other drugs:

  Antipsychotics: these drugs antagonize the action of apomorphine and their own effects are antagonized by apomorphine.

Proprietary preparation: Britaject.

apraclonidine A *sympathomimetic drug, similar to *brimonidine, that stimulates alpha *adrenoceptors. It is used to reduce the pressure inside the eye in the short-term treatment of chronic (open-angle) *glaucoma and following some types of eye surgery: it is thought to act by reducing the production of aqueous fluid and also by aiding the drainage of fluid from the eye. Unlike brimonidine, it may dilate the pupil. Its benefits usually diminish after one month. Apraclonidine is available as eye drops on *prescription only.

Side effects: include allergic reactions in the eye, dry mouth, and taste disturbances.

Precautions: apraclonidine should be used with caution by people with a history of angina or severe heart disease, those with liver or kidney disease, and by women who are pregnant or breastfeeding. It should not be used by those who wear soft contact lenses.

Interactions with other drugs:

  Adrenaline <epinephrine> and noradrenaline <norepinephrine>: there is a possible risk of high blood pressure.

  MAOIs: should not be used with apraclonidine.

  Tricyclic antidepressants: should not be used with apraclonidine.

Proprietary preparation: Iopidine.

Apresoline (Alliance Pharmaceuticals) *See* HYDRALAZINE HYDROCHLORIDE.

Aprinox (Knoll) *See* BENDROFLUAZIDE <BENDROFLUMETHIAZIDE>.

aprotinin An antifibrinolytic drug (*see* HAEMOSTATIC DRUGS) that inhibits the action of certain enzymes (including plasmin) that dissolve blood clots in the circulation. It is used for preventing haemorrhage in people who are at high risk of major blood loss during open-heart surgery and for preventing severe bleeding due to a high concentration of plasmin in the blood, which occurs in certain cancers (such as leukaemia) and may occur after therapy with *fibrinolytic drugs. Aprotinin is given by intravenous injection or infusion and is available on *prescription only.
Side effects: aprotinin occasionally causes allergic reactions and localized thrombophlebitis (inflammation and thrombosis in a vein).
Proprietary preparation: Trasylol.

Aprovel (Bristol-Myers Squibb; Sanofi Winthrop) *See* IRBESARTAN.

Apsin (APS-Berk) *See* PHENOXYMETHYLPENICILLIN.

Apsolol (APS-Berk) *See* PROPRANOLOL HYDROCHLORIDE.

Apstil (APS-Berk) *See* STILBOESTROL <DIETHYLSTILBESTROL>.

Aquadrate (Procter & Gamble) *See* UREA.

Aquasept (Seton Scholl Healthcare) *See* TRICLOSAN.

arachis oil (peanut oil) An oil extracted from peanuts. It is an ingredient of emulsions used in nutrition. It is also used in an enema, as a *faecal softener for the treatment of constipation and impacted faeces, as an *emollient in creams, and as an ingredient of ear drops for softening earwax.
Precautions: arachis oil should not be used by people allergic to peanuts.
Proprietary preparations: Fletchers' Arachis Oil Retention Enema; Oilatum Cream (emollient); CERUMOL (combined with paradichlorobenzene and chlorbutol <chlorobutanol>); EAREX EAR DROPS (combined with camphor and almond oil); HYDROMOL CREAM (combined with isopropyl myristate, liquid paraffin, sodium lactate, and sodium pyrrolidone); POLYTAR (combined with tar, coal tar, and oleyl alcohol).

Aramine (Merck Sharp & Dohme) *See* METARAMINOL.

Arbralene (APS-Berk) *See* METOPROLOL TARTRATE.

Aredia (Novartis Pharmaceuticals) *See* DISODIUM PAMIDRONATE.

Aricept (Eisai; Pfizer) *See* DONEPEZIL HYDROCHLORIDE.

Aridil (CP Pharmaceuticals) *See* CO-AMILOFRUSE.

Arimidex (AstraZeneca) *See* ANASTROZOLE.

Arnica Ointment (Weleda) A proprietary preparation of the traditional herbal remedy arnica, used for the relief of muscular pain, stiffness, sprains, and bruises. It is freely available *over the counter. *Side effects and precautions:* see RUBEFACIENTS.

aromatase inhibitors A class of drugs that inhibit the action of aromatase, an enzyme required for the conversion of *androgens to *oestrogens. Aromatase inhibitors thus decrease the concentrations of oestrogens in the body and are effective against tumours that depend on oestrogen for growth. They are usually used as second-line therapy (after *tamoxifen) for the treatment of breast cancer in postmenopausal women (*see* CANCER). The aromatase inhibitors include *anastrozole, *formestane, *letrozole, and *aminoglutethimide.

Arpicolin (Rosemont Pharmaceuticals) *See* PROCYCLIDINE.

Arpimycin (Rosemont Pharmaceuticals) *See* ERYTHROMYCIN.

Arret (Janssen-Cilag) *See* LOPERAMIDE HYDROCHLORIDE.

arrhythmia An abnormal heartbeat that may be slower or faster than normal, or just irregular. Normally, electrical impulses originate in the sinoatrial node (natural pacemaker) of the heart and pass along conducting pathways to coordinate the pumping action of the two atria and the two ventricles – the four chambers of the heart. If this coordination breaks down, arrhythmias occur. There are four major types of arrhythmia: **atrial fibrillation**, the most common, when the atria contract irregularly and too rapidly for the ventricles to keep pace; **ventricular tachycardia**, when abnormal electrical activity causes the ventricles to contract too rapidly; **supraventricular tachycardia**, when extra electrical signals arise in the atria, stimulating the ventricles to contract rapidly; and **heart block**, when signals are not conducted from the atria to the ventricles, so that the ventricles beat slowly. Minor disturbances of heart rhythm are common and do not normally require treatment. However, if the pumping action of the heart is seriously altered the circulation of the blood may be compromised and treatment with *anti-arrhythmic drugs is necessary. Arrhythmias may be due to a birth defect (congenital), to coronary heart disease, or to other less common heart disorders. Overactivity of the thyroid gland and some drugs can disturb heart rhythm.

Arthrofen (Ashbourne Pharmaceuticals) *See* IBUPROFEN.

Arthrosin (Ashbourne Pharmaceuticals) *See* NAPROXEN.

Arthrotec (Searle) A proprietary combination of *diclofenac sodium (an NSAID) and *misoprostol (a prostaglandin analogue), used for the treatment of rheumatoid arthritis and osteoarthritis; the misoprostol is added to prevent the gastric bleeding and ulceration that may result from the use of diclofenac alone. Arthrotec is available, on *prescription only, as tablets of two strengths of diclofenac (**Arthrotec 50** and **Arthrotec 70**).

Side effects and precautions: see NSAIDS; MISOPROSTOL.

Interactions with other drugs: see NSAIDS.

Arthroxen (CP Pharmaceuticals) *See* NAPROXEN.

Arythmol (Knoll) *See* PROPAFENONE HYDROCHLORIDE.

Asacol (SmithKline Beecham Pharmaceuticals) *See* MESALAZINE.

Asasantin Retard (Boehringer Ingelheim) A proprietary combination of *dipyridamole and *aspirin (both antiplatelet drugs), used to prevent the recurrence of strokes in people who have already had a stroke. It is available as *modified-release capsules on *prescription only.

Side effects, precautions, and interactions with other drugs: see DIPYRIDAMOLE; ASPIRIN.

Ascarbiol (Rhône-Poulenc Rorer) *See* BENZYL BENZOATE.

ascorbic acid *See* VITAMIN C.

Asendis (Wyeth Laboratories) *See* AMOXAPINE.

Aserbine (Goldshield Pharmaceuticals) A proprietary combination of *malic acid, *benzoic acid, and *salicylic acid (all keratolytics), used to remove dead tissue from wounds and promote the healing of ulcers, burns, pressure sores, and traumatic injuries and to cleanse wounds. It is available as a cream or solution and can be obtained without a prescription, but only from pharmacies.

Side effects and precautions: see SALICYLIC ACID.

Asilone Heartburn (Seton Scholl Healthcare) A proprietary combination of *alginic acid, *aluminium hydroxide, *magnesium trisilicate, and *sodium bicarbonate, used as an antacid for the relief of indigestion, heartburn, gastritis, flatulence, and peptic ulceration (*see* ACID-PEPTIC DISEASES). It is freely available *over the counter in the form of a suspension (**Asilone Heartburn Liquid**) or tablets (**Asilone Heartburn Tablets**); it cannot be prescribed on the NHS.

Side effects, precautions, and interactions with other drugs: see ANTACIDS.

Asilone Suspension (Seton Scholl Healthcare) A proprietary combination of *aluminium hydroxide and *magnesium oxide (antacids) and activated *dimethicone <dimeticone> (an antifoaming agent), used for the treatment of indigestion, heartburn, gastritis, flatulence, and peptic ulceration (*see* ACID-PEPTIC DISEASES). It is freely available *over the counter. This combination is also available as **Asilone Antacid Liquid** and **Asilone Antacid Tablets**, which cannot be prescribed on the NHS.

Side effects and interactions with other drugs: see ANTACIDS.

Precautions: Asilone is not recommended for children under 12 years old.

Askit (Roche Products) A proprietary combination of *aspirin and *aloxiprin (analgesics and antipyretics) and *caffeine (a stimulant), used for the treatment of mild to moderate pain (including headache, neuralgia, toothache, and period pains) and fever and to relieve the symptoms of influenza and colds. It is freely available *over the counter in the form of capsules or powders.

Side effects and interactions with other drugs: see ASPIRIN.

Precautions: Askit should not be given to children, except on medical advice. *See also* ASPIRIN; CAFFEINE.

Asmabec Clickhaler (Medeva) *See* BECLOMETHASONE <BECLOMETASONE> DIPROPIONATE.

Asmabec Spacehaler (Medeva) *See* BECLOMETHASONE <BECLOMETASONE> DIPROPIONATE.

Asmasal Clickhaler (Medeva) *See* SALBUTAMOL.

Asmaven (APS-Berk) *See* SALBUTAMOL.

Aspav (Hoechst Marion Roussel) A proprietary combination of *aspirin (an analgesic) and *papaveretum (a mixture of opioids), used for the relief of moderate to severe pain. It is available as dispersible tablets on *prescription only.

Side effects and precautions: see ASPIRIN; MORPHINE.

Interactions with other drugs: see ASPIRIN; OPIOIDS.

aspirin (acetylsalicylic acid) An *analgesic drug that also reduces fever (i.e. it is antipyretic). It is the most common of the group of drugs known as *salicylates and is also classed as a non-steroidal anti-inflammatory drug (*see* NSAIDS), although other drugs of this class are usually preferred to aspirin for treating chronic inflammatory conditions because of its adverse side effects (see below). Aspirin is widely used for treating mild to moderate pain – particularly headache, period pains, and painful (but short-lasting) conditions of muscles and joints – and feverish conditions (such as influenza and colds). Aspirin is also a valuable *antiplatelet drug, used to prevent the formation of blood clots (*thrombosis). Low doses of aspirin (75–100 mg/day) are given to people who have had a heart attack or stroke to prevent a recurrence of these conditions; they are also used to prevent thrombosis in people who are at high risk, for example following bypass surgery.

Aspirin is available in a variety of forms – tablets (including *enteric-coated tablets), dispersible tablets, powders, and suppositories – and can be obtained without a prescription, although there are restrictions on the quantities of tablets that can be supplied. Packs containing 16 tablets are freely available *over the counter; packs containing up to 32 (or exceptionally up to 100) tablets can only be obtained from pharmacies. Larger quantities are available on *prescription only. Aspirin is combined with paracetamol, codeine, or other ingredients in a variety of compound analgesic preparations and cold remedies. *See also* BENORYLATE; CO-CODAPRIN.

Side effects: aspirin can irritate the lining of the stomach, causing indigestion, stomach pain, nausea and vomiting, and (rarely) gastrointestinal bleeding. Rashes, wheezing, or breathing problems may develop in people who are allergic to NSAIDs. *See also* SALICYLATES.

Precautions: aspirin should not be given to children under 12 years old (unless specifically prescribed by a doctor) because it has been associated with Reye's syndrome (a disorder causing liver and brain damage); *paracetamol is the recommended alternative. Aspirin should not be taken by people who are allergic to it or to other NSAIDs or who have an active peptic ulcer, severe liver or kidney disease, or haemophilia, or by women who are breastfeeding. Aspirin should be used with caution in pregnant women and in people with asthma or a history of peptic ulceration.

Interactions with other drugs:

Anticoagulants: the risk of bleeding is increased if aspirin is taken with anticoagulants (especially warfarin).

Methotrexate: aspirin increases the side effects of methotrexate.

NSAIDs: aspirin should not be taken with other NSAIDs as this increases the likelihood of stomach irritation and bleeding.

Proprietary preparations: Alka-Seltzer; Angettes 75 (antiplatelet); Aspro, Aspro Clear; Bayer Aspirin; Beechams Lemon Tablets; Boots Back Pain Relief; Caprin (standard and antiplatelet); Dispirin, Dispirin Direct; Dispirin CV (antiplatelet); Fynnon Calcium Aspirin; Maximum Strength Aspro Clear; Nu-Seals Aspirin (standard and antiplatelet); PostMI 75EC (antiplatelet). For details of these and other preparations of which aspirin is an ingredient, see Appendix.

Aspro, **Aspro Clear** (Roche Products) *See* ASPIRIN.

astemizole   One of the newer (non-sedating) *antihistamines, used to relieve the symptoms of such allergic conditions as hay fever, perennial allergic rhinitis, urticaria, and other allergic skin conditions. It is available as tablets or a suspension on *prescription only.

Side effects: *see* ANTIHISTAMINES. Astemizole may also occasionally cause weight gain, and at high doses there is a risk of an abnormal heartbeat (*see* ARRHYTHMIA); a doctor should be informed if this occurs.

Precautions: *see* ANTIHISTAMINES.

Interactions with other drugs: the following drugs should not be given with astemizole, as this increases the risk of arrhythmias: anti-arrhythmic drugs; antipsychotic drugs; clarithromycin; diuretics;

erythromycin; imidazole antifungals (e.g. itraconazole, ketoconazole); monoamine oxidase inhibitors; sotalol; tricyclic antidepressants (e.g. dothiepin <dosulepin>, lofepramine, amitriptyline, imipramine). *Proprietary preparation:* Hismanal.

asthma A condition marked by widespread narrowing of the bronchial airways, which changes in severity over short periods of time (either spontaneously or under treatment) and leads to cough, wheezing, and difficulty in breathing. Bronchial asthma may be precipitated by exposure to one or more of a wide range of stimuli, including allergens, drugs (such as aspirin and other NSAIDs), exertion, emotion, infections, and air pollution.

Treatment of asthma is with sympathomimetic drugs that stimulate beta receptors, such as *salbutamol or *terbutaline (*see* BRONCHODILATORS), with or without *corticosteroids (such as *beclomethasone <beclometasone> dipropionate and *budesonide); all these drugs are usually administered via aerosol or dry-powder *inhalers, or – if the condition is more severe – via a *nebulizer. Other drugs that can be used for the prevention of asthmatic attacks include *sodium cromoglycate <cromoglicate> or *nedocromil, *theophylline, the antimuscarinic drugs *oxitropium bromide or *ipratropium bromide, and the *leukotriene receptor antagonists. Oral corticosteroids are reserved for those patients who fail to respond adequately to these measures. Severe asthmatic attacks may need large doses of oral corticosteroids (such as *prednisolone).

astringents Drugs that cause cells to shrink by precipitating proteins on their surfaces, making the surface less permeable to liquids, especially water. The cells therefore dry up but do not die. Astringents in various dilutions are used in soothing preparations to treat haemorrhoids (*see* BISMUTH OXIDE; BISMUTH SUBGALLATE; HAMAMELIS), in eye drops to treat watering eyes (*see* ZINC SULPHATE), in lotions to treat weeping skin conditions (*see* ALUMINIUM ACETATE; POTASSIUM PERMANGANATE), and in ear drops to clean the ear canal (aluminium acetate). Other salts of zinc and aluminium are used in antiperspirants (*see* ALUMINIUM CHLORIDE) or skin creams and lotions (*see* ZINC OXIDE; CALAMINE). *See also* ALLANTOIN.

AT 10 (Sanofi Winthrop) *See* DIHYDROTACHYSTEROL.

Atarax (Pfizer) *See* HYDROXYZINE HYDROCHLORIDE.

Atenix (Ashbourne Pharmaceuticals) *See* ATENOLOL.

Atenix-Co (Ashbourne Pharmaceuticals) *See* CO-TENIDONE.

atenolol A cardioselective *beta blocker used for the treatment and prevention of cardiac *arrhythmias and *angina and the treatment of *hypertension. It is available on *prescription only as tablets, syrup, or a solution for injection.

Side effects, precautions, and interactions with other drugs: see BETA BLOCKERS.

Proprietary preparations: Antipressan; Atenix, Tenormin; Totamol; BETA-ADALAT (combined with nifedipine); KALTEN (combined with amiloride hydrochloride and hydrochlorothiazide); TENBEN (combined with bendrofluazide <bendroflumethiazide>); TENIF (combined with nifedipine); Tenoret 50 (*see* CO-TENIDONE); Tenoretic (*see* CO-TENIDONE). *See also* ANTI-ARRHYTHMIC DRUGS; ANTIHYPERTENSIVE DRUGS.

atherosclerosis A disease of the arteries in which their inner walls degenerate with the formation of fatty plaques and scar tissue, which obstructs the flow of blood and predisposes to arterial *thrombosis. It is associated with high concentrations of *cholesterol in the blood (*see* HYPERLIPIDAEMIA), which may require treatment with *lipid-lowering drugs.

Ativan (Wyeth Laboratories) *See* LORAZEPAM.

atorvastatin A *statin used for the treatment of primary hypercholesterolaemia (*see* HYPERLIPIDAEMIA) that has not responded to dietary measures. It is available as tablets on *prescription only. *Side effects, precautions, and interactions with other drugs:* see STATINS. *Proprietary preparation:* Lipitor.

atovaquone An *antibiotic with activity against certain types of protozoa. Atovaquone is used for the treatment of mild to moderate pneumonia caused by *Pneumocystis carinii* (which is most common in people with AIDS); it is prescribed for people who cannot tolerate *co-trimoxazole, and it should be taken with food. It is available as a suspension on *prescription only. Atovaquone is also used in combination with *proguanil hydrochloride for the treatment of falciparum *malaria.
Side effects: include diarrhoea, nausea, and vomiting (which may hinder its absorption), headache, insomnia, rash, and fever.
Precautions: atovaquone should be used with caution by elderly people, pregnant women, and people with liver or kidney disease. It should not be taken by women who are breastfeeding.
Interactions with other drugs:
  Antibiotics: rifampicin and tetracycline may reduce the plasma concentration of atovaquone to the extent that it is not effective.
  Metoclopramide: reduces the plasma concentration (and possibly the effectiveness) of atovaquone.
Proprietary preparations: Wellvone; MALARONE (combined with proguanil).

atrial fibrillation *See* ARRHYTHMIA.

Atromid-S (AstraZeneca) *See* CLOFIBRATE.

atropine sulphate An *antimuscarinic drug; atropine is one of the components of *belladonna. Atropine sulphate is applied to the eye to dilate the pupil before examination of the interior of the eye, especially in young children. Since its action is long-lasting and it paralyses the ciliary muscles (which control the focusing ability of the eye) as well as the muscle of the iris (which controls the size of the pupil), it is also used for treating inflammation of the ciliary muscles and iris. Atropine is taken by mouth for the relief of gut spasms (*see* ANTISPASMODICS). Injections of atropine are occasionally used during surgery for drying up secretions in the airways and for preventing or reversing the effects of *neostigmine in slowing the heart rate; atropine injections are also given to patients who have a slow heart rate associated with *arrhythmias after a heart attack. Atropine is available as eye drops or ointment, tablets, or an injection on *prescription only; compound antispasmodic preparations containing atropine are available from pharmacies without a prescription.

Side effects: for *systemic effects, *see* ANTIMUSCARINIC DRUGS. Eye drops or ointment can cause transient stinging and an increase in pressure in the eye; with prolonged use, local irritation and conjunctivitis can occur.

Precautions: see ANTIMUSCARINIC DRUGS. Eye ointment (rather than drops) should be used in children under three months, since they are more likely to develop systemic effects with eye drops.

Interactions with other drugs: see ANTIMUSCARINIC DRUGS.

Proprietary preparations: Isopto Atropine (eye drops); Minims Atropine Sulphate (single-dose eye drops); Min-I-Jet Atropine (injection); ACTONORM POWDER (combined with antacids and peppermint oil).

Atrovent (Boehringer Ingelheim) *See* IPRATROPIUM BROMIDE.

attapulgite A purified form of magnesium aluminium silicate. It is highly adsorbent and is used in pharmaceutical preparations, especially in preparations to treat diarrhoea (*see* ANTIDIARRHOEAL DRUGS).

Proprietary preparations: DIOCALM DUAL ACTION (combined with morphine); ENTROTABS (combined with aluminium hydroxide).

Audax (Seton Scholl Healthcare) A proprietary combination of *choline salicylate (an analgesic) and *glycerin, used for the relief of pain in ear infections and for softening earwax to aid its removal. Audax is available as ear drops and can be obtained without a prescription, but only from pharmacies; it cannot be prescribed on the NHS.

Precautions: Audax should not be used in children under one year old without a doctor's advice. *See also* CHOLINE SALICYLATE.

Audicort (Wyeth Laboratories) A proprietary combination of *triamcinolone acetonide (a potent steroid) and *neomycin (an antibiotic), used for the treatment of acute and chronic bacterial infections of the outer ear. It is available as ear drops on *prescription only.

Side effects: there may be local irritation and secondary infection. *See also* TOPICAL STEROIDS.

Precautions: Audicort should not to be used on perforated eardrums and it should be used with caution by women who are pregnant or breastfeeding. *See also* TOPICAL STEROIDS.

Augmentin (SmithKline Beecham Pharmaceuticals) *See* CO-AMOXICLAV.

auranofin A salt of gold that is taken by mouth for the treatment of active progressive rheumatoid arthritis when *NSAIDs alone are inadequate. Unlike NSAIDs, auranofin does not have an immediate therapeutic effect and it may take 4–6 months to obtain a full response. It is available as tablets on *prescription only.

Side effects: see SODIUM AUROTHIOMALATE. In addition, diarrhoea may occur, which can be treated with bran or other bulking agents.

Precautions and interactions with other drugs: see SODIUM AUROTHIOMALATE.

Proprietary preparation: Ridaura.

Aureocort (Wyeth Laboratories) A proprietary combination of *triamcinolone acetonide (a potent steroid) and *chlortetracycline (an antibiotic), used for the treatment of inflammatory skin conditions when infection is present. It is available as a cream on *prescription only.

Side effects and precautions, and interactions with other drugs: see TOPICAL STEROIDS; TETRACYCLINES.

Aureomycin (Wyeth Laboratories) *See* CHLORTETRACYCLINE.

aurothiomalate *See* SODIUM AUROTHIOMALATE.

Aveeno (Bioglan Laboratories) A proprietary preparation consisting of an extract of oatmeal, used as an *emollient for the relief of *eczema and dry skin conditions, including those associated with itching. It is available as an oil, to be added to the bath or applied directly to the skin before bathing, or as a cream to be rubbed into the skin. **Aveeno Oilated**, containing added mineral oil, is a powder to be added to the bath. All preparations are freely available *over the counter.

Avloclor (AstraZeneca) *See* CHLOROQUINE.

Avoca (Bray Health & Leisure) *See* SILVER NITRATE.

Avomine (Rhône-Poulenc Rorer) *See* PROMETHAZINE THEOCLATE <TEOCLATE>.

Avonex (Biogen) *See* INTERFERON-BETA.

Axid (Eli Lilly & Co) *See* NIZATIDINE.

Axsain (Euroderma) *See* CAPSAICIN.

Azactam (Bristol-Myers Squibb) *See* AZTREONAM.

azapropazone An *NSAID that is used only for the treatment of rheumatoid arthritis, ankylosing spondylitis (a type of arthritis that affects the spine), and acute gout, but only when these conditions have failed to respond to other NSAIDs. It is available as capsules or tablets on *prescription only.

Side effects: azapropazone is more likely than other NSAIDs to cause severe gastrointestinal bleeding and ulceration. Other side effects include rashes, sensitivity to sunlight (people taking azapropazone should avoid exposure to sunlight or use a sunblock), fluid retention, and (rarely) inflammation of the lungs and blood disorders. *See also* NSAIDS.

Precautions: azapropanone must not be taken by people with a history of peptic ulcers or blood disorders. *See also* NSAIDS.

Interactions with other drugs: see NSAIDS. In addition:

  Methotrexate: should not be taken with azapropazone, as its excretion is reduced by azapropazone, causing amounts of methotrexate to build up and have adverse effects.

  Phenytoin: should not be taken with azapropazone as its effects are enhanced by azapropazone.

  Warfarin: should not be taken with azapropazone as its anticoagulant effects are greatly enhanced by azapropazone.

Proprietary preparation: Rheumox.

azatadine maleate An *antihistamine that also has some activity against serotonin, a transmitter that, like histamine, acts on receptors in the skin to produce the weals and flares seen after nettle or insect stings. Azatadine is used for the treatment of hay fever, bites and stings, urticaria, and other itching skin conditions. It is available in the form of a syrup or tablets and can be bought from pharmacies without a prescription.

Side effects: include drowsiness, impaired reactions, increased appetite, *antimuscarinic effects, nausea, and headache.

Precautions: alcohol enhances the drowsiness caused by azatadine. Azatadine should be used with caution by people with an enlarged prostate gland or peptic ulcers.

Interactions with other drugs:

  MAOIs: increase the sedative effects of azatadine. *See also* ANTIHISTAMINES.

Proprietary preparation: Optimine.

azathioprine An *immunosuppressant that is a powerful *cytotoxic drug. It is used to prevent the rejection of transplants (and to minimize the use of *corticosteroids for this purpose) and also to treat a number of autoimmune conditions, usually when corticosteroids have been inadequate, including myasthenia gravis and rheumatoid arthritis. It is also used in the treatment of ulcerative colitis. Azathioprine is available as tablets on *prescription only.

Side effects: include nausea and vomiting, loss of appetite, malaise, dizziness, fever, muscular aches and pains, rashes, and hair loss. Azathioprine can suppress production of white blood cells and platelets in the bone marrow, leading to increased susceptibility to infections and unusual bruising or bleeding.

Precautions: azathioprine should only be taken under specialist supervision, and blood counts should be monitored during the treatment period. Any evidence of infection or unusual bruising or bleeding should be reported to a doctor immediately.

Interactions with other drugs:

  Allopurinol: increases the toxic effects of azathioprine, whose dosage will therefore need to be reduced.

  Rifampicin: increases the metabolism of azathioprine and may lead to transplant rejection.

Proprietary preparations: Immunoprin; Imuran; Oprisine.

azelaic acid An antibacterial drug used for the *topical treatment of mild to moderate *acne. It is available as a cream on *prescription only.

Side effects: azelaic acid may irritate the skin and (rarely) make the skin more sensitive to sunlight.

Precautions: azelaic acid should not be applied near the eyes. It should be used with caution by women who are pregnant or breastfeeding.

Proprietary preparation: Skinoren.

azelastine hydrochloride An *antihistamine used to relieve the symptoms of allergic rhinitis, including hay fever, and allergic conjunctivitis. It is available in a metered-dose pump spray and as eye drops on *prescription only; a nasal spray specifically for the treatment of hay fever is available from pharmacies without a prescription.

Side effects: include local irritation and taste disturbances.

Precautions: azelastine should be used with caution by women who are pregnant or breastfeeding.

Interactions with other drugs: see ANTIHISTAMINES.

Proprietary preparations: Optilast (eye drops); Rhinolast (nasal spray); Rhinolast Hayfever (nasal spray).

azidothymidine (AZT) *See* ZIDOVUDINE.

azithromycin A *macrolide antibiotic used for the treatment of infections of the respiratory tract, ear, skin, and soft tissues and for genital infections. It is similar to *erythromycin, but has a longer duration of action and can be taken only once daily. It is available, on *prescription only, as capsules, tablets, or a suspension.

Side effects, precautions, and interactions with other drugs: see
ERYTHROMYCIN.
Proprietary preparation: Zithromax.

azlocillin A broad-spectrum *penicillin that is active against *Pseudomonas* and *Proteus* bacteria. It is used for the treatment of systemic (generalized) and local infections (such as infected wounds or burns) and respiratory and urinary-tract infections. Given by injection or infusion, it is available on *prescription only. It is used sometimes in conjunction with an *aminoglycoside antibiotic.
Side effects, precautions, and interactions with other drugs: see
BENZYLPENICILLIN.
Proprietary preparation: Securopen.

AZT 1. (azidothymidine) *See* ZIDOVUDINE. 2. An abbreviation sometimes used for *azathioprine and *azithromycin.

aztreonam A beta-lactam *antibiotic that is similar to the *penicillins but may be less likely to produce allergic reactions in people sensitive to pencillins. It is used for the treatment of infections of the lower respiratory tract, including lung infections in patients with cystic fibrosis. It is also used to treat bone, skin, and soft-tissue infections, abdominal and gynaecological infections, septicaemia, and meningitis. It is given by *intramuscular or *intravenous injection and is available on *prescription only.
Side effects: may include nausea, vomiting, diarrhoea, abdominal cramps, mouth ulcers, altered taste, jaundice, hepatitis, blood disorders, and rashes.
Precautions: aztreonam should not be taken by women who are pregnant or breastfeeding or by anyone who is allergic to it, and it should be used with caution in those who have liver or kidney disease.
Interactions with other drugs:

 Anticoagulants: the effects of warfarin and nicoumalone
  <acenocoumarol> may be increased by aztreonam.
Proprietary preparation: Azactam.

B

Baby Meltus (Seton Scholl Healthcare) *See* ACETIC ACID.

bacitracin zinc An *antibiotic used for the treatment of bacterial infections of the skin and eyes. It is available, on *prescription only, in the form of compound preparations with other antibiotics.
Side effects and precautions: see entries for individual compound preparations.
Proprietary preparations: CICATRIN (combined with neomycin sulphate); POLYFAX (combined with polymyxin B sulphate)

baclofen A skeletal *muscle relaxant used to relieve muscle spasm, especially when due to trauma or disease of the central nervous system, such as multiple sclerosis, meningitis, or cerebral palsy. Dosages should be increased slowly to avoid side effects. It is available, on *prescription only, as tablets or a sugar-free liquid.
Side effects: sedation, drowsiness, and nausea are the most common. Less common side effects include confusion, dizziness, headache, insomnia, tremor, loss of sensation in the extremities, muscle pain and weakness, and (rarely) hallucinations and convulsions.
Precautions: baclofen should not be taken by people with peptic ulcer and it should be used with caution in those with psychiatric illness, liver or kidney disease, stroke, diabetes, epilepsy, and porphyria and in women who are pregnant or breastfeeding. The drug should be withdrawn gradually at the end of treatment.
Interactions with other drugs:
  Anti-arrhythmic drugs: procainamide and quinidine increase the effect of baclofen.
  Antihypertensives: baclofen increases their effect in lowering blood pressure.
  Tricyclic antidepressants: increase the effect of baclofen.
Proprietary preparations: Baclospas; Balgifen; Lioresal.

Baclospas (Ashbourne Pharmaceuticals) *See* BACLOFEN.

Bactroban, Bactroban Nasal (SmithKline Beecham Pharmaceuticals) *See* MUPIROCIN.

BAL *See* DIMERCAPROL.

balanced salt solution A sterile solution of *sodium chloride, sodium acetate, *sodium citrate, *calcium chloride, and magnesium chloride, used to wash out the eyes to remove foreign bodies or harmful

substances. It is also used for irrigating the eyes during surgery. The solution is available without a prescription, but only from pharmacies.
Proprietary preparation: Iocare.

Balgifen (APS-Berk) *See* BACLOFEN.

Balmosa (Pharmax) A proprietary combination of *methyl salicylate, *camphor, *menthol, and *capsicum oleoresin, used for the relief of rheumatic, muscular and mild arthritic pain, lumbago, and sciatica (*see* RUBEFACIENTS). It is freely available *over the counter in the form of a cream.
Side effects and precautions: see RUBEFACIENTS; SALICYLATES.

Balneum (Crookes Healthcare) *See* SOYA OIL.

Balneum Plus Cream (Crookes Healthcare) A proprietary combination of *urea (an emollient) and *lauromacrogols (antipruritic agents), used for soothing dry skin conditions associated with scaling and itching. It is freely available *over the counter.

Balneum Plus Oil (Crookes Healthcare) A proprietary combination of *soya oil (an emollient) and *lauromacrogols (antipruritic agents), used for soothing dry skin conditions, including those associated with itching. It is freely available, in the form of a bath oil, *over the counter.

balsalazide sodium An *aminosalicylate that is used for the treatment of mild to moderate ulcerative colitis; it is converted to *mesalazine in the body. Balsalazide is available as capsules on *prescription only.
Side effects: include abdominal pain and vomiting; *see also* AMINOSALICYLATES.
Precautions: see AMINOSALICYLATES.
Proprietary preparation: Colazide.

balsam of Peru *See* PERU BALSAM.

Bambec (Novex Pharma) *See* BAMBUTEROL HYDROCHLORIDE.

bambuterol hydrochloride A drug that is converted to *terbutaline in the body; it is used as a *bronchodilator for the treatment of asthma attacks and the relief of wheezing and breathlessness in bronchitis and emphysema. Bambuterol is available as tablets on *prescription only.
Side effects, precautions, and interactions with other drugs: see SALBUTAMOL.
Proprietary preparation: Bambec.

Bansor Mouth Antiseptic (Thornton & Ross) *See* CETRIMIDE.

Baratol (Monmouth Pharmaceuticals) *See* INDORAMIN HYDROCHLORIDE.

barbiturates A class of drugs that depress activity of the central nervous system; they are classified into three groups according to their duration of action: short-, intermediate-, and long-acting. Barbiturates were formerly widely used as *hypnotic drugs but have largely been superseded by the *benzodiazepines; they should now only be prescribed for patients who are already taking them (*see* AMYLOBARBITONE <AMOBARBITAL>; BUTOBARBITONE <BUTOBARBITAL>; QUINALBARBITONE <SECOBARBITAL>). They produce *tolerance and *dependence; abrupt withdrawal causes severe effects similar to those seen in alcoholics deprived of alcohol. Toxic effects leading to coma and death are common after overdose, especially when accompanied by alcohol. The long-acting barbiturates *phenobarbitone <phenobarbital> and *methylphenobarbitone <methylphenobarbital> are occasionally used in the treatment of epilepsy, and the short-acting drugs **thiopentone <thiopental> sodium** and **methohexitone <methohexital> sodium** are used to induce general anaesthesia. Barbiturates are *controlled drugs; they are available as tablets, capsules, or solutions for injection.

Side effects: include 'hangover' effects with drowsiness, dizziness, shaky movements, unsteady gait, depression of breathing, headache, paradoxical excitement, and confusion. Tolerance and dependence may develop.

Precautions: barbiturates should not be used to treat insomnia caused by uncontrolled pain; they should not be taken by women who are pregnant or breastfeeding, by people with a history of drug or alcohol abuse, or by children, young adults, or elderly people. Barbiturates should be used with caution in people who have liver or kidney disease.

Interactions with other drugs:

  Anticoagulants: the anticoagulant effects of warfarin and nicoumalone <acenocoumarol> are reduced by barbiturates.

  Antidepressants: reduce the anticonvulsant effects of barbiturates used to treat epilepsy; the effects of mianserin and tricyclic antidepressants are reduced by barbiturates.

  Antiepileptic drugs: taking phenobarbitone <phenobarbital> with other antiepileptic drugs may increase their adverse effects without enhancing their anticonvulsant actions.

  Antipsychotics: reduce the anticonvulsant effects of barbiturates used to treat epilepsy.

  Antiviral drugs: the plasma concentrations of indinavir, nelfinavir, and saquinavir may be reduced by barbiturates.

  Calcium antagonists: the effects of diltiazem, felodipine, isradipine, verapamil, and probably nicardipine and nifedipine are reduced by barbiturates.

  Corticosteroids: their effects are reduced by barbiturates.

  Cyclosporin: its effects are reduced by barbiturates.

  Oral contraceptives: their effects are reduced by barbiturates.

barrier preparations Creams, ointments, or sprays used to protect the skin against water-soluble irritants (e.g. detergents, breakdown products of urine). Barrier preparations often contain a silicone (such as *dimethicone <dimeticone>). They are used for preventing and treating such conditions as napkin rash and pressure sores and for protecting the skin around a *stoma.

Baxan (Bristol-Myers Squibb) *See* CEFADROXIL.

Baycaron (Bayer) *See* MEFRUSIDE.

BCNU *See* CARMUSTINE.

Beclazone Easi-Breathe, **Beclazone 250 Easi-Breathe** (Norton Healthcare) *See* BECLOMETHASONE <BECLOMETASONE> DIPROPIONATE.

Becloforte (Allen & Hanburys) *See* BECLOMETHASONE <BECLOMETASONE> DIPROPIONATE.

beclomethasone dipropionate <beclometasone dipropionate> A *corticosteroid used mainly for the prevention of *asthma attacks and the treatment of allergic rhinitis (including hay fever). It may be used in conjunction with *bronchodilators and/or *sodium cromoglycate <cromoglicate>. Beclomethasone is also used to treat inflammatory skin conditions. It is administered by aerosol or powder inhalation (for asthma), by nasal spray (for rhinitis), or as a cream (for skin conditions), and most preparations are available on *prescription only.

Side effects: the most common side effects with an inhaler are hoarseness (due to weakness of the vocal muscles), fungal (*Candida*) infections of the mouth or throat (which can be reduced by rinsing out the mouth after doses), nasal discomfort, or irritation. Disturbances in taste and smell may occur with nasal sprays. There may be local effects with the cream. *See also* CORTICOSTEROIDS; TOPICAL STEROIDS.

Precautions: beclomethasone should be taken with caution by people who have (or have had) tuberculosis. *See also* CORTICOSTEROIDS.

Interactions with other drugs: see CORTICOSTEROIDS.

Proprietary preparations: AeroBec Autohaler (breath-activated metered-dose aerosol inhaler); AeroBec Forte (high-dose inhaler); Asmabec Clickhaler (standard-dose and high-dose dry powder for inhalation); Asmabec Spacehaler (metered-dose inhaler with spacer device); Beclazone Easi-Breathe (aerosol inhaler); Beclazone 250 Easi-Breathe (a stronger preparation); Becodisks (discs containing powder blisters, of varying strengths, for use in a breath-activated inhaler); Beconase (nasal spray available from pharmacies without a prescription); Becotide Inhaler; Becotide Rotacaps (capsules containing powder for use in a breath-activated inhaler); Filair (inhaler); Nasobec (nasal spray); Propaderm (skin cream); Qvar (aerosol inhalation); Qvar Autohaler (breath-activated inhaler); Zonivent (nasal atomizer); VENTIDE (combined with salbutamol).

Becodisks (Allen & Hanburys) *See* BECLOMETHASONE <BECLOMETASONE> DIPROPIONATE.

Beconase (Allen & Hanburys) *See* BECLOMETHASONE <BECLOMETASONE> DIPROPIONATE.

Becotide Inhaler (Allen & Hanburys) *See* BECLOMETHASONE <BECLOMETASONE> DIPROPIONATE.

Becotide Rotacaps (Allen & Hanburys) *See* BECLOMETHASONE <BECLOMETASONE> DIPROPIONATE.

Bedranol SR (Lagap Pharmaceuticals) *See* PROPRANOLOL HYDROCHLORIDE.

Beechams All-in-One (SmithKline Beecham Consumer Healthcare) A proprietary combination of *paracetamol (an analgesic and antipyretic), *guaiphenesin <guaifenesin> (an expectorant), and *phenylephrine (a decongestant), used to relieve the symptoms of colds, chills, and influenza. It is freely available *over the counter in the form of a liquid.
Side effects: see GUAIPHENESIN <GUAIFENESIN>; PHENYLEPHRINE.
Precautions: this medicine should not be given to children under six years old except on medical advice. *See also* PARACETAMOL; GUAIPHENESIN <GUAIFENESIN>; PHENYLEPHRINE.
Interactions with other drugs: see PHENYLEPHRINE.

Beechams Flu-Plus Caplets (SmithKline Beecham Consumer Healthcare) A proprietary combination of *paracetamol (an analgesic and antipyretic), *caffeine (a stimulant), and *phenylephrine (a decongestant), used to relieve the symptoms of colds and influenza. including chills, fever, headache, aches and pains, nasal congestion, sinus pain, and sore throat. It is freely available *over the counter in the form of tablets.
Side effects and interactions with other drugs: see PHENYLEPHRINE.
Precautions: this medicine should not be given to children, except on medical advice. *See also* PARACETAMOL; PHENYLEPHRINE; CAFFEINE.

Beechams Flu-Plus Hot Lemon, **Beechams Flu-Plus Hot Berry Fruits** (SmithKline Beecham Consumer Healthcare) Proprietary combinations of *paracetamol (an analgesic and antipyretic), *phenylephrine (a decongestant), and ascorbic acid (*vitamin C), used to relieve the symptoms of influenza. **Beechams Warmers Lemon**, **Beechams Warmers Lemon and Honey**, and **Beechams Warmers Hot Berry Fruits** are lower-strength preparations appropriate for treating colds. All are freely available *over the counter in the form of powders to be dissolved in hot water.
Side effects and interactions with other drugs: see PHENYLEPHRINE.

Precautions: these powders should not be given to children, except on medical advice. *See also* PARACETAMOL; PHENYLEPHRINE.

Beechams Lemon Tablets (SmithKline Beecham Consumer Healthcare) *See* ASPIRIN.

Beechams Pills (SmithKline Beecham Consumer Healthcare) *See* ALOIN.

Beechams Powders (SmithKline Beecham Consumer Healthcare) A proprietary combination of *aspirin (an analgesic and antipyretic) and *caffeine (a stimulant), used to relieve the symptoms of influenza, chills, and colds. It is also be used for the treatment of mild to moderate pain, such as headache, neuralgia, toothache, rheumatic pains, sore throat, and period pains. It is freely available *over the counter.
Side effects and interactions with other drugs: see ASPIRIN.
Precautions: Beechams Powders should not be given to children, except on medical advice. *See also* ASPIRIN; CAFFEINE.

Beechams Powders Capsules (SmithKline Beecham Consumer Healthcare) A proprietary combination of *paracetamol (an analgesic and antipyretic), *caffeine (a stimulant), and *phenylephrine (a decongestant), used to relieve the symptoms of influenza, fevers, chills, and colds, including nasal congestion, sinus pain, and catarrh. It is freely available *over the counter.
Side effects and interactions with other drugs: see PHENYLEPHRINE.
Precautions: these capsules should not be given to children, except on medical advice. *See also* PARACETAMOL; CAFFEINE; PHENYLEPHRINE.

Beechams Throat-Plus Lozenges (SmithKline Beecham Consumer Healthcare) A proprietary combination of the antiseptics *hexylresorcinol and *benzalkonium chloride, used for the relief of sore throats. It is freely available *over the counter.
Precautions: these lozenges are not recommended for children under seven years old.

Beechams Veno's Expectorant (SmithKline Beecham Consumer Healthcare) *See* GUAIPHENESIN <GUAIFENESIN>.

Beechams Veno's Honey and Lemon (SmithKline Beecham Consumer Healthcare) A proprietary combination of lemon juice, honey, and liquid glucose used as a *demulcent for the relief of dry irritating coughs. It is freely available *over the counter as a syrup.

Beechams Warmers *See* BEECHAMS FLU-PLUS HOT LEMON.

belladonna extract A collection of *alkaloids extracted from deadly nightshade (*Atropa belladonna*): they include *atropine sulphate, *hyoscine hydrobromide, and *hyoscine butylbromide, which are *antimuscarinic drugs. Belladonna is used as an *antispasmodic that is included in preparations for the treatment of diarrhoea and also in plasters for the relief of aches, pains, and stiffness.

Side effects and precautions: see ANTIMUSCARINIC DRUGS.

Proprietary preparations: Cuxson Gerrard Belladonna Plasters; ENTEROSAN (combined with morphine and kaolin); OPAZIMES (combined with kaolin, aluminium hydroxide, and morphine).

Benadon (Roche Products) *See* PYRIDOXINE.

Benadryl Allergy Relief (Warner-Lambert Consumer Healthcare) *See* ACRIVASTINE.

bendrofluazide <bendroflumethiazide> A *thiazide diuretic used to treat *oedema and *hypertension. It is available as tablets on *prescription only.

Side effects, precautions, and interactions with other drugs: see THIAZIDE DIURETICS.

Proprietary preparations: Aprinox; Berkozide; Neo-Bendromax; Neo-Naclex; CORGARETIC 40, CORGARETIC 80 (combined with nadolol); INDERETIC and INDEREX (combined with propranolol); NEO-NACLEX-K (combined with potassium chloride); PRESTIM (combined with timolol); TENBEN (combined with atenolol).

See also ANTIHYPERTENSIVE DRUGS; DIURETICS.

bendroflumethiazide *See* BENDROFLUAZIDE.

Benemid (Merck Sharp & Dohme) *See* PROBENECID.

Benerva (Roche Products) *See* THIAMINE.

Benoral (Sanofi Winthrop) *See* BENORYLATE.

benorilate *See* BENORYLATE.

benorylate <benorilate> A combination of *aspirin (an analgesic, antipyretic, and anti-inflammatory drug) and *paracetamol (an analgesic and antipyretic), used for the treatment of pain and inflammation in rheumatic disease and other muscular disorders. It is also used to relieve other types of mild to moderate pain and to reduce fever. Benorylate is available as tablets, granules, or a suspension and can be obtained from pharmacies without a prescription.

Side effects: similar to those of *aspirin, but benorylate causes less gastrointestinal bleeding than aspirin.

Precautions and interactions with other drugs: see ASPIRIN; PARACETAMOL.

Proprietary preparation: Benoral.

benperidol A butyrophenone *antipsychotic drug used for the treatment of patients with unacceptable deviant sexual behaviour. It is available as tablets on *prescription only.

Side effects: as for *chlorpromazine, but benperidol has more pronounced *extrapyramidal reactions, fewer antimuscarinic effects, and is less sedating.

Precautions: *see* CHLORPROMAZINE HYDROCHLORIDE.

Interactions with other drugs:

Anaesthetics: their effect in lowering blood pressure is enhanced.

Antidepressants: there is an increased risk of antimuscarinic effects and arrhythmias if benperidol is taken with tricyclic antidepressants.

Antiepileptic drugs: their anticonvulsant effects are antagonized by benperidol.

Antihistamines: there is an increased risk of arrhythmias if benperidol is taken with astemizole or terfenadine.

Halofantrine: there is an increased risk of arrhythmias if this drug is taken with benperidol.

Ritonavir: may increase the effects of benperidol.

Sedatives: the sedative effects of benperidol are increased if it is taken with anxiolytic or hypnotic drugs, or any other drug that causes sedation.

Proprietary preparation: Anquil.

benserazide hydrochloride A drug that inhibits the enzyme that breaks down *levodopa (an antiparkinsonian drug) to *dopamine in the peripheral tissues. Given in combination with levodopa (*see* CO-BENELDOPA), it increases the amount of levodopa available to cross into the brain and also helps prevent the side effects of nausea, vomiting, and low blood pressure seen with levodopa therapy.

Proprietary preparations: Madopar and Madopar CR (*see* CO-BENELDOPA).

Benylin Chesty Coughs Non Drowsy (Warner-Lambert Consumer Healthcare) A proprietary combination of *guaiphenesin <guaifenesin> (an expectorant) and *menthol, used for the relief of productive coughs. It is freely available *over the counter in the form of a syrup.

Side effects and precautions: *see* GUAIPHENESIN <GUAIFENESIN>. This medicine is not recommended for children under six years old.

Benylin Chesty Coughs Original (Warner-Lambert Consumer Healthcare) A proprietary combination of *diphenhydramine (a sedative antihistamine), *ammonium chloride (an expectorant), and *menthol, used for the relief of productive coughs and other symptoms of congestion. It is available as a syrup without a prescription, but only from pharmacies. It cannot be prescribed on the NHS.

Side effects and interactions with other drugs: *see* ANTIHISTAMINES.

Precautions: this syrup is not recommended for children under six years old. *See also* ANTIHISTAMINES.

Benylin Children's Chesty Coughs (Warner-Lambert Consumer Healthcare) *See* GUAIPHENESIN <GUAIFENESIN>.

Benylin Children's Coughs and Colds (Warner-Lambert Consumer Healthcare) A proprietary combination of *dextromethorphan (a cough suppressant) and *triprolidine (an antihistamine), used to relieve the symptoms of dry unproductive coughs. It is available as a liquid without a prescription, but only from pharmacies.
Side effects and interactions with other drugs: see DEXTROMETHORPHAN; ANTIHISTAMINES.
Precautions: this medicine is not recommended for children under one year old. *See also* ANTIHISTAMINES; OPIOIDS.

Benylin Children's Dry Coughs (Warner-Lambert Consumer Healthcare) *See* PHOLCODINE.

Benylin Children's Night Coughs (Warner-Lambert Consumer Healthcare) A proprietary combination of *diphenhydramine (a sedative antihistamine) and *menthol, used for the relief of coughs in children that interfere with sleep. It is available as a syrup without a prescription, but only from pharmacies.
Side effects and interactions with other drugs: see ANTIHISTAMINES.
Precautions: this medicine should not normally be given to children under one year old. *See also* ANTIHISTAMINES.

Benylin Cough & Congestion (Warner-Lambert Consumer Healthcare) A proprietary combination of *dextromethorphan (a cough suppressant), *diphenhydramine (a sedative antihistamine), *pseudoephedrine (a decongestant), and *menthol, used for the relief of coughs and symptoms of congestion associated with colds. It is available as a syrup without a prescription, but only from pharmacies.
Side effects and interactions with other drugs: see DEXTROMETHORPHAN; OPIOIDS; COUGH SUPPRESSANTS; ANTIHISTAMINES; EPHEDRINE HYDROCHLORIDE; DECONGESTANTS.
Precautions: this medicine is not recommended for children under six years old. *See also* OPIOIDS; ANTIHISTAMINES; EPHEDRINE HYDROCHLORIDE; DECONGESTANTS.

Benylin Day & Night Tablets (Warner-Lambert Consumer Healthcare) A proprietary combination of *paracetamol (an analgesic and antipyretic), and *phenylpropanolamine (a decongestant) in day tablets, and paracetamol and *diphenhydramine (a sedative antihistamine) in night tablets, used to relieve the symptoms of colds and influenza (the night tablets facilitate sleep). The tablets are available without a prescription, but only from pharmacies.
Side effects, precautions, and interactions with other drugs: see PARACETAMOL; EPHEDRINE HYDROCHLORIDE; DECONGESTANTS; ANTIHISTAMINES.

Benylin Dry Coughs Non Drowsy (Warner-Lambert Consumer Healthcare) *See* DEXTROMETHORPHAN.

Benylin Dry Coughs Original (Warner-Lambert Consumer Healthcare) A proprietary combination of *dextromethorphan (a cough suppressant), *diphenhydramine (a sedative antihistamine), and *menthol, used for the relief of dry persistent coughs. It is available as a syrup without a prescription, but only from pharmacies. It cannot be prescribed on the NHS.

Side effects and interactions with other drugs: see DEXTROMETHORPHAN; OPIOIDS; COUGH SUPPRESSANTS; ANTIHISTAMINES.

Precautions: this medicine is not recommended for children under six years old. *See also* OPIOIDS; ANTIHISTAMINES.

Benylin 4 Flu (Warner-Lambert Consumer Healthcare) A proprietary combination of *paracetamol (an analgesic and antipyretic), *pseudoephedrine (a decongestant), and *diphenhydramine (a sedative antihistamine), used to relieve the symptoms of colds and influenza. It is available as tablets or a liquid and can be obtained without a prescription, but only from pharmacies.

Side effects: see EPHEDRINE HYDROCHLORIDE; ANTIHISTAMINES.

Precautions: this preparation is not recommended for children under six years old. *See also* PARACETAMOL; EPHEDRINE HYDROCHLORIDE; DECONGESTANTS; ANTIHISTAMINES.

Interactions with other drugs: see EPHEDRINE HYDROCHLORIDE; ANTIHISTAMINES.

Benylin with Codeine (Warner-Lambert Consumer Healthcare) A proprietary combination of *codeine (an analgesic and cough suppressant), *diphenhydramine (a sedative antihistamine), and *menthol, used for the relief of persistent dry coughs. It is available as a syrup without a prescription, but only from pharmacies.

Side effects: see CODEINE; ANTIHISTAMINES.

Precautions: this medicine is not recommended for children under six years old. *See also* CODEINE; ANTIHISTAMINES.

Interactions with other drugs: see ANTIHISTAMINES.

benzalkonium chloride An *antiseptic that is used in the form of lozenges for treating mouth ulcers, gum disease, and infections of the mouth and throat. It is also an ingredient in creams, paints, and lotions for treating a variety of skin conditions. Benzalkonium is included as a preservative in eye drops. Some preparations containing benzalkonium can be obtained without a prescription, but some combined preparations can only be bought from pharmacies.

Precautions: eye drops containing benzalkonium should not be used by wearers of soft contact lenses.

Proprietary preparations: Bradosol (lozenges); BEECHAMS THROAT-PLUS LOZENGES (combined with hexylresorcinol); CONOTRANE (combined with

dimethicone <dimeticone>); DERMOL (combined with liquid paraffin,
isopropyl myristate, and chlorhexidine hydrochloride); DETTOL
ANTISEPTIC PAIN RELIEF SPRAY (combined with lignocaine <lidocaine>
hydrochloride); DRAPOLENE CREAM (combined with cetrimide);
EMULSIDERM (combined with liquid paraffin and isopropyl myristate);
IONAX SCRUB (combined with an abrasive); IONIL T (combined with
salicylic acid and coal tar); OILATUM PLUS (combined with liquid paraffin
and triclosan); TIMODINE (combined with nystatin, hydrocortisone, and
dimethicone <dimeticone>).

Benzamycin (Bioglan Laboratories) A proprietary combination of
*erythromycin (an antibiotic) and *benzoyl peroxide (a keratolytic), used
for the treatment of acne. It is available as a gel on *prescription only.
Side effects: there may be mild local irritation.
Precautions: Benzamycin should not come into contact with the eyes,
mouth, or other mucous membranes. It should be used with caution by
women who are pregnant or breastfeeding.

benzatropine mesilate *See* BENZTROPINE MESYLATE.

benzhexol hydrochloride <trihexyphenidyl hydrochloride> An
*antimuscarinic drug used for the treatment of Parkinson's disease and
for the reversal of drug-induced *extrapyramidal reactions (*see*
ANTIPARKINSONIAN DRUGS). It is available, on *prescription only, as
tablets or a syrup.
Side effects: dry mouth, gastrointestinal disturbances, dizziness, and
blurred vision are common; less common side effects are difficulty in
urinating, slow heart rate, and nervousness. In high doses and in
susceptible patients, mental confusion, excitement, and psychiatric
disturbances can occur.
Precautions: benzhexol should not be taken by people with acute
glaucoma, gastrointestinal obstruction, or enlargement of the prostate. It
should be used with caution in those with heart, liver, or kidney disease.
Interactions with other drugs:
  Antihistamines: increase the adverse effects of benzhexol.
Proprietary preparation: Broflex.

benzocaine A *local anaesthetic applied to the skin or mucous
membranes, particularly around the mouth and throat, for the relief of
pain. It is available, alone or combined with other drugs, in the form of
sprays, creams, gels, lotions, suppositories, or lozenges and can be
obtained without a prescription, but only from pharmacies.
Precautions: benzocaine should be used with caution by women who are
pregnant or breastfeeding.
Proprietary preparations: AAA Spray; Burneze Spray; Lanacane Creme;
Vicks Ultra Chloraseptic (spray); DEQUACAINE (combined with
dequalinium chloride); INTRALGIN (combined with salicylamide);
MEROCAINE (combined with cetylpyridinium chloride); RINSTEAD ADULT

GEL (combined with chloroxylenol); SOLARCAINE (combined with triclosan); TYROZETS (combined with tyrothricin); WASP-EZE SPRAY (combined with mepyramine).

benzodiazepines A group of drugs that are used in the short-term treatment of anxiety and insomnia (*see* ANXIOLYTIC DRUGS; HYPNOTIC DRUGS). They are also used to relax patients before surgery or diagnostic procedures. Benzodiazepines should only be used to relieve anxiety or insomnia that is severe, disabling, or causing unacceptable distress. The lowest effective dosage should be used for the shortest possible time (preferably no more than 2 weeks for insomia, 2–4 weeks for anxiety); the drug should then be withdrawn gradually. Physical and psychological *dependence can develop with prolonged use, and sudden withdrawal can produce 'rebound' insomnia and anxiety. Benzodiazepines have a low incidence of side effects and are relatively safe in overdose when compared with older drugs, such as *barbiturates, although a paradoxical increase in hostility and aggression has been reported by some people taking benzodiazepines (see below); dosage adjustment usually overcomes this problem.

Benzodiazepines vary in their duration of action. Short-acting benzodiazepines, such as *lorazepam and *oxazepam, are effective for 6–10 hours; they have mild residual effects but carry a greater risk of withdrawal reactions. Long-acting drugs include *diazepam, *alprazolam, *bromazepam, *chlordiazepoxide, *clobazam, and *clorazepate. They have a prolonged action, with persistent sedative effects, but withdrawal reactions are less of a problem. Benzodiazepines are available, on *prescription only, as tablets, capsules, syrups, or injections. Drug abuse with benzodiazepines, especially *temazepam and *flunitrazepam, has increased recently. Many benzodiazepines can no longer be prescribed on the NHS, and temazepam and flunitrazepam are now *controlled drugs.

Side effects and precautions: side effects include drowsiness and light-headedness (which may persist the next day), confusion, shaky movements, and unsteady gait (especially in elderly people), amnesia, and a paradoxical increase in hostility and aggression. This may range from talkativeness and excitement to aggressive and antisocial acts; increased anxiety, hallucinations, and delusions may also occur. Dependence can develop, and it is important that benzodiazpines are stopped gradually to avoid withdrawal reactions; these can include worsening of insomnia and anxiety, sweating, tremor, and weight loss. Drowsiness can impair judgment and dexterity, and the sedative effects of benzodiazepines are increased by alcohol.

Interactions with other drugs: the sedative effects of benzodiazepines are increased by a number of other drugs, including anaesthetics, opioid analgesics, antidepressants, antihistamines, antipsychotics, cimetidine, and most importantly ritonavir, which may in some cases cause profound sedation (see entries for individual drugs).

benzoic acid An antifungal and antibacterial agent that is used mainly as a preservative in medicines and foods. In combination with *salicylic acid, it is used in the form of an ointment for treating fungal infections of the skin, such as ringworm; it is also included in some soothing preparations for *haemorrhoids. Benzoic acid also has *keratolytic properties and is used in combination with *malic acid and salicylic acid for removing dead skin from ulcers, burns, and wounds.

Proprietary preparations: ASERBINE (combined with malic acid and salicylic acid); HEMOCANE (combined with lignocaine <lidocaine>, cinnamic acid, zinc oxide, and bismuth oxide).

benzoin tincture compound (friar's balsam) A combination of balsamic acids in the form of a *tincture, used as an aromatic inhalation to relieve nasal congestion or soothe bronchitis. The tincture is added to hot water and the vapour is inhaled. Benzoin tincture compound is available without a prescription, but only from pharmacies.

benzoyl peroxide A mild *keratolytic that also has some antibacterial and antifungal activity and is used mainly for the treatment of *acne. It is available as a gel, lotion, solution, or cream and can be obtained without a prescription, but only from pharmacies.

Side effects: benzoyl peroxide may cause transient irritation and peeling of the skin.

Precautions: benzoyl peroxide should not come into contact with the eyes, mouth, or other mucous membranes.

Proprietary preparations: Acnecide (gel); Clearasil Max 10 (cream); Nericur (gel); Oxy 5, Oxy 10 (lotions); Oxy On-the-Spot (cream); PanOxyl (gel, cream, lotion, or wash); ACNIDAZIL (combined with miconazole nitrate); BENZAMYCIN (combined with erythromycin); QUINODERM (combined with hydroxyquinoline sulphate); QUINOPED (combined with hydroxyquinoline sulphate).

benzthiazide A *thiazide diuretic given in combination with *triamterene for the treatment of *oedema associated with heart failure, liver disease, or kidney disease. It is available as capsules on *prescription only.

Side effects, precautions, and interactions with other drugs: see THIAZIDE DIURETICS.

Proprietary preparation: DYTIDE (combined with triamterene).

See also DIURETICS.

benztropine mesylate <benzatropine mesilate> An *antimuscarinic drug used for the treatment of Parkinson's disease and for the reversal of drug-induced *extrapyramidal reactions (*see* ANTIPARKINSONIAN DRUGS). It is available as tablets on *prescription only.

Side effects: dry mouth, gastrointestinal disturbances, dizziness, and blurred vision are common; less common side effects are difficulty in urinating, slow heart rate, and nervousness. This drug has a sedative effect, which may be useful in treating patients adversely affected by antimuscarinics that cause excitement.

Precautions: see BENZHEXOL <TRIHEXYPHENIDYL> HYDROCHLORIDE. In addition, benztropine should not be given to children under three years old.

Interactions with other drugs: see BENZHEXOL <TRIHEXYPHENIDYL> HYDROCHLORIDE.

Proprietary preparation: Cogentin.

benzydamine hydrochloride An *NSAID used for the relief of painful conditions of the mouth and throat associated with inflammation and ulceration. Benzydamine is available as a mouthwash, a throat and mouth spray, and a cream; it can be obtained without a prescription, but only from pharmacies.

Side effects: the mouthwash may occasionally cause stinging or numbness. *See also* NSAIDS.

Precautions: the mouthwash is not recommended for children under 12 years old. *See* NSAIDS.

Proprietary preparation: Difflam.

benzyl alcohol An antimicrobial preservative. It is included in many pharmaceutical preparations to keep them free of bacteria. It is also mildly anaesthetic and possesses antipruritic activity (i.e. it relieves itching) and is used as an ingredient in some topical preparations.

Side effects: benzyl alcohol may cause local irritation.

benzyl benzoate A drug used in the treatment of *scabies. It is available as an emulsion to be applied to the body and can be obtained without a prescription, but only from pharmacies.

Side effects: benzyl benzoate can irritate the skin and produces a burning sensation when applied to the genital area or to scratched skin. Rashes may rarely occur.

Precautions: benzyl benzoate should not be used to treat children and should be used with caution by women who are pregnant or breastfeeding. It should not come into contact with the eyes, mucous membranes, or broken skin.

Proprietary preparation: Ascarbiol.

benzylpenicillin (penicillin G) The first *antibiotic of the *penicillin group to be used therapeutically. It is active against a number of bacteria, including streptococci, gonococci, and meningococci, and is used for the treatment of infections of the skin, soft tissues, respiratory tract, ear, nose, or throat, septicaemia, meningitis, endocarditis (inflammation of the membranes surrounding the heart), and gonorrhoea. It is also effective against anthrax, diphtheria, gas gangrene, leptospirosis, syphilis, tetanus, yaws, and Lyme disease. Benzylpenicillin is inactivated by pencillinases and therefore can only be used to treat infections caused by bacteria that do not produce penicillinase. It is given by injection and is available on *prescription only.

Side effects: allergic reactions may occur, including nettle rash, fever, joint pain, oedema (swelling) of the face, and *anaphylaxis.

Precautions: benzylpenicillin should not be taken by people allergic to penicillins because of the risk of anaphylaxis (*see* PENICILLINS). It should be used with caution in those with impaired kidney function.

Interactions with other drugs:

 Methotrexate: concentrations of methotrexate in the blood are increased, which may cause adverse effects.

Proprietary preparations: Crystapen; BICILLIN (combined with procaine penicillin <procaine benzylpenicillin>).

beractant A synthetic pulmonary *surfactant that is used to treat breathing difficulties in premature babies who are receiving mechanical ventilation (*see* VENTILATOR). Beractant is available, on *prescription only, as a suspension that is administered through a tube placed in the trachea (windpipe).

Side effects: beractant may cause bleeding in the lungs.

Precautions: constant monitoring of heart rate and blood gases is necessary during treatment as beractant can cause a rapid improvement in the baby's condition and high concentrations of oxygen in the tissues have toxic effects.

Proprietary preparation: Survanta.

Berkatens (APS-Berk) *See* VERAPAMIL HYDROCHLORIDE.

Berkmycin (APS-Berk) *See* OXYTETRACYCLINE.

Berkolol (APS-Berk) *See* PROPRANOLOL HYDROCHLORIDE.

Berkozide (APS-Berk) *See* BENDROFLUAZIDE <BENDROFLUMETHIAZIDE>.

Berotec 100 (Boehringer Ingelheim) *See* FENOTEROL HYDROBROMIDE.

Beta-Adalat (Bayer) A proprietary combination of *atenolol (a *beta blocker) and *nifedipine (a *calcium antagonist), used for the treatment of *angina or *hypertension, usually when either of these drugs singly has been inadequate. It is available as tablets on *prescription only.

Side-effects, precautions, and interactions with other drugs: see BETA BLOCKERS; CALCIUM ANTAGONISTS.

See also ANTIHYPERTENSIVE DRUGS.

beta agonists (beta stimulants) *See* SYMPATHOMIMETIC DRUGS.

beta blockers (β-blockers; in full **beta-adrenoceptor blockers**) Drugs that act on the heart, reducing its force and speed of contraction, and on blood vessels, preventing *vasodilatation. They produce their effects by blocking the stimulation of beta-adrenergic receptors by noradrenaline <norepinephrine> in the *sympathetic nervous system (*see*

ADRENOCEPTORS). There are two types of beta receptors: 1 and 2. Beta 1 receptors are located mainly in the heart muscle; beta 2 receptors are found in the airways and blood vessels. Drugs acting only on the beta 1 receptors are described as **cardioselective**; drugs acting on both types of receptor are called **non-cardioselective**. Beta blockers are used to control abnormal heartbeats (*arrhythmias), to treat *angina, and to reduce high blood pressure (*hypertension). (Although they prevent the dilatation of blood vessels, beta blockers are used in the treatment of hypertension as their action on the heart is usually sufficient to correct raised blood pressure.) They are useful for treating people who have both hypertension and arrhythmias. They are also used after a heart attack to prevent a recurrence and may be used to improve heart function in the heart disorders known as cardiomyopathies. Beta blockers reduce symptoms of anxiety (such as palpitations) and are sometimes taken by performers to make them feel more calm. They can also be taken to prevent *migraine headaches. In the form of eye drops, beta blockers are used to reduce fluid pressure inside the eyes in people with *glaucoma. Drugs whose name ends in '-alol' or '-olol' (with the exception of stanozolol) are usually beta blockers.

See ACEBUTOLOL; ATENOLOL; BISOPROLOL FUMARATE; BETAXOLOL HYDROCHLORIDE; CARTEOLOL HYDROCHLORIDE; CARVEDILOL; CELIPROLOL HYDROCHLORIDE; ESMOLOL HYDROCHLORIDE; LABETALOL HYDROCHLORIDE; LEVOBUNOLOL HYDROCHLORIDE; METOPROLOL TARTRATE; NADOLOL; OXPRENOLOL HYDROCHLORIDE; PINDOLOL; PROPRANOLOL HYDROCHLORIDE; SOTALOL HYDROCHLORIDE; TIMOLOL MALEATE.

Side effects: beta blockers may reduce the capacity for strenuous exercise or cause tiredness; many people experience cold hands and/or feet due to restriction of the blood supply to the limbs. Temporary reversible impotence and odd dreams may occur.

Precautions: beta blockers cause constriction of the air passages, although cardioselective beta blockers are less likely to cause such problems. For this reason, non-cardioselective beta blockers should not be taken by people with obstructive airways disease (such as asthma, chronic bronchitis, or emphysema), and cardioselective drugs should be used with extreme care and only when no alternative treatment is available. Beta blockers reduce the ability of the liver to release sugar when blood sugar is low and may mask some of the signs of *hypoglycaemia; they should therefore be used with caution in people with diabetes. Beta blockers should not be stopped suddenly after prolonged use as this may provoke sudden and severe recurrence of original symptoms and even a heart attack.

Interactions with other drugs:

  Anaesthetics: their effect in lowering blood pressure is increased by beta blockers.

  Anti-arrhythmic drugs: the risk of bradycardia (slow heart rate) and depression of heart function is increased if these drugs are taken with beta blockers.

  Antihypertensive drugs: their effect in lowering blood pressure is enhanced by beta blockers; there is an increased risk of hypertension with clonidine if beta blockers are stopped suddenly.

Calcium antagonists: taking these drugs with beta blockers can have adverse effects on the heart.

Sympathomimetic drugs: severe hypertension can result if adrenaline <epinephrine> or noradrenaline <norepinephrine> are taken with beta blockers.

Thymoxamine <moxisylyte>: may cause a severe fall in blood pressure on standing up.

For other interactions, see entries for individual beta blockers.

See also ANTI-ARRHYTHMIC DRUGS; ANTIHYPERTENSIVE DRUGS.

Betacap (Dermal Laboratories) *See* BETAMETHASONE.

Beta-Cardone (Medeva) *See* SOTALOL HYDROCHLORIDE.

Betadine (Seton Scholl Healthcare) *See* POVIDONE–IODINE.

Betaferon (Schering Health Care) *See* INTERFERON-BETA.

Betagan (Allergan) *See* LEVOBUNOLOL HYDROCHLORIDE.

betahistine An *analogue of *histamine that increases blood flow through the inner ear and is used to reduce the build-up of pressure that is thought to cause the vertigo and tinnitus (ringing in the ears) associated with Ménière's disease. It is available as tablets on *prescription only.

Side effects: include indigestion, headache, and itching or rashes.

Precautions: betahistine should not be taken by people with phaeochromocytoma (a tumour of the adrenal glands) and should be used with caution by people with asthma or peptic ulcers and by women who are pregnant or breastfeeding.

Proprietary preparation: Serc.

betaine hydrochloride A salt that is used as a source of chloride ions and is also included in some oral *potassium supplements.

Proprietary preparation: KLOREF (combined with potassium chloride, potassium benzoate, and potassium bicarbonate).

beta-lactam antibiotics *See* ANTIBIOTICS.

Betaloc, Betaloc SA (AstraZeneca) *See* METOPROLOL TARTRATE.

betamethasone A *corticosteroid with potent anti-inflammatory activity, used for the treatment of severe asthma, allergic conditions, rheumatoid arthritis, and connective-tissue diseases. It is also applied topically to treat infections or inflammation of the eyes and ears, rhinitis and hay fever, and a variety of eczematous inflammations and other skin conditions. Betamethasone and its salts (the dipropionate, the valerate, and the sodium phosphate) are available, on *prescription only, in the form of tablets, an injection, *suppositories, eye, ear, and nose drops, and ointments, creams, and lotions.

Side effects, precautions, and interactions with other drugs: see CORTICOSTEROIDS; TOPICAL STEROIDS.

Proprietary preparations: Betacap (scalp lotion); Betnelan; Betnesol; Betnovate; Bettamousse (scalp mousse); Diprosone; Vista-Methasone (eye or nose drops); BETNESOL-N (combined with neomycin); BETNOVATE-C (combined with clioquinol); BETNOVATE-N (combined with neomycin); BETNOVATE RECTAL (combined with phenylephrine and lignocaine <lidocaine>); DIPROSALIC (combined with salicylic acid); FUCIBET (combined with fusidic acid); LOTRIDERM (combined with clotrimazole); VISTA-METHASONE N (combined with neomycin).

Beta-Prograne (Tillomed Laboratories) *See* PROPRANOLOL HYDROCHLORIDE.

beta stimulants (beta agonists) *See* SYMPATHOMIMETIC DRUGS.

betaxolol hydrochloride A cardioselective *beta blocker used for the treatment of *hypertension and chronic (open-angle) *glaucoma. It is available, on *prescription only, as tablets or (for glaucoma) as eye drops.
Side effects, precautions, and interactions with other drugs: see BETA BLOCKERS.
Proprietary preparations: Betoptic (eye drops); Kerlone (tablets).
See also ANTIHYPERTENSIVE DRUGS.

bethanechol chloride A *cholinergic drug that enhances motility of the intestines and contraction of the bladder and has been used in the treatment of reflux oesophagitis and urinary retention (it is now seldom used). Bethanechol is available as tablets on *prescription only.
Side effects: include nausea, vomiting, sweating, blurred vision, and slowing of the heart rate.
Precautions: bethanechol chloride should not be taken by people with intestinal or urinary obstruction or when increased muscular activity of the urinary or gastrointestinal tract would be harmful.
Proprietary preparation: Myotonine.

bethanidine sulphate <betanidine sulphate> A drug that prevents the release of noradrenaline <norepinephrine> from nerve endings in the *sympathetic nervous system. It is used in the treatment of *hypertension that is resistant to standard *antihypertensive therapy and is available as tablets on *prescription only.
Side effects: include low blood pressure, particularly on standing up, failure of ejaculation, nasal congestion, headache, diarrhoea, and drowsiness.
Precautions: bethanidine should not be taken by people with

phaeochromocytoma (a tumour of the adrenal gland). It should be used with caution by people with kidney disease.

Interactions with other drugs:

Anaesthetics: their effect in lowering blood pressure is increased by bethanidine.

Sympathomimetic drugs: some cough and cold remedies (e.g. ephedrine) and methylphenidate antagonize the blood-pressure-lowering effect of bethanidine.

Tricyclic antidepressants: antagonize the blood-pressure-lowering effect of bethanidine.

Betim (Leo Pharmaceuticals) *See* TIMOLOL MALEATE.

Betnelan (Medeva) *See* BETAMETHASONE.

Betnesol (Medeva) *See* BETAMETHASONE.

Betnesol-N (Medeva) A proprietary combination of *betamethasone (a corticosteroid) and *neomycin sulphate (an antibiotic), used for the treatment of infected allergic conditions of the eyes or ears. It is available, on *prescription only, as eye drops or an ointment.

Side effects: allergic reactions may develop; *see also* TOPICAL STEROIDS; NEOMYCIN SULPHATE.

Precautions: *see* TOPICAL STEROIDS; NEOMYCIN SULPHATE. In addition, soft contact lenses should not be worn during treatment.

Betnovate (GlaxoWellcome) *See* BETAMETHASONE.

Betnovate-C (GlaxoWellcome) A proprietary combination of *betamethasone (a corticosteroid) and *clioquinol (an antifungal agent), used for the treatment of inflammatory conditions of the skin when candidal and/or bacterial infection is present. It is available as a cream or ointment on *prescription only.

Side effects and precautions: *see* TOPICAL STEROIDS; CLIOQUINOL.

Betnovate-N (GlaxoWellcome) A proprietary combination of *betamethasone (a corticosteroid) and *neomycin sulphate (an antibiotic), used for the treatment of inflammatory conditions of the skin when infection is present. It is available as a cream or ointment on *prescription only.

Side effects, precautions, and interactions with other drugs: *see* TOPICAL STEROIDS; NEOMYCIN SULPHATE.

Betnovate Rectal (GlaxoWellcome) A proprietary combination of *betamethasone (a corticosteroid), *phenylephrine hydrochloride (a sympathemimetic drug), and *lignocaine <lidocaine> hydrochloride (a local anaesthetic), used for the treatment of haemorrhoids and mild

proctitis (inflammation of the rectum). It is available as an ointment on
*prescription only.
Precautions: Betnovate Rectal should not be used when viral or fungal
infection is present and should not be used for longer than seven days.

Betoptic (Alcon Laboratories) *See* BETAXOLOL HYDROCHLORIDE.

Bettamousse (Medeva) *See* BETAMETHASONE.

bezafibrate A *fibrate used for the treatment of a wide variety of
*hyperlipidaemias that have not responded to dietary modification and
other appropriate measures. It is available as tablets and *modified-
release tablets on *prescription only.
Side effects and precautions: see FIBRATES.
Interactions with other drugs:
  Anticoagulants: the effects of warfarin, phenindione, and nicoumalone
    <acenocoumarol> are enhanced.
  Antidiabetic agents: the effects of these drugs are enhanced.
  See also FIBRATES.
Proprietary preparations: Bezalip; Bezalip-Mono (modified-release tablets
twice the strength of Bezalip).

Bezalip, Bezalip-Mono (Roche Products) *See* BEZAFIBRATE.

bicalutamide An *anti-androgen used for the treatment of advanced
*cancer of the prostate gland, usually in conjunction with an analogue of
*gonadorelin. It is available as tablets on *prescription only.
Side effects: include hot flushes, itching, breast tenderness and
enlargement, diarrhoea, nausea, weakness, and (more rarely) jaundice,
angina, heart failure, irregularities in heart rhythm, and blood disorders.
Other side effects, which are more common in the elderly, include loss of
appetite, dry mouth, indigestion, constipation, impotence,
breathlessness, and rashes.
Precautions: liver function should be monitored in people with liver
disease.
Interactions with other drugs:
  Warfarin: its anticoagulant effect may be enhanced.
Proprietary preparation: Casodex.

bicarbonate *See* POTASSIUM BICARBONATE; SODIUM BICARBONATE.

Bicillin (Yamanouchi Pharma) A proprietary combination of the
penicillins *procaine penicillin <procaine benzylpenicillin> and
*benzylpenicillin, used in the treatment of syphilis. It is available, on
*prescription only, as an intramuscular injection.
Side effects, precautions, and interactions with other drugs: see
BENZYLPENICILLIN.

BiCNU (Bristol-Myers Squibb) *See* CARMUSTINE.

biguanides *See* METFORMIN HYDROCHLORIDE.

bile acids A group of acidic compounds that are normally secreted by the gall bladder and aid the digestion and absorption of fats. The bile acids *chenodeoxycholic acid and *ursodeoxycholic acid are used in the treatment of gallstone disease, but are suitable only for those who have small or medium-sized stones. Treatment may take months to complete (typically 3–18 months), and after the stones have dissolved some people may need to take long-term medication in order to prevent recurrence. People taking bile acids should restrict their intake of foods rich in cholesterol and calories.

bile-acid sequestrants A class of *lipid-lowering drugs. They are resins that combine with bile acids and decrease the absorption of fats, thus increasing the amount of fat excreted in the faeces and lowering plasma *cholesterol concentrations. The main drugs in this class are *cholestyramine <colestyramine> and *colestipol. They can reduce plasma LDL-cholesterol by up to 25% (*see* LIPOPROTEINS).
Side effects: bile-acid sequestrants have effects on the gastrointestinal tract, causing discomfort, flatulence, dyspepsia, and constipation, which makes high doses hard to tolerate. The taste and texture of resins is often unacceptable; many people mix them with fruit juice to overcome this problem, but with limited success.
Precautions: the intestinal absorption of fat-soluble vitamins is reduced by resins, so that supplemental vitamins A, D, K, and possibly E may need to be taken by those receiving long-term treatment.
Interactions with other drugs: other drugs should be taken at least 1 hour before or 4–6 hours after resins to reduce possible interference with drug absorption.
  Anticoagulants: the anticoagulant effects of warfarin, nicoumalone <acenocoumarol>, and phenindione may be increased.
  Sodium valproate: absorption of this drug may be reduced.
  Thiazide diuretics: absorption of these drugs is reduced; resins and thiazides should be taken at least two hours apart.

BiNovum (Janssen-Cilag) A proprietary combination of *ethinyloestradiol <ethinylestradiol> and *norethisterone used as an *oral contraceptive of the biphasic type. These tablets are packaged in two phases, which differ in the amounts of the active ingredients they contain. BiNovum is available on *prescription only.
Side effects, precautions, and interactions with other drugs: see ORAL CONTRACEPTIVES.

Bioplex (Cortecs Healthcare) *See* CARBENOXOLONE SODIUM.

Bioral Gel (SmithKline Beecham Consumer Healthcare) *See* CARBENOXOLONE SODIUM.

Biorphen (Bioglan Laboratories) *See* ORPHENADRINE.

biotin *See* VITAMIN B COMPLEX.

biperiden An *antimuscarinic drug used for the treatment of Parkinson's disease and for the reversal of drug-induced *extrapyramidal reactions (*see* ANTIPARKINSONIAN DRUGS). It is available, on *prescription only, as tablets or as a solution for injection.
Side effects: see BENZTROPINE MESYLATE <BENZATROPINE MESILATE>. Injections may cause low blood pressure.
Precautions and interactions with other drugs: see BENZHEXOL <TRIHEXYPHENIDYL> HYDROCHLORIDE.
Proprietary preparation: Akineton.

biphasic insulins *See* INSULIN.

BIPP *See* BISMUTH SUBNITRATE AND IODOFORM.

Birleys (Torbet Laboratories) A proprietary combination of the antacids *aluminium hydroxide, *magnesium trisilicate, and *magnesium carbonate, used for the relief of indigestion and other minor stomach upsets. It is freely available *over the counter in the form of a powder to be dissolved in water.
Side effects, precautions, and interactions with other drugs: see ANTACIDS.

bisacodyl A *stimulant laxative used to treat constipation and to clear the bowel before surgery, childbirth, or X-ray examination. It is available as *enteric-coated tablets and suppositories and can be obtained without a prescription, but only from pharmacies.
Side effects and precautions: see STIMULANT LAXATIVES.
Proprietary preparations: Dulco-Lax Suppositories; Dulco-Lax Suppositories for Children; Dulco-Lax Tablets.

Bismag Tablets (Whitehall Laboratories) A proprietary combination of the antacids *sodium bicarbonate and *magnesium carbonate, used for the relief of upset stomach, heartburn, indigestion, and trapped wind (*see* ACID-PEPTIC DISEASES). It is freely available *over the counter.
Side effects and interactions with other drugs: see MAGNESIUM SALTS; ANTACIDS.
Precautions: these tablets are not recommended for children. *See also* MAGNESIUM SALTS.

bismuth aluminate An insoluble salt of bismuth that is included in some *antacid preparations. Although it has no ability to neutralize stomach acid, it may protect the stomach lining from mechanical or chemical irritation.

Proprietary preparation: MOORLAND (combined with magnesium trisilicate, aluminium hydroxide, magnesium carbonate, calcium carbonate, and light kaolin).

bismuth oxide An *astringent that is used to relieve the discomfort of *haemorrhoids and the pain, soreness, or itching of other disorders of the anus or rectum. It is included as an ingredient in a variety of creams, ointments, and suppositories.

Proprietary preparations: ANUGESIC-HC (combined with hydrocortisone acetate, zinc oxide, pramoxine <pramocaine> hydrochloride, Peru balsam, and benzyl benzoate); ANUGESIC-HC SUPPOSITORIES (combined with benzyl benzoate, pramoxine <pramocaine> hydrochloride, hydrocortisone acetate, zinc oxide, Peru balsam, and bismuth subgallate); ANUSOL (combined with bismuth subgallate, Peru balsam, and zinc oxide); ANUSOL-HC (combined with hydrocortisone acetate, benzyl benzoate, bismuth subgallate, Peru balsam, and zinc oxide); HEMOCANE (combined with zinc oxide, benzoic acid, cinnamic acid, and lignocaine <lidocaine>).

bismuth subgallate An *astringent that is used to relieve the discomfort of *haemorrhoids and the pain, soreness, or itching of other disorders of the anus or rectum. It is included as an ingredient in a variety of creams, ointments, and suppositories.

Proprietary preparations: ANUSOL (combined with bismuth oxide, Peru balsam, and zinc oxide); ANUSOL-HC (combined with hydrocortisone acetate, benzyl benzoate, bismuth oxide, Peru balsam, and zinc oxide); ANUGESIC-HC SUPPOSITORIES (combined with benzyl benzoate, pramoxine <pramocaine> hydrochloride, hydrocortisone acetate, zinc oxide, Peru balsam, and bismuth oxide).

bismuth subnitrate and iodoform An *astringent and *antiseptic mixture that is used for packing cavities after ear, nose, or throat operations and for stopping nosebleeds. It is available as **bismuth iodoform paraffin paste** (BIPP), which is applied to gauze packing, or as BIPP-impregnated gauze and is freely available *over the counter.

Proprietary preparations: OxBipp; OxBipp-G (impregnated gauze).

bismuth subsalicylate An insoluble salt of bismuth used for the treatment of diarrhoea, stomach upsets, nausea, and indigestion (*see* ANTACIDS). It is available as a suspension and can be obtained without a prescription, but only from pharmacies.

Side effects: bismuth subsalicylate causes blackening of the stools. If large quantities are taken, salicylate may be absorbed and produce the adverse effects associated with *salicylates.

Proprietary preparation: Pepto-Bismol.

Bisodol Antacid Powder (Whitehall Laboratories) A proprietary combination of *sodium bicarbonate and *magnesium carbonate, used for the relief of upset stomach, heartburn, indigestion, and trapped wind (see ACID-PEPTIC DISEASES). It is freely available *over the counter.
Side effects and interactions with other drugs: see ANTACIDS.
Precautions: this powder is not recommended for children.

Bisodol Antacid Tablets, **Bisodol Extra Strong Mint** (Whitehall Laboratories) Proprietary combinations of *sodium bicarbonate, *calcium carbonate, and *magnesium carbonate, used for the relief of upset stomach, heartburn, indigestion, and trapped wind (see ACID-PEPTIC DISEASES). They are freely available *over the counter in the form of chewable tablets.
Side effects and interactions with other drugs: see ANTACIDS.
Precautions: these tablets are not recommended for children.

Bisodol Extra Tablets (Whitehall Laboratories) A proprietary combination of *sodium bicarbonate, *calcium carbonate, and *magnesium carbonate (antacids) and activated *dimethicone <dimeticone> (an antifoaming agent), used for the relief of upset stomach, heartburn, indigestion, and trapped wind (see ACID-PEPTIC DISEASES). It is freely available *over the counter.
Side effects and interactions with other drugs: see ANTACIDS.
Precautions: these tablets are not recommended for children.

bisoprolol fumarate A cardioselective *beta blocker used for the treatment of *angina. It is available as tablets on *prescription only.
Side effects and precautions: see BETA BLOCKERS.
Interactions with other drugs:
  Rifampicin: reduces the plasma concentration of bisoprolol.
  For other interactions, *see* BETA BLOCKERS.
Proprietary preparations: Emcor; Emcor LS; Monocor; MONOZIDE 10 (combined with hydrochlorothiazide).

bisphosphonates A group of drugs that prevent the loss of calcium from bone and its transfer to the bloodstream. They are used to strengthen the bones in the treatment of Paget's disease (in which the bones become deformed and fracture easily), to lower high concentrations of calcium in the blood in patients with bone cancer, and to treat or prevent osteoporosis. *See* ALENDRONIC ACID; DISODIUM ETIDRONATE; DISODIUM PAMIDRONATE; SODIUM CLODRONATE; TILUDRONIC ACID.

Blemix (Ashbourne Pharmaceuticals) *See* MINOCYCLINE.

bleomycin A *cytotoxic antibiotic that is injected into a vein or a muscle for the treatment of lymphomas, certain solid tumours, and squamous cell carcinoma (a form of skin cancer). It can be injected directly into the chest or abdomen to treat metastases in accumulations of fluid caused by certain *cancers. It is available as a form for injection on *prescription only.

Side effects: bleomycin causes little *bone marrow suppression. The most likely side effects are increased pigmentation of the skin, especially between the toes and fingers, inside the elbows and knees, and in the groin, hard swellings beneath the skin, and inflammation of the mucous membranes. Allergic reactions, including chills and fevers, are common a few hours after administration of bleomycin. These can be treated with corticosteroids (such as hydrocortisone), antihistamines, and/or antipyretics. Fibrosis (thickening) of the lung tissue, which can have effects on breathing, may occur with long-term use. *See also* CYTOTOXIC DRUGS.

Precautions: see CYTOTOXIC DRUGS. Bleomycin is irritant to skin and must be handled with caution.

Blocadren (Merck Sharp & Dohme) *See* TIMOLOL MALEATE.

BN Liniment (3M Health Care) A proprietary combination of *turpentine oil, strong *ammonia solution, and *ammonium chloride, used as a *rubefacient for the relief of muscular aches and pains, sprains, and pulled muscles. It is available freely *over the counter.

Side effects and precautions: see RUBEFACIENTS.

Bocasan (Oral-B Laboratories) A proprietary combination of *sodium perborate (an antiseptic) and sodium hydrogen tartrate (which reduces the acidity of sodium perborate), used as a mouthwash for cleaning the gums in the treatment of gingivitis (inflammation of the gums) or stomatitis (inflammation of the lining of the mouth). It is available as granules to be dissolved in water and can be obtained without a prescription, but only from pharmacies.

Precautions: Bocasan should not be taken by children under five years old or by people with kidney disease. It should not be used for more than seven days except on medical advice.

Bonefos (Boehringer Ingelheim) *See* SODIUM CLODRONATE.

bone marrow suppression A reduction in the activity of the bone marrow, the tissue contained within the internal cavities of the bones that produces blood cells. Many drugs, especially *cytotoxic drugs, suppress the activity of this tissue, resulting in a decrease in the number of white cells, red cells, and platelets in the blood. A loss of white blood cells leaves the individual susceptible to infection; decreased numbers of red blood cells causes *anaemia and tiredness; loss of platelets causes spontaneous bruising and prolonged bleeding after injury. Bone marrow suppression is usually reversible once the drug responsible is stopped, but it may take a couple of weeks for the bone marrow to return to its normal activity.

Bonjela (Reckitt & Colman) A proprietary combination of *cetalkonium chloride (an antiseptic) and *choline salicylate (a local analgesic), used for the relief of pain and discomfort of mouth ulcers, cold sores, sores caused by dentures, and teething problems. It is freely available *over the counter.

Precautions: Bonjela is not recommended for children under four months old. *See also* CETALKONIUM CHLORIDE; CHOLINE SALICYLATE.

Boots Allergy Relief Antihistamine Tablets (Boots) *See* CHLORPHENIRAMINE <CHLORPHENAMINE> MALEATE.

Boots Avert (Boots) *See* ACICLOVIR.

Boots Bite and Sting Antihistamine Cream (Boots) *See* MEPYRAMINE.

Boots Bronchial Cough Mixture (Boots) A proprietary combination of ammonium carbonate, *ammonium chloride, and *guaiphenesin <guaifenesin> (all *expectorants), used for the relief of productive coughs with congestion. It is available as a syrup without a prescription, but only from Boots.

Side effects and precautions: see GUAIPHENESIN <GUAIFENESIN>.

Boots Catarrh Cough Syrup (Boots) A proprietary combination of *codeine (an analgesic and cough suppressant) and creosote (an antiseptic), used for the relief of productive coughs and congestion. It is available without a prescription, but only from Boots.

Side effects, precautions, and interactions with other drugs: see CODEINE; COUGH SUPPRESSANTS; OPIOIDS.

Boots Catarrh Syrup for Children (Boots) A proprietary combination of *diphenhydramine (a sedative antihistamine) and *pseudoephedrine (a decongestant), used for the relief of congestion associated with colds and hay fever in children. It is available without a prescription, but only from Boots.

Side effects, precautions, and interactions with other drugs: see ANTIHISTAMINES; DECONGESTANTS; EPHEDRINE.

Boots Children's 1 Year Plus Night Time Cough Syrup (Boots) A proprietary combination of *diphenhydramine (a sedative antihistamine) and *pholcodine (a cough suppressant), used for the relief of dry irritating coughs in children. It is available without a prescription, but only from Boots.

Side effects, precautions, and interactions with other drugs: see ANTIHISTAMINES; PHOLCODINE; COUGH SUPPRESSANTS.

Boots Children's Pain Relief Syrup (Boots) *See* PARACETAMOL.

Boots Cold and 'Flu Relief Tablets (Boots) A proprietary combination of *paracetamol (an analgesic and antipyretic), *caffeine (a stimulant), *phenylephrine (a decongestant), and ascorbic acid (*vitamin C), used to relieve the symptoms of colds and influenza. It is available without a prescription, but only from Boots.
Side effects and precautions: see PARACETAMOL; CAFFEINE; PHENYLEPHRINE.
Interactions with other drugs: see PHENYLEPHRINE.

Boots Cold Relief Hot Blackcurrant, **Boots Cold Relief Hot Lemon** (Boots) *See* PARACETAMOL.

Boots Cold Relief Hot Lemon with Decongestant (Boots) A proprietary combination of *paracetamol (an analgesic and antipyretic) and *phenylephrine (a decongestant), used to relieve the symptoms of colds, including fever and nasal congestion. **Boots Cold Relief Hot Blackcurrant with Decongestant** is a similar preparation. Both are powders to be dissolved in hot water; they are available *over the counter, but only from Boots.
Side effects and precautions: see PARACETAMOL; PHENYLEPHRINE.
Interactions with other drugs: see PHENYLEPHRINE.

Boots Compound Laxative (Boots) A proprietary combination of *senna and figs, used as a *stimulant laxative for the treatment of constipation. It is available without a prescription, but only from Boots.
Side effects and precautions: see STIMULANT LAXATIVES.

Boots Cystitis Relief (Boots) *See* SODIUM CITRATE.

Boots Day Cold Comfort (Boots) A proprietary combination of *paracetamol (an analgesic and antipyretic), *pseudoephedrine (a decongestant), and *pholcodine (a cough suppressant), used to relieve the symptoms of colds and influenza. It is available as capsules without a prescription, but only from Boots.
Side effects and precautions: see PARACETAMOL; EPHEDRINE HYDROCHLORIDE; DECONGESTANTS; CODEINE.
Interactions with other drugs: see EPHEDRINE HYDROCHLORIDE; OPIOIDS.

Boots Daytime Cough Relief (Boots) *See* PHOLCODINE.

Boots Decongestant Tablets (Boots) *See* PSEUDOEPHEDRINE.

Boots Diareze (Boots) *See* LOPERAMIDE HYDROCHLORIDE.

Boots Excess Acid Control (Boots) *See* FAMOTIDINE.

Boots Haemorrhoid Ointment (Boots) A proprietary combination of *zinc oxide (an astringent) and *lignocaine <lidocaine> (a local anaesthetic), used to relieve the discomfort and pain of *haemorrhoids. It can be obtained without a prescription, but only from Boots.

Boots Hayfever Relief (Boots) *See* LORATADINE.

Boots IBS Relief (Boots) *See* MEBEVERINE HYDROCHLORIDE.

Boots Infant Pain Relief (Boots) *See* PARACETAMOL.

Boots Infant Sugar Free Cough and Congestion Syrup

(Boots) A proprietary combination of *ephedrine (a decongestant), and *ipecacuanha (an expectorant), used for the relief of coughs and nasal congestion in young children. It is available without a prescription, but only from Boots.

Side effects, precautions, and interactions with other drugs: see EPHEDRINE HYDROCHLORIDE; DECONGESTANTS; IPECACUANHA.

Boots Migraine Relief (Boots) A proprietary combination of *paracetamol (a non-opioid analgesic) and *codeine (an opioid analgesic), used for the relief of *migraine. It is available as tablets and can be bought without a prescription, but only from Boots.

Side effects and precautions: see PARACETAMOL; CODEINE.
Interactions with other drugs: see OPIOIDS.

Boots Muscular Pain Relief Gel (Boots) *See* KETOPROFEN.

Boots Night Cold Comfort (Boots) A proprietary combination of *paracetamol (an analgesic and antipyretic), *pseudoephedrine (a decongestant), *diphenhydramine (a sedative antihistamine), and *pholcodine (a cough suppressant), taken at night to relieve the symptoms of colds and influenza. It is available as tablets without a prescription, but only from Boots.

Side effects and precautions: see PARACETAMOL; EPHEDRINE HYDROCHLORIDE; ANTIHISTAMINES; CODEINE.

Interactions with other drugs: see EPHEDRINE HYDROCHLORIDE; ANTIHISTAMINES; OPIOIDS.

Boots Night-time Cough Relief (Boots) A proprietary combination of *diphenhydramine (a sedative antihistamine) and *pholcodine (a cough suppressant), used for the relief of dry coughs that interfere with sleep. It is available as a syrup without a prescription, but only from Boots.

Side effects, precautions, and interactions with other drugs: see ANTIHISTAMINES; PHOLCODINE; OPIOIDS.

Boots Pain Relief Balm (Boots) A proprietary combination of the rubefacients *ethyl nicotinate, glycol monosalicylate (*see* GLYCOL SALICYLATE), and *nonylic acid vanillylamide in the form of a cream, used for the relief of muscular and rheumatic pains and stiffness, including backache, sciatica, lumbago, and fibrositis. It is available *over the counter, but only from Boots.

Side effects and precautions: see RUBEFACIENTS; SALICYLATES.

Boots Pain Relief Embrocation (Boots) A proprietary combination of *camphor and *turpentine oil, used as a *rubefacient for the relief of muscular and rheumatic pains and stiffness, including backache, sciatica, lumbago, and fibrositis. It is available *over the counter, but only from Boots.

Side effects and precautions: see RUBEFACIENTS.

Boots Pain Relief Extra Caplets (Boots) A proprietary combination of *paracetamol and *caffeine, used as an analgesic for the relief of mild to moderate pain. **Boots Pain Relief Extra Soluble** is in the form of soluble tablets. Both preparations are available *over the counter, but only from Boots.

Side effects and precautions: see PARACETAMOL; CAFFEINE.

Boots Pain Relief Warming Spray (Boots) A proprietary combination of *camphor, *ethyl nicotinate, and *methyl salicylate, used as a *rubefacient for the relief of muscular and rheumatic pains and stiffness, including backache, sciatica, lumbago, fibrositis, and sprains. It is available *over the counter, but only from Boots.

Side effects and precautions: see RUBEFACIENTS; SALICYLATES.

Boots Senna Tablets (Boots) *See* SENNA.

Boots Suppositories for Haemorrhoids (Boots) A proprietary combination of *zinc oxide (an astringent), *benzyl alcohol (an antipruritic agent), and glycol monosalicylate (*see* GLYCOL SALICYLATE) and *methyl salicylate (salicylates), used to relieve the pain and discomfort of *haemorrhoids. It can be obtained without a prescription, but only from Boots.

Boots Tension Headache Relief (Boots) A proprietary combination of *paracetamol and *codeine (analgesics), *caffeine (a stimulant), and *doxylamine (an antihistamine), used for the relief of headaches brought on by stress. It is available as tablets and can be obtained without a prescription, but only from Boots.

Side effects and precautions: see PARACETAMOL; CAFFEINE; CODEINE; ANTIHISTAMINES.

Interactions with other drugs: see OPIOIDS; ANTIHISTAMINES.

Boots Threadworm Treatment (Boots) *See* MEBENDAZOLE.

Botox (Allergan) *See* BOTULINUM A TOXIN-HAEMAGGLUTININ COMPLEX.

botulinum A toxin-haemagglutinin complex   A biological product used in minute doses as a *muscle relaxant for the treatment of blepharospasm (a tight contraction of the eyelids), one-sided facial spasms, and torticollis (twisting of the neck). It is administered by local injection by specialists trained in its use; as its duration of action is only 8–12 weeks, repeated injections are usually necessary. Botulinum toxin is available on *prescription only.

Side effects: there may be weakness and pain in the injected muscle and some jitter in other muscles; a transient burning sensation can occur after injection and a rash may develop. Reduced response may occur after repeated injections due to the formation of antibodies against botulinum toxin.

Precautions: botulinum toxin should not be used in people who have myasthenia gravis or in women who are pregnant or breastfeeding.

Interactions with other drugs:
  Antibiotics: aminoglycosides and spectinomycin should not be used with botulinum toxin as they increase the risk of its toxic effects.

Proprietary preparations: Botox; Dysport.

bowel-cleansing solutions   Preparations used to evacuate the bowel before exploratory procedures, surgery, or radiography. Containing osmotic or stimulant *laxatives, they are available as solutions, or powders to be dissolved in water, and are taken by mouth at regular intervals until the bowel effluent does not contain any solid material.

Side effects: include nausea, bloating, and (less commonly) abdominal cramps and vomiting.

Precautions: bowel-cleansing solutions should not be taken by people with gastrointestinal obstruction or ulceration and should be used with caution in pregnant women and in people with heart disease, ulcerative colitis, diabetes mellitus, or reflux oesophagitis.

Proprietary preparations: Citramag (*see* MAGNESIUM CITRATE); FLEET PHOSPHO-SODA (phosphate laxatives); KLEAN-PREP (macrogol '3340' and salts); PICOLAX (sodium picosulphate <picosulfate> and magnesium citrate).

Bradosol (Novartis Consumer Health) *See* BENZALKONIUM CHLORIDE.

Bradosol Plus (Novartis Consumer Health) A proprietary combination of *domiphen bromide (an antiseptic) and *lignocaine <lidocaine> hydrochloride (a local anaesthetic), used to relieve the pain and other symptoms of sore throats. It is available as lozenges and can be obtained without a prescription, but only from pharmacies.

Precautions: these lozenges are not recommended for children under 12 years old. *See also* LOCAL ANAESTHETICS.

bran   The fibrous outer layers of cereal grain. Wheat or oat bran is an effective *bulk-forming laxative. Wheat bran is freely available *over the counter in the form of a powder.

Side effects and precautions: see ISPAGHULA HUSK.
Proprietary preparation: Trifyba.

Brasivol (Stiefel Laboratories) *See* ALUMINIUM OXIDE.

breath-activated inhaler (breath-acuated inhaler) *See* INHALER.

Bretylate (GlaxoWellcome) *See* BRETYLIUM TOSYLATE <BRETYLIUM TOSILATE>.

bretylium tosylate <bretylium tosilate> An *anti-arrhythmic drug used to correct disordered heartbeats, especially ventricular *arrhythmias, during cardiac arrest. It is available, on *prescription only, as a solution for intravenous or intramuscular injection.
Side effects: include hypotension (low blood pressure), nausea, and vomiting.
Precautions: the injection site should be changed frequently to avoid local tissue damage. *See also* ANTI-ARRHYTHMIC DRUGS.
Interactions with other drugs:
  Anaesthetics: their effect in lowering blood pressure is increased by bretylium.
  Cisapride: should not be taken with bretylium as this combination increases the risk of ventricular arrhythmias.
  Sympathomimetic drugs: the effect of bretylium in lowering blood pressure is antagonized by some sympathomimetics, including ephedrine and methylphenidate.
Proprietary preparation: Bretylate.

Brevibloc (Gensia Automedics) *See* ESMOLOL HYDROCHLORIDE.

Brevinor (Searle) A proprietary combination of *ethinyloestradiol <ethinylestradiol> and *norethisterone used as an *oral contraceptive. It is available as tablets on *prescription only.
Side effects, precautions, and interactions with other drugs: see ORAL CONTRACEPTIVES.

Bricanyl (AstraZeneca) *See* TERBUTALINE SULPHATE.

brimonidine tartrate A *sympathomimetic drug, similar to *apraclonidine, that stimulates alpha *adrenoceptors. It is used primarily in the treatment of *glaucoma, in which it is thought to act by reducing the amount of fluid produced in the eye and also by aiding the drainage of the fluid from the eye. It may be used in conjunction with a *beta blocker. Brimonidine is available as eye drops on *prescription only.
Side effects: include bloodshot eyes, stinging, itching, allergic reactions, dry mouth, headache, fatigue, and drowsiness.
Precautions: brimonidine is not recommended for children. It should be used with caution in people with severe heart disease, depression,

Raynaud's syndrome, or impaired kidney or liver function and in women who are pregnant or breastfeeding. People who wear soft contact lenses should wait at least 15 minutes after applying the drops before inserting their lenses.

Interactions with other drugs:

Adrenaline <epinephrine> and noradrenaline <norepinephrine>: there is a possible risk of high blood pressure.

MAOIs: should not be used with brimonidine.

Tricyclic antidepressants: should not be used with brimonidine.

Proprietary preparation: Alphagan.

Britaject (Britannia Pharmaceuticals) *See* APOMORPHINE HYDROCHLORIDE.

BritLofex (Britannia Pharmaceuticals) *See* LOFEXIDINE HYDROCHLORIDE.

Broflex (Bioglan Laboratories) *See* BENZHEXOL <TRIHEXYPHENIDYL> HYDROCHLORIDE.

Brolene (Rhône-Poulenc Rorer) *See* PROPAMIDINE ISETHIONATE <ISETIONATE>.

bromazepam A long-acting *benzodiazepine used for the short-term treatment of anxiety. It is available as tablets on *prescription only and cannot be prescribed on the NHS.

Side effects and precautions: *see* DIAZEPAM; BENZODIAZEPINES.

Interactions with other drugs: *see* BENZODIAZEPINES.

Proprietary preparation: Lexotan.

bromocriptine A drug that stimulates dopamine receptors in the brain (i.e. it is a *dopamine receptor agonist) and is used for the treatment of parkinsonism (*see* ANTIPARKINSONIAN DRUGS). As it is longer acting than *levodopa, bromocriptine may be useful for patients who have early-morning disability. However, it should only be used when treatment with levodopa (with benserazide or carbidopa) has failed. Bromocriptine inhibits the secretion of prolactin and is therefore also used to treat disorders associated with overproduction of this hormone, including cyclical benign breast disease and prolactinoma (a tumour of the prolactin-secreting cells in the pituitary gland), as well as to prevent or suppress lactation in women who do not wish to breastfeed and to treat certain types of infertility in both men and women. It also inhibits the release of *growth hormone and is used to treat acromegaly (enlargement of the hands, feet, and face due to overproduction of this hormone). A *prescription only medicine, bromocriptine is available as tablets or capsules.

Side effects: include nausea, vomiting, constipation, headache, dizziness, and low blood pressure on standing. High doses of bromocriptine can cause confusion, excitation, hallucinations, involuntary abnormal movements, dry mouth, leg cramps, and fluid on the lungs (in which case treatment may need to be stopped). In rare cases bromocriptine can cause stomach ulcers.

Precautions: bromocriptine should be used with caution in people with a history of psychiatric illness or severe heart disease. Women should undergo regular gynaecological assessment. Any breathing or lung problems should be reported to a doctor. Alcohol should be avoided as it increases the likelihood of bromocriptine causing adverse effects.

Interactions with other drugs:

Antiemetics: metoclopramide and domperidone reduce the effect of bromocriptine in inhibiting prolactin secretion.

Antipsychotics: reduce the effects of bromocriptine in treating parkinsonism and overproduction of prolactin.

Erythromycin: increases the plasma concentration of bromocriptine (and therefore its potential for toxicity).

Sympathomimetic drugs: there is an increased risk of adverse effects when phenylpropanolamine or isometheptene are taken with bromocriptine.

Proprietary preparation: Parlodel.

brompheniramine maleate One of the original (sedating) *antihistamines, used to relieve the symptoms of such allergic conditions as hay fever and urticaria. It is available as tablets, *modified-release tablets, a solution, or an *elixir and can be bought from pharmacies without a prescription.

Side effects, precautions, and interactions with other drugs: *see* ANTIHISTAMINES.

Proprietary preparations: Dimotane LA (modified-release tablets), Dimotane Tablets; Dimotane Elixir; DIMOTANE CO (combined with codeine and pseudoephedrine); DIMOTANE EXPECTORANT (combined with guaiphenesin <guaifenesin> and pseudoephedrine); DIMOTANE PLUS (combined with pseudoephedrine); DIMOTAPP (combined with phenylephrine and phenylpropanolamine).

Bronalin Dry Cough (Seton Scholl Healthcare) A proprietary combination of *dextromethorphan (a cough suppressant) and *pseudoephedrine (a decongestant), used to relieve the symptoms of dry irritating coughs and colds. It is available as a syrup without a prescription, but only from pharmacies.

Side effects and interactions with other drugs: *see* DEXTROMETHORPHAN; OPIOIDS; EPHEDRINE HYDROCHLORIDE; DECONGESTANTS.

Precautions: this medicine is not recommended for children under six years old. *See also* OPIOIDS; EPHEDRINE HYDROCHLORIDE; DECONGESTANTS.

Bronalin Expectorant (Seton Scholl Healthcare) A proprietary combination of *ammonium chloride (an expectorant) and *diphenhydramine (a sedative antihistamine), used to relieve the symptoms of productive coughs and colds. It is available without a prescription, but only from pharmacies.

Side effects and interactions with other drugs: see ANTIHISTAMINES.

Precautions: this medicine is not recommended for children under six years old. *See also* ANTIHISTAMINES.

Bronalin Paediatric (Seton Scholl Healthcare) *See* DIPHENHYDRAMINE.

Bronchodil (ASTA Medica) *See* REPROTEROL HYDROCHLORIDE.

bronchodilators Drugs that cause widening of the airways by relaxing bronchial smooth muscle. *Sympathomimetic drugs that stimulate beta *adrenoceptors, such as *salbutamol, *terbutaline, and *salmeterol, are potent bronchodilators used for the relief of *asthma and chronic bronchitis. These drugs are often administered in aerosols to give rapid relief, but in high doses they may stimulate the heart, increasing heart rate. Other drugs used as bronchodilators are the *antimuscarinic drugs *ipratropium and *oxitropium and the *xanthines, including *theophylline.

See also BAMBUTEROL HYDROCHLORIDE; EFORMOTEROL <FORMOTEROL> FUMARATE; FENOTEROL HYDROBROMIDE; ORCIPRENALINE SULPHATE; REPROTEROL HYDROCHLORIDE; TULOBUTEROL HYDROCHLORIDE.

Brufen, **Brufen Retard** (Knoll) *See* IBUPROFEN.

buccal Relating to the mouth or mouth cavity. Buccal tablets are designed to be dissolved in the mouth – between the upper lip and gum.

Buccastem (Reckitt & Colman) *See* PROCHLORPERAZINE.

buclizine hydrochloride An *antihistamine that is used as an *antiemetic in preparations for the treatment of *migraine.

Side effects, precautions, and interactions with other drugs: see ANTIHISTAMINES.

Proprietary preparation: MIGRALEVE (pink tablets: combined with paracetamol and codeine phosphate).

budesonide A *corticosteroid used for the prevention of *asthma attacks and the treatment of rhinitis (including hay fever). It is given by inhalation or nasal spray and may be used in conjunction with *bronchodilators and/or *sodium cromoglycate <cromoglicate>. Budesonide is also used to treat inflammatory bowel disease, being given by mouth for the treatment of Crohn's disease and rectally for ulcerative colitis. All preparations are available on *prescription only.

Side effects: when taken by inhalation or nasally, the most common side effects are hoarseness (due to weakness of the vocal muscles) and fungal (*Candida*) infections of the mouth or throat. For side effects when taken orally or rectally, *see* CORTICOSTEROIDS.

Precautions: budesonide inhalers or nasal sprays should be used with caution by people who have (or have had) tuberculosis and by pregnant women. For precautions when taken orally or rectally, *see* CORTICOSTEROIDS.

Proprietary preparations: Entocort CR (modified-release capsules); Entocort Enema; Pulmicort Inhaler; Pulmicort Turbohaler (disks of powder, of varying strengths, for use with an inhaler); Pulmicort Respules (ampoules for use with a nebulizer); Rhinocort Aqua (nasal spray).

bulk-forming laxatives (bulking agents) *Laxatives that act by absorbing water, increasing the bulk and softening the consistency of the stools. They consist either of plant fibre (e.g. *bran, *ispaghula husk, *sterculia) or of a synthetic agent (e.g. *methylcellulose). Bulking agents are usually effective 12–24 hours after being taken, but it can take some days for their full effect to develop. They are useful for encouraging bowel movements in people with a colostomy, ileostomy, haemorrhoids, or anal fissure and for treating chronic diarrhoea in people with irritable bowel syndrome or diverticular disease, when their ability to absorb water in the gut is exploited to decrease the liquidity of the stools.

Bulk-forming laxatives that swell in water should always be swallowed with plenty of water and should not be taken immediately before going to bed.

bumetanide A *loop diuretic used to treat *oedema resulting from congestive heart failure, kidney disease, or cirrhosis of the liver. It can be injected in emergencies to relieve pulmonary oedema (fluid in the spaces of the lungs causing breathing difficulties). Bumetanide is usually given with a *potassium supplement or a *potassium-sparing diuretic. A *prescription only medicine, it can be taken orally as tablets or liquid and is also available as a solution for injection.

Side effects, precautions, and interactions with other drugs: see LOOP DIURETICS.

Proprietary preparations: Burinex; BURINEX A (combined with amiloride hydrochloride); BURINEX K (combined with potassium chloride).

See also DIURETICS.

bupivacaine *See* LOCAL ANAESTHETICS.

buprenorphine An *opioid analgesic used for the treatment of moderate to severe pain, including pain relief before and during surgery. Buprenorphine is a *controlled drug; it is available as tablets to be dissolved under the tongue and as an injection.

Side effects and precautions: see MORPHINE. Buprenorphine may give rise to mild withdrawal symptoms in people who are regularly taking other opioids since it antagonizes their action.

Interactions with other drugs: see OPIOIDS.

Proprietary preparation: Temgesic.

Burinex (Leo Pharmaceuticals) *See* BUMETANIDE.

Burinex A (Leo Pharmaceuticals) A proprietary combination of
*bumetanide (a loop diuretic) and *amiloride hydrochloride (a potassium-
sparing diuretic), used for the treatment of *oedema or *hypertension. It
is available as tablets on *prescription only.
Side effects, precautions, and interactions with other drugs: see LOOP
DIURETICS; POTASSIUM-SPARING DIURETICS.
See also ANTIHYPERTENSIVE DRUGS; DIURETICS.

Burinex K (Leo Pharmaceuticals) A proprietary combination of
*bumetanide (a loop diuretic) and *potassium chloride. Available on
prescription only, it is taken orally in the form of *modified-release
tablets for the treatment of *oedema associated with congestive heart
failure, liver disease, or kidney disease.
Side effects, precautions, and interactions with other drugs: see LOOP
DIURETICS.
See also DIURETICS.

Burneze Spray (Seton Scholl Healthcare) *See* BENZOCAINE.

Buscopan (Boehringer Ingelheim) *See* HYOSCINE BUTYLBROMIDE.

buserelin An analogue of *gonadorelin used to treat *endometriosis
and to suppress the release of gonadotrophins by the pituitary gland
before inducing ovulation in women undergoing fertility treatment. It is
also used to reduce concentrations of testosterone in the treatment of
prostate cancer that requires testosterone for growth (*see* LEUPRORELIN).
Buserelin is available, on *prescription only, as a nasal spray or a solution
for injection.
Side effects: include hot flushes, loss of libido, headache, and depression;
the spray may cause transient nasal irritation. In women there may also
be vaginal dryness, emotional upset, changes in breast size, breast
tenderness, and ovarian cysts; men may rarely experience enlargement
of the breasts.
Precautions: buserelin should not be taken by women who are pregnant
or breastfeeding or who have undiagnosed vaginal bleeding; a
nonhormonal method of contraception should be used during treatment.
The drug should be used with caution in women with osteoporosis or
depression.
Proprietary preparations: Suprecur (nasal spray for endometriosis);
Suprefact (nasal spray for prostate cancer).

Buspar (Bristol-Myers Squibb) *See* BUSPIRONE.

buspirone An *anxiolytic drug used for the short-term treatment of
anxiety. Although some beneficial effects may be seen during the first
week, the response to buspirone treatment can take up to two weeks. It

produces less sedation than the *benzodiazepines and less dependence and potential for abuse. If benzodiazepines are being replaced by buspirone, treatment with the benzodiazepine needs to be tapered off gradually, since buspirone will not alleviate the withdrawal symptoms associated with stopping benzodiazepines. Buspirone is available as tablets on *prescription only.

Side effects: include nausea, dizziness, headache, nervousness, lightheadedness, excitement, and (rarely) a fast heart rate, palpitations, chest pain, drowsiness, confusion, dry mouth, fatigue, and sweating.

Precautions: buspirone should not be taken by people with epilepsy, severe liver or kidney disease, or by women who are pregnant or breastfeeding. Alcohol enhances the sedative effect of buspirone.

Interactions with other drugs: the sedative effect of buspirone is increased by a number of drugs, including anaesthetics, opioid analgesics, antidepressants, antihistamines, and antipsychotic drugs.

   MAOIs: should not be taken with buspirone.

Proprietary preparation: Buspar.

busulfan *See* BUSULPHAN.

busulphan <busulfan> An *alkylating drug used for the treatment of chronic myeloid leukaemia (*see* CANCER). It is available as tablets on *prescription only.

Side effects: include *bone marrow suppression and increased pigmentation of the skin. *See also* CYTOTOXIC DRUGS.

Precautions: see CYTOTOXIC DRUGS.

Proprietary preparation: Myleran.

Butacote (Novartis Consumer Health) *See* PHENYLBUTAZONE.

butobarbital *See* BUTOBARBITONE.

butobarbitone <butobarbital> An intermediate-acting *barbiturate used for the short-term treatment of severe insomnia in patients who are already taking barbiturates. A *controlled drug, it is available as tablets.

Side effects, precautions, and interactions with other drugs: see BARBITURATES.

Proprietary preparation: Soneryl.

Buttercup Honey and Lemon (Pfizer Consumer Healthcare) *See* SQUILL.

Buttercup Infant Cough Syrup (Pfizer Consumer Healthcare) *See* IPECACUANHA.

Buttercup Syrup Traditional (Pfizer Consumer Healthcare) *See* SQUILL.

C

Cabaser (Pharmacia & Upjohn) *See* CABERGOLINE.

Cabdrivers (Merck Consumer Health) A proprietary combination of
*dextromethorphan (a cough suppressant) and *menthol, used for the
relief of coughs. It is available as a syrup and as a sugar-free mixture
(**Cabdrivers Sugar Free**) without a prescription, but only from
pharmacies.

Side effects and interactions with other drugs: see DEXTROMETHORPHAN;
OPIOIDS.

Precautions: this medicine is not recommended for children. *See also*
OPIOIDS.

cabergoline A *dopamine agonist, very similar to *bromocriptine,
that is used as an *adjunct to *levodopa (with carbidopa or benserazide)
in the treatment of Parkinson's disease (*see* ANTIPARKINSONIAN DRUGS). It
is also used to reduce high concentrations of the hormone prolactin in
certain types of infertility. It is available as tablets on *prescription only.

Side effects: include dizziness, vertigo, nausea, headache, fatigue, breast
pain, gastrointestinal upsets, hot flushes, and depression.

Precautions: cabergoline should be used with caution in people who have
liver, kidney, or heart disease, Raynaud's syndrome, or gastrointestinal
ulcers or bleeding. It should be discontinued for one month before trying
to conceive.

Interactions with other drugs:

Antiemetics: metoclopramide and domperidone reduce the effect of
cabergoline in inhibiting prolactin secretion.

Antipsychotics: reduce the effects of cabergoline.

Erythromycin: increases the plasma concentration of cabergoline (and
therefore its potential for toxicity).

Proprietary preparations: Cabaser; Dostinex.

Cacit (Procter & Gamble) *See* CALCIUM CARBONATE.

Cacit D3 (Procter & Gamble) A proprietary combination of *calcium
carbonate and *cholecalciferol <colecalciferol> (vitamin D3), used to treat
*vitamin D deficiency and as an *adjunct in the treatment of
osteoporosis. It is available as effervescent granules and can be obtained
without a prescription, but only from pharmacies.

Side effects: nausea, vomiting, and other stomach upsets may occur. *See*
VITAMIN D.

Precautions: this medicine should be taken with caution by people with
kidney disease or a history of kidney stones.

Interactions with other drugs:

Antiepileptic drugs: carbamazepine, phenobarbitone <phenobarbital>, phenytoin, and primidone reduce the effects of Cacit D3.

Thiazide diuretics: increase the risk of high concentrations of calcium in the blood; *see* VITAMIN D.

cade oil (juniper tar) An oil extracted from the wood of *Juniperus oxycedrus*, a species of juniper. It is an ingredient of several topical preparations for the treatment of scaling conditions of the scalp, such as *psoriasis.

Proprietary preparations: GELCOTAR (combined with strong coal tar solution; POLYTAR (combined with tar, coal tar extract, and other ingredients); POLYTAR AF (combined with tar, coal tar extract, and other ingredients).

cadexomer iodine An antibacterial substance (*see* ANTIBIOTICS) used to absorb the liquid that exudes from ulcers and infected wounds. It is available as a paste, powder, or ointment on *prescription only.

Precautions: cadexomer iodine should not be used by women who are pregnant or breastfeeding or by people with diseases of the thyroid gland.

Proprietary preparations: Iodoflex (paste); Iodosorb (powder or ointment).

Caelyx (Schering-Plough) *See* DOXORUBICIN.

Cafergot (Alliance Pharmaceuticals) *See* ERGOTAMINE TARTRATE.

caffeine A mild *stimulant that is found in tea and coffee. It is often included, in small doses, in analgesic preparations, and is claimed to increase analgesic effects. However, there is considerable scepticism as to whether it actually contributes to pain control.

Side effects and precautions: the alerting effect of caffeine in analgesic preparations may not always be wanted, and the caffeine may worsen a headache. Overconsumption of caffeine can cause feelings of anxiety and restlessness, and very large doses, or sudden withdrawal, can cause headaches.

Proprietary preparations: ALKA-SELTZER XS (combined with aspirin and paracetamol); ANADIN (combined with aspirin); ANADIN EXTRA, ANADIN EXTRA SOLUBLE (combined with aspirin and paracetamol); ANDREWS SELTZER EXTRA (combined with paracetamol and sodium bicarbonate); ASKIT (combined with aloxiprin and aspirin); BEECHAMS FLU-PLUS CAPLETS (combined with paracetamol and phenylephrine); BEECHAMS POWDERS (combined with aspirin); BEECHAMS POWDERS CAPSULES (combined with paracetamol and phenylephrine); BOOTS COLD AND 'FLU RELIEF TABLETS (combined with paracetamol, phenylephrine, and ascorbic acid); BOOTS PAIN RELIEF TABLETS (combined with paracetamol); CATARRH-EX (combined with paracetamol and phenylephrine); DE WITT'S ANALGESIC PILLS (combined with paracetamol); DRISTAN DECONGESTANT TABLETS (combined with aspirin, phenylephrine, and chlorpheniramine <chlophenamine>); FEMINAX (combined with paracetamol, codeine, and hyoscine); HEDEX EXTRA (combined with paracetamol); LEMSIP COLD + FLU COMBINED RELIEF CAPSULES (combined with paracetamol and phenylephrine); NURSE SYKES POWDERS (combined with aspirin and paracetamol); PANADOL EXTRA (combined with paracetamol); PARACLEAR EXTRA STRENGTH (combined with paracetamol); PHENSIC (combined with aspirin); PROPAIN (combined with paracetamol, codeine, and diphenhydramine); SOLPADEINE (combined with paracetamol and codeine); SP COLD RELIEF CAPSULES (combined with paracetamol and phenylephrine); SYNDOL (combined with paracetamol, codeine, and doxylamine); TOPTABS (combined with aspirin); VEGANIN (combined with paracetamol and aspirin).

cajuput oil An aromatic oil distilled from the leaves of *Melaleuca cajuputi*, a tree native to southeast Asia and Australia. It is mildly antiseptic and acts as a *rubefacient, being included as an ingredient in preparations for the relief of muscular aches and pains. It is also included in inhalations to relieve the congestion associated with colds and catarrh.

Proprietary preparations: OLBAS INHALER (combined with menthol, eucalyptus oil, and peppermint oil); OLBAS OIL (combined with menthol, eucalyptus oil, clove oil, juniper berry oil, and oil of wintergreen); TIGER BALM (combined with camphor, clove oil, peppermint oil, and menthol); TIGER BALM RED EXTRA STRENGTH (combined with camphor, menthol, clove oil, cinnamon oil, and peppermint oil).

Calabren (APS-Berk) *See* GLIBENCLAMIDE.

Caladryl (Warner-Lambert Consumer Healthcare) A proprietary combination of *calamine (an antipruritic), *diphenhydramine hydrochloride (an antihistamine), and *camphor (a rubefacient), used to relieve irritation of the skin, sunburn, and insect stings and bites. It is available as a cream or lotion and can be obtained without a prescription, but only from pharmacies.

Precautions: Caladryl should not be applied to broken skin, the mouth lining or other mucous membranes, measles or chickenpox rashes, or weeping skin conditions.

calamine A preparation of zinc carbonate, coloured with ferric oxide. It is used in the form of a lotion or cream as a mild *astringent to relieve itching. It is also an ingredient of other skin preparations. Preparations containing calamine can be obtained without a prescription.

Proprietary preparations: CALADRYL (combined with diphenhydramine and camphor); VASOGEN CREAM (combined with zinc oxide and dimethicone <dimeticone>).

Calanif (APS-Berk) *See* NIFEDIPINE.

Calazem (Norton Healthcare) *See* DILTIAZEM HYDROCHLORIDE.

Calceos (Cortecs Healthcare) A proprietary combination of *calcium carbonate and *cholecalciferol <colecalciferol> (vitamin D₃), used to treat *vitamin D deficiency and as an *adjunct in the treatment of osteoporosis. It is available as chewable tablets and can be obtained without a prescription, but only from pharmacies.

Side effects: nausea, vomiting, and other stomach upsets may occur. *See* VITAMIN D.

Precautions: this medicine should be taken with caution by people with kidney disease or a history of kidney stones.

Interactions with other drugs:

 Antiepileptic drugs: carbamazepine, phenobarbitone <phenobarbital>, phenytoin, and primidone reduce the effects of Calceos.

 Thiazide diuretics: increase the risk of high concentrations of calcium in the blood; *see* VITAMIN D.

Calcicard CR (Norton Healthcare) *See* DILTIAZEM HYDROCHLORIDE.

Calcichew (Shire Pharmaceuticals) *See* CALCIUM CARBONATE.

Calcichew D3 (Shire Pharmaceuticals) A proprietary combination of *calcium carbonate and *cholecalciferol <colecalciferol> (vitamin D₃), used for the treatment of *vitamin D deficiency and as an *adjunct in the treatment of osteoporosis. **Calcichew D3 Forte** is a similar preparation but contains twice as much cholecalciferol <colecalciferol>. Both preparations are available as chewable tablets and can be obtained from pharmacies without a prescription.

Side effects: include constipation and flatulence. *See also* VITAMIN D.

Precautions and interactions with other drugs: *see* VITAMIN D.

Calcidrink (Shire Pharmaceuticals) *See* CALCIUM CARBONATE.

calciferol A high-strength formulation of *cholecalciferol <colecalciferol> or *ergocalciferol that is used to treat vitamin D deficiency caused by poor absorption of calcium from the intestines or liver disease. It is available as tablets, which can be obtained without a prescription, but only from pharmacies, or as a solution for injection, which is available on *prescription only.

Side effects, precautions, and interactions with other drugs: *see* VITAMIN D.

Calcijex (Abbott Laboratories) *See* CALCITRIOL.

Calciparin (Sanofi Winthrop) *See* HEPARIN.

calcipotriol An *analogue of *vitamin D that is used in the treatment of *psoriasis. It acts by slowing down the division of skin cells whose overgrowth causes the formation of scaly patches seen in this disease.

Calcipotriol is available, on *prescription only, as an ointment, a cream, or a scalp lotion.

Side effects: calcipotriol may irritate the skin, causing itching or reddening; rarely, it may cause a rash on the face or around the mouth.

Precautions: calcipotriol should not be used by people with disorders of calcium metabolism and it should not be applied to the face. It should be used with caution by people with peeling psoriasis and by pregnant women.

Proprietary preparations: Dovonex (ointment); Dovonex Cream; Dovonex Scalp Lotion.

Calcisorb (3M Health Care) *See* SODIUM CELLULOSE PHOSPHATE.

Calcitare (Rhône-Poulenc Rorer) *See* CALCITONIN.

calcitonin A hormone, secreted by the thyroid gland, that lowers circulating concentrations of calcium by promoting the uptake of calcium into bone. A form of the hormone extracted from pig thyroid is used to reduce abnormally high concentrations of calcium in the blood and to relieve pain in Paget's disease (in which the bones become deformed and fracture easily). Calcitonin can cause allergic reactions; less allergenic is *salcatonin <calcitonin (salmon)>, a synthetic form of the hormone. Calcitonin is available as an injection on *prescription only.

Side effects: include nausea, vomiting, and flushing (which diminish with use); less common side effects are tingling of hands, an unpleasant taste, rash, and inflammation at the injection site.

Precautions: some people are allergic to calcitonin and a scratch test may be necessary before taking the drug. It should be used with caution in women who are pregnant or breastfeeding.

Proprietary preparation: Calcitare.

calcitonin (salmon) *See* SALCATONIN.

calcitriol A *vitamin D derivative used to prevent and treat the bone disease that may occur in kidney dialysis patients and to treat postmenopausal osteoporosis. It is available as capsules or an injection on *prescription only.

Side effects, precautions, and interactions with other drugs: see VITAMIN D.

Proprietary preparations: Calcijex (injection); Rocaltrol (capsules).

calcium A metallic element essential for the normal development and functioning of the body. It is required for many metabolic processes, including nerve function, muscle contraction, and blood clotting, and it is an important constituent of bones and teeth. Calcium is maintained at the correct concentration in the blood by the action of hormones (*see* CALCITONIN; PARATHYROID HORMONE). The uptake of calcium from the gut and its deposition in bone is facilitated by *vitamin D; deficiency of this vitamin may therefore result in bone disorders, such as rickets in children and osteoporosis or osteomalacia in adults. Deficiency of calcium in the blood leads to tetany (spasm and twitching of the muscles). Conversely, high plasma concentrations of calcium may lead to the deposition of calcium in soft tissues and cause 'hardening' of the tissues (calcification).

Calcium supplements are given to prevent or treat calcium deficiency. Extra calcium may be required by growing children, pregnant or breastfeeding women, women who have reached the menopause, and elderly people; it reduces bone loss in people with osteoporosis. Supplementary calcium may also be required by people who cannot tolerate milk. Oral calcium supplements are available in the form of crystalline bone extract (*see* HYDROXYAPATITE) or as a variety of calcium salts, including *calcium carbonate, *calcium gluconate, *calcium lactate, *calcium lactate gluconate, *calcium phosphate, **calcium glubionate**, and **calcium lactobionate**, which are readily absorbed. They are often packaged with *vitamin D. Calcium gluconate and *calcium chloride can be given intravenously. Calcium salts are also used in *antacid preparations.

Side effects: include constipation and flatulence. Injections may cause slowing of the heart rate, irregular heartbeat, and irritation.

Precautions: calcium supplements should not be taken by people with conditions associated with high plasma calcium concentrations or tissue calcification (including some forms of cancer and kidney disease) or by those who are immobile for long periods (since prolonged immobilization causes resorption of calcium from bone and high plasma calcium concentrations).

Interactions with other drugs:

Antibiotics: the absorption of tetracyclines and ciprofloxacin is reduced by calcium salts.

Bisphosphonates: their absorption is reduced by calcium salts.

Digoxin and digitoxin: calcium given by intravenous injection can cause irregular heartbeats.

Thiazide diuretics: the risk of high blood calcium concentrations is increased.

Calcium 500 (Martindale Pharmaceuticals) *See* CALCIUM CARBONATE.

calcium acetate A salt of *calcium that is used as a *phosphate-binding agent. It is available as tablets and can be obtained without a prescription.

Precautions: calcium acetate should not be taken by people with low concentrations of phosphate in the blood or high concentrations of calcium in the blood or urine. Plasma *electrolytes and albumin may therefore need to be monitored.

Interactions with other drugs: see CALCIUM.

Proprietary preparation: Phosex.

calcium antagonists Drugs that inhibit the influx of calcium into heart muscle and the smooth muscle of blood vessels. They are often called **calcium-channel blockers** (which is a more correct description of their action), but the term calcium antagonist is more widely used. Muscles need calcium to contract; these drugs therefore reduce the force of heart-muscle contractions and cause *vasodilatation in the blood vessels. Some of them also slow the passage of nerve signals through the heart, which can be helpful in correcting certain types of abnormal heartbeat (*see* ARRHYTHMIA). Dilating the blood vessels decreases the work done by the heart and so relieves the strain on the heart that gives rise to *angina. Calcium antagonists are classified into three groups (I, II, and III) depending on the way in which they act. Class I drugs (e.g. *verapamil hydrochloride) act mainly on the heart, reducing the force of contractions and the conduction of nerve impulses. Class II drugs (e.g. *nifedipine, *nimodipine, *amlodipine, *felodipine, *isradipine, *lacidipine, *lercanidipine, *nicardipine, *nisoldipine) have actions mainly on the blood vessels and not on the heart. They are used for various cardiovascular disorders, such as *angina, and *hypertension, but have little anti-arrhythmic activity. They may be used in conjunction with *beta blockers, which prevent the reflex increase in heart rate that they cause, but they are also useful for people who cannot tolerate beta blockers. Class III drugs (e.g. *diltiazem) have actions mainly on the coronary arteries.

Side effects: dizziness and sometimes fainting, headaches at the start of treatment, and flushing of the face are quite common. Palpitations and ankle *oedema may occur with class II drugs.

Precautions: people taking calcium antagonists (except amlodipine and diltiazem) should avoid grapefruit juice, as this interferes with their metabolism by increasing their plasma concentrations.

Interactions with other drugs:

 Anaesthetics: the general anaesthetic isoflurane increases the effect of the class II calcium antagonists in lowering blood pressure.

 Antihypertensive drugs: their effects in lowering blood pressure are increased by calcium antagonists.

 Beta blockers: should not be used with class I drugs (verapamil) as this combination causes severe hypotension (low blood pressure) and can precipitate heart failure. This is less likely to happen with class II drugs, which can be given with beta blockers if monitored closely.

 Ritonavir: may increase the plasma concentrations of calcium antagonists.

 For other interactions, see entries for individual drugs.

calcium carbonate A *calcium salt with a variety of uses. It is taken as a calcium supplement, and is often packaged with *vitamin D for the treatment of osteoporosis. It is used as a *phosphate-binding agent in people with kidney failure, especially if they are on dialysis. Calcium carbonate is a common ingredient in *antacid preparations, for the relief of indigestion, heartburn, and similar conditions, and is also included in some *antidiarrhoeal preparations. It is also used with sodium perborate as a tooth powder. Calcium carbonate is available as chewable tablets, effervescent tablets, or granules and can be obtained without a prescription, but only from pharmacies. Antacid preparations containing calcium carbonate are usually freely available *over the counter.

Side effects, precautions, and interactions with other drugs: see CALCIUM.

Proprietary preparations: Cacit (effervescent tablets); Calcichew (chewable tablets); Calcichew Forte (chewable tablets); Calcidrink (granules); Calcium 500 (tablets); Tums (antacid); Rap-Eze (antacid); Remegel (antacid); Rennie Rap-Eze (antacid); Settlers Antacid Peppermint Tablets; ANDREWS ANTACID (combined with magnesium carbonate); BISODOL ANTACID TABLETS (combined with sodium bicarbonate and magnesium carbonate); BISODOL EXTRA TABLETS (combined with sodium bicarbonate, magnesium carbonate, and simethicone); CACIT D3 (combined with vitamin D_3); CALCEOS (combined with vitamin D_3); CALCICHEW D3 (combined with vitamin D_3); DE WITT'S ANTACID POWDER (combined with sodium bicarbonate, magnesium carbonate, magnesium trisilicate, kaolin, and peppermint oil); GAVISCON LIQUID (combined with sodium alginate and sodium bicarbonate); J COLLIS BROWNE'S TABLETS (combined with kaolin and morphine); KAO-C (combined with kaolin); MOORLAND (combined with aluminium hydroxide, bismuth aluminate, magnesium trisilicate, magnesium carbonate, and kaolin); PEPTAC (combined with alginic acid and sodium bicarbonate); RENNIE (combined with magnesium carbonate); RENNIE DEFLATINE (combined with simethicone and magnesium carbonate); TITRALAC (combined with glycine).

calcium-channel blockers *See* CALCIUM ANTAGONISTS.

calcium chloride A *calcium salt that is given intravenously to resuscitate patients who have suffered a heart attack associated with high levels of *potassium in the blood. It is also included as an ingredient in artifical saliva preparations and in *balanced salt solution for washing out the eyes. Calcium chloride injection is available on *prescription only.

Side effects, precautions, and interactions with other drugs: see CALCIUM.
Proprietary preparation: Min-I-Jet Calcium Chloride.

calcium folinate *See* FOLINIC ACID.

calcium glubionate *See* CALCIUM; CALCIUM-SANDOZ.

calcium gluconate A *calcium salt used to treat calcium deficiency or to prevent osteoporosis. It is available as tablets or effervescent tablets, which can be obtained without a prescription from pharmacies, and as an injection (for treating tetany), which is available on *prescription only.
Side effects, precautions, and interactions with other drugs: see CALCIUM.

calcium lactate A *calcium salt used to correct calcium deficiency or to prevent osteoporosis. It is also combined with *ergocalciferol (as **calcium and ergocalciferol**) for the treatment of vitamin D deficiency. Calcium lactate is available as tablets and can be obtained without a prescription, but only from pharmacies.
Side effects, precautions, and interactions with other drugs: see CALCIUM.

calcium lactate gluconate A *calcium salt used to correct calcium deficiency or to prevent osteoporosis. It is available as effervescent tablets and can be obtained without a prescription, but only from pharmacies.
Side effects, precautions, and interactions with other drugs: see CALCIUM.
Proprietary preparations: SANDOCAL 400 and SANDOCAL 1000 (combined with calcium carbonate).

calcium lactobionate *See* CALCIUM; CALCIUM-SANDOZ.

calcium leucovorin *See* FOLINIC ACID.

calcium levofolinate (calcium levoleucovorin) *See* FOLINIC ACID.

calcium phosphate A *calcium salt used to correct calcium deficiency or to prevent osteoporosis. It is also combined with *ergocalciferol (as **calcium and ergocalciferol**) for the treatment of vitamin D deficiency. Calcium phosphate is available as a powder to be dissolved in water and taken by mouth and can be obtained without a prescription, but only from pharmacies.
Side effects, precautions, and interactions with other drugs: see CALCIUM.
Proprietary preparation: Ostram.

calcium polystyrene sulphonate A resin that exchanges potassium ions for calcium ions in the intestine when it is taken by mouth or by enema. It is used to reduce high concentrations of potassium in blood associated with failure of the kidneys to produce sufficient urine or in patients on dialysis (*see* ELECTROLYTE). It is available as a powder and can be obtained without a prescription, but only from pharmacies.
Side effects: include high plasma calcium concentrations, low plasma potassium concentrations, loss of appetite, nausea and vomiting, constipation, and diarrhoea. If constipation occurs, treatment should be stopped and magnesium-containing laxatives avoided. Intestinal obstruction has been occasionally reported.
Precautions: calcium polystyrene sulphonate should not be taken by people with overactive parathyroid glands (*see* PARATHYROID HORMONE), myeloma (cancer of the bone marrow), metastatic cancer (secondaries) involving kidney failure, or obstructive bowel disease. It should be used with caution in women who are pregnant or breastfeeding. Plasma electrolytes may need to be monitored.
Proprietary preparation: Calcium Resonium.

Calcium Resonium (Sanofi Winthrop) *See* CALCIUM POLYSTYRENE SULPHONATE.

Calcium-Sandoz (Novartis Consumer Health) A proprietary combination of the salts calcium glubionate and calcium lactobionate, used as a *calcium supplement. It is available as a syrup and can be obtained without a prescription, but only from pharmacies.
Side effects, precautions, and interactions with other drugs: see CALCIUM.

Calcort (Hoechst Marion Roussel) *See* DEFLAZACORT.

Calgel (Warner-Lambert Consumer Healthcare) A proprietary combination of *cetylpyridinium chloride (an antiseptic) and *lignocaine <lidocaine> hydrochloride (a local anaesthetic) in the form of a gel, used to relieve teething pain and soothe the gums. It is freely available *over the counter.
Precautions: Calgel is not recommended for babies under three months old.

Califig California Syrup of Figs (Merck Consumer Health) A proprietary combination of *senna and figs, used as a *stimulant laxative for the treatment of constipation. It is freely available *over the counter.
Precautions: this syrup should not be taken by children under one year old. *See* STIMULANT LAXATIVES.

Calimal (Sussex Pharmaceutical *See* CHLORPHENIRAMINE <CHLORPHENAMINE> MALEATE.

Calmurid (Galderma) A proprietary combination of *urea (a moisturizing agent) and *lactic acid (a keratolytic and antibiotic), used for the treatment of chronic dry and itching skin conditions. It is available as a cream and can be obtained without a prescription, but only from pharmacies.

Calmurid HC (Galderma) A proprietary combination of *hydrocortisone (a corticosteroid), *urea (a hydrating agent), and *lactic acid (a keratolytic and antibiotic), used for the treatment of dry *eczema and similar skin conditions. It is available as a cream on *prescription only.
Side effects and precautions: see TOPICAL STEROIDS.

Calpol (Warner-Lambert Consumer Healthcare) *See* PARACETAMOL.

Calsalettes (Torbet Laboratories) *See* ALOIN.

Calsynar (Rhône-Poulenc Rorer) *See* SALCATONIN <CALCITONIN (SALMON)>.

CAM (Shire Pharmaceuticals) *See* EPHEDRINE HYDROCHLORIDE.

Camcolit (Norgine) *See* LITHIUM CARBONATE.

camphor An aromatic substance obtained from the wood of a southeast Asian tree (*Cinnamomum camphora*) or manufactured synthetically. When applied to the skin it produces a cooling effect. Camphor is used in *rubefacient preparations to relieve the pain of sprains and strains, backache, rheumatic pains, and neuralgia. It is also used in some *emollient skin preparations to relieve the itching associated with such conditions as eczema. Camphor is also an ingredient in cough remedies, ear drops, and preparations for the removal of corns and verrucas.

Proprietary preparations: BALMOSA (combined with menthol, methyl salicylate, and capsicum oleoresin); BOOTS PAIN RELIEF EMBROCATION (combined with turpentine oil); BOOTS PAIN RELIEF WARMING SPRAY (combined with ethyl nicotinate and methyl salicylate); CORN AND CALLUS REMOVAL LIQUID (combined with salicylic acid); EAREX EAR DROPS (combined with arachis oil and almond oil); PR HEAT SPRAY (combined with methyl salicylate and ethyl nicotinate); RADIAN-B MUSCLE LOTION (combined with menthol, ammonium salicylate, and salicylic acid); RADIAN-B MUSCLE RUB (combined with capsicin, menthol, and methyl salicylate); SALONAIR (combined with benzyl nicotinate, glycol salicylate, menthol, methyl salicylate and squalane); SALONPAS PLASTERS (combined with methyl salicylate, glycol salicylate, and menthol); SEAL AND HEAL VERRUCA REMOVAL GEL (combined with salicylic acid); TIGER BALM (combined with cajuput oil, clove oil, peppermint oil, and menthol); TIGER BALM RED EXTRA STRENGTH (combined with menthol, cajuput oil, clove oil, cinnamon oil, and peppermint oil); TIXYLIX INHALANT (combined with turpentine oil, eucalyptus oil, and menthol); VICKS VAPORUB (combined with eucalyptus oil, turpentine oil, and menthol).

Campral EC (Merck Pharmaceuticals) *See* ACAMPROSATE CALCIUM.

Campto (Rhône-Poulenc Rorer) *See* IRINOTECAN.

cancer Any one of a group of diseases characterized by unregulated cell division that gives rise to malignant tumours. Such tumours invade and destroy the tissues in which they originate and can spread to other parts of the body via the blood or lymphatic system or across a body cavity, such as the abdomen or chest. These secondary tumours, or **metastases**, are usually the cause of death, not the primary tumour. Tumours may be classified as solid tumours (usually occurring in an organ, such as the lung, stomach, or ovary), soft-tissue tumours (occurring in such tissue as muscle), **leukaemias** (cancers of the blood-producing tissue in the bone marrow characterized by overproduction of abnormal or immature forms of white blood cells), and **lymphomas** (cancers of the lymphatic system). Leukaemias are further classified according to the rate of progression of the disease (acute or chronic) and the type of white cell involved (e.g.

hairy cell leukaemia, lymphoblastic leukaemia). Lymphomas are divided into Hodgkin's disease and non-Hodgkin's lymphomas, according to their appearance under the microscope.

Cancer can occur at any age, but the incidence of most cancers rises sharply after the age of 60 years. In the Western world the most common cancers are those of the lung, breast, skin, gut, and prostate gland. Cancer is treated by a combination of surgery, radiotherapy, and/or chemotherapy (*see* CYTOTOXIC DRUGS), depending on the site and type of tumour.

candesartan cilexetil An *angiotensin II inhibitor used in the treatment of *hypertension. It is available as tablets on *prescription only.

Side effects: include infections of the upper respiratory tract, influenza-like symptoms, and (less commonly) back pain, fluid retention, and nausea.

Precautions: candesartan should not be taken during pregnancy or by people with severe liver disease or some types of jaundice. It should be used with caution in people with kidney disease and some types of heart disease.

Interactions with other drugs: see ACE INHIBITORS.
Proprietary preparation: Amias.

candidiasis *See* ANTIFUNGAL DRUGS.

Canesten (Bayer) *See* CLOTRIMAZOLE.

Canesten-Combi (Bayer) *See* CLOTRIMAZOLE.

Canesten HC (Bayer) A proprietary combination of *hydrocortisone (a corticosteroid), and *clotrimazole (an antifungal drug), used for the treatment of fungal infections of the skin accompanied by inflammation. It is available as a cream on *prescription only.

Side effects, precautions, and interactions with other drugs: see TOPICAL STEROIDS; CLOTRIMAZOLE.

Canusal (CP Pharmaceuticals) *See* HEPARIN.

Capasal (Dermal Laboratories) A proprietary combination of *salicylic acid and *coal tar (both keratolytics), used for the treatment of seborrhoeic *eczema (including cradle cap in babies) and *psoriasis of the scalp. It is available as a shampoo and can be obtained without a prescription, but only from pharmacies.

Side effects and precautions: see SALICYLIC ACID.

Capastat (Dista) *See* CAPREOMYCIN.

Caplenal (APS-Berk) *See* ALLOPURINOL.

Capoten (Bristol-Myers Squibb) *See* CAPTOPRIL.

Capozide (Bristol-Myers Squibb) A proprietary combination of
*captopril (an ACE inhibitor) and *hydrochlorothiazide (a thiazide
diuretic), used in the treatment of mild to moderate *hypertension. It is
available as tablets on *prescription only. **Capozide LS** is a similar
preparation half the strength of Capozide.
Side effects, precautions, and interactions with other drugs: see ACE
INHIBITORS; THIAZIDE DIURETICS.
See also ANTIHYPERTENSIVE DRUGS; DIURETICS.

capreomycin An *antibiotic reserved for treating *tuberculosis
resistant to first-line antituberculosis drugs. It is available as an injection
on *prescription only.
Side effects: include itching and rash, kidney impairment, and hearing
loss with tinnitus and vertigo.
Precautions: capreomycin should be used with caution in patients who
have liver, kidney, or hearing impairment and in women who are
pregnant or breastfeeding.
Proprietary preparation: Capastat.

Caprin (Sinclair Pharmaceuticals) *See* ASPIRIN.

capsaicin The active ingredient of *capsicum oleoresin; it is the
chemical in chillies and peppers that is responsible for their 'hot' taste.
Capsaicin is used as a *rubefacient to relieve the pain that follows an
attack of shingles (it should not be applied until the rash has healed) and
the pain associated with nerve damage in people with diabetes. It is also
used in the treatment of osteoarthritis. Capsaicin is available as a cream
on *prescription only.
Side effects and precautions: see RUBEFACIENTS.
Proprietary preparations: Axsain; Zacin (for osteoarthritis).

capsicin *See* CAPSICUM OLEORESIN.

capsicum oleoresin (capsicin) A resinous extract from sweet peppers
and chillies that contains the active ingredient *capsaicin. It is used in
the form of an ointment as a *rubefacient for the relief of muscular
aches, pains, and stiffness, such as backache, sciatica, lumbago, and
rheumatism. It is also an ingredient of various other ointments and
creams. Preparations containing capsicum oleoresin are usually freely
available *over the counter.
Side effects and precautions: see RUBEFACIENTS.
Proprietary preparations: Fiery Jack Ointment; ALGIPAN RUB (combined
with glycol salicylate and methyl nicotinate); BALMOSA (combined with
camphor, menthol, and methyl salicylate); CREMALGIN (combined with
glycol salicylate and methyl nicotinate); FIERY JACK CREAM (combined
with diethylamine salicylate, glycol salicylate, and methyl nicotinate);

RADIAN-B MUSCLE RUB (combined with camphor, menthol, and methyl salicylate); RALGEX CREAM (combined with glycol monosalicylate and methyl nicotinate); RALGEX STICK (combined with ethyl salicylate, methyl salicylate, glycol salicylate, and menthol).

capsule A soluble case, usually made of gelatin, containing a drug (usually in powdered form) for oral administration.

Capsuvac (Galen) *See* CO-DANTHRUSATE.

captopril An *ACE inhibitor used as an adjunct to *diuretics for the treatment of *heart failure. It is also used to treat *hypertension, and kidney disease in people with insulin-dependent (type I) diabetes. Captopril is available as tablets on *prescription only.
Side effects, precautions, and interactions with other drugs: see ACE INHIBITORS.
Proprietary preparations: Acepril; Capoten; Kaplon; ACEZIDE (combined with hydrochlorothiazide); CAPOZIDE and CAPOZIDE LS (combined with hydrochlorothiazide).
See also ANTIHYPERTENSIVE DRUGS.

Carace (Du Pont Pharmaceuticals) *See* LISINOPRIL.

Carace Plus (Du Pont Pharmaceuticals) A proprietary combination of *lisinopril (an ACE inhibitor) and *hydrochlorothiazide (a thiazide diuretic), used in the treatment of mild to moderate *hypertension. A *prescription only medicine, it is available as tablets of two strengths: **Carace 20 Plus** is twice the strength of **Carace 10 Plus**.
Side effects, precautions, and interactions with other drugs: see ACE INHIBITORS; THIAZIDE DIURETICS.
See also ANTIHYPERTENSIVE DRUGS; DIURETICS.

carbachol A *cholinergic drug that improves the drainage of fluid from the front chamber of the eye (*see* MIOTICS) and is therefore used to reduce the pressure inside the eye in the treatment of *glaucoma. It is available, on *prescription only, as eye drops.
Side effects: include blurred vision and difficulty in seeing in dim light.
Precautions: carbachol eye drops are not recommended for children. They should not be used by people with abrasions of the cornea or inflammation of the iris or by those who wear soft contact lenses.
Proprietary preparation: ISOPTO CARBACHOL (combined with hypromellose).

Carbalax (Pharmax) A proprietary combination of *sodium acid phosphate (an osmotic laxative) and *sodium bicarbonate (which provides effervescence), used for the treatment of constipation or to evacuate the bowel before investigative procedures or surgery. It is freely available *over the counter in the form of suppositories.

Precautions: Carbalax is not recommended for children. *See also* PHOSPHATE LAXATIVES.

carbamazepine An *anticonvulsant drug used for the treatment of most types of epilepsy except absence seizures. It is also used to relieve the stabbing pains that may occur along the course of certain nerves, especially trigeminal neuralgia (a searing pain in the face) and phantom limb pain, and to treat manic-depressive illness resistant to *lithium. It is available, on *prescription only, as tablets, *modified-release tablets, or a liquid for oral use and as *suppositories.

Side effects: include dizziness, drowsiness, nausea and vomiting, double vision, headache, and unsteady gait. Mild allergic skin reactions occur quite frequently; less common side effects are blood disorders, jaundice, hepatitis, kidney failure, depression, and impotence.

Precautions: carbamazepine should be used with caution in people who have liver, kidney, or heart disease and in women who are breastfeeding; women who are planning to become pregnant, or who are already pregnant, should seek specialist advice.

Interactions with other drugs:

Antibacterials: the effect of doxycycline is reduced; the concentration of carbamazepine in the blood is increased by clarithromycin, erythromycin, and isoniazid.

Anticoagulants: the effects of warfarin and nicoumalone <acenocoumarol> are reduced; dosages of these drugs may need to be adjusted.

Anticonvulsants: taking two or more anticonvulsants together may increase their adverse effects.

Antidepressants: reduce the anticonvulsant effect of carbamazepine.

Antipsychotics: reduce the anticonvulsant effect of carbamazepine; carbamazepine reduces the plasma concentrations of haloperidol, olanzapine, and sertindole.

Calcium antagonists: diltiazem and verapamil increase the effect of carbamazepine.

Cimetidine: may increase the effects of carbamazepine.

Dextropropoxyphene: increases the effect of carbamazepine.

Oral contraceptives: carbamazepine may reduce the effect of oral contraceptives; an alternative form of contraception may be required.

Proprietary preparations: Epimaz; Tegretol; Tegretol Retard (modifed-release tablets); Teril CR (modified-release tablets); Timonil Retard (modified-release tablets).

carbaryl A pesticide that is used clinically to kill head and crab *lice. It is available as a lotion, which may be left on for 12 hours or overnight. Some lotions contain alcohol; these are not recommended for treating crab lice (see also precautions below). Hair treated with carbaryl preparations should be allowed to dry naturally. Carbaryl is a *prescription only medicine.

Side effects: carbaryl may irritate the skin.

Precautions: carbaryl should not be applied near the eyes or on broken skin; treatment of children under six months should be supervised by a doctor. Lotions containing alcohol should not be used to treat crab lice; they should also not be used for treating head lice in young children or people with asthma (since inhalation of the fumes can be dangerous).

Proprietary preparation: Carylderm.

Carbellon (Torbet Laboratories) A proprietary combination of *magnesium hydroxide (an antacid), charcoal (*see* ACTIVATED CHARCOAL), and *peppermint oil (an antispasmodic), used for the relief of indigestion and flatulence. It is available as tablets that can be obtained without a prescription, but only from pharmacies.

Side effects and precautions: see MAGNESIUM SALTS.

Interactions with other drugs: see ANTACIDS.

carbenoxolone sodium A drug with *cytoprotectant action that, in combination with *antacids, is used for the treatment of inflammation and ulceration of the oesophagus. Because of its side effects (see below), other treatments for these conditions are usually preferred. Alone, carbenoxolone is used topically to treat mouth ulcers. For treating oesophageal disease carbenoxolone (combined with antacids) is supplied as tablets or a liquid on *prescription only. For treating mouth ulcers it is available as a mouthwash (on prescription only) or as a gel (without a prescription).

Side effects (of tablets and liquid only): carbenoloxone commonly causes sodium and water retention and occasionally hypokalaemia (low concentrations of *potassium in the blood). These effects may cause or worsen hypertension (high blood pressure) and heart failure.

Precautions (with tablets and liquid only): carbenoloxone should not be used by people with hypokalaemia, heart failure, or impaired liver or kidney function, or by pregnant women.

Interactions with other drugs (tablets and liquid only):

  Antihypertensive drugs: carbenoloxone inhibits their effects in lowering blood pressure.

  Cardiac glycosides: their toxicity is increased if plasma potassium concentrations are lowered by carbenoloxone.

  Spironolactone: reduces the activity of carbenoloxone.

Proprietary preparations: Bioplex (mouthwash); Bioral Gel; PYROGASTRONE (combined with magnesium trisilicate, aluminium hydroxide, sodium bicarbonate, and alginic acid).

carbidopa A drug that inhibits the enzyme that breaks down *levodopa (an antiparkinsonian drug) to *dopamine in the peripheral tissues. Given in combination with levodopa (*see* CO-CARELDOPA), it increases the amount of levodopa available to cross into the brain and also helps to minimize the side effects of vomiting and low blood pressure seen with levodopa therapy.

carbimazole An antithyroid drug that blocks the synthesis of *thyroid hormones. It is used for the long-term treatment of thyrotoxicosis (overproduction of thyroid hormones) and may also be given to decrease hormone concentrations before surgery to remove part of an overactive thryroid gland. Carbimazole is available as tablets on *prescription only.

Side effects: include rashes, nausea, stomach upsets, headache, joint pain, hair loss, and suppression of blood-cell production by the bone marrow (increasing the risk of infection). A sore throat, mouth ulcers, or fever should be reported to a doctor immediately, as these may indicate a serious effect on blood cells.

Precautions: carbimazole should be used with caution in people with a large goitre or liver disorders and in women who are pregnant or breastfeeding.

Proprietary preparation: Neo-Mercazole.

carbocisteine A *mucolytic drug that reduces the viscosity of bronchial secretions by liquefying mucus and is used to relieve congestion of the airways. It is also used to liquefy the viscous fluid that accumulates in glue ear. Carbocisteine is available, on *prescription only, as capsules or a syrup. It cannot be prescribed on the NHS unless it is to be used by children under 18 years old with a tracheostomy.

Side effects: include stomach and bowel upsets, nausea, and rash.

Precautions: carbocisteine should not be taken by people with an active peptic ulcer and should be used with caution in those with a history of peptic ulcers and in pregnant women.

Proprietary preparation: Mucodyne.

Carbo-Dome (Lagap Pharmaceuticals) *See* COAL TAR.

carbomer (polyacrylic acid) An agent used in the treatment of dry eyes to thicken and strengthen the natural film of tears that covers the eyes. It is available as a liquid gel in eye drops and can be obtained without a prescription, but only from pharmacies.

Side effects: there may be transient irritation and blurred vision on application.

Precautions: carbomer should not be used with soft contact lenses.

Proprietary preparations: Geltears; Viscotears.

Carbomix (Penn Pharmaceuticals) *See* ACTIVATED CHARCOAL.

carbonic anhydrase inhibitors Drugs that inhibit the action of carbonic anhydrase, an enzyme in the red blood cells that controls the formation of carbonic acid or bicarbonate from carbon dioxide and is therefore important in maintaining the acid-base balance of the blood. Carbonic anhydrase inhibitors include *acetazolamide and *dorzolamide; they have a weak *diuretic action but are used mainly in the treatment of *glaucoma.

carboplatin A *cytotoxic drug that is an *analogue of *cisplatin but is less toxic. It is active against the types of *cancer that are sensitive to cisplatin, including ovarian cancer and a form of lung cancer, but is less effective than cisplatin for treating testicular cancer. A *prescription only medicine, it is given by intravenous infusion in specialist oncology centres.

Side effects: the main side effect is *bone marrow suppression. Other adverse effects are those of *cisplatin, including nausea and vomiting, kidney damage, and hearing loss, but these are much less severe than with cisplatin.

Precautions: see CISPLATIN; CYTOTOXIC DRUGS.

Proprietary preparation: Paraplatin.

carboprost A *prostaglandin used to control the bleeding that occurs after delivery of a baby if the mother's uterus fails to contract normally. It is given by deep intramuscular injection by a doctor and is available on *prescription only.

Side effects: include nausea, vomiting, diarrhoea, high body temperature and flushing, and constriction of the airways; less frequently, pain at the injection site, raised blood pressure, breathlessness, chills, headache, and dizziness may occur.

Precautions: carboprost should not be given to women with acute pelvic inflammatory disease or heart, kidney, lung, or liver disease. It should be used with caution in women with a history of glaucoma, asthma, high or low blood pressure, anaemia, jaundice, diabetes, or epilepsy.

Proprietary preparation: Hemabate.

carboxymethylcellulose *See* CARMELLOSE.

Cardene, Cardene SR (Roche Products) *See* NICARDIPINE.

cardiac glycosides A group of drugs used in the treatment of congestive *heart failure and *arrhythmias. Also known as **digitalis drugs**, they were originally extracted from the foxglove plant. These drugs slow down the heart so that each beat is more effective in pumping blood. They are also used to help reduce tiredness, breathlessness, and fluid retention in heart failure. *See* DIGOXIN.

Cardilate MR (Norton Healthcare) *See* NIFEDIPINE.

Cardinol (CP Pharmaceuticals) *See* PROPRANOLOL HYDROCHLORIDE.

Cardura (Pfizer) *See* DOXAZOSIN.

Carisoma (Pharmax) *See* CARISOPRODOL.

carisoprodol A *muscle relaxant used for the short-term relief of muscle spasm. It is available as tablets on *prescription only.

Side effects: include drowsiness, dizziness, nausea, lassitude, flushes, headache, constipation, and rash.

Precautions: carisoprodol should not be taken by people with porphyria or by breastfeeding women. It should be used with caution in those with liver or kidney disease or a history of drug or alcohol abuse and in pregnant women. Treatment should be stopped gradually.

Proprietary preparation: Carisoma.

carmellose A substance used as an agent in which to suspend active ingredients, as an emulsifying and thickening agent, and as a coating for tablets. It is also used to make artificial saliva solutions for the relief of dry mouth caused by such treatments as radiotherapy and *antimuscarinic drugs. Carmellose is an ingredient of protective agents used in the fitting of ileostomy or colostomy appliances (*see* STOMA) and a component of thick pastes that adhere to the lining of the mouth to provide protection from mechanical damage. It is also an ingredient of *laxative preparations. Carmellose is available, in the form of **carmellose sodium** or **carmellose calcium** (also called **carboxymethylcellulose**), without a prescription.

Proprietary preparations: Luborant (carboxymethylcellulose; artificial saliva aerosol spray); ADCORTYL IN ORABASE (combined with triamcinolone); GLANDOSANE (combined with electrolytes); ORABASE (combined with pectin and gelatin); SALIVACE (combined with electrolytes and xylitol).

carmustine (BCNU; bis-chloroethylnitrosourea) An *alkylating drug used for the treatment of myeloma (cancer of the plasma cells of the bone marrow), lymphoma, and brain tumours (*see* CANCER). It is available as an injection on *prescription only.

Side effects: include nausea and vomiting, which may be moderately severe, and pain at the injection site. *See also* CYTOTOXIC DRUGS.

Precautions: see CYTOTOXIC DRUGS.

Proprietary preparation: BiCNU.

Carnation Corn Caps, Carnation Verruca Treatment (Cuxson, Gerrard & Co) *See* SALICYLIC ACID.

carteolol hydrochloride A *beta blocker used for the treatment of chronic (open-angle) *glaucoma and some secondary types of glaucoma. It is available as eye drops on *prescription only.

Side effects: include irritation, stinging, burning, and pain in the eye, blurred vision, and bloodshot or dry eyes. The drops can trickle into the back of the nose and be swallowed, causing *systemic effects and possibly interactions with other drugs (*see* BETA BLOCKERS).

Precautions: carteolol should not be used by people who wear soft contact lenses, by pregnant women, or by people with heart failure or asthma.

Interactions with other drugs:
  Beta blockers: other beta blockers taken by mouth can enhance the effect of these eye drops. *See also* BETA BLOCKERS.
Proprietary preparation: Teoptic.

carvedilol A combined *alpha and *beta blocker used in the treatment of *hypertension and angina. It is also used, under hospital supervision, in the treatment of some forms of chronic heart failure. Carvedilol is available as tablets on *prescription only.
Side effects: include low blood pressure on standing, dizziness, headache, fatigue, gastrointestinal upsets, and a slow heart rate. *See also* BETA BLOCKERS.
Precautions and interactions with other drugs: see BETA BLOCKERS.
Proprietary preparation: Eucardic.
See also ANTIHYPERTENSIVE DRUGS.

Carylderm (Seton Scholl Healthcare) *See* CARBARYL.

cascara A powerful *stimulant laxative extracted from the bark of the tree *Rhamnus purshiana*. It is usually active 6–8 hours after administration. Although no longer recommended as a laxative, it is still included as an ingredient of various *over the counter preparations for the treatment of constipation.
Side effects and precautions: see STIMULANT LAXATIVES.
Proprietary preparations: POTTER'S CLEANSING HERB (combined with aloes and senna); RHUAKA (combined with rhubarb and senna).

Casodex (AstraZeneca) *See* BICALUTAMIDE.

Catapres (Boehringer Ingelheim) *See* CLONIDINE HYDROCHLORIDE.

Catarrh-Ex (Thompson Medical Company) A proprietary combination of *paracetamol (an analgesic and antipyretic), *caffeine (a stimulant), and *phenylephrine (a decongestant), used to relieve catarrh and other symptoms of colds and influenza. It is freely available *over the counter in the form of capsules.
Side effects and interactions with other drugs: see PHENYLEPHRINE.
Precautions: Catarrh-Ex is not recommended for children. *See also* PARACETAMOL; CAFFEINE; PHENYLEPHRINE.

cathartics *See* LAXATIVES.

caustics *See* KERATOLYTICS.

Caverject (Pharmacia & Upjohn) *See* ALPROSTADIL.

CCNU (Medac) *See* LOMUSTINE.

Ceanel Concentrate (Quinoderm) A proprietary combination of *cetrimide (an antiseptic), phenylethyl alcohol (an antibiotic), and *undecenoic acid (an antifungal agent), used as a shampoo for the treatment of psoriasis and seborrhoea of the scalp and dandruff; it may be applied directly to treat psoriasis of the trunk and limbs. Ceanel is available as a liquid without a *prescription, but only from pharmacies. *Precautions:* the liquid should not be allowed to come into contact with the eyes.

Cedax (Schering-Plough) *See* CEFTIBUTEN.

Cedocard Retard (Pharmacia & Upjohn) *See* ISOSORBIDE DINITRATE.

cefaclor A second-generation *cephalosporin used for the treatment of infections of the urinary tract, respiratory tract, skin, and soft tissues. It is available, on *prescription only, as capsules, *modified-release tablets, or a suspension.
Side effects: diarrhoea and, rarely, antibiotic-associated inflammation of the colon may occur (both are more likely with higher doses); other possible side effects are nausea and vomiting, abdominal discomfort, headache, blood disorders, nervousness, sleep disturbances, confusion, and dizziness. Allergic reactions include rashes, itching, fever, and muscle aches.
Precautions: cefaclor should not be taken by people who are allergic to cephalosporins and should be used with caution in those who are allergic to penicillins.
Proprietary preparations: Distaclor; Distaclor MR (modified-release tablets).

cefadroxil A first-generation *cephalosporin used for the treatment of infections of the urinary tract, respiratory tract, skin, and soft tissues. It is available, on *prescription only, as capsules or a suspension.
Side effects and precautions: see CEFACLOR.
Proprietary preparation: Baxan.

cefalexin *See* CEPHALEXIN.

cefamandole *See* CEPHAMANDOLE.

cefazolin *See* CEPHAZOLIN.

cefixime A third-generation *cephalosporin used for the treatment of infections of the urinary tract, respiratory tract, skin, and soft tissues. It is available, on *prescription only, as tablets or as a suspension for children.
Side effects and precautions: see CEFACLOR.
Proprietary preparation: Suprax.

cefodizime A third-generation *cephalosporin used for the treatment

of infections of the urinary tract, respiratory tract, skin, and soft tissues. It is available, on *prescription only, as an injection.
Side effects and precautions: see CEFACLOR.
Proprietary preparation: Timecef.

cefotaxime A third-generation *cephalosporin used for the treatment of infections of the urinary tract, respiratory tract, skin, and soft tissues. It is also used to treat meningitis. Cefotaxime is given by intramuscular or intravenous injection and is available on *prescription only.
Side effects and precautions: see CEFACLOR.
Proprietary preparation: Claforan.

cefoxitin A second-generation cephalosporin used for the treatment of infections of the urinary tract, respiratory tract, skin, and soft tissues. It is also used to prevent infections after surgery. It is given by intramuscular or intravenous injection or intravenous infusion and is available on *prescription only.
Side effects and precautions: see CEFACLOR.
Proprietary preparation: Mefoxin.

cefpirome A third-generation *cephalosporin used for the treatment of infections of the urinary tract, respiratory tract, skin, and soft tissues. It is also used to prevent infections after surgery. It is given by *intravenous injection or infusion and is available on *prescription only.
Side effects and precautions: see CEFACLOR.
Proprietary preparation: Cefrom.

cefpodoxime A third-generation *cephalosporin used for the treatment of infections of the respiratory tract, pharyngitis, and tonsillitis. Cefpodoxime is usually reserved for infections that are chronic, recurrent, or resistant to other antibiotics. It is available, on *prescription only, as tablets or an oral suspension.
Side effects and precautions: see CEFACLOR.
Proprietary preparation: Orelox.

cefprozil A second-generation *cephalosporin used for the treatment of infections of the upper respiratory tract, outer ear, skin, and soft tissues, and chronic bronchitis. It is available as tablets or a suspension on *prescription only.
Side effects and precautions: see CEFACLOR.
Proprietary preparation: Cefzil.

cefradine *See* CEPHRADINE.

Cefrom (Hoechst Marion Roussel) *See* CEFPIROME.

ceftazidime A third-generation *cephalosporin used for the treatment of infections of the urinary tract, respiratory tract, skin, and soft tissues.

It is given by *intramuscular or *intravenous injection or intravenous infusion and is available on *prescription only.

Side effects and precautions: see CEFACLOR.

Proprietary preparations: Fortum; Kefadim.

ceftibuten A third-generation *cephalosporin used for the treatment of infections of the respiratory tract, pharyngitis, tonsillitis, bronchitis, and ear infections in children. It is available, on *prescription only, as tablets or an oral suspension.

Side effects and precautions: see CEFACLOR.

Proprietary preparation: Cedax.

ceftriaxone A third-generation *cephalosporin used for the treatment of pneumonia, septicaemia, meningitis, infections of bones, skin, and soft tissues, and gonorrhoea. It is also used to prevent infections after surgery. It is given by *intramuscular or *intravenous injection or intravenous infusion and is available on *prescription only.

Side effects: see CEFACLOR.

Precautions: see CEFACLOR. In addition, ceftriaxone should be used with caution in patients with liver disease.

Proprietary preparation: Rocephin.

cefuroxime A second-generation *cephalosporin used for the treatment of infections of the urinary tract, respiratory tract, skin, and soft tissues, meningitis, and gonorrhoea. It is also used to prevent infections after surgery. Cefuroxime sodium is given by *intramuscular or *intravenous injection or intravenous infusion; cefuroxime axetil can be taken by mouth as tablets, a suspension, or sachets. Cefuroxime is available on *prescription only.

Side effects and precautions: see CEFACLOR.

Proprietary preparations: Zinacef; Zinnat.

Cefzil (Bristol-Myers Squibb) *See* CEFPROZIL.

Celance (Eli Lilly & Co) *See* PERGOLIDE.

Celectol (Rhône-Poulenc Rorer) *See* CELIPROLOL HYDROCHLORIDE.

Celevac (Monmouth Pharmaceuticals) *See* METHYLCELLULOSE.

celiprolol hydrochloride A cardioselective *beta blocker that also has some *vasodilator action on peripheral blood vessels. It is used to treat mild to moderate *hypertension. It is available as tablets on *prescription only.

Side effects, precautions, and interactions with other drugs: see BETA BLOCKERS.

Proprietary preparation: Celectol.

See also ANTIHYPERTENSIVE DRUGS.

CellCept (Roche Products) *See* MYCOPHENOLATE MOFETIL.

Centrapryl (Opus) *See* SELEGILINE.

cephalexin <cefalexin> A first-generation *cephalosporin used for the
treatment of infections of the urinary tract, respiratory tract, skin, and
soft tissues, and gonorrhoea. It is available, on *prescription only, as
capsules, tablets, a suspension, or a syrup.
Side effects and precautions: see CEFACLOR.
Proprietary preparations: Ceporex; Keflex; Kiflone; Tenkorex.

cephalosporins A group of broad-spectrum beta-lactam *antibiotics.
They have a similar action to *penicillins in that they inhibit bacterial
cell wall formation and are also susceptible to degradation by enzymes
produced by bacteria (penicillinases or beta-lactamases). The drug
*probenecid may be given with cephalosporins to prevent their excretion
by the kidneys and thus increase their concentrations in the body.
Cephalosporins are used for the treatment of septicaemia, pneumonia,
meningitis, biliary-tract infections, peritonitis, and urinary-tract
infections. All act against the same types of bacteria, although individual
drugs have differing activity against specific organisms. The principal
side effects are allergic reactions; about 10% of people who are allergic to
penicillins will also be allergic to cephalosporins. Modification of the
chemical structure of cephalosporins has produced the second- and third-
generation cephalosporins, which have activity against a wider range of
bacteria. The older (first generation) cephalosporins include *cephradine
<cefradine>, *cephazolin <cefalozin>, *cephalexin <cefalexin>, and
*cefadroxil; second-generation cephalosporins include *cefuroxime,
*cephamandole <cefamandole>, *cefaclor, *cefprozil, and *cefoxitin.
Third-generation drugs include *cefotaxime, *ceftazidime, *cefodizime,
*ceftriaxone, *cefixime, *cefpodoxime, *ceftibuten, and *cefpirome.

cephamandole <cefamandole> A second-generation *cephalosporin
used for the treatment of serious and life-threatening infections. It is also
used to prevent infections after surgery. It is given by *intramuscular or
*intravenous injection or intravenous infusion and is available on
*prescription only.
Side effects and precautions: see CEFACLOR.
Proprietary preparation: Kefadol.

cephazolin <cefazolin> One of the original *cephalosporins, used for
the treatment of infections of the urinary tract, respiratory tract, skin,
and soft tissues. It is also used to treat septicaemia and to prevent
infections after surgery. Cephazolin is given by *intramuscular or
*intravenous injection or intravenous infusion and is available on
*prescription only.
Side effects and precautions: see CEFACLOR.
Proprietary preparation: Kefzol.

cephradine <cefradine> One of the original (first-generation) *cephalosporins, used for the treatment of infections of the urinary and respiratory tracts, skin and soft tissues, bones, and joints. It is also used to prevent infections after surgery. Cephradine is available, on *prescription only, as capsules or a syrup for oral use and as an injection.
Side effects and precautions: see CEFACLOR.
Proprietary preparation: Velosef.

Ceporex (GlaxoWellcome) *See* CEPHALEXIN <CEFALEXIN>.

Cerebrovase (Ashbourne Pharmaceuticals) *See* DIPYRIDAMOLE.

Ceredase (Genzyme Therapeutics) *See* ALGLUCERASE.

Cerezyme (Genzyme Therapeutics) *See* IMIGLUCERASE.

cerivastatin A *statin used for the treatment of primary hypercholesterolaemia (*see* HYPERLIPIDAEMIA) that has not responded to dietary measures. It is available as tablets on *prescription only.
Side effects, precautions, and interactions with other drugs: see STATINS.
Proprietary preparation: Lipobay.

certoparin A *low molecular weight heparin used for the prevention of deep-vein *thrombosis, particularly following surgery. It is available as a solution for subcutaneous injection on *prescription only.
Side effects, precautions, and interactions with other drugs: see HEPARIN.
Proprietary preparation: Alphaparin.

Cerubidin (Rhône-Poulenc Rorer) *See* DAUNORUBICIN.

Cerumol (Laboratories for Applied Biology) A proprietary combination of *arachis oil, *chlorbutol <chlorobutanol> (an antiseptic), and paradichlorobenzene (which reduces the viscosity of the preparation so that it penetrates better), used for the softening and removal of earwax. It is available as ear drops and can be obtained without a *prescription, but only from pharmacies.
Precautions: Cerumol should not be used by people with otitis externa (inflammation of the outer ear), a perforated eardrum, dermatitis, or an allergy to peanuts. It should be used for a maximum of three days.

cetalkonium chloride An *antiseptic similar to *benzalkonium chloride. It is used in a variety of *topical preparations for the treatment of minor infections of the eye, mouth, and throat; most of these preparations are freely available *over the counter.
Precautions: cetalkonium should not be swallowed as it can cause nausea and vomiting, and strong solutions can cause damage to the oesophagus (gullet). Very large doses can depress breathing, which can be dangerous.

Proprietary preparations: BONJELA (combined with choline salicylate); DINNEFORDS TEEJEL (combined with choline salicylate).

Cetavlex (AstraZeneca) *See* CETRIMIDE.

cetirizine hydrochloride One of the newer (non-sedating) *antihistamines, used to relieve the symptoms of such allergic conditions as hay fever and urticaria. It is available as tablets on *prescription, and packs containing no more than 10 days' supply may be purchased from pharmacies without a prescription.
Side effects, precautions, and interactions with other drugs: see ANTIHISTAMINES.
Proprietary preparations: Zirtek; Zirtek 7.

cetrimide (cetrimonium bromide) An *antiseptic with detergent properties and variable activity against different types of bacteria and some fungi. It is used alone or in combination with *chlorhexidine for cleansing and disinfecting the skin and for treating minor wounds, burns, and napkin rash. A very dilute solution is applied topically for the relief of sore gums. It is also used as an ingredient of shampoos for treating seborrhoea and psoriasis. Cetrimide liquid or cream is freely available *over the counter, but some combined preparations can only be bought from pharmacies.
Side effects: cetrimide may cause local irritation or allergic reactions; if swallowed, it may cause nausea and vomiting.
Proprietary preparations: Bansor Mouth Antiseptic; Cetavlex; JW Cetrimide Cream; CEANEL CONCENTRATE (combined with phenylethyl alcohol and undecenoic acid); HIBICET HOSPITAL CONCENTRATE (combined with chlorhexidine); SAVLON ANTISEPTIC CREAM (combined with chlorhexidine); STERIPOD YELLOW (combined with chlorhexidine); TISEPT, TISEPT CONCENTRATE (combined with chlorhexidine); TRAVASEPT 100 (combined with chlorhexidine).

cetylpyridinium chloride An antiseptic used alone or in combination with other drugs for cleansing the mouth and treating minor throat or mouth infections and teething problems. Used alone, cetylpyridinium is freely available *over the counter in the form of a solution or lozenges, but some combined preparations can only be bought from pharmacies.
Proprietary preparations: Merocet (gargle or mouthwash); Merocets (lozenges); ANBESOL (combined with chlorocresol and lignocaine <lidocaine>); CALGEL (combined with lignocaine <lidocaine>); DENTINOX TEETHING GEL (combined with lignocaine <lidocaine>); JUNIOR MELTUS EXPECTORANT (combined with guaiphenesin <guaifenesin>); MEROCAINE (combined with benzocaine); ORAGARD (combined with lignocaine <lidocaine>); RINSTEAD TEETHING GEL (combined with lignocaine <lidocaine>); WOODWARD'S TEETHING GEL (combined with lignocaine <lidocaine>).

charcoal *See* ACTIVATED CHARCOAL.

chemotherapy *See* CYTOTOXIC DRUGS.

Chemotrim Paediatric (Rosemont Pharmaceuticals) *See* CO-TRIMOXAZOLE.

chenodeoxycholic acid A *bile acid used in the treatment of gallstones or to prevent recurrence after they have dissolved. It is suitable for people with mild symptoms who cannot be treated by other means. Treatment should not be stopped without consulting a doctor, even when symptoms are under control. Chenodeoxycholic acid is available as capsules on *prescription only.
Side effects: include diarrhoea (particularly at the start of treatment and if a high dosage is used) and itching; abnormalities of liver function have been reported.
Precautions: chenodeoxycholic acid should not be taken by women who are pregnant or planning to become pregnant, or by people with chronic liver disease or inflammatory bowel disease. Blood tests may be necessary to check liver function.
Interactions with other drugs:
  Clofibrate: reduces the beneficial effect of chenodeoxycholic acid.
  Oral contraceptives: oestrogens reduce the effect of chenodeoxycholic acid; women should use nonhormonal methods of contraception while undergoing treatment.

Chimax (Chiron) *See* FLUTAMIDE.

Chloractil (DDSA Pharmaceuticals) *See* CHLORPROMAZINE HYDROCHLORIDE.

chloral betaine <cloral betaine> A *hypnotic drug that is a derivative of *chloral hydrate and is used for the short-term treatment of insomnia. It is available as tablets on *prescription only.
Side effects, precautions, and interactions with other drugs: see CHLORAL HYDRATE.
Proprietary preparation: Welldorm.

chloral hydrate A *hypnotic drug used for the short-term treatment of insomnia. It is available, on *prescription only, as a mixture (oral solution) and as an elixir for children.
Side effects: include nausea and vomiting, abdominal distension, flatulence, vertigo, shaky movements and unsteady gait, excitement, nightmares, headache, light-headedness, and allergic rashes.
Precautions: chloral hydrate should not be taken by people with heart disease, gastritis (inflammation of the stomach), or liver or kidney disease, or by women who are pregnant or breastfeeding. It should be used with caution in people with respiratory diseases and by those with a

history of drug or alcohol abuse. Prolonged use can lead to *dependence and should be avoided; treatment should be stopped gradually. *See also* HYPNOTIC DRUGS.

Interactions with other drugs: the sedative effects of chloral hydrate are increased by a number of other drugs, including anaesthetics, opioid analgesics, antidepressants, antihistamines, and antipsychotic drugs.

Proprietary preparation: Welldorm Elixir.

chlorambucil An *alkylating drug that is used mainly for the treatment of chronic lymphocytic leukaemia, non-Hodgkin's lymphoma, Hodgkin's disease, and ovarian cancer (*see* CANCER). It is available as tablets on *prescription only.

Side effects: *bone marrow suppression is the most common side effect. Occasionally a widespread severe rash develops: if this occurs, the prescribing doctor should be informed and treatment stopped. *See also* CYTOTOXIC DRUGS.

Precautions: chlorambucil should not be taken by people with porphyria or by pregnant women. *See also* CYTOTOXIC DRUGS.

Proprietary preparation: Leukeran.

chloramphenicol A potent *antibiotic that is effective against many microorganisms but is reserved for the treatment of life-threatening *systemic infections, such as bacterial meningitis and typhoid, because it has serious side effects when given systemically. However, it may be used safely as a topical treatment for local infections of the eyes or ears. A *prescription only medicine, it is available as eye drops or ointment, ear drops, capsules, or a solution for *intramuscular or *intravenous injection or infusion.

Side effects: when given by mouth or injection, chloramphenicol may cause blood disorders, inflammation of peripheral or optic nerves, nausea, vomiting, diarrhoea, and sore mouth. Topical preparations may sting.

Precautions (apply only to systemic preparations): chloramphenicol should not be taken by women who are pregnant or breastfeeding or by people with porphyria. It should be used with caution in people with liver or kidney disease. Repeated courses or prolonged administration should be avoided, and regular blood counts should be carried out.

Interactions with other drugs (with systemic preparations only):

Anticoagulants: the effects of warfarin and nicoumalone <acenocoumarol> are enhanced.

Phenobarbitone <phenobarbital>: reduces the effect of chloramphenicol.

Phenytoin: the effect of this antiepileptic drug is enhanced.

Rifampicin: reduces the effect of chloramphenicol.

Tolbutamide: the effects of this and other oral antidiabetic drugs are enhanced.

Proprietary preparations: Chloromycetin (eye drops or ointment); Kemicetine (injection); Minims Chloramphenicol (single-dose eye drops);

Sno Phenicol (eye drops); ACTINAC (combined with hydrocortisone acetate, butoxyethyl nicotinate, and allantoin).

chlorbutol <chlorobutanol> An *antiseptic that is active against bacteria and fungi and is used in preparations for the treatment of mouth ulcers. It is also used as a preservative in solutions for injection, eye drops, and ear drops. Chlorbutol is available without a prescription, but some preparations can only be obtained from pharmacies.

Proprietary preparations: CERUMOL (combined with arachis oil and paradichlorobenzene); ELUDRIL MOUTHWASH (combined with chlorhexidine); FRADOR (combined with menthol, styrax, and balsamic benzoin); KARVOL (combined with aromatic oils); MONPHYTOL (combined with methyl undecenoate, salicylic acid, methyl salicylate, propyl salicylate, and propyl undecenoate).

chlordiazepoxide A long-acting *benzodiazepine used for the short-term treatment of anxiety. It is also used to relieve the symptoms of alcohol withdrawal. It is available as tablets or capsules on *prescription only. Proprietary preparations cannot be prescribed on the NHS.

Side effects and precautions: see DIAZEPAM; BENZODIAZEPINES.
Interactions with other drugs: see BENZODIAZEPINES.
Proprietary preparations: Librium; Tropium.

chlorhexidine An antiseptic and disinfectant that is widely used for dressing minor skin wounds and burns to prevent infection and in oral preparations for treating sore gums and mouth ulcers, cleansing the mouth, and preventing the formation of plaque on teeth. It is used before surgery and obstetrical procedures to cleanse and disinfect the skin of the patient and the hands of the surgeon. Chlorhexidine is also used for washing out catheters and may be instilled into the bladder for treating bladder infections. It is used in the form of gluconate, acetate, or hydrochloride, either alone or in combination with other drugs, and is available as a liquid, mouthwash, dental gel, spray, cream, or powder. Preparations in which it is the sole ingredient are usually freely available *over the counter, but some combined preparations can only be bought from pharmacies.

Side effects: very rarely chlorhexidine may cause local irritation or allergic reactions. Dental preparations may cause local discoloration, taste disturbances, and bleeding of the gums.

Proprietary preparations: Acriflex Cream; Chlorohex; Corsodyl; Corsodyl Mint Mouthwash; Corsodyl Dental Gel; CX Powder; Hibicet; Hibiscrub; Hibisol; Hibitane; Hibitane Cream; Hibitane Obstetric; pHiso-Med; Savlon Antiseptic Wound Wash; Sterexidine; Steripod Pink; Unisept; Uriflex C (solution for catheters); Uro-Tainer Chlorhexidine (solution for catheters); DERMOL (combined with liquid paraffin, isopropyl myristate, and benzalkonium chloride); ELUDRIL MOUTHWASH (combined with chlorbutol <chlorobutanol>); GERMOLENE CREAM (combined with phenol); HIBICET HOSPITAL CONCENTRATE (combined with cetrimide); INSTILLAGEL (combined with lignocaine <lidocaine> hydrochloride); MYCIL POWDER (combined with tolnaftate); NASEPTIN (combined with neomycin sulphate); NYSTAFORM (combined with nystatin); NYSTAFORM-HC (combined with nystatin and hydrocortisone); SAVLON ANTISEPTIC CREAM, SAVLON CONCENTRATED ANTISEPTIC (combined with cetrimide); STERIPOD YELLOW (combined with cetrimide); TISEPT, TISEPT CONCENTRATE (combined with cetrimide); TRAVASEPT 100 (combined with cetrimide); XYLOCAINE ANTISEPTIC GEL (combined with lignocaine <lidocaine> hydrochloride).

chlormethiazole <clomethiazole> A *hypnotic drug that does not have the hangover effects of *benzodiazepines and is therefore suitable for the treatment of insomnia in elderly people. However, it should only be taken in the short term as *dependence can occur. It is also used to treat status epilepticus (prolonged epileptic seizures) and the symptoms of alcohol withdrawal. Chlormethiazole is available, on *prescription only, as capsules, a syrup, or a solution for intravenous infusion.
Side effects: include nasal congestion and irritation, conjunctival (eye) irritation, headache, and (rarely) paradoxical excitement, confusion, dependence, nausea, vomiting, and rash. Excessive sedation can occur with high doses.
Precautions: chlormethiazole should not be taken by people with severe lung disease or by those who are dependent on alcohol and continue drinking. It should be used with caution in people with heart or lung disease, a history of drug abuse, or marked personality disorder. The sedative effects of chlormethiazole are enhanced by alcohol. *See also* HYPNOTIC DRUGS.
Interactions with other drugs: the sedative effects of chlormethiazole are increased by a number of drugs, including anaesthetics, opioid analgesics, antidepressants, antihistamines, antipsychotics, cimetidine, and possibly ritonavir.
Proprietary preparation: Heminevrin.

chlormethine hydrochloride *See* MUSTINE HYDROCHLORIDE.

chlorocresol An *antiseptic and disinfectant active against a wide range of bacteria and fungi. It is used in various preparations for disinfecting skin and wounds and as a preservative in many creams, lotions, and solutions for injection.

Chlorohex (Colgate-Palmolive) *See* CHLORHEXIDINE.

Chloromycetin (Parke-Davis Medical) *See* CHLORAMPHENICOL.

chloroquine A drug used for the treatment of benign *malarias, although resistance to it has developed in some areas, and for the prevention of malaria (when it may be used in conjunction with *proguanil hydrochloride). It is also used in the long-term treatment of active rheumatoid arthritis, to slow down the progress of the disease; it may take 4–6 months to have a full effect. Chloroquine can also be used for the eradication of the parasites causing amoebic hepatitis. It is available, on *prescription only, as tablets, a syrup, or as a solution for injection.

Side effects: include nausea, diarrhoea, abdominal pain, headache, and (more rarely) rash, blurred vision, loss of pigmentation in the hair, and hair loss. Occasionally, with long-term use, irreversible damage to the retina may occur.

Precautions: eye examinations should be performed regularly in people taking chloroquine on a long-term basis. The drug should be used with caution in people who have liver or kidney disease and in women who are pregnant or breastfeeding. It can exacerbate psoriasis and neurological disorders and should not be used for the prevention of malaria in anyone with epilepsy. It may aggravate myasthenia gravis and severe gastrointestinal disorders.

Interactions with other drugs:
 Antacids: reduce the absorption of chloroquine.
 Antiepileptics: chloroquine reduces their anticonvulsant effect.
 Antimalarials: there is a risk of convulsions with mefloquine.
 Cimetidine: increases plasma concentrations of chloroquine.
 Cyclosporin: the likelihood of toxic effects of cyclosporin is increased.
 Digoxin: its plasma concentration is increased by chloroquine.
 Halofantrine: increases the risk of abnormal heartbeats.

Proprietary preparations: Avloclor; Nivaquine; PALUDRINE/AVLOCLOR (packaged with proguanil).

chlorothiazide A *thiazide diuretic used for the treatment of *hypertension and *oedema associated with heart failure, liver disease, or kidney disease. It is available as tablets on *prescription only.

Side effects, precautions, and interactions with other drugs: see THIAZIDE DIURETICS.

Proprietary preparation: Saluric.

See also ANTIHYPERTENSIVE DRUGS; DIURETICS.

chloroxylenol A *disinfectant with antibacterial activity. It is used diluted as an *antiseptic for treating minor wounds, bites, stings, etc., and is included as an ingredient in many preparations for treating minor skin conditions (its activity may be enhanced by edetic acid). Chloroxylenol is freely available *over the counter.

Side effects: chloroxylenol may rarely cause local allergic reactions.

Proprietary preparations: Dettol Liquid; DETTOL ANTISEPTIC CREAM (combined with triclosan and edetic acid); RINSTEAD ADULT GEL (combined with benzocaine); RINSTEAD SUGAR FREE PASTILLES (combined with menthol); TCP FIRST AID ANTISEPTIC CREAM (combined with triclosan and TCP Liquid Antiseptic); ZEASORB (combined with aldioxa).

chlorpheniramine maleate <chlorphenamine maleate> One of the original (sedating) *antihistamines, used to relieve the symptoms of such allergic conditions as hay fever and urticaria. It is also used for the emergency treatment of anaphylactic shock (an extreme and potentially life-threatening allergic reaction). It is also an ingredient in many cough medicines and decongestants. Chlorpheniramine is available as tablets or syrup from pharmacies without a prescription or as an injection on *prescription only.

Side effects, precautions, and interactions with other drugs: see ANTIHISTAMINES.

Proprietary preparations: Boots Allergy Relief Antihistamine Tablets; Calimal; Piriton; CONTAC 400 (combined with phenylpropanolamine); DRISTAN DECONGESTANT TABLETS (combined with aspirin, phenylephrine, and caffeine); EXPULIN (combined with menthol, pholcodine, and pseudoephedrine); EXPULIN DECONGESTANT FOR BABIES AND CHILDREN (combined with ephedrine and menthol); EXPULIN PAEDIATRIC (combined with menthol and pholcodine); GALPSEUD PLUS (combined with pseudoephedrine); HAYMINE (combined with ephedrine); TIXYLIX COUGH & COLD (combined with pholcodine and pseudoephedrine).

chlorpromazine hydrochloride A phenothiazine *antipsychotic drug used for the treatment of schizophrenia and other psychoses. It has a pronounced sedative effect and is effective in calming violent or agitated patients. Chlorpromazine is also used as an *antiemetic for controlling nausea and vomiting in patients who are terminally ill and have not responded to other antiemetics, and is occasionally used for the treatment of severe hiccups. It is available, on *prescription only, as tablets, an oral solution, syrup, or suspension, an injection, or as suppositories.

Side effects: include marked drowsiness and apathy, pallor, nightmares, insomnia, depression, antimuscarinic effects (such as dry mouth, difficulty in passing urine, constipation, and blurred vision), *extrapyramidal reactions, nasal stuffiness, low blood pressure, hypothermia, a fast heart rate, and abnormal heartbeats (*arrhythmias). Other side effects can include weight gain, enlargement of the breasts, menstrual changes, jaundice, blood disorders, sensitivity to sunlight, dermatitis, and (with prolonged high dosage) eye changes.

Precautions: chlorpromazine should not be given to comatose patients, to people whose bone marrow function is impaired, or to people with phaeochromocytoma (a tumour of the adrenal gland). It should be used with caution in people with disorders of circulation affecting the heart or brain, chest diseases, parkinsonism, epilepsy, an underactive thyroid gland, an enlarged prostate gland, glaucoma, liver disease or a history of jaundice, kidney disease, or myasthenia gravis. It should be used with care in elderly people (especially in very hot or very cold weather) and in women who are pregnant or breastfeeding. Drowsiness can affect driving or the performance of other skilled tasks and is increased by alcohol.

Interactions with other drugs:

Anaesthetics: their effect in lowering blood pressure is enhanced.

Antidepressants: there is an increased risk of antimuscarinic effects and arrhythmias if chlorpromazine is taken with tricyclic antidepressants.

Antiepileptic drugs: their anticonvulsant effects are antagonized by chlorpromazine.

Antihistamines: there is an increased risk of arrhythmias if chlorpromazine is taken with astemizole or terfenadine.

Beta blockers: the risk of arrhythmias is increased if sotalol is taken with chlorpromazine; if propranolol is taken with chlorpromazine, the plasma concentrations of both drugs may be increased.

Cisapride: should not be taken with chlorpromazine as this combination increases the risk of arrhythmias.

Halofantrine: there is an increased risk of arrhythmias if this drug is taken with chlorpromazine.

Ritonavir: may increase the effects of chlorpromazine.

Sedatives: the sedative effects of chlorpromazine are increased if it is taken with anxiolytic or hypnotic drugs, or any other drug that causes sedation.

Proprietary preparations: Chloractil; Largactil.

chlorpropamide A long-acting *sulphonylurea used for the treatment of noninsulin-dependent (type II) *diabetes mellitus. It has more side effects than the other sulphonylureas and is not usually given to elderly people. Chlorpropamide is also used in the treatment of diabetes insipidus (*see* VASOPRESSIN). It is available as tablets on *prescription only.

Side effects: include flushing of the face after drinking alcohol and *hypoglycaemia. *See also* SULPHONYLUREAS.

Precautions and interactions with other drugs: *see* SULPHONYLUREAS.

chlorquinaldol *See* LOCOID C.

chlortalidone *See* CHLORTHALIDONE.

chlortetracycline A tetracycline antibiotic used for the treatment of eye infections, bacterial skin infections, and severe inflammatory skin conditions. It is also used in combination with other *tetracyclines to treat chronic bronchitis, brucellosis, chlamydial infections, and infections caused by mycoplasmas and rickettsias. It is available, on *prescription only, as an ointment.

Side effects, precautions, and interactions with other drugs: *see* TETRACYCLINES.

Proprietary preparations: Aureomycin; AUREOCORT (combined with triamcinolone); DETECLO (combined with tetracycline hydrochloride and demeclocycline hydrochloride).

chlorthalidone <chlortalidone> A thiazide-like diuretic (*see* THIAZIDE DIURETICS) used for the treatment of *hypertension and *oedema associated with heart failure, liver disease, or kidney disease. It is available as tablets on *prescription only.

Side effects, precautions, and interactions with other drugs: see THIAZIDE DIURETICS.

Proprietary preparations: Hygroton; KALSPARE (combined with triamterene); Tenoret 50 (*see* CO-TENIDONE); Tenoretic (*see* CO-TENIDONE). *See also* ANTIHYPERTENSIVE DRUGS; DIURETICS.

cholecalciferol <colecalciferol> (vitamin D₃) One of the D vitamins (*see* VITAMIN D), which is used for the treatment of simple vitamin D deficiency, such as that caused by lack of sunlight. Combined with *calcium carbonate, it is available as tablets without a prescription, but only from pharmacies; a solution for injection is available on *prescription only (*see* CALCIFEROL).

Side effects, precautions, and interactions with other drugs: see VITAMIN D.

Proprietary preparations: CACIT D3 (combined with calcium carbonate); CALCEOS (combined with calcium carbonate); CALCICHEW D3 (combined with calcium carbonate).

cholesterol A complex molecule that has a core structure similar to that of a *steroid molecule; it is attached to a fatty acid to form cholesterol ester. Cholesterol is vital to life, being an essential component of all animal cell membranes (plants do not contain cholesterol), and is required to make bile acids (needed for fat absorption), adrenal hormones *corticosteroids, sex hormones (*androgens, *oestrogens), and *vitamin D. Cholesterol forms part of the diet and is also synthesized in the body, mainly in the liver. It is carried in the blood by *lipoproteins. Too much cholesterol in the bloodstream (**hypercholesterolaemia**: *see* HYPERLIPIDAEMIA) can lead to deposits (plaques) on the inner wall of the arteries, giving rise to *atherosclerosis. In the advanced stage, usually when a vessel is more than 50% blocked, atherosclerosis can result in thrombosis, causing a stroke or heart attack. A high circulating concentration of low-density lipoprotein (LDL) cholesterol is one of the most important risk factors for developing coronary heart disease. It enhances the adverse effects of other risk factors, such as smoking, *obesity, *hypertension, and *diabetes. Reducing circulating cholesterol lowers the incidence of heart attacks and other events related to coronary artery disease. Cholesterol reduction is achieved by dietary modification (reducing the intake of saturated fats and increasing consumption of fibre, oats, and pulses), which is the usual first-line treatment, or by *lipid-lowering drugs. It is important that other cardiovascular risk factors are also addressed.

cholestyramine <colestyramine> A *bile-acid sequestrant used to lower plasma *cholesterol in *hyperlipidaemia and for the prevention of coronary heart disease in men with high plasma cholesterol concentrations that are unresponsive to diet and other appropriate measures. It is also used for the relief of diarrhoea associated with surgical removal of part of the small intestine, Crohn's disease, or radiation. A *prescription only medicine, it is available as a powder to be dissolved in liquid.

Side effects and precautions: see BILE-ACID SEQUESTRANTS.

Interactions with other drugs:

Acarbose: its effect in lowering blood sugar is increased by cholestyramine.

Paracetamol and phenylbutazone: absorption of these analgesics is reduced by cholestyramine.

Vancomycin: its effect is antagonized by cholestyramine.

See also BILE-ACID SEQUESTRANTS.

Proprietary preparations: Questran; Questran Light.

cholinergic drugs Drugs whose actions resemble those of *acetylcholine. Because they have the effect of stimulating the *parasympathetic nervous system they are also called **parasympathomimetic drugs**. These effects include stimulating secretions of the salivary glands, tear ducts, and bronchi, slowing the heart rate, increasing movements of the bowel, contracting the bladder, and constricting the iris of the eye and thus reducing the size of the pupil. Cholinergic drugs produce their effects in various ways and with varying intensity, which determines which conditions they are used to treat. Cholinergic drugs include alkaloids (such as *pilocarpine), *anticholinesterases (such as neostigmine and pyridostigmine), and choline esters (such as *carbachol and *bethanechol).

choline salicylate An *analgesic used in *topical preparations for the relief of pain in ear infections, mouth ulcers, cold sores, denture irritation, and infant teething. It is available, in the form of solutions or gels, without a prescription, but some preparations can only be obtained from pharmacies.

Precautions: frequent applications, especially in children, should be avoided, since this could give rise to salicylate poisoning (*see* SALICYLATES).

Proprietary preparations: AUDAX (combined with glycerin); BONJELA (combined with cetalkonium chloride); DINNEFORDS TEEJEL (combined with cetalkonium chloride); EAREX PLUS EAR DROPS (combined with glycerin).

Choragon (Ferring Pharmaceuticals) *See* HUMAN CHORIONIC GONADOTROPHIN.

chorionic gonadotrophin *See* HUMAN CHORIONIC GONADOTROPHIN.

chromones A group of anti-allergic drugs that are thought to act by preventing the release of *histamine, an important mediator of the allergic response; they also inhibit the release of other body chemicals that promote the allergic response. Because they act in this way (unlike

the *antihistamines, which antagonize the action of histamine once it
has been released), chromones are best used to prevent an attack before
contact with the allergen occurs. When used to treat hay fever it is often
necessary to continue taking the chromone even during symptom-free
days. Chromones can be used regularly to prevent recurrent *asthma or
exercise-induced asthma (but not to treat asthma attacks) and allergic
conditions in the lungs, nose, eyes (including vernal keratoconjunctivitis),
and intestines (e.g. food allergies). The main chromones are *sodium
cromoglycate <cromoglicate> and *nedocromil sodium.

Chymol Emollient Balm (Anglian Pharma) A proprietary
combination of *eucalyptus oil, *terpineol, *methyl salicylate, and
*phenol, used as a *rubefacient for the relief of chapped and sore skin,
chilblains, bruises, and sprains. It is freely available *over the counter.
Side effects and precautions: see RUBEFACIENTS.

Cicatrin (GlaxoWellcome) A proprietary combination of the antibiotics
*neomycin sulphate and *bacitracin zinc, used for the treatment of
superficial bacterial infections of the skin. It is available as a cream on
*prescription only.
Side effects: hearing may be affected; allergic reactions may occur.
Precautions: Cicatrin should not be used on very large areas of damaged
skin.

cidofovir An *antiviral drug that inhibits DNA polymerase, the enzyme
within human cells that is required by the virus to replicate itself.
Cidofovir is used for the treatment of cytomegalovirus retinitis (a serious
eye infection that can cause blindness) in AIDS patients when other drugs
are unsuitable. It is given in combination with *probenecid to prevent its
adverse effects on the kidneys. Cidofovir is available as a solution for
injection on *prescription only.
Side effects: include protein in the urine, a low white-blood-cell count,
fever, hair loss, nausea, vomiting, and rash.
Precautions: cidofovir should not be given to people with kidney disease
or to women who are pregnant or breastfeeding. Women should avoid
becoming pregnant during treatment and for a month after treatment
stops; men should not father a child during, or for three months after,
treatment. Cidofovir should be used with caution in diabetics. Blood tests
to monitor kidney function may be necessary.
Interactions with other drugs:
  Zidovudine: interacts with probenecid, which may be given with
  cidofovir; zidovudine may therefore be stopped, or its dosage reduced,
  before treatment with cidofovir and probenecid.
Proprietary preparation: Vistide.

Cidomycin (Hoechst Marion Roussel) *See* GENTAMICIN.

cilastatin An agent that inhibits the activity of an enzyme in the

kidneys that partially breaks down the antibiotic *imipenem. It is used in combination with imipenem to enhance the activity of this antibiotic.
Proprietary preparation: Primaxin (*see* IMIPENEM).

cilazapril An *ACE inhibitor used as an adjunct to *diuretics for the treatment of *heart failure. It is also used to treat essential *hypertension. It is available as tablets on *prescription only.
Side effects, precautions, and interactions with other drugs: *see* ACE INHIBITORS.
Proprietary preparation: Vascace.
See also ANTIHYPERTENSIVE DRUGS.

Cilest (Janssen-Cilag) A proprietary combination of *ethinyloestradiol <ethinylestradiol> and *norgestimate used as an *oral contraceptive. It is available as tablets on *prescription only.
Side effects, precautions, and interactions with other drugs: *see* ORAL CONTRACEPTIVES.

Ciloxan (Alcon Laboratories) *See* CIPROFLOXACIN.

cimetidine An *H$_2$-receptor antagonist used in the treatment of gastric and duodenal ulcers, reflux oesophagitis, Zollinger-Ellison syndrome, and all other types of *acid-peptic disease. It is available, as tablets, effervescent tablets, a syrup, or an injection, on *prescription only; packs containing no more than two weeks' supply of tablets, for the relief of indigestion and heartburn in people over 16 years old, can be obtained from pharmacies without a prescription.
Side effects: side effects, which are uncommon, include diarrhoea, dizziness, rash, tiredness, and reversible liver damage; rarely, reversible confusion, blood disorders, and muscle or joint pain may occur. In high doses cimetidine can cause breast pain and enlargement in men.
Precautions: cimetidine should be used with caution in people with poor kidney or liver function and in women who are pregnant or breastfeeding.
Interactions with other drugs: cimetidine can inhibit the metabolism (and therefore may increase the effects) of a number of drugs, most importantly the following:

Anti-arrhythmic drugs: cimetidine increases the plasma concentrations of amiodarone, flecainide, lignocaine <lidocaine>, procainamide, propafenone, and quinidine.

Anticoagulants: cimetidine enhances the anticoagulant properties of warfarin and nicoumalone <acenocoumarol>.

Antiepileptic drugs: cimetidine increases the plasma concentrations of carbamazepine, phenytoin, and valproate.

Cyclosporin: cimetidine increases the plasma concentration of cyclosporin.

Theophylline and aminophylline: cimetidine increases the plasma concentrations of these drugs.

Proprietary preparations: Acid-Eze; Acitak; Dyspamet; Galenamet; Peptimax; Phimetin; Tagamet; Ultec; Zita; ALGITEC (combined with alginic acid).

Cinazière (Ashbourne Pharmaceuticals) *See* CINNARIZINE.

cinchocaine hydrochloride A *local anaesthetic that is included in creams, ointments, and suppositories for the relief of *haemorrhoids and other painful or itching anorectal conditions.
Proprietary preparations: PROCTOSEDYL (combined with hydrocortisone); SCHERIPROCT (combined with prednisolone hexanoate); ULTRAPROCT (combined with fluocortolone); UNIROID-HC (combined with hydrocortisone).

cineole *See* EUCALYPTUS OIL.

cinnarizine An *antihistamine used for the treatment of nausea and vomiting, especially that associated with disorders of the ear (such as Ménière's disease) and motion sickness. A stronger preparation is used for the treatment of disorders of the peripheral arteries, especially intermittent claudication (pain in the calf on walking) and Raynaud's disease (poor circulation of the hands and fingers), but is not established as being effective. Cinnarizine is available as tablets and can be obtained from pharmacies without a prescription.
Side effects: include drowsiness and allergic skin reactions; *see also* ANTIHISTAMINES.
Precautions and interactions with other drugs: *see* ANTIHISTAMINES.
Proprietary preparations: Stugeron; Cinazière; Stugeron Forte (for vascular disorders).

Cinobac (Eli Lilly & Co) *See* CINOXACIN.

cinoxacin A *quinolone antibiotic, similar to *ciprofloxacin, that is used for the treatment of urinary-tract infections. It is available as capsules on *prescription only.
Side effects, precautions, and interactions with other drugs: *see* QUINOLONES.
Proprietary preparation: Cinobac.

Cipramil (Lundbeck) *See* CITALOPRAM.

ciprofibrate A *fibrate used for the treatment of a wide variety of *hyperlipidaemias that have not responded to dietary modification and other appropriate measures. It is available as tablets on *prescription only.
Side effects and precautions: *see* FIBRATES.
Interactions with other drugs: *see* BEZAFIBRATE.
Proprietary preparation: Modalim.

ciprofloxacin A *quinolone antibiotic used for the treatment of
infections of the respiratory and urinary tracts and of the gastrointestinal
system, typhoid, gonorrhoea, and septicaemia. It is also used to treat skin
infections, although many of the causative organisms are now resistant,
and corneal ulcers. It is used to prevent infections after gastrointestinal
surgery. Ciprofloxacin is available, on *prescription only, as tablets, an
intravenous infusion, or eye drops.

Side effects: see QUINOLONES. Local irritation may occur with eye drops.

Precautions and interactions with other drugs: see QUINOLONES.

Proprietary preparations: Ciloxan (eye drops); Ciproxin.

Ciproxin (Bayer) *See* CIPROFLOXACIN.

cisapride A *prokinetic drug that stimulates emptying of the stomach
and increases motility of the large bowel. It is used in the treatment of
gut motility disorders, gastro-oesophageal reflux, and indigestion that is
not due to peptic ulceration. Cisapride should be taken 15–30 minutes
before a meal, or at bedtime for nocturnal symptoms. It is available as
tablets or as a suspension on *prescription only.

Side effects: include abdominal cramps, diarrhoea, and (occasionally)
headaches, light-headedness, and allergic reactions.

Precautions: cisapride should not be used in people at risk of developing
ventricular *arrhythmias, in those with gastrointestinal bleeding or
obstruction, or in women who are breastfeeding. It should be used with
caution in people with impaired liver or kidney function, the elderly, and
pregnant women.

Interactions with other drugs: the following drugs should not be taken
with cisapride since they increase the risk of serious ventricular
arrhythmias: amiodarone, astemizole, bretylium, clarithromycin,
disopyramide, erythromycin, fluconazole, halofantrine, haloperidol,
itraconazole, ketoconazole, lithium, miconazole, nefazodone,
pentamidine isethionate <isetionate>, phenothiazines, pimozide,
procainamide, protease inhibitors, quinidine, quinine, sertindole, sotalol,
terfenadine, and tricyclic antidepressants.

Proprietary preparations: Prepulsid; Prepulsid Quicklet (tablets that
dissolve on the tongue).

cis-diamminedichloroplatinum *See* CISPLATIN.

cisplatin (cisplatinum; cis-diamminedichloroplatinum) A platinum-
containing compound that is a powerful *cytotoxic drug: it acts by
binding to DNA and thus preventing cell replication. It is highly effective
in the treatment of testicular *cancer, usually in combination with
*vinblastine and *bleomycin. It is also used for the treatment of cancer of
the ovary and bladder, lymphomas, a form of lung cancer, and some
cancers of the head and neck. It is, however, highly toxic (see side effects
below) and this limits its use. A *prescription only medicine, cisplatin is
given by intravenous infusion in specialist oncology units.

Side effects: cisplatin causes severe nausea and vomiting that may persist for several days. It also has adverse effects on the kidneys and when given in high doses must be accompanied by large volumes of fluid to prevent kidney damage. It can damage the nerves to the ears, resulting in some hearing loss and tinnitus (the sensation of noises in the ears), and the nerves in the arms and legs, causing numbness and tingling in the fingers and toes. Other side effects include *bone marrow suppression (which is not severe) and a reduction in magnesium concentrations in the blood. *See also* CYTOTOXIC DRUGS.

Precautions: cisplatin should not be given to people with kidney disease or to women who are pregnant or breastfeeding. *See also* CYTOTOXIC DRUGS.

Interactions with other drugs:

 Antibiotics: aminoglycosides and capreomycin increase the risk of damage to the kidneys and possibly hearing.

 Diuretics: increase the risk of damage to the kidneys and possibly to hearing.

citalopram An *antidepressant drug of the *SSRI group that is used for the treatment of depressive illness and panic disorder. It is available as tablets on *prescription only.

Side effects and precautions: see SSRIS.

Interactions with other drugs:

 Terfenadine: there is an increased risk of *arrhythmias and citalopram should not be taken with terfenadine.

 For other interactions, *see* SSRIS.

Proprietary preparation: Cipramil.

Citanest (AstraZeneca) *See* PRILOCAINE.

Citramag (Bioglan Laboratories) *See* MAGNESIUM CITRATE.

citric acid An acid found in citrus fruits that is included in pharmaceutical preparations to produce effervescent formulations (e.g. tablets or granules). Preparations containing citric acid are also used to dissolve small kidney stones, to treat cystitis and other infections of the urinary tract, or to prevent the encrustation of urinary catheters. Citric acid is also included in some anticoagulant preparations and in preparations used for the relief of gastrointestinal upsets.

Proprietary preparations: DIORALYTE TABLETS (combined with sodium bicarbonate, glucose, sodium chloride, and potassium chloride); ENO (combined with sodium bicarbonate and sodium carbonate); MICTRAL (combined with nalidixic acid, sodium citrate, and sodium bicarbonate); URIFLEX G (combined with sodium bicarbonate, magnesium oxide, and disodium edetate).

cladribine A potent but rather toxic *antimetabolite that is used for the treatment of hairy cell leukaemia and for treating chronic

lymphocytic leukaemia (*see* CANCER) that has not responded to
*alkylating drugs. It is available, on *prescription only, as a solution for
intravenous infusion.

Side effects: see CYTOTOXIC DRUGS: *bone marrow suppression may be
severe and nerve damage may occur rarely.

Precautions: see CYTOTOXIC DRUGS.

Proprietary preparation: Leustat.

Claforan (Hoechst Marion Roussel) *See* CEFOTAXIME.

Clariteyes (Schering-Plough) *See* SODIUM CROMOGLYCATE
<CROMOGLICATE>.

clarithromycin A *macrolide antibiotic, similar to *erythromycin,
that is used for the treatment of respiratory-tract infections and mild to
moderate skin and soft-tissue infections and to eradicate causative
bacteria in the treatment of duodenal ulcers (*see* ACID-PEPTIC DISEASES). It
is available, on *prescription only, as tablets, granules, *modified-release
tablets, a suspension for children, and an *intravenous injection.

Side effects and precautions: see ERYTHROMYCIN.

Interactions with other drugs:

 Zidovudine: clarithromycin reduces the absorption of zidovudine.

 For other interactions, *see* ERYTHROMYCIN.

Proprietary preparations: Klaricid; Klaricid XL (modifed-release tablets).

Clarityn (Schering-Plough) *See* LORATADINE.

clavulanic acid An agent that inhibits the activity of beta-lactamases,
enzymes that are produced by bacteria and destroy *penicillins. It is
given in combination with some penicillins to prevent their destruction.
See CO-AMOXICLAV; TIMENTIN.

Clearasil Max 10 (Procter & Gamble) *See* BENZOYL PEROXIDE.

Clearasil Treatment Cream Regular (Procter & Gamble) A
proprietary combination of the antiseptics *triclosan and *sulphur, used
for the treatment and prevention of spots and acne. It is freely available
*over the counter.

clemastine One of the original (sedating) *antihistamines, used to
relieve the symptoms of such allergic conditions as hay fever and
urticaria. It is available as tablets or an elixir from pharmacies without a
prescription.

Side effects, precautions, and interactions with other drugs: see
ANTIHISTAMINES.

Proprietary preparations: Aller-eze; Tavegil; ALLER-EZE PLUS (combined
with phenylpropanolamine).

Clexane (Rhône-Poulenc Rorer) *See* ENOXAPARIN.

Climagest (Novartis Pharmaceuticals) A proprietary preparation of
*oestradiol <estradiol> tablets and *norethisterone tablets used as
sequential combined *hormone replacement therapy for the relief of
menopausal symptoms in women who have not had a hysterectomy. The
tablets, which are available on *prescription only, must be taken in the
prescribed order.
Side effects, precautions, and interactions with other drugs: *see* HORMONE
REPLACEMENT THERAPY.

Climaval (Novartis Pharmaceuticals) *See* OESTRADIOL <ESTRADIOL>;
HORMONE REPLACEMENT THERAPY.

Climesse (Novartis Pharmaceuticals) A proprietary combination of
*oestradiol <estradiol> and *norethisterone used as continuous combined
*hormone replacement therapy for the relief of menopausal symptoms
and prevention of osteoporosis in women who have not had a
hysterectomy and who have not had a period for a year. It is available as
tablets on *prescription only.
Side effects, precautions, and interactions with other drugs: *see* HORMONE
REPLACEMENT THERAPY.

clindamycin An *antibiotic used for the treatment of infections of the
bones and joints and the membranes or valves of the heart. It is also
applied topically to treat bacterial infections of the vagina and *acne. It is
available, on *prescription only, as capsules, a suspension for children, a
solution for *intravenous or *intramuscular injection, and as a cream or
lotion. Because of its serious side effects clindamycin is not widely used.
Side effects: clindamycin can cause overgrowth of the microbes normally
found in the gut resulting in pseudomembranous colitis, a condition
associated with severe diarrhoea that can in extreme cases be fatal. This
complication is most common in middle-aged and elderly women,
especially following surgery. Any signs of diarrhoea, particularly if
accompanied by blood, should be reported to a doctor and treatment
discontinued. Other possible side effects are abdominal discomfort,
nausea, vomiting, rash, and jaundice. There may be a local reaction after
intramuscular injection.
Precautions: clindamycin should be used with caution in people who
have liver or kidney disease and in women who are pregnant or
breastfeeding.
Proprietary preparations: Dalacin (cream); Dalacin C; Dalacin T (lotion).

Clinitar Cream (Shire Pharmaceuticals) *See* COAL TAR.

Clinoril (Merck Sharp & Dohme) *See* SULINDAC.

clioquinol An *antibiotic with activity against fungi, used for the treatment of *Candida* infections of the skin and outer ear. It is combined with other drugs in creams, ointments, and ear drops that are available on *prescription only.

Side effects: local allergic reactions may occur; clioquinol stains skin and clothing.

Precautions: clioquinol should not be applied to perforated eardrums.

Proprietary preparations: BETNOVATE-C (combined with betamethasone); LOCORTEN-VIOFORM (combined with flumethasone <flumetasone> pivalate); SYNALAR C (combined with fluocinolone acetonide); VIOFORM-HYDROCORTISONE (combined with hydrocortisone).

clobazam A long-acting *benzodiazepine used in the treatment of epilepsy and for the short-term treatment of anxiety. It is available as tablets on *prescription only and cannot be prescribed on the NHS.

Side effects and precautions: see DIAZEPAM; BENZODIAZEPINES.

Interactions with other drugs: see BENZODIAZEPINES.

Proprietary preparation: Frisium.

clobetasol propionate A very potent *topical steroid used to treat *psoriasis, *eczema that is unresponsive to other treatments, and other inflammatory conditions of the skin. It is available, on *prescription only, as a cream, ointment, or scalp lotion.

Side effects and precautions: see TOPICAL STEROIDS.

Proprietary preparations: Dermovate; Dermovate Scalp; DERMOVATE-NN (combined with neomycin sulphate and nystatin).

clobetasone butyrate A moderately potent *topical steroid used for the treatment of a variety of skin conditions and inflammatory conditions of the eyes. It is available, on *prescription only, as a cream, ointment, or eye drops.

Side effects and precautions: see TOPICAL STEROIDS.

Proprietary preparations: Cloburate (eye drops); Eumovate; TRIMOVATE (combined with nystatin and oxytetracycline). *See also* corticosteroids.

Cloburate (Dominion Pharma) *See* CLOBETASONE BUTYRATE.

clofazimine An *antibiotic used for the treatment of leprosy. It is available as capsules on *prescription only.

Side effects: include nausea, vomiting, abdominal pain, headache, tiredness, and discoloration of skin exposed to light and also of hair, urine, faeces, and body fluids; discoloration of soft contact lenses may occur. Other possible side effects are rash, itching, acne-like eruptions, and loss of appetite.

Precautions: clofazimine should be used with caution in people with liver or kidney disease and in women who are pregnant or breastfeeding.

Proprietary preparation: Lamprene.

clofibrate A *fibrate used for the treatment of *hyperlipidaemia and for the prevention of coronary heart disease in middle-aged men with high concentrations of plasma lipids that are unresponsive to dietary modification and other appropriate measures. It is available as capsules on *prescription only.

Side effects: see FIBRATES.

Precautions: see FIBRATES. In addition, clofibrate can predispose to gallstones and may cause weight gain.

Interactions with other drugs:

Anticoagulants: the effects of warfarin, nicoumalone <acenocoumarol>, and phenindione are enhanced.

Phenytoin: its effect is increased.

Antidiabetic agents: the effects of these drugs are enhanced.

Proprietary preparation: Atromid-S.

clomethiazole *See* CHLORMETHIAZOLE.

Clomid (Hoechst Marion Roussel) *See* CLOMIPHENE CITRATE <CLOMIFENE CITRATE>.

clomiphene citrate <clomifene citrate> An *oestrogen antagonist used for the treatment of infertility in women caused by failure of the ovaries to produce egg cells; it acts by stimulating the secretion of *gonadotrophins by the pituitary gland. Clomiphene, which is sometimes used in conjunction with *human chorionic gonadotrophin, is available as tablets on *prescription only.

Side effects: the most common are hot flushes and abdominal discomfort; more rare side effects are ovarian enlargement and hyperstimulation (the uncontrolled production of large numbers of follicles in the ovaries), visual disturbances (in which case treatment should be stopped), nausea, vomiting, depression, insomnia, breast tenderness, headache, weight gain, and hair loss. There is a risk of multiple pregnancy, cysts in the ovaries, fibroids, ectopic pregnancy, and convulsions.

Precautions: clomiphene should not be used during pregnancy or by women who have liver disease, ovarian cysts, hormone-dependent tumours, or undiagnosed vaginal bleeding.

Proprietary preparation: Clomid.

clomipramine hydrochloride A *tricyclic antidepressant drug used for the treatment of depressive illness, phobias, and obsessional states and as an adjunct for treating narcolepsy (an extreme tendency to fall asleep). It is available, on *prescription only, as capsules, *modified-release tablets, or a syrup.

Side effects, precautions, and interactions with other drugs: see AMITRIPTYLINE HYDROCHLORIDE; TRICYCLIC ANTIDEPRESSANTS.

Proprietary preparations: Anafranil; Anafranil SR (modified-release tablets); Tranquax.

clonazepam A *benzodiazepine used for the treatment of all forms of epilepsy (*see* ANTICONVULSANT DRUGS). It is available, on *prescription only, as tablets for oral use and as a form for injection or infusion for treating status epilepticus. Intravenous infusion of clonazepam may be hazardous and should only be performed in specialist centres where intensive care facilities are available.

Side effects: include drowsiness, fatigue, dizziness, lack of coordination, and behavioural changes, such as paradoxical aggression and irritability (*see also* BENZODIAZEPINES). There is increased salivation in babies.

Precautions: clonazepam should not be taken by patients with severe lung problems and should be used with caution in people who have liver or kidney disease and in women who are pregnant or breastfeeding; women who are planning to become pregnant should seek specialist advice. Dosage of the drug should be reduced gradually at the end of treatment (*see* BENZODIAZEPINES).

Interactions with other drugs: see BENZODIAZEPINES.

Proprietary preparation: Rivotril.

clonidine hydrochloride An alpha stimulant (*see* SYMPATHOMIMETIC DRUGS) that acts centrally (on receptors in the brain). It is used in the treatment of all grades of *hypertension, sometimes in combination with *diuretics, and may also be used to prevent *migraine attacks. Clonidine is available, on *prescription only, as tablets, *modified-release capsules, or a solution for injection.

Side effects: include drowsiness, dry mouth, dizziness, and fluid retention.

Precautions: abrupt withdrawal of clonidine can cause severe hypertension; treatment must therefore be stopped gradually. Drowsiness may affect driving ability and may be increased by alcohol.

Interactions with other drugs:

  Antidepressants: may reduce the effects of clonidine and increase the risk of rebound hypertension if clonidine is stopped.

  Beta blockers: the risk of hypertension is increased if beta blockers are stopped suddenly.

Proprietary preparations: Catapres; Catapres Perlongets (modified-release capsules); Dixarit (for migraine prophylaxis).

See also ANTIHYPERTENSIVE DRUGS.

clopamide *See* VISKALDIX.

clopidogrel An *antiplatelet drug used to prevent strokes or heart attacks occurring in people at risk, particularly in those who have had a previous stroke or heart attack. It is available as tablets on *prescription only.

Side effects: bleeding from the stomach, intestines, or elsewhere can occur; other side effects may include nausea, vomiting, abdominal discomfort, constipation, diarrhoea, headache, dizziness, and rashes.

Precautions: clopidogrel should not be taken by people with bleeding peptic ulcers or bleeding from other sites or by women who are breastfeeding, and it is not recommended for people with severe angina or for those who have had coronary-artery surgery. It should be used with caution in pregnant women and in people with liver or kidney disease.

Interactions with other drugs:

Anticoagulants: their effects are enhanced by clopidogrel; warfarin should not be used with clopidogrel.

NSAIDS (including aspirin): may increase the risk of gastrointestinal bleeding.

Proprietary preparation: Plavix.

Clopixol, **Clopixol Acuphase**, **Clopixol Conc.** (Lundbeck) *See* ZUCLOPENTHIXOL.

cloral betaine *See* CHLORAL BETAINE.

clorazepate dipotassium A long-acting *benzodiazepine used for the short-term treatment of anxiety. It is available as capsules on *prescription only and cannot be prescribed on the NHS.

Side effects and precautions: *see* DIAZEPAM; BENZODIAZEPINES.

Interactions with other drugs:

Ritonavir: increases the plasma concentration of clorazepate, causing profound sedation; these drugs should therefore not be taken together.

See also BENZODIAZEPINES.

Proprietary preparation: Tranxene.

Clotam (Cortecs Healthcare) *See* TOLFENAMIC ACID.

clotrimazole An imidazole *antifungal drug used for the treatment of candidiasis (thrush) of the vagina and tinea (ringworm) of the ear, skin, and nails. It is available as a solution, cream, pessaries, powder, or spray for topical application and can be obtained without a prescription, but only from pharmacies (compound preparations containing corticosteroids are *prescription only medicines).

Side effects: local mild burning or irritation is the most common side effect.

Proprietary preparations: Canesten; Canesten 10% (vaginal cream); Canesten AF (cream or powder for athlete's foot); Canesten Cream; Canesten Pessaries (Canesten 1); Canesten Powder; Canesten Spray; Canesten-Combi (pessaries and cream); Masnoderm (cream); Mycil Gold (cream); CANESTEN HC (combined with hydrocortisone); LOTRIDERM (combined with betamethasone).

clove oil An oil produced from the distillation of cloves. It can produce local anaesthesia when applied topically and is used as a home remedy for toothache. It is also an ingredient of mixtures used for the treatment of flatulent colic, of preparations to relieve the congestion of colds and catarrh, and of *rubefacient preparations for the relief of minor muscular aches and pains. Preparations containing clove oil are freely available *over the counter.

Proprietary preparations: NELLA RED OIL (combined with methyl nicotinate and mustard oil); OLBAS OIL (combined with eucalyptus oil, menthol, cajuput oil, juniper berry oil, and oil of wintergreen); OLBAS PASTILLES (combined with eucalyptus oil, menthol, peppermint oil, juniper berry oil, and oil of wintergreen); TIGER BALM (combined with cajuput oil, camphor, peppermint oil, and menthol); TIGER BALM RED EXTRA STRENGTH (combined with camphor, menthol, cajuput oil, cinnamic acid, and peppermint oil).

clozapine An atypical *antipsychotic drug used for the treatment of schizophrenia in patients who have not responded to or cannot tolerate conventional antipsychotic drugs. Because it can cause a severe deficiency of certain white blood cells, people taking clozapine must be registered with the Clozaril Patient Monitoring Service. Clozapine is available as tablets on *prescription only.

Side effects: include headache, dizziness, weight gain, low blood pressure on standing, increased salivation, urinary incontinence and retention, fever, and a decrease in the number of white blood cells. Less frequently it can cause sedation and *extrapyramidal reactions (which are usually mild and transient).

Precautions: clozapine should not be taken by people who have bone marrow disorders or who have previously had low white cell counts due to drug treatment, or by people with severe heart failure, liver disease, severe kidney disease, psychosis due to alcohol or drugs, or uncontrolled epilepsy, or by women who are pregnant or breastfeeding. It should be used with caution in people with kidney disease, acute glaucoma, or an enlarged prostate gland. Therapy should be started in hospital and blood counts must be monitored regularly (weekly at the start of treatment).

Interactions with other drugs: clozapine should not be used with drugs that cause *bone marrow suppression, especially carbamazepine, co-trimoxazole, chloramphenicol, sulphonamides, azapropazone, penicillamine, cytotoxic drugs, or antipsychotic drugs given by *depot injection.

Anaesthetics: their effect in lowering blood pressure is enhanced.

Antidepressants: fluoxetine and fluvoxamine may increase the plasma concentration of clozapine; the effects of MAOIs on the central nervous system may be increased by clozapine.

Antiepileptic drugs: their anticonvulsant effects are antagonized by clozapine; the effects of clozapine are reduced by carbamazepine and phenytoin.

Antihistamines: there is an increased risk of arrhythmias if clozapine is taken with astemizole or terfenadine.

Erythromycin: may possibly increase the plasma concentration of clozapine and the risk of convulsions.

Halofantrine: there is an increased risk of arrhythmias if this drug is taken with clozapine.

Phenytoin: reduces the effects of clozapine.

Ritonavir: increases the plasma concentration (and the risk of adverse effects) of clozapine: the two drugs should therefore not be taken together.

Sedatives: the sedative effects of clozapine are increased if it is taken with anxiolytic or hypnotic drugs, or any other drug that causes sedation.

Proprietary preparation: Clozaril.

Clozaril (Novartis Pharmaceuticals) *See* CLOZAPINE.

coal tar A complex mixture of substances obtained from the distillation of coal. Crude coal tar is potent but may be irritating and stains clothing; coal tar extract is usually milder and more acceptable. Coal tar is a *keratolytic that also relieves inflammation and itching and has *antiseptic properties. It also has a photosensitizing action (i.e. it makes skin more susceptible to the effects of sunlight). Coal tar is used for the treatment or relief of a variety of skin disorders, including *psoriasis (in which it also stops proliferation of skin cells), *eczema, and dandruff. It is an ingredient of many lotions, creams, and shampoos and is usually freely available *over the counter, but some combined preparations can only be obtained from pharmacies.

Side effects: include local irritation and an acne-like rash; the skin may become more sensitive to sunlight.

Precautions: coal tar should not be applied to broken or inflamed skin and should not come into contact with the eyes; it should be used with caution on the face and genitals. It may stain the skin and clothing.

Proprietary preparations: Alphosyl 2-in-1 Shampoo; Carbo-Dome (cream); Clinitar Cream; Exorex (lotion); Pentrax (shampoo); Psoriderm (cream and scalp lotion); PsoriGel (gel); T/Gel (shampoo); ALPHOSYL (combined with allantoin); ALPHOSYL HC (combined with allantoin and hydrocortisone); CAPASAL (combined with salicylic acid and coconut oil); COCOIS (combined with sulphur and salicylic acid); DENOREX ANTI-DANDRUFF SHAMPOO (combined with menthol); GELCOSAL (combined with tar and salicylic acid); GELCOTAR (combined with tar); IONIL T (combined with salicylic acid and benzalkonium chloride); PRAGMATAR (combined with sulphur and salicylic acid); POLYTAR (combined with tar, cade oil, oleyl alcohol, and polypeptide); TARCORTIN (combined with hydrocortisone).

co-amilofruse A mixture of *frusemide <furosemide> (a loop diuretic) and *amiloride hydrochloride (a potassium-sparing diuretic), used for the treatment of *oedema (fluid retention) associated with cirrhosis of the liver, heart failure, or other conditions. It is available as tablets on *prescription only.

Side effects, precautions, and interactions with other drugs: *see* LOOP DIURETICS; THIAZIDE DIURETICS.

Proprietary preparations: Aridil; Froop-Co; Fru-Co; Frumil; Frumil LS; Frumil Forte; Lasoride.

co-amilozide A mixture of *hydrochlorothiazide (a thiazide diuretic) and *amiloride hydrochloride (a potassium-sparing diuretic), used for the treatment of *oedema and *hypertension. It is available as tablets or an oral solution on *prescription only.

Side effects, precautions, and interactions with other drugs: see THIAZIDE DIURETICS; POTASSIUM-SPARING DIURETICS.

Proprietary preparations: Amilmaxco 5/50; Amil-Co; Delvas; Moduret 25; Moduretic; Zida-Co.

co-amoxiclav A mixture of *amoxycillin <amoxicillin> (a penicillin) and *clavulanic acid (a beta-lactamase inhibitor). It is used for the treatment of infections of the respiratory tract, ear, nose, throat, skin and soft tissues, bones, joints, and the urinary tract and for dental infections. It is available, on *prescription only, as tablets, dispersible tablets, and a syrup for oral use and as an injection.

Side effects: see AMPICILLIN. Additional side effects may include jaundice and hepatitis.

Precautions: co-amoxiclav should not be taken by those who are allergic to penicillins. It should be used with caution in people with liver or kidney disease and in pregnant women.

Interactions with other drugs: see AMPICILLIN.

Proprietary preparation: Augmentin.

Cobadex (Cox Pharmaceuticals) A proprietary combination of *hydrocortisone (a corticosteroid) and *dimethicone <dimeticone> (a water repellent), used for the treatment of inflammatory skin conditions and itching of the anus or vulva. It is available as a cream on *prescription only.

Side effects and precautions: see TOPICAL STEROIDS.

Cobalin-H (Link Pharmaceuticals) *See* HYDROXOCOBALAMIN.

co-beneldopa A combination of *levodopa and *benserazide hydrochloride, used for the treatment of Parkinson's disease (*see* ANTIPARKINSONIAN DRUGS). It is available as capsules, *modified-release capsules, or dispersible tablets on *prescription only.

Side effects, precautions, and interactions with other drugs: see LEVODOPA.

Proprietary preparations: Madopar; Madopar CR (modified-release capsules).

Co-Betaloc (AstraZeneca) A proprietary combination of *metoprolol tartrate (a cardioselecetive beta blocker) and *hydrochlorothiazide (a thiazide diuretic), used in the treatment of mild to moderate *hypertension. It is available as tablets on *prescription only. **Co-Betaloc SA** is a similar preparation twice the strength of Co-Betaloc.

Side effects, precautions, and interactions with other drugs: see BETA BLOCKERS; THIAZIDE DIURETICS.

See also ANTIHYPERTENSIVE DRUGS; DIURETICS.

cocaine A drug that stimulates the central nervous system and produces a feeling of euphoria or exhilaration. It is addictive and is a commonly used drug of abuse. Cocaine is a *controlled drug; in clinical medicine it is now used only as a *local anaesthetic in ear, nose, and throat operations, being applied in the form of a solution or paste to the mucous membranes of the nasal passages (which it readily penetrates) before surgery. Because it constricts small blood vessels at the site of application (which prolongs its action), cocaine does not need to be given with adrenaline <epinephrine> (*see* LOCAL ANAESTHETICS). Care must be used when it is applied since it can cause *arrhythmias if absorbed. Cocaine is now little used in eye surgery, because it has toxic effects on the cornea. Formerly cocaine was used as an ingredient of soothing and painkilling mixtures for the terminally ill, but this practice has been discontinued.

co-careldopa A combination of *levodopa and *carbidopa used for the treatment of Parkinson's disease (*see* ANTIPARKINSONIAN DRUGS). It is available as tablets or *modified-release tablets on *prescription only.
Side effects, precautions, and interactions with other drugs: see LEVODOPA.
Proprietary preparations: Half Sinemet CR (modified-release tablets); Sinemet; Sinemet CR (modified-release tablets); Sinemet LS; Sinemet Plus.

co-codamol A mixture of *paracetamol (a non-opioid analgesic) and *codeine phosphate (an opioid analgesic), used for the relief of mild to moderate pain. **Co-codamol 8/500** contains 8 mg of codeine and is available as tablets, capsules, or dispersible (effervescent) tablets; it is a *prescription only medicine, but under certain circumstances can be obtained from pharmacies without a prescription. Preparations containing a higher dosage of codeine are **co-codamol 30/500** and **co-codamol 60/1000** (which also contains a higher dosage of paracetamol). They are available on *prescription only.
Side effects and precautions: see CODEINE; PARACETAMOL. Higher strength preparations are not recommended for children and the dosage should be reduced for elderly people.
Interactions with other drugs: see OPIOIDS.
Proprietary preparations: Kapake (higher strength); Kapake Insts (sachets, higher strength); Panadeine; Paracodol (capsules and effervescent tablets); Parake; Solpadol (higher strength); Tylex (higher strength).

co-codaprin A mixture of *aspirin (a non-opioid analgesic) and *codeine phosphate (an opioid analgesic), used for the relief of mild to moderate pain. It is available as tablets or dispersible tablets and can be obtained without a prescription provided that packs contain no more

than 32 (or exceptionally 100) tablets; larger quantities are available on
*prescription only.
Side effects, precautions, and interactions with other drugs: see ASPIRIN;
CODEINE; OPIOIDS.

Cocois (Medeva) A proprietary combination of *coal tar, *sulphur, and
*salicylic acid (all keratolytics), used in the form of an ointment for
treating *psoriasis and *eczema of the scalp and dandruff. It is freely
available *over the counter.
Side effects and precautions: see COAL TAR; SALICYLIC ACID.

Codafen Continus (Napp Pharmaceuticals) A proprietary combination
of *ibuprofen (an NSAID) and *codeine phosphate (an opioid analgesic),
used for the treatment of rheumatoid arthritis and other disorders of
joints or muscles, postoperative pain, and period pains. It is available as
*modified-release tablets on *prescription only.
Side effects and precautions: see NSAIDS; CODEINE; OPIOIDS. These tablets
are not recommended for children.
Interactions with other drugs: see NSAIDS; OPIOIDS.

Codalax, Codalax Forte (Napp Pharmaceuticals) *See* CO-DANTHRAMER.

Codanin (Whitehall Laboratories) A proprietary combination of
*paracetamol (a non-opioid analgesic) and *codeine (an opioid analgesic),
used for the relief of mild to moderate pain, including headache,
neuralgia, migraine, period pains, rheumatic pains, and toothache. It is
available as tablets and can be obtained without a prescription, but only
from pharmacies.
Side effects and precautions: Codanin is not recommended for children
under six years old. *See also* PARACETAMOL; CODEINE.
Interactions with other drugs: see OPIOIDS.

co-danthramer A mixture of *danthron <dantron> (a stimulant
laxative) and poloxamer '188' (a *faecal softener). It is used for the
treatment of constipation produced by analgesic drugs in the terminally
ill, and for constipation in the elderly and in people with heart failure or
coronary thrombosis. Co-danthramer is available as a suspension or
capsules on *prescription only.
Side effects: see DANTHRON <DANTRON>.
Precautions: co-danthramer should not be taken by people with
gastrointestinal obstruction or acute painful conditions of the abdomen
or by babies in napkins.
Proprietary preparations: Ailax (suspension); Ailax Forte (a strong
suspension); Codalax (suspension); Codalax Forte (a strong suspension).

co-danthrusate A mixture of *danthron <dantron> and *docusate
sodium, used as a stimulant laxative and faecal softener for the treatment
of constipation in elderly patients and in those with heart failure or

coronary thrombosis and constipation caused by analgesics in terminally ill patients. Co-danthrusate is available as capsules or a suspension on *prescription only.

Side effects: *see* DANTHRON <DANTRON>.

Precautions: co-danthrusate should not be taken by people with intestinal obstruction and should be used with caution by women who are pregnant or breastfeeding.

Proprietary preparations: Capsuvac; Normax.

codeine A weak *opioid that is usually used for the relief of mild to moderate pain and is an ingredient in many *analgesic medications. It is also used as a *cough suppressant, being included in many cough medicines. Codeine slows down the movements of the intestines, causing constipation, and is therefore used as an *antidiarrhoeal drug. Codeine hydrochloride and codeine phosphate are available as tablets, a linctus, or a solution for injection. At lower dosages codeine is available without a prescription, but only from pharmacies; at higher dosages and as a form for injection it is available on *prescription only. *See also* CO-CODAMOL; CO-CODAPRIN.

Side effects: constipation is the most common side effect. In therapeutic doses codeine is unlikely to produce the other adverse effects associated with opioids, such as nausea, vomiting, and drowsiness, although respiratory depression can occur in sensitive individuals. Dependence is unusual.

Precautions: cough suppressants and antidiarrhoeal preparations are generally not recommended for children. Cough suppressants should be used with caution by people with asthma, and antidiarrhoeal preparations should not be used in acute conditions or when abdominal distension is present.

Interactions with other drugs: *see* OPIOIDS.

Proprietary preparations: Galcodeine and Galcodeine Paediatric (liquids); ASPAV (combined with aspirin and papaveretum); BENYLIN WITH CODEINE (combined with diphenhydramine and menthol); BOOTS CATARRH COUGH SYRUP (combined with creosote); BOOTS MIGRAINE RELIEF (combined with paracetamol); BOOTS TENSION HEADACHE RELIEF (combined with paracetamol, caffeine, and doxylamine); CODAFEN CONTINUS (combined with ibuprofen); CODANIN (combined with paracetamol); CODIS 500 (combined with aspirin); DIARREST (combined with dicyclomine <dicycloverine> hydrochloride, potassium chloride, sodium chloride, and sodium citrate); DIMOTANE CO (combined with brompheniramine and pseudoephedrine); FAMEL ORIGINAL (combined with creosote); FEMINAX (combined with caffeine, hyoscine, and paracetamol); KAODENE (combined with kaolin); Kapake (*see* CO-CODAMOL); MIGRALEVE (combined with buclizine hydrochloride and/or paracetamol); Panadeine (*see* CO-CODAMOL); PANADOL ULTRA (combined with paracetamol); Paracodol (*see* CO-CODAMOL); Parake (*see* CO-CODAMOL); PROPAIN (combined with caffeine, diphenhydramine, and paracetamol); PULMO BAILLY (combined with guaiacol); ROBITUSSIN NIGHT-TIME (combined with brompheniramine and pseudoephedrine); SOLPADEINE (combined with caffeine and paracetamol); Solpadol (see CO-CODAMOL); SYNDOL (combined with caffeine, doxylamine, and paracetamol); Tylex (see CO-CODAMOL); UNIFLU WITH GREGOVITE C (combined with diphenhydramine, paracetamol, and phenylephrine); VEGANIN (combined with aspirin and paracetamol).

co-dergocrine mesylate <co-dergocrine mesilate> An *alkaloid used as an *adjunct in the treatment of elderly patients with mild to moderate dementia. It is claimed to improve mental functioning by increasing blood flow to the brain, but its efficacy in dementia has not been proved. Co-dergocrine mesylate is available as tablets on *prescription only.
Side effects: include nausea, vomiting, flushes, rash, and nasal congestion.
Precautions: co-dergocrine should be used with caution in patients with severe bradycardia (slowing of the heart).
Proprietary preparation: Hydergine.

Codis 500 (Reckitt & Colman) A proprietary combination of *aspirin (an analgesic and antipyretic) and *codeine (an opioid analgesic), used for the treatment of mild to moderate pain (including headache, neuralgia, toothache, and period pains) and fever and to relieve the symptoms of influenza and colds. It is freely available *over the counter as dispersible tablets.
Side effects: see ASPIRIN; CODEINE.
Precautions: these tablets should not be given to children, except on medical advice. *See also* ASPIRIN; OPIOIDS.
Interactions with other drugs: see ASPIRIN; OPIOIDS.

co-dydramol A mixture of *paracetamol (a non-opioid analgesic) and *dihydrocodeine tartrate (a weak opioid analgesic), used for the relief of mild to moderate pain. It is available as tablets on *prescription only.
Side effects and precautions: see PARACETAMOL; MORPHINE. Co-dydramol is not recommended for children.
Interactions with other drugs: see OPIOIDS.
Proprietary preparation: Galake.

co-fluampicil A mixture of *ampicillin and *flucloxacillin (both broad-spectrum *antibiotics), used for the treatment of infections caused by more than one type of bacterium (e.g. skin infections) when the exact type of bacterium is unknown. It is available, on *prescription only, as capsules, a syrup, and as a solution for injection.
Side effects, precautions, and interactions with other drugs: see AMPICILLIN; FLUCLOXACILLIN.
Proprietary preparations: Flu-Amp; Magnapen.

co-flumactone A mixture of *spironolactone (a potassium-sparing diuretic) and *hydroflumethiazide (a thiazide diuretic), used to treat congestive *heart failure. It is available as tablets on *prescription only.

Side effects, precautions, and interactions with other drugs: see POTASSIUM-SPARING DIURETICS; THIAZIDE DIURETICS.

Proprietary preparations: Aldactide 25; Aldactide 50 (higher-strength tablets).

Cogentin (Merck Sharp & Dohme) *See* BENZTROPINE MESYLATE <BENZATROPINE MESILATE>.

Colazide (AstraZeneca) *See* BALSALAZIDE SODIUM.

colchicine A drug that is used for the treatment of acute attacks of gout and to prevent attacks of gout in people who are taking *allopurinol. It is usually given to people who have been unable to tolerate *NSAIDs. Unlike NSAIDs, colchicine does not cause fluid retention, and can therefore be taken by people with heart failure. However, its use is limited because it has toxic effects at higher dosages (see below). Colchicine is available as tablets on *prescription only.

Side effects: nausea, vomiting, and abdominal pain are the most common effects; high doses can cause profuse diarrhoea, gastrointestinal bleeding, rashes, and damage to the kidneys and liver.

Precautions: colchicine should not be taken by women who are pregnant or breastfeeding and should be used with caution in the elderly and in people with heart, liver, or kidney disease.

Interactions with other drugs:

  Cyclosporin: the risk of kidney and muscle damage is increased if cyclosporin is taken with colchicine.

Coldrex Blackcurrant Powders, **Coldrex Hot Lemon Powders** (Schering Health Care) Proprietary combinations of *paracetamol (an analgesic and antipyretic) and *phenylephrine (a decongestant), used to relieve the symptoms of colds and influenza. They are available without a prescription.

Side effects, precautions, and interactions with other drugs: see PARACETAMOL; PHENYLEPHRINE.

Coldrex Tablets (Schering Health Care) A proprietary combination of *paracetamol (an analgesic and antipyretic), *caffeine (a stimulant), and *phenylephrine (a decongestant), used to relieve the symptoms of colds and influenza. It is freely available *over the counter.

Side effects: see PHENYLEPHRINE; CAFFEINE.

Precautions and interactions with other drugs: see PARACETAMOL; PHENYLEPHRINE.

colecalciferol *See* CHOLECALCIFEROL.

Colestid (Pharmacia & Upjohn) *See* COLESTIPOL.

colestipol A *bile-acid sequestrant that is used to lower plasma *cholesterol in the treatment of certain types of *hyperlipidaemia. It is available, on *prescription only, as granules or a powder to be dissolved in liquid.

Side effects, precautions, and interactions with other drugs: see BILE-ACID SEQUESTRANTS.

Proprietary preparation: Colestid.

colestyramine *See* CHOLESTYRAMINE.

colfosceril palmitate A synthetic pulmonary *surfactant that is used to treat breathing difficulties in premature babies who are receiving mechanical ventilation (*see* VENTILATOR). It is also used to prevent breathing problems in premature babies. Colfosceril is available, on *prescription only, as a suspension that is administered through a tube placed in the trachea (windpipe).

Side effects: colfosceril may cause bleeding in the lungs and the secretion of mucus that can obstruct the tube.

Precautions: constant monitoring of heart rate and blood gases is necessary during treatment as colfosceril can cause a rapid improvement in the baby's condition and high concentrations of oxygen in the tissues have toxic effects.

Proprietary preparation: Exosurf Neonatal.

Colifoam (Stafford-Miller) *See* HYDROCORTISONE.

colistin An *antibiotic that is applied topically as a solution to treat skin infections, burns, and wounds. It is not absorbed from the gut but may be taken orally in the form of tablets, syrup, or a suspension to sterilize the bowel before surgery. It can also be inhaled via a *nebulizer as an *adjunct to standard antibiotics. Although available as an injection, it is very toxic by this route and therefore rarely used. Colistin is available on *prescription only.

Side effects: include numbness around the mouth, vertigo, muscle weakness, breathlessness, and kidney damage. Rare side effects are slurred speech, visual disturbances, and confusion.

Precautions: colistin should not be taken by people with myasthenia gravis or by women who are pregnant or breastfeeding. It should be used with caution in people who have kidney disease or porphyria.

Interactions with other drugs: see GENTAMICIN.

Proprietary preparation: Colomycin.

collodion A syrupy solution of nitrocellulose in a mixture of alcohol and ether. When applied to the surface of the body it evaporates to leave a thin clear transparent skin, useful for the protection of minor wounds. Flexible collodion also contains camphor and castor oil, which allow the skin to stretch a little more.

Colofac (Solvay Healthcare) *See* MEBEVERINE HYDROCHLORIDE.

Colomycin (Pharmax) *See* COLISTIN.

Colpermin (Pharmacia & Upjohn) *See* PEPPERMINT OIL.

co-magaldrox A mixture of *aluminium hydroxide and *magnesium hydroxide, used as an *antacid for the relief of digestive disorders (*see* ACID-PEPTIC DISEASES). It is freely available *over the counter in the form of a suspension or tablets.
Side effects and interactions with other drugs: see ANTACIDS.
Precautions: see ALUMINIUM HYDROXIDE; MAGNESIUM SALTS.
Proprietary preparations: Maalox (sugar-free suspension); Maalox TC (tablets or sugar-free suspension); Mucogel (sugar-free suspension).

Combivent (Boehringer Ingelheim) A proprietary combination of the bronchodilators *salbutamol (a sympathomimetic drug) and *ipratropium bromide (an antimuscarinic drug), used to relieve constriction of the airways associated with chronic bronchitis or emphysema. It is available as a metered-dose aerosol *inhaler; **Combivent UDV** is a solution for use in a *nebulizer. Both preparations are *prescription only medicines.
Side effects, precautions, and interactions with other drugs: see SALBUTAMOL; IPRATROPIUM BROMIDE.

Combivir (GlaxoWellcome) A proprietary combination of the antiviral drugs *zidovudine and *lamivudine, used to delay the progression of disease in *HIV-infected patients. It is available as tablets on *prescription only.
Side effects, precautions, and interactions with other drugs: see ZIDOVUDINE; LAMIVUDINE.

co-methiamol *See* PARADOTE.

Comixco (Ashbourne Pharmaceuticals) *See* CO-TRIMOXAZOLE.

compound gentian infusion A liquid obtained from the root of the plant *Gentiana lutea*. It is used in *tonics to stimulate the appetite (*see* GENTIAN MIXTURE) and is also an ingredient in homeopathic medicines.
Proprietary preparation: EFFICO (combined with nicotinamide, caffeine, and thiamine).

Comtess (Orion Pharma) *See* ENTACAPONE.

Concordin (Merck Sharp & Dohme) *See* PROTRIPTYLINE HYDROCHLORIDE.

Condrotec (Searle) A proprietary combination of *naproxen (an NSAID) and *misoprostol (a prostaglandin analogue), used for the treatment of rheumatoid arthritis, osteoarthritis, and ankylosing spondylitis; the misoprostil is added to prevent the bleeding and ulceration of stomach or duodenum that may result from the use of naproxen alone. Condrotec is available as tablets on *prescription only.

Side effects and precautions: see NSAIDS; MISOPROSTOL.
Interactions with other drugs: see NSAIDS.

Condyline (Nycomed Amersham) *See* PODOPHYLLOTOXIN.

congestive heart failure *See* HEART FAILURE.

Conotrane (Yamanouchi Pharma) A proprietary combination of *benzalkonium chloride (an antiseptic) and *dimethicone <dimeticone> (a water repellent), used in the form of a cream as a *barrier preparation for the treatment of napkin rash and pressure sores. It is freely available *over the counter.

Contac 400 (SmithKline Beecham Consumer Healthcare) A proprietary combination of *phenylpropanolamine (a decongestant) and *chlorpheniramine <chlorphenamine> (an antihistamine), used for the relief of nasal congestion and other symptoms of colds, hay fever, and sinusitis. It is available as capsules without a prescription, but only from pharmacies.

Side effects and interactions with other drugs: see ANTIHISTAMINES; EPHEDRINE HYDROCHLORIDE.
Precautions: this medicine is not recommended for children. *See also* ANTIHISTAMINES; EPHEDRINE HYDROCHLORIDE.

Contac CoughCaps (SmithKline Beecham Consumer Healthcare) *See* DEXTROMETHORPHAN.

Contimin (APS-Berk) *See* OXYBUTYNIN HYDROCHLORIDE.

continuous-release preparation *See* MODIFIED-RELEASE PREPARATION.

contraceptives *See* DEPOT CONTRACEPTIVES; ORAL CONTRACEPTIVES.

Contraflam (APS-Berk) *See* MEFENAMIC ACID.

controlled drugs Drugs that can only be prescribed under the guidelines of the Misuse of Drugs Act (1971) and Regulations (1973, 1985). These are usually drugs that have the potential for *dependence and abuse and they are divided into three classes; the most serious drugs of addiction (class A) include *cocaine, *diamorphine (heroin), *morphine, and the synthetic *opioids. The Regulations specify the categories of persons who may supply these drugs and lay down rules for writing prescriptions (including the requirement that the prescription must be in the prescriber's own handwriting). There are also regulations relating to manufacture, supply, and record keeping.

Convulex (Pharmacia & Upjohn) *See* VALPROIC ACID.

co-phenotrope A mixture of diphenoxylate hydrochloride (an *opioid that reduces gut motility) and *atropine sulphate (an antispasmodic drug), used for the treatment of diarrhoea (*see* ANTIDIARRHOEAL DRUGS). It is available as tablets on *prescription only.

Side effects: include allergic skin reactions and abdominal cramp and bloating. *See also* ANTIMUSCARINIC DRUGS; OPIOIDS.

Precautions: co-phenotrope should not be used by people with intestinal obstruction, acute ulcerative colitis, antibiotic-induced colitis, or jaundice. It should not be taken until severe dehydration or *electrolyte imbalance has been corrected.

Proprietary preparations: Diarphen; Lomotil; Tropergen.

Coppertone (Seton Scholl Healthcare) A proprietary *sunscreen preparation consisting of a cream containing ethylhexyl *p*-methoxycinnamate, oxybenzone, and padimate-O. It protects against both UVA and UVB (SPF 23) and can be prescribed on the NHS or obtained without a prescription.

co-proxamol A mixture of *paracetamol (a non-opioid analgesic) and *dextropropoxyphene hydrochloride (a weak opioid analgesic), used for the relief of mild to moderate pain. It is available as tablets on *prescription only.

Side effects and precautions: overdosage with co-proxamol can cause respiratory depression and heart failure (due to dextropropoxyphene) and liver damage (due to paracetamol), which requires rapid emergency treatment. Co-proxamol should therefore not be given to those who are suicidal or otherwise at risk. It is not recommended for children, and the dosage should be reduced for elderly people.

Interactions with other drugs: see DEXTROPROPOXYPHENE HYDROCHLORIDE; OPIOIDS.

Proprietary preparations: Cosalgesic; Distalgesic.

Coracten (Medeva) *See* NIFEDIPINE.

Cordarone X (Sanofi Winthrop) *See* AMIODARONE.

Cordilox (Norton Healthcare) *See* VERAPAMIL HYDROCHLORIDE.

Corgard (Sanofi Winthrop) *See* NADOLOL.

Corgaretic 40, **Corgaretic 80** (Sanofi Winthrop) Proprietary combinations of *nadolol (a beta blocker) and *bendrofluazide

<bendroflumethiazide> (a thiazide diuretic), used in the treatment of
*hypertension. It is available as tablets on *prescription only.
Side effects, precautions, and interactions with other drugs: see BETA
BLOCKERS; THIAZIDE DIURETICS.
See also ANTIHYPERTENSIVE DRUGS; DIURETICS.

Corlan (Medeva) *See* HYDROCORTISONE.

Corn and Callus Removal Liquid (Seton Scholl Healthcare) A
proprietary combination of *salicylic acid (a keratolytic) and *camphor,
used for the treatment of corns and calluses. It is freely available *over
the counter.
Precautions: this preparation is not recommended for children.

Corn Removal Pads, **Corn Removal Plasters** (Seton Scholl
Healthcare) *See* SALICYLIC ACID.

Coroday MR (Generics) *See* NIFEDIPINE.

Coro-Nitro Pump Spray (Roche Products) *See* GLYCERYL TRINITRATE.

Corsodyl (SmithKline Beecham Consumer Healthcare) *See*
CHLORHEXIDINE.

corticosteroids Steroid hormones that are secreted by the outer layer
(cortex) of the adrenal glands, or semisynthetic substances that closely
resemble the natural products. There are two main types of
corticosteroids: **mineralocorticoids** and **glucocorticoids**
Mineralocorticoids (e.g. aldosterone) assist in the maintenance of salt and
water balance. Glucocorticoids (e.g. cortisol, cortisone) affect the
metabolism of glucose, protein, and fat and inhibit inflammation.
   Synthetic mineralocorticoids (e.g. *fludrocortisone acetate) are used for
replacement therapy in people who lack the natural hormone as a result
of disease or surgical removal of the adrenal glands. Drugs with
glucocorticoid activity (e.g. *hydrocortisone, *betamethasone,
*prednisolone) may be used as replacement therapy but are more
commonly employed for their anti-inflammatory activity. They are used
to treat a wide range of inflammatory conditions, including asthma,
rheumatoid arthritis, inflammatory bowel disease (e.g. Crohn's disease,
ulcerative colitis), and connective tissue disorders (such as systemic lupus
erythematosus). They are also included in the therapy for some cancers
and to prevent the rejection of organ and tissue transplants (*see*
IMMUNOSUPPRESSANTS). Corticosteroids may be given by mouth or
intravenous injection. They can be applied topically for the treatment of
inflammatory conditions of the skin, eyes, ears, and nose (*see* TOPICAL
STEROIDS). They may also be administered in enemas, by direct injection
into joints or around tendons, or by inhalation. Inhaled steroids are used
for the prevention of *asthma attacks; they must be inhaled regularly,
even when no symptoms are present.

Because the concentration of corticosteroids required to produce anti-inflammatory activity is higher than that normally present in the body, corticosteroid therapy can have adverse effects on metabolism. When given in high doses or during long-term treatment, *systemic corticosteroids are associated with a number of side effects (see below). Steroids administered locally or topically have, in general, fewer and less serious side effects: the severity of these will depend on the strength of the steroid, the area of the body that is exposed to the steroid, and the duration of treatment. Long-term use of systemic corticosteroids leads to adrenal suppression, in which the adrenal glands fail to produce the normal amount of hormones. For this reason, withdrawal of treatment after long-term use must always be gradual; sudden withdrawal can lead to severe lowering of the blood pressure and may even be fatal. Increased amounts of corticosteroids are normally produced by the adrenal glands in response to stress (e.g. injury, surgery, or infection). Because normal production is suppressed in those taking long-term corticosteroid therapy, increased doses must be given to cope with episodes of stress.

See also BECLOMETHASONE <BECLOMETASONE> DIPROPIONATE; BUDESONIDE; DEFLAZACORT; DEXAMETHASONE; FLUNISOLIDE; FLUTICASONE PROPIONATE; METHYLPREDNISOLONE; TRIAMCINOLONE ACETONIDE.

Side effects: long-term use of systemic corticosteroids in high doses can lead to decreased activity of the immune system and susceptibility to infection; the inflammatory response is reduced, which can mask signs of infection. Disturbance in calcium metabolism results in loss of bone tissue, which can retard growth in children and exacerbate osteoporosis in adults. Salt and water balance is affected, especially with mineralocorticoids, resulting in retention of *sodium and water (and loss of *potassium), with consequent fluid retention and high blood pressure. Glucocorticoids also affect protein metabolism, causing muscle weakness and thinning of the skin, with delayed wound healing and stretch marks (striae); glucose metabolism, resulting in diabetes mellitus; and the metabolism of fat, which is deposited in the face ('moon face'), on the shoulders ('buffalo hump'), and in the abdomen. These signs of excess glucocorticoids are sometimes called 'Cushingoid features'. Long-term use of steroids leads to adrenal suppression, in which the response to stress is reduced (see above). Other side effects include indigestion (which is common) and possibly peptic ulceration; increased appetite and weight gain; acne; increased growth of facial and body hair; mood changes, ranging from euphoria to depression and paranoia; insomnia; and menstrual irregularities. Inhaled steroids commonly cause hoarseness or huskiness of the voice, due to weakening of the vocal muscles, and a sore throat, due to fungal (*Candida*) infection. Rinsing the mouth out after each inhaled dose helps to prevent the latter complication. *See also* TOPICAL STEROIDS.

Precautions: people taking steroids should always mention this fact to their doctor, dentist, or chiropodist when undergoing other treatment. People taking corticosteroids by mouth for more than one month are advised to carry a warning card; higher doses may be required during periods of illness or stress. Withdrawal of treatment after long-term use should be gradual (see above). Corticosteroids should not be taken by people with systemic infections unless active treatment of the infection is given at the same time. People taking systemic corticosteroids for purposes other than replacement therapy should avoid contact with those suffering from chickenpox or shingles while taking the steroids and up to three months after treatment; anyone taking systemic steroids who has been in close contact with someone suffering from chickenpox should see a doctor. People taking high doses of corticosteroids systemically should not be given vaccinations with live vaccines. Corticosteroids reduce the effect of insulin and care must be taken by people with diabetes. Dosage may need to be reduced in the elderly, in whom side effects may be more pronounced. Corticosteroids should be used with caution during pregnancy.

Interactions with other drugs (systemic corticosteroids):

Antidiabetic drugs: their effect is reduced to a small extent.

Antiepileptics: carbamazepine, phenobarbitone <phenobarbital>, phenytoin, and primidone reduce the effects of corticosteroids.

Antihypertensive drugs: their effect in lowering blood pressure is antagonized.

Digoxin: there is an increased risk of toxicity from digoxin if plasma potassium concentrations fall.

Diuretics: there is an increased risk of reduced plasma potassium concentrations, and steroids (especially mineralocorticoids) tend to cause water retention.

Rifampicin: reduces the effects of corticosteroids.

cortisol *See* CORTICOSTEROIDS; HYDROCORTISONE.

cortisone acetate A *corticosteroid used mainly as replacement therapy when the adrenal glands are functioning poorly or have been surgically removed. It is available as tablets on *prescription only.
Side effects, precautions, and interactions with other drugs: see CORTICOSTEROIDS.
Proprietary preparation: Cortisyl.

Cortisyl (Hoechst Marion Roussel) *See* CORTISONE ACETATE.

Corwin (AstraZeneca) *See* XAMOTEROL.

Cosalgesic (Cox Pharmaceuticals) *See* CO-PROXAMOL.

co-simalcite *See* ALTACITE PLUS.

Cosmegen Lyovac (Merck Sharp & Dohme) *See* DACTINOMYCIN.

Cosopt (Merck Sharp & Dohme) A proprietary combination of *dorzolamide (a carbonic anhydrase inhibitor) and *timolol maleate (a beta blocker), used for the treatment of chronic (open-angle) *glaucoma that has not responded to beta blockers alone. It is available as eye drops on *prescription only.

Side effects, precautions, and interactions with other drugs: see DORZOLAMIDE; BETA BLOCKERS.

Cosuric (DDSA Pharmaceuticals) *See* ALLOPURINOL.

co-tenidone A mixture of *atenolol (a cardioselective beta blocker) and *chlorthalidone <chlortalidone> (a thiazide diuretic), used for the treatment of *hypertension. It is available as tablets on *prescription only.

Side effects, precautions, and interactions with other drugs: see BETA BLOCKERS; THIAZIDE DIURETICS.

Proprietary preparations: Atenix-Co; Tenchlor; Tenoret 50; Tenoretic (contains twice the amount of atenolol as Tenoret 50); Totaretic.

See also ANTIHYPERTENSIVE DRUGS; DIURETICS.

co-trimoxazole A mixture of *trimethoprim (an antibacterial drug) and sulphamethoxazole <sulfamethoxazole> (a *sulphonamide antibiotic) in the proportions 1:5; the effect of this combination is greater than the sum of the effects of its two constituent drugs given singly. It is the drug of choice for treating pneumonia caused by *Pneumocystis carinii*; it is also used to treat toxoplasmosis (a protozoal disease that can cause blindness and mental retardation in a fetus) and nocardiasis (a bacterial infection of the lungs, skin, and brain, causing abscesses). Co-trimoxazole is available, on *prescription only, as tablets, dispersible tablets, a suspension, or a paediatric syrup for oral use and as a solution for intravenous infusion.

Side effects: include nausea, vomiting, rash, and blood disorders; if the last two effects occur, the treatment should be discontinued immediately. More rarely, allergic reactions, diarrhoea, sore mouth, loss of appetite, and muscle and joint pains may occur.

Precautions: co-trimoxazole should not be taken by patients with liver or kidney failure or porphyria, and it should be used with caution in those who have impaired liver or kidney function or blood disorders and in women who are pregnant or breastfeeding.

Interactions with other drugs:

Anticoagulants: the effects of warfarin and nicoumalone <acenocoumarol> are increased.

Cyclosporin: there is an increased risk of adverse effects on the kidneys.

Methotrexate: the effect of this drug is increased.

Phenytoin: the plasma concentration of this drug is increased.

Pyrimethamine: there is an increased risk of folate deficiency, which may lead to megaloblastic anaemia.

Sulphonylureas: the effects of these oral antidiabetic drugs are enhanced.

Proprietary preparations: Chemotrim Paediatric; Comixco; Fectrim; Fectrim Forte; Septrin.

cough suppressants (antitussives) Drugs that act on the brain to suppress the cough reflex; they do not treat the underlying cause of the coughing. Cough suppressants are used to relieve dry persistent coughs. The most commonly used drugs are *dextromethorphan, *codeine, and *pholcodine, all of which are *opioids; they tend to cause constipation. *See also* EXPECTORANTS; DEMULCENTS.

counterirritants *See* RUBEFACIENTS.

Coversyl (Servier Laboratories) *See* PERINDOPRIL.

Covonia Bronchial Balsam (Thornton & Ross) A proprietary combination of *dextromethorphan (a cough suppressant) and *menthol, used for the relief of dry coughs, such as those associated with colds and bronchitis. It is available as a syrup without a prescription, but only from pharmacies.
Side effects and interactions with other drugs: see DEXTROMETHORPHAN; OPIOIDS.
Precautions: this medicine is not recommended for children under six years old. *See also* OPIOIDS.

Covonia Night Time Formula (Thornton & Ross) A proprietary combination of *dextromethorphan (a cough suppressant) and *diphenhydramine (a sedative antihistamine), used to relieve dry coughs that interfere with sleep. It is available as a syrup without a prescription, but only from pharmacies.
Side effects and interactions with other drugs: see DEXTROMETHORPHAN; OPIOIDS.
Precautions: this medicine is not recommended for children. *See also* OPIOIDS.

Cozaar (Merck Sharp & Dohme) *See* LOSARTAN POTASSIUM.

Cozaar-Comp (Merck Sharp & Dohme) A proprietary combination of *losartan potassium (an angiotensin II inhibitor) and *hydrochlorothiazide (a thiazide diuretic), used in the treatment of *hypertension. It is available as tablets on *prescription only.
Side effects, precautions, and interactions with other drugs: see ANGIOTENSIN II INHIBITORS; THIAZIDE DIURETICS.
See also ANTIHYPERTENSIVE DRUGS; DIURETICS.

Crampex (Seton Scholl Healthcare) A proprietary combination of *nicotinic acid, vitamin D$_3$ (*see* CHOLECALCIFEROL <COLECALCIFEROL>), and *calcium gluconate, used for the relief of muscle cramps at night. It is available as tablets that can be obtained without a prescription, but only from pharmacies.
Precautions: Crampex is not recommended for children.

cream A medicinal preparation consisting of an oil-in-water emulsion that is applied to the skin. Less greasy than *ointments and easier to apply, creams are usually readily absorbed into the skin. *See* EMOLLIENTS.

Cremalgin (Co-Pharma) A proprietary combination of the rubefacients *capsicum oleoresin, *glycol salicylate, and *methyl nicotinate in the form of a cream, used for the relief of muscular and rheumatic pains and stiffness, including backache, sciatica, lumbago, and fibrositis. It is freely available *over the counter.
Side effects and precautions: see RUBEFACIENTS.

Creon, Creon 10 000, Creon 25 000 (Solvay Healthcare) *See* PANCREATIN.

cretinism *See* THYROID HORMONES.

Crinone (Wyeth Laboratories) *See* PROGESTERONE.

crisantaspase An enzyme preparation (asparaginase) used as a *cytotoxic drug for the treatment of acute lymphoblastic leukaemia (*see* CANCER). It is given by intramuscular or subcutaneous injection in specialist units and is available on *prescription only.
Side effects: include nausea, vomiting, depression of central nervous activity, and changes in liver function and blood lipids (fats); severe allergic reactions (*see* ANAPHYLAXIS) may occur. *See also* CYTOTOXIC DRUGS.
Precautions: tests for liver function, blood lipids, and concentrations of glucose in the urine should be performed throughout treatment. *See also* CYTOTOXIC DRUGS.
Proprietary preparation: Erwinase.

Crixivan (Merck Sharp & Dohme) *See* INDINAVIR.

Cromogen (Norton Healthcare) *See* SODIUM CROMOGLYCATE <CROMOGLICATE>.

cromoglicate *See* SODIUM CROMOGLYCATE <CROMOGLICATE>.

cromoglycate <cromoglicate> *See* SODIUM CROMOGLYCATE <CROMOGLICATE>.

crotamiton A drug that is used to relieve itching, including that associated with *scabies. It is freely available *over the counter in the form of a cream or lotion.
Precautions: crotamiton should not be used to treat weeping skin conditions. It should not be used near the eyes or on broken skin.
Proprietary preparations: Eurax; Eurax Lotion.

Crystacide (Medeva) *See* HYDROGEN PEROXIDE.

crystal violet (gentian violet, methyl violet, methylrosanilinium chloride) A purple dye that has *antiseptic properties. Diluted in purified water, it is used to disinfect unbroken skin in the treatment of burns, boils, and minor bacterial or fungal infections. It is also used to cleanse the skin before surgery. Crystal violet is available as a paint that can be obtained without a prescription, but only from pharmacies.
Side effects and precautions: crystal violet should not be applied to mucous membranes (because it causes ulceration) or to open wounds. It stains skin and clothing.

Crystapen (Britannia Pharmaceuticals) *See* BENZYLPENICILLIN.

Cultivate (GlaxoWellcome) *See* FLUTICASONE PROPIONATE.

Cuplex (Smith & Nephew Healthcare) A proprietary combination of *salicylic acid and *lactic acid (keratolytics) and copper acetate (an astringent), used for the treatment of warts, verrucas, corns, and calluses. It is available as a gel and can be obtained without a prescription, but only from pharmacies.
Side effects and precautions: see SALICYLIC ACID.

Cuprofen, Cuprofen Ibutop Gel, Cuprofen Maximum Strength (Seton Scholl Healthcare) *See* IBUPROFEN.

Curatoderm (Crookes Healthcare) *See* TACALCITOL.

Curosurf (Serono Laboratories) *See* PORACTANT ALFA.

Cuxson Gerrard Belladonna Plasters (Cuxson, Gerrard & Co) *See* BELLADONNA EXTRACT.

CX Powder (Adams Healthcare) *See* CHLORHEXIDINE.

cyanocobalamin A form of vitamin B_{12} (*see* VITAMIN B COMPLEX) that is used to treat or prevent deficiency of this vitamin (such as occurs in strict vegetarians). For treating pernicious anaemia, cyanocobalamin has been replaced by *hydroxocobalamin. Cyanocobalamin is available as tablets or a liquid, which can be obtained from pharmacies without a prescription, or as an injection, which is available on *prescription only.
Side effects: cyanocobalamin may rarely cause allergic reactions.
Proprietary preparations: Cytacon; Cytamen (injection).

Cyclimorph (GlaxoWellcome) A proprietary combination of *morphine tartrate (an opioid analgesic) and *cyclizine tartrate (an antiemetic antihistamine). It is used for the treatment of moderate to severe pain; the cyclizine is included to prevent the nausea and vomiting associated with opioids. Cyclimorph is available as an injection; it is a *controlled drug.

Side effects: include drowsiness, dry mouth, blurred vision, and dependence (*see* MORPHINE).

Precautions: Cyclimorph is not recommended for terminally ill patients. In people who have had a heart attack it may aggravate severe heart failure.

Interactions with other drugs: see ANTIHISTAMINES; OPIOIDS.

cyclizine An *antihistamine used for the treatment of nausea, vomiting, vertigo, motion sickness, and disorders of the inner ear affecting balance. When used alone, it is available as tablets without a prescription.

Side effects: drowsiness is the most common side effect; dry mouth and blurred vision may occasionally occur (*see* ANTIHISTAMINES).

Precautions and interactions with other drugs: see ANTIHISTAMINES.

Proprietary preparations: Valoid; CYCLIMORPH (combined with morphine); DICONAL (combined with dipipanone); FEMIGRAINE (combined with aspirin); MIGRIL (combined with ergotamine).

Cyclodox (APS-Berk) *See* DOXYCYCLINE.

Cyclogest (Shire Pharmaceuticals) *See* PROGESTERONE.

Cyclomin (APS-Berk) *See* MINOCYCLINE.

cyclopenthiazide A *thiazide diuretic used for the treatment of *hypertension and *oedema associated with heart failure, liver disease, or kidney disease. It is available as tablets on *prescription only.

Side effects, precautions, and interactions with other drugs: see THIAZIDE DIURETICS.

Proprietary preparations: Navidrex; NAVISPARE (combined with amiloride hydrochloride); TRASIDREX (combined with oxprenolol).

See also ANTIHYPERTENSIVE DRUGS; DIURETICS.

cyclopentolate hydrochloride An *antimuscarinic drug that is applied to the eye before examination of the interior in order to dilate the pupil and paralyse the ciliary muscles (which control the focusing ability of the eye). It is particularly useful for examining the eyes of young children. Cyclopentolate is available as eye drops on *prescription only.

Side effects: cyclopentolate may cause transient stinging and an increase in pressure in the eye; with prolonged use, local irritation and conjunctivitis can occur. Systemic effects may occur in very young children and elderly people (*see* ANTIMUSCARINIC DRUGS).

Precautions and interactions with other drugs: see ANTIMUSCARINIC DRUGS.

Proprietary preparations: Mydrilate; Minims Cyclopentolate (single-dose eye drops).

cyclophosphamide An *alkylating drug used to treat a wide variety of *cancers. In the body it is converted to phosphoramide mustard (the active agent) and a substance called acrolein. Acrolein can cause irritation and bleeding in the bladder. Cyclophosphamide is therefore often given with *mesna, an agent that binds to acrolein and prevents this problem. Fluid intake must also be increased to reduce the time acrolein is present in the bladder. Cyclophosphamide may be given intravenously or as tablets and is available on *prescription only.

Side effects: include nausea and vomiting (which are more severe when the drug is given intravenously), hair loss, *bone marrow suppression, blood in the urine, lack of periods in women, and decreased fertility in men. Cyclophosphamide can also have adverse effects on the heart. *See also* CYTOTOXIC DRUGS.

Precautions: cyclophosphamide should not be taken by people who are already passing blood in their urine, by those who have a urinary-tract infection or porphyria, or by women who are pregnant or breastfeeding. *See also* CYTOTOXIC DRUGS.

Interactions with other drugs:

Allopurinol: may enhance bone marrow suppression.

Antidiabetic drugs: their control of diabetes can be disturbed in people given cyclophosphamide.

Proprietary preparation: Endoxana.

Cyclo-Progynova 1 mg (ASTA Medica) A proprietary preparation of *oestradiol <estradiol> (1-milligram tablets) and combined oestradiol (1 mg)/*levonorgestrel tablets used as sequential combined *hormone replacement therapy for the relief of menopausal symptoms in women who have not had a hysterectomy. **Cyclo-Progynova 2 mg**, in which the tablets contain 2 milligrams of oestradiol <estradiol>, also provides protection against osteoporosis. Both preparations are available on *prescription only and the tablets must be taken in the prescribed order.

Side effects, precautions, and interactions with other drugs: see HORMONE REPLACEMENT THERAPY.

cycloserine A drug that is used in combination with other drugs for the treatment of *tuberculosis that is resistant to the standard therapy. It is available as capsules on *prescription only.

Side effects: include headache, dizziness, vertigo, drowsiness, tremor, convulsions, confusion, depression, rashes, and megaloblastic *anaemia.

Precautions: cycloserine should not be taken by people with kidney disease, epilepsy, depression, severe anxiety, psychotic illness, or alcohol dependence (alcohol increases the risk of convulsions).

Interactions with other drugs:

Phenytoin: cycloserine increases the plasma concentration of phenytoin and therefore the risk of side effects associated with it.

cyclosporin An *immunosuppressant drug used to limit rejection after organ or bone-marrow transplant surgery. It is also used for the treatment of active rheumatoid arthritis and certain skin conditions, including atopic *eczema and *psoriasis. Unlike many immunosuppressants, it does not affect the blood-cell-producing capacity of the bone marrow, but it can damage the kidneys. It is available, on *prescription only, as capsules or a solution for oral use and as a form for intravenous infusion.

Side effects: the most common side effects are nausea, gum swelling, excessive hair growth, and tremor; liver and kidney function may be impaired. Other side effects may include diarrhoea, headache, high blood pressure, fluid retention, fatigue, muscle weakness or cramps, burning sensations in the hands and feet, rashes, and itching.

Precautions: kidney function must be monitored closely; liver function and blood pressure should also be monitored. Grapefruit juice can increase the plasma concentration of cyclosporin and therefore increase its toxic effects.

Interactions with other drugs:

ACE inhibitors: increase the risk of high concentrations of *potassium in the blood.

Antibacterial drugs: increase plasma concentrations of cyclosporin.

Antiepileptics: reduce plasma concentrations of cyclosporin.

Antifungal drugs: amphotericin increases the risk of toxic effects on the liver; itraconazole and ketoconazole increase plasma concentrations of cyclosporin.

Calcium antagonists: increase plasma concentrations of cyclosporin.

Cimetidine: may increase plasma concentrations of cyclosporin.

Chloroquine: increases plasma concentrations of cyclosporin (and the risk of toxic effects).

Colchicine: increases plasma concentrations of cyclosporin (and the risk of toxic effects on the kidneys and muscles).

Corticosteroids: increase plasma concentrations of cyclosporin.

Cytotoxic drugs: there is an increased risk of toxic effects with methotrexate, doxorubicin, and melphalan.

Danazol: increases plasma concentrations of cyclosporin.

NSAIDs: increase the risk of toxic effects on the kidneys and liver; cyclosprorin increases plasma concentrations of diclofenac.

Potassium-sparing diuretics: increase the risk of high concentrations of potassium in the blood.

Progestogens: increase plasma concentrations of cyclosporin.

Ritonavir: may increase plasma concentrations of cyclosporin.

Statins: increase the risk of muscle weakness.

Tacrolimus: increases the risk of toxic effects.

Proprietary preparations: Neoral; Sandimmun (available for named patients only).

Cyklokapron (Pharmacia & Upjohn) *See* TRANEXAMIC ACID.

Cymalon (Seton Scholl Healthcare) *See* SODIUM CITRATE.

Cymevene (Roche Products) *See* GANCICLOVIR.

cyproheptadine hydrochloride One of the original (sedating)
*antihistamines, used to relieve the symptoms of such allergic conditions
as hay fever and urticaria (nettle rash). Cyproheptadine also antagonizes
the action of *serotonin and is used for the prevention of *migraine
attacks in people who have not responded to other prophylactic
treatments. It is available as tablets and can be obtained from pharmacies
without a prescription.
Side effects: see ANTIHISTAMINES. Additional side effects may include
weight gain, an increase in appetite, and fatigue.
Precautions and interactions with other drugs: see ANTIHISTAMINES.
Proprietary preparation: Periactin.

Cyprostat (Schering Health Care) *See* CYPROTERONE ACETATE.

cyproterone acetate An *anti-androgen used to treat hypersexuality
and sexual deviation in men; it is also used in the treatment of cancer of
the prostate. Cyproterone produces a temporary infertility. Combined
with ethinyloestradiol <ethinylestradiol>, it is used to treat severe acne in
women. It is available, on *prescription only, as *transdermal (skin)
patches or tablets.
Side effects: include fatigue and lassitude, breathlessness, weight
changes, reduced sebum production, changes in hair pattern, and breast
enlargement. High-dose treatment (for prostate cancer) may cause liver
damage (jaundice, hepatitis).
Precautions: cyproterone should not be taken by people with liver
disease, severe diabetes, sickle-cell anaemia, wasting disease, severe
depression, or a history of thromboembolism or by boys under 18 years
old (except when used for treating prostate cancer).
Proprietary preparations: Androcur; Cyprostat; DIANETTE (combined with
ethinyloestradiol <ethinylestradiol>).

Cystemme (Abbott Laboratories) *See* SODIUM CITRATE.

Cystoleve (Seton Scholl Healthcare) *See* SODIUM CITRATE.

Cystopurin (Roche Products) *See* POTASSIUM CITRATE.

Cystrin (Lorex Synthélabo) *See* OXYBUTYNIN HYDROCHLORIDE.

Cytacon (Goldshield Pharmaceuticals) *See* CYANOCOBALAMIN.

Cytamen (Medeva) *See* CYANOCOBALAMIN.

cytarabine An *antimetabolite that is used predominantly for the

treatment of acute myeloblastic leukaemia but is also used to treat
leukaemias and lymphoma (*see* CANCER). It is available as a solution for
injection on *prescription only.
Side effects and precautions: see CYTOTOXIC DRUGS.
Proprietary preparation: Cytosar.

cytoprotectant Describing the action of certain drugs in protecting
the lining of the stomach. Such drugs act by various mechanisms to form
a barrier between the stomach wall and the acid contents of the stomach,
which relieves the symptoms or prevents the formation of gastric ulcers.
They may increase the secretion of protective mucus in the stomach, or
they may coat the ulcer and thus prevent contact with stomach acid.
Drugs with cytoprotectant actions include *sucralfate, *misoprostol, and
salts of bismuth (including *tripotassium dicitratobismuthate).

Cytosar (Pharmacia & Upjohn) *See* CYTARABINE.

Cytotec (Searle) *See* MISOPROSTOL.

cytotoxic antibiotics A group of antibiotics that are used for the
treatment of *cancer because they interfere with DNA replication and
protein synthesis (*see* CYTOTOXIC DRUGS). They mimic the action of
radiation and should not be used together with radiotherapy. The
common cytotoxic antibiotics are *aclarubicin, *bleomycin,
*dactinomycin, *daunorubicin, *doxorubicin, *epirubicin, *idarubicin,
*mitomycin, and *mitozantrone <mitoxantrone>. With the exception of
bleomycin and mitozantrone, these antibiotics are derived or synthesized
from *Streptomyces* bacteria and are known as **anthracyclines**.

cytotoxic drugs A group of drugs that are toxic to cells and cause cell
death or prevent cell replication. These drugs are used mainly to treat
*cancer, although some have other uses. Cancer treatment with cytotoxic
drugs is known as **chemotherapy** and has a variety of purposes. The
drugs may be used to shrink a tumour before surgery (neoadjuvant
chemotherapy); they may be used after the primary tumour has been
treated with surgery or radiotherapy to prevent the spread and growth of
secondary tumours (adjuvant chemotherapy), or they may be the main
treatment for the disease. Chemotherapy may be given to cure the
disease or, if cure is not possible, to control its symptoms (palliative
chemotherapy). Not every type of cancer responds to cytotoxic drugs, and
some cancers are unresponsive to them (e.g. pancreatic cancer). Because
cytotoxic drugs also attack healthy cells they can cause a variety of
adverse effects, and a balance has to be struck between the likely benefit
and the severity of the adverse effects (see below).
   The main classes of cytotoxic drugs are: *alkylating drugs,
*antimetabolites, *vinca alkaloids, *cytotoxic antibiotics, and a
miscellaneous group, which includes platinum compounds (e.g.
*carboplatin), *taxanes, *topoisomerase inhibitors, *procarbazine,
*crisantaspase, and *hydroxyurea. *Rituximab (a monoclonal antibody)

and *aldesleukin (an interleukin) are recently introduced cytotoxic drugs (*see also* INTERFERONS). Sex hormones are also used to treat cancer. Tumours of the prostate gland are often stimulated by male sex hormones (the androgens) and so these cancers may be treated with *oestrogens (to oppose the androgens) or with *anti-androgens. Analogues of gonadorelin, such as *buserelin, *goserelin, *leuprorelin, and *triptorelin, are also used. Some breast cancers are stimulated by oestrogens; such cancers respond to the *oestrogen antagonists *tamoxifen and *toremifene or to *aromatase inhibitors. Cytotoxic drugs are usually only prescribed by cancer specialists (oncologists) and administered in a hospital. They may be taken by mouth or given by injection or infusion, by specially trained nurses or doctors. Quite often a combination of two, three, or more drugs will be given. The effects of cytotoxic drugs are carefully monitored and blood tests are carried out regularly.

Side effects: the cells most susceptible to the actions of cytotoxic drugs are those that are rapidly dividing: the cells lining the gut, the cells of the mucous membranes, the cells of the bone marrow, and the hair follicles. The resultant side effects are: nausea and vomiting; inflammation and soreness of the mucous membranes (mucositis), especially the mouth; *bone marrow suppression, which will make the patient extremely susceptible to infection (due to loss of white cells) and bleeding (due to loss of platelets); and hair loss. With some drugs, nausea and vomiting can be particularly severe and can last for several days, which may cause patients to refuse further treatment. Some people experience these symptoms when going for their treatment, even before the drugs are administered. It is important, therefore, that people who are likely to be sick are given *antiemetics and have antiemetics to take after they have left hospital. Some drugs, especially the vinca alkaloids, can cause pain and local tissue damage if they leak out (extravasation) during intravenous infusion.

Precautions: most cytotoxic drugs can cause malformations in a fetus and should not be given during pregnancy, although severe circumstances may make this unavoidable. Contraception should be used during treatment by both men and women. Treatment with some drugs may result in irreversible infertility; counselling is necessary, and the possibility of storing sperm or eggs to allow the patient to try to have children at a later date may be discussed.

dacarbazine A *cytotoxic drug used for the treatment of melanoma (a type of skin cancer) and cancers of soft tissue (e.g. muscle). In combination with doxorubicin, bleomycin, and vinblastine, it is also used to treat Hodgkin's disease (*see* CANCER). Dacarbazine is available as a form for intravenous injection on *prescription only.

Side effects: the main side effects are severe nausea and vomiting and *bone marrow suppression. Dacarbazine is irritant to skin and other tissues. *See also* CYTOTOXIC DRUGS.

Precautions: dacarbazine should not be given to people with severely impaired liver or kidney function; the dosage may need to be reduced in people with lesser degrees of impairment. *See also* CYTOTOXIC DRUGS.

Proprietary preparation: DTIC-Dome.

dactinomycin (actinomycin D) A *cytotoxic antibiotic used for the treatment of cancers in children. It is available as a form for intravenous injection on *prescription only.

Side effects: similar to those of *doxorubicin, except that dactinomycin does not have adverse effects on the heart.

Precautions: *see* CYTOTOXIC DRUGS.

Proprietary preparation: Cosmegen Lyovac.

Daktacort (Janssen-Cilag) A proprietary combination of *miconazole (an antifungal drug) and *hydrocortisone (a mild topical steroid), used for the treatment of fungal and bacterial infections accompanied by inflammation. It is available as a cream or ointment on *prescription only.

Side effects, precautions, and interactions with other drugs: *see* MICONAZOLE; TOPICAL STEROIDS.

Daktarin (Janssen-Cilag) *See* MICONAZOLE.

Dalacin, **Dalacin C**, **Dalacin T** (Pharmacia & Upjohn) *See* CLINDAMYCIN.

Dalivit (Eastern Pharmaceuticals) A proprietary combination of *vitamin A, vitamins of the B group (*see* VITAMIN B COMPLEX), *vitamin C, and *vitamin D, used as a multivitamin supplement. It is freely available *over the counter in the form of drops.

Dalmane (Roche Products) *See* FLURAZEPAM.

dalteparin sodium A *low molecular weight heparin used for the prevention and treatment of deep-vein *thrombosis and in the treatment of unstable *angina. It is also used in patients undergoing kidney dialysis, in order to prevent the formation of blood clots. Dalteparin is available as a solution for subcutaneous or intravenous injection on *prescription only.

Side effects, precautions, and interactions with other drugs: *see* HEPARIN.

Proprietary preparation: Fragmin.

danaparoid sodium A *heparinoid used for the prevention of deep-vein *thrombosis in patients undergoing surgery. It may sometimes be used in place of *heparin in those patients who develop low platelet counts as a side effect of heparin therapy, although it does not have a *licence for this purpose. Danaparoid is available as a solution for subcutaneous or intravenous injection on *prescription only.

Side effects, precautions, and interactions with other drugs: *see* HEPARIN.

Proprietary preparation: Orgaran.

danazol A drug that inhibits the release of *gonadotrophins from the pituitary gland and therefore reduces the secretion of oestrogen and progesterone by the ovaries. It is used for the treatment of heavy periods, *endometriosis, severe breast pain associated with periods, breast cysts, and enlargement of the breasts in men. It has also been used for the treatment of hereditary angioedema (*see* ANAPHYLAXIS), although it does not have a *licence for this use. Danazol is available as capsules on *prescription only.

Side effects: include nausea, dizziness, rashes or other skin reactions, fluid retention and weight gain, acne, unusual hair growth or hair loss, voice changes, mood changes, reduction in breast size, backache, flushing, muscle spasm, menstrual disturbances, headache, and emotional upset.

Precautions: danazol should not be taken by women who are pregnant (it must be stopped if pregnancy occurs) or breastfeeding or by women who have severe liver, kidney, or heart disease.

Interactions with other drugs:

Anticoagulants: the effects of warfarin and nicoumalone <acenocoumarol> are enhanced.

Carbamazepine: its side effects are increased.

Cyclosporin: its side effects are increased.

Proprietary preparation: Danol.

Danol (Sanofi Winthrop) *See* DANAZOL.

danthron <dantron> A *stimulant laxative that is used for the prevention and treatment of constipation in the elderly; constipation in terminally ill patients caused by analgesics, especially *opioids; and constipation in people with heart failure and coronary thrombosis, when it is important to avoid straining. Danthron is no longer widely used since animal studies have indicated that it has a potential for causing cancer. A *prescription only medicine, it is available (combined with other laxatives) in the form of capsules or a suspension (*see* CO-DANTHRAMER; CO-DANTHRUSATE).

Side effects: danthron may cause abdominal cramps and colour the urine red; prolonged contact with the skin (for example in incontinent patients) may cause irritation.

Precautions: see CO-DANTHRAMER; CO-DANTHRUSATE; STIMULANT LAXATIVES.

Proprietary preparations: Ailax (*see* CO-DANTHRAMER); Capsuvac (*see* CO-DANTHRUSATE); Codalax (*see* CO-DANTHRAMER); Normax (*see* CO-DANTHRUSATE).

Dantrium (Procter & Gamble) *See* DANTROLENE SODIUM.

dantrolene sodium A *muscle relaxant used for the treatment of chronic severe spasms of voluntary muscles. It is available, on *prescription only, as capsules or as a solution for injection.

Side effects: include transient drowsiness, dizziness, weakness, malaise, fatigue, diarrhoea (treatment should be stopped if this is severe), loss of appetite, nausea, headache, and rash.

Precautions: drowsiness may impair the performance of skilled tasks, and this is exacerbated by alcohol. Dantrolene should not be taken by people with liver disease or acute muscle spasms and should be used with caution in those with heart or lung disease.

Proprietary preparation: Dantrium.

dantron *See* DANTHRON.

Daonil (Hoechst Marion Roussel) *See* GLIBENCLAMIDE.

dapsone An *antibiotic used for the treatment of leprosy and *malaria. It is given in combination with *pyrimethamine to prevent travellers contracting malaria. It is also used for treating dermatitis herpetiformis (an itchy blistering rash). A *prescription only medicine, dapsone is available as tablets or an injection.

Side effects: include blood disorders, rashes, gastrointestinal upset, headache, and psychiatric disturbances.

Precautions: dapsone should be used only under specialist supervision and should not be taken by people with severe anaemia or porphyria. It should be used with caution in women who are breastfeeding, and folate supplements should be taken during pregnancy.

Interactions with other drugs:

Probenecid: increases the risk of side effects of dapsone.

Rifampicin: reduces plasma concentrations of dapsone.

Proprietary preparation: MALOPRIM (combined with pyrimethamine).

Daraprim (GlaxoWellcome) *See* PYRIMETHAMINE.

daunorubicin A *cytotoxic antibiotic that is similar to *doxorubicin. It is used for the treatment of acute leukaemias (*see* CANCER) and advanced AIDS-related Kaposi's sarcoma (a tumour of blood vessels in the skin). A *prescription only medicine, it is available as a solution for intravenous infusion; a lipid formulation, which enhances its uptake by the tumour cells, is used for the treatment of Kaposi's sarcoma.

Side effects and precautions: see DOXORUBICIN; CYTOTOXIC DRUGS.

Proprietary preparations: Cerubidin; DaunoXome (lipid formulation).

DaunoXome (NeXstar Pharmaceuticals) *See* DAUNORUBICIN.

Day Nurse (SmithKline Beecham Consumer Healthcare) A proprietary combination of *paracetamol (an analgesic and antipyretic), *phenylpropanolamine (a decongestant), and *dextromethorphan (a cough suppressant), used to relieve the symptoms of colds and influenza, including nasal congestion, cough, and running nose. It is available as capsules or a liquid (the liquid is twice the strength of the capsules) and can be obtained without a prescription, but only from pharmacies.

Side effects: see EPHEDRINE HYDROCHLORIDE; DEXTROMETHORPHAN.

Precautions: Day Nurse is not recommended for children under six years old. *See also* PARACETAMOL; EPHEDRINE HYDROCHLORIDE; OPIOIDS.

Interactions with other drugs: see PHENYLPROPANOLAMINE; EPHEDRINE HYDROCHLORIDE; OPIOIDS.

DDAVP (Ferring Pharmaceuticals) *See* DESMOPRESSIN.

Debrisan (Pharmacia & Upjohn) *See* DEXTRANOMER.

debrisoquine A drug that prevents the release of noradrenaline <norepinephrine> in the *sympathetic nervous system. It may be used, in conjunction with other drugs, in the treatment of *hypertension that is resistant to standard *antihypertensive therapy. Debrisoquine is available as tablets on *prescription only.

Side effects, precautions, and interactions with other drugs: see BETHANIDINE <BETANIDINE> SULPHATE.

Decadron, **Decadron Injection**, **Decadron Shock-Pak** (Merck Sharp & Dohme) *See* DEXAMETHASONE.

Deca-Durabolin 100 (Organon Laboratories) *See* NANDROLONE DECANOATE.

De-capeptyl sr (Ipsen) *See* TRIPTORELIN.

decongestants Drugs that are administered to relieve or reduce congestion of the airways and the nose. Nasal decongestants are used for the treatment of colds. They may be applied locally, in the form of nose drops or sprays, or given orally; they are a common ingredient in proprietary cold remedies. Decongestants may also be used to relieve congestion due to hay fever and similar allergic reactions, but *antihistamines are usually preferred for treating these conditions. Most decongestants are *sympathomimetic drugs that act by constricting the blood vessels in the membranes lining the nose and airways. This reduces the swelling associated with congestion and therefore improves drainage. However, when given by mouth these drugs also act on other blood vessels and the heart, increasing heart rate and blood pressure. In addition, most sympathomimetic drugs interact with *monoamine oxidase inhibitors (a class of antidepressants) to cause a dangerous rise in blood pressure. For these reasons medicines containing sympathomimetic drugs should be used with caution by people with heart disease, high blood pressure, an overactive thyroid gland, or diabetes mellitus. Nasal drops and sprays are less likely to cause these adverse effects because little of the drug is absorbed into the body. However, if drops or sprays are used for more than a few days nasal congestion can increase (rebound congestion) as the effect of the drug wears off. *See also* EPHEDRINE HYDROCHLORIDE; PHENYLEPHRINE; PHENYLPROPANOLAMINE; PSEUDOEPHEDRINE; TRAMAZOLINE HYDROCHLORIDE; XYLOMETAZOLINE.

Deep Freeze Cold Gel (The Mentholatum Co) *See* MENTHOL.

Deep Heat Massage Liniment (The Mentholatum Co) A proprietary combination of *menthol and *methyl salicylate, used as a rubefacient for the relief of muscular and rheumatic pains and stiffness, including backache, sciatica, lumbago, and fibrositis. **Deep Heat Maximum** is a stronger cream formulation. Both preparations are freely available *over the counter.
Side effects and precautions: see RUBEFACIENTS; SALICYLATES.

Deep Heat Maximum (The Mentholatum Co) *See* DEEP HEAT MASSAGE LINIMENT.

Deep Heat Rub (The Mentholatum Co) A proprietary combination of *menthol, *turpentine oil, *eucalyptus oil, and *methyl salicylate in the form of a cream, used as a rubefacient for the relief of muscular and rheumatic aches, pains, and stiffness (including backache, sciatica, lumbago, and fibrositis), bruises, sprains, and chilblains. It is freely available *over the counter.
Side effects and precautions: see RUBEFACIENTS.

Deep Heat Spray (The Mentholatum Co) A proprietary combination of *methyl salicylate, *methyl nicotinate, *ethyl salicylate, and *glycol salicylate, used as a rubefacient for the relief of muscular and rheumatic aches and pains, including fibrositis, lumbago, and sciatica. It is freely available *over the counter.
Side effects and precautions: see RUBEFACIENTS; SALICYLATES.

Deep Relief (Eastern Pharmaceuticals) A proprietary combination of *ibuprofen (an NSAID) and *menthol, applied to the skin for the relief of rheumatic pain, muscular pain, strains, and sprains. It is available as a gel and can be obtained from pharmacies without a prescription.
Side effects and precautions: see NSAIDS.

DEET *See* DIETHYLTOLUAMIDE.

deferoxamine mesilate *See* DESFERRIOXAMINE MESYLATE.

deflazacort A *corticosteroid used for the treatment of inflammatory conditions. It is available as tablets on *prescription only.
Side effects, precautions, and interactions with other drugs: see
CORTICOSTEROIDS.
Proprietary preparation: Calcort.

Delfen (Janssen-Cilag) *See* NONOXINOL-9.

Deltacortril Enteric (Pfizer) *See* PREDNISOLONE.

Deltastab (Knoll) *See* PREDNISOLONE.

Delvas (APS-Berk) *See* CO-AMILOZIDE.

demeclocycline hydrochloride A tetracycline antibiotic used for the treatment of chronic bronchitis, brucellosis, chlamydial infections, and infections caused by mycoplasmas and rickettsias (*see*
TETRACYCLINES). It is also used to treat mouth ulcers and acne. It is available as tablets or capsules on *prescription only.
Side effects, precautions, and interactions with other drugs: see
TETRACYCLINES.
Proprietary preparations: Ledermycin; DETECLO (combined with tetracycline hydrochloride and chlortetracycline).

Demix (Ashbourne Pharmaceuticals) *See* DOXYCYCLINE.

Demser (Merck Sharp & Dohme) *See* METIROSINE.

demulcents Soothing preparations that protect mucous membranes and relieve irritation. Demulcents are included in proprietary medicines for relieving dry irritating coughs and in mouthwashes and gargles, as they protect and soothe the membranes lining the throat and mouth. They include *glycerin, syrup, and **simple linctus** (citric acid monohydrate).

Dencyl (SmithKline Beecham Pharmaceuticals) A proprietary combination of *ferrous sulphate, *folic acid, and *zinc sulphate monohydrate, used to prevent deficiencies of iron and folic acid during

pregnancy. It is available as *modified-release capsules and can be obtained without a prescription, but only from pharmacies.
Side effects, precautions, and interactions with other drugs: see IRON.

De-Nol (Yamanouchi Pharma) *See* TRIPOTASSIUM DICITRATOBISMUTHATE.

De-Noltab (Yamanouchi Pharma) *See* TRIPOTASSIUM DICITRATOBISMUTHATE.

Denorex Anti-Dandruff Shampoo, **Denorex Anti-Dandruff Shampoo Plus Conditioner** (Whitehall Laboratories) Proprietary combinations of *coal tar (a keratolytic) and *menthol, used to treat dandruff, *psoriasis of the scalp, and seborrhoeic *eczema. It is available without a prescription, but only from pharmacies.
Side effects and precautions: see COAL TAR.

Dentinox Infant Colic Drops (DDD) *See* DIMETHICONE <DIMETICONE>.

Dentinox Teething Gel (DDD) A proprietary combination of *cetylpyridinium chloride (an antiseptic) and *lignocaine <lidocaine> hydrochloride (a local anaesthetic), used to relieve teething pain and soothe the gums. It is suitable for use from birth onwards and is freely available *over the counter.

Dentomycin (Wyeth Laboratories) *See* MINOCYCLINE.

dependence The physical and/or psychological effects produced by the habitual taking of certain drugs, characterized by a compulsive need for the drug. In **physical dependence** withdrawal of the drug causes specific symptoms (**withdrawal symptoms**), such as sweating, vomiting, or tremors, that are reversed by further doses. Drugs that induce physical dependence include alcohol, morphine, diamorphine (heroin), and cocaine. **Psychological dependence** is the condition in which repeated use of a drug induces reliance on it for a state of well-being and contentment, but there are no physical withdrawal symptoms if use of the drug is stopped. Psychological dependence is produced by such drugs as nicotine (in tobacco), cannabis, and amphetamines. The term **addiction** is used synonymously with dependence, although some would argue that addiction should refer to the state in which both physical and psychological dependence are present.

Depixol (Lundbeck) *See* FLUPENTHIXOL <FLUPENTIXOL>.

Depo-Medrone (Pharmacia & Upjohn) *See* METHYLPREDNISOLONE.

Depo-Medrone with Lidocaine (Pharmacia & Upjohn) A proprietary combination of *methylprednisolone (a corticosteroid) and *lignocaine <lidocaine> hydrochloride (a local anaesthetic), which is injected into a joint to relieve pain and increase mobility in the treatment of

rheumatoid arthritis and other inflammatory diseases of joints. It is available on *prescription only.
Side effects, precautions, and interactions with other drugs: see CORTICOSTEROIDS.

Deponit (Schwartz Pharma) *See* GLYCERYL TRINITRATE.

Depo-Provera (Pharmacia & Upjohn) *See* MEDROXYPROGESTERONE.

Depostat (Cambridge Laboratories) *See* GESTRONOL <GESTONORONE> HEXANOATE.

depot contraceptives Preparations of synthetic *progestogens that are designed to release the hormone over a prolonged period (which may range from weeks to years) to provide long-term reversible contraception. Formulations given by intramuscular injection are Depo-Provera (*see* MEDROXYPROGESTERONE), which provides contraceptive cover for up to three months, and Noristerat (*see* NORETHISTERONE), which lasts up to eight weeks. *Levonorgestrel is available in two depot formulations: implants (Norplant), which can remain in place for up to five years; and an intrauterine system (Mirena), which lasts for up to three years.

depot injection A formulation of a drug that is injected into a muscle, where it resides and releases the active ingredient(s) slowly over a period of days, weeks, or years. Depot injection is most often used to deliver hormones for long-term contraception (*see* DEPOT CONTRACEPTIVES).

depression *See* ANTIDEPRESSANT DRUGS.

Dequacaine (Crookes Healthcare) A proprietary combination of *dequalinium chloride (an antiseptic) and *benzocaine (a local anaesthetic), used for the relief of sore throats. It is available as lozenges and can be obtained without a prescription, but only from pharmacies.

Dequadin (Crookes Healthcare) *See* DEQUALINIUM CHLORIDE.

dequalinium chloride A mild *antiseptic with weak antifungal properties, used for the treatment of bacterial or fungal infections of the mouth and throat. It is available as lozenges or pastilles and can be obtained without a prescription, but only from pharmacies.
Precautions: dequalinium chloride is not usually given to children under 10 years old.
Proprietary preparations: Dequadin (lozenges); Labosept (pastilles); DEQUACAINE (combined with benzocaine).

Derbac-M (Seton Scholl Healthcare) *See* MALATHION.

Dermacort (Sankyo Pharma) *See* HYDROCORTISONE.

Dermalex (Sanofi Winthrop) A proprietary combination of
*hexachlorophane <hexachlorophene> (an antiseptic), *allantoin (an
astringent), and *squalane, used mainly to prevent pressure sores and
incontinence rashes. It is available as a lotion without a prescription, but
only from pharmacies.
Precautions: Dermalex should not be used during pregnancy or
breastfeeding and should not be applied to broken skin or to mucous
membranes.

Dermamist (Yamanouchi Pharma) A proprietary combination of
*white soft paraffin and *liquid paraffin (both emollients), used to relieve
*eczema and dry skin conditions, including those associated with itching.
It is available as a spray and can be obtained without a prescription, but
only from pharmacies.
Precautions: Dermamist should not be used on broken skin.

dermatitis *See* ECZEMA.

Dermestril (Sanofi Winthrop) *See* OESTRADIOL <ESTRADIOL>; HORMONE
REPLACEMENT THERAPY.

Dermidex (Seton Scholl Healthcare) A proprietary combination of
*lignocaine <lidocaine> (a local anaesthetic), *chlorbutol <chlorobutanol>
and *cetrimide (antiseptics), and aluminium chlorhydroxyallantoinate
(an astringent; a derivative of *allantoin), used to relieve the pain of
stings, grazes, and dermatitis. It is available as a cream that can be
obtained without a prescription, but only from pharmacies.
Precautions: Dermidex should not be used for longer than seven days and
should not be applied to mucous membranes; it is not recommended for
children under four years old.

Dermol (Dermal Laboratories) A proprietary combination of the
antiseptics *benzalkonium chloride and *chlorhexidine hydrochloride
and the emollients *liquid paraffin and *isopropyl myristate, used for the
relief of dry and itching skin conditions, such as eczema. It may be
applied directly to the skin or used in the bath or shower. Dermol is
available as a lotion and may be bought without a *prescription, but only
from pharmacies.
Precautions: the lotion should not be used in or around the eyes.

Dermovate, Dermovate Scalp (GlaxoWellcome) *See* CLOBETASOL
PROPIONATE.

Dermovate-NN (GlaxoWellcome) A proprietary combination of
*clobetasol propionate (a very potent topical steroid), *neomycin
sulphate (an antibiotic), and *nystatin (an antifungal agent), used for the
treatment of psoriasis, eczema that is unresponsive to other treatments,

and other inflammatory conditions of the skin when infection is present. It is available as a cream or an ointment on *prescription only.

Side effects and precautions: see TOPICAL STEROIDS.

Deseril (Alliance Pharmaceuticals) *See* METHYSERGIDE.

Desferal (Novartis Pharmaceuticals) *See* DESFERRIOXAMINE MESYLATE <MESILATE>.

desferrioxamine mesylate (<desferrioxamine mesilate>; deferoxamine mesilate)
A drug that binds to iron and is used to treat iron poisoning, which most commonly occurs in children as a result of accidental ingestion and causes nausea, vomiting, abdominal pain, diarrhoea, and rectal bleeding. Desferrioxamine can also be used to bind to excessive amounts of iron in the body that can occur in patients with certain types of anaemias as a result of repeated blood transfusions, and it may be used for treating haemochromatosis (iron-storage disease), in which there is excessive absorption and storage of iron. Desferrioxamine is available in a form for infusion on *prescription only.

Side effects: include generalized allergic reactions, low blood pressure (if given too rapidly), dizziness, convulsions, disturbances of hearing or vision, and pain at the injection site.

Precautions: desferrioxamine should be used with caution in people with kidney disease. Eye and ear examinations may be necessary before treatment and at three-monthly intervals during treatment.

Interactions with other drugs:

Prochlorperazine: should not be taken with desferrioxamine.

Proprietary preparation: Desferal.

desmopressin
An analogue of *vasopressin that has a longer duration of action than vasopressin and does not cause constriction of blood vessels. It is used for the treatment of diabetes insipidus and for those who have problems with bedwetting, including people with multiple sclerosis. Desmopressin is available, on *prescription only, as tablets or a nasal spray.

Side effects: include abdominal cramps, nausea, an urge to defecate, and headache; nasal congestion and irritation may occur with use of a nasal spray.

Precautions: see VASOPRESSIN.

Interactions with other drugs:

Carbamazepine: may increase the effect of desmopressin.

Chlorpropamide: may increase the effect of desmopressin.

Indomethacin <indometacin>: may increase the effect of desmopressin.

Proprietary preparations: DDAVP; Desmotabs; Desmospray.

Desmospray (Ferring Pharmaceuticals) *See* DESMOPRESSIN.

Desmotabs (Ferring Pharmaceuticals) *See* DESMOPRESSIN.

desogestrel A synthetic *progestogen used as an ingredient in combined *oral contraceptives. There is a higher risk of thromboembolism with this progestogen than with certain others. It is available on *prescription only.
Side effects and interactions with other drugs: see ORAL CONTRACEPTIVES.
Precautions: desogestrel should not be taken by women who are at risk of developing thromboembolism, for example because they are very overweight or have varicose veins or a history of thrombosis. It should therefore only be taken by women who cannot tolerate other brands and who are prepared to accept the increased risk. *See also* ORAL CONTRACEPTIVES.
Proprietary preparations: MARVELON (combined with ethinyloestradiol <ethinylestradiol>); MERCILON (combined with ethinyloestradiol <ethinylestradiol>).

desoxymethasone <desoximetasone> A moderately potent *topical steroid used for the treatment of a variety of skin disorders. It is available as an oily cream on *prescription only.
Side effects and precautions: see TOPICAL STEROIDS.
Proprietary preparations: Stiedex LP; STIEDEX LOTION (combined with salicylic acid).

Destolit (Norgine) *See* URSODEOXYCHOLIC ACID.

Deteclo (Wyeth Laboratories) A proprietary combination of the antibiotics *tetracycline hydrochloride, *chlortetracycline, and *demeclocycline hydrochloride, used for the treatment of chronic bronchitis, brucellosis, chlamydial infections, and infections caused by mycoplasmas and rickettsias (*see* TETRACYCLINES). It is also used to treat mouth ulcers and acne. Deteclo is available as tablets on *prescription only.
Side effects, precautions, and interactions with other drugs: see TETRACYCLINES.

Detrunorm (Schering-Plough) *See* PROPIVERINE HYDROCHLORIDE.

Detrusitol (Pharmacia & Upjohn) *See* TOLTERODINE TARTRATE.

Dettol Antiseptic Cream (Reckitt & Colman) A proprietary combination of *triclosan and *chloroxylenol (both antiseptics) and edetic acid (an agent that enhances the activity of chloroxylenol), used for the treatment of cuts, bites, stings, and abrasions. It is freely available *over the counter.

Dettol Antiseptic Pain Relief Spray (Reckitt & Colman) A proprietary combination of *benzalkonium chloride (an antiseptic) and *lignocaine <lidocaine> hydrochloride (a local anaesthetic), used for the relief of pain from minor wounds, such as cuts and grazes, insect bites and stings, small burns, and scalds. It is available without a prescription, but only from pharmacies.

Dettol Liquid (Reckitt & Colman) *See* CHLOROXYLENOL.

De Witt's Analgesic Pills (E. C. De Witt & Co) A proprietary combination of *paracetamol (an analgesic and antipyretic) and *caffeine (a stimulant), used to relieve rheumatic aches and pains and the symptoms of colds and influenza. It is available without a prescription, but larger packs can only be obtained from pharmacies.

Precautions: these pills are not recommended for children under 12 years old. *See also* PARACETAMOL; CAFFEINE.

De Witt's Antacid Powder (E. C. De Witt & Co) A proprietary combination of *sodium bicarbonate, *calcium carbonate, *magnesium carbonate, *magnesium trisilicate, *kaolin, and *peppermint oil, used for the relief of upset stomach, heartburn, indigestion, excess acidity, and trapped wind (*see* ACID-PEPTIC DISEASES). It is freely available *over the counter.

Side effects and interactions with other drugs: see ANTACIDS.
Precautions: this powder is not recommended for children.

De Witt's Antacid Tablets (E. C. De Witt & Co) A proprietary combination of *calcium carbonate, *magnesium carbonate, *magnesium trisilicate, and *peppermint oil, used for the relief of upset stomach, heartburn, indigestion, and trapped wind (*see* ACID-PEPTIC DISEASES). It is freely available *over the counter.

Side effects and interactions with other drugs: see ANTACIDS.
Precautions: these tablets are not recommended for children.

De Witt's Worm Syrup (E. C. De Witt & Co) *See* PIPERAZINE.

dexamethasone A *corticosteroid with anti-inflammatory activity. It is used for the treatment of inflammatory conditions (including rheumatic disease) and it is injected intravenously to treat shock and cerebral oedema (swelling of the brain). Dexamethasone is also used in the diagnosis of Cushing's disease. A *prescription only medicine, it is available as tablets, as a solution for intravenous injection or local injection into joints or around tendons, as eye drops or ointment, and as ear drops.

Side effects: see CORTICOSTEROIDS. In addition, perineal or scrotal irritation and pain can occur if intravenous injections are given too rapidly.

Precautions and interactions with other drugs: see CORTICOSTEROIDS.

Proprietary preparations: Decadron, Decadron Injection, Decadron Shock-Pak (injection); Maxidex (eye drops); Minims Dexamethasone (single-dose eye drops); DEXA-RHINASPRAY DUO (combined with tramazoline hydrochloride); MAXITROL (combined with neomycin, polymyxin B sulphate, and hypromellose); OTOMIZE (combined with acetic acid and neomycin sulphate); SOFRADEX (combined with framycetin sulphate and gramicidin).

dexamphetamine sulphate <dexamfetamine sulphate> A drug that acts directly on the brain as a *stimulant (*see* AMPHETAMINES). In adults it is used to treat narcolepsy (an extreme tendency to fall asleep). Paradoxically it has a sedative effect in children and can be used to treat attention deficit disorder. A *controlled drug, it is available as tablets and is potentially addictive.

Side effects: include insomnia, irritability, restlessness, night terrors, euphoria, tremor, dizziness, headache, loss of appetite and stomach upsets, and raised blood pressure and a fast heart rate. Growth retardation may occur in children.

Precautions: *tolerance to the effects of dexamphetamine develops with prolonged use, and *dependence can occur. Dexamphetamine should only be given to children under specialist supervision, owing to its effects on growth and lack of knowledge of its effects with long-term use. It should not be taken by people with heart disease, high blood pressure, thyroid disease, glaucoma, or liver or kidney disease; by those with states of hyperexcitability or with a history of drug or alcohol abuse; or by women who are pregnant or breastfeeding. It may affect driving ability.

Interactions with other drugs:

  MAOIs: there is a risk of a dangerous rise in blood pressure.

Proprietary preparation: Dexedrine.

Dexa-Rhinaspray Duo (Boehringer Ingelheim) A proprietary combination of *tramazoline hydrochloride (a decongestant) and *dexamethasone (a corticosteroid), used for the treatment of hay fever. It is available as a nasal spray on *prescription only.

Side effects: see TOPICAL STEROIDS; DECONGESTANTS.

Precautions: prolonged use should be avoided; *see also* TOPICAL STEROIDS; DECONGESTANTS.

Dexedrine (Medeva) *See* DEXAMPHETAMINE <DEXAMFETAMINE> SULPHATE.

Dexomon SR, **Dexomon Retard 100** (Hillcross Pharmaceuticals) *See* DICLOFENAC SODIUM.

dextran A carbohydrate that strengthens the natural film of tears that covers the eyes and is used as an ingredient of eye drops to treat dry eyes. It is also used in intravenous infusions to increase blood volume in some conditions of shock.

Proprietary preparation: TEARS NATURALE (combined with hypromellose).

dextranomer A substance used to absorb the liquid that exudes from ulcers and infected wounds. It is available as beads or a paste and can be obtained without a prescription, but only from pharmacies.

Proprietary preparation: Debrisan.

dextromethorphan An *opioid that acts as a *cough suppressant; it has no analgesic or sedative properties. Dextromethorphan is used for the relief of dry irritating persistent coughs, either alone or in combination with other drugs in linctuses, syrups, and lozenges. It can be bought from pharmacies without a prescription.

Side effects: side effects, such as dizziness, drowsiness, constipation, nausea, and vomiting, are rare and there is no evidence of dependence. Confusion and depression of breathing may occur after overdosage. *See also* OPIOIDS.

Precautions and interactions with other drugs: see OPIOIDS.

Proprietary preparations: Benylin Dry Coughs Non Drowsy (liquid); Contac CoughCaps (*modified-release capsules); Meltus Cough Control (capsules); Nirolex Lozenges; Robitussin Dry Cough; Robitussin Junior Persistent Cough; Vicks Vaposyrup Children's Dry Cough; Vicks Vaposyrup Dry Cough; ACTIFED COMPOUND LINCTUS (combined with pseudoephedrine and triprolidine); ACTIFED JUNIOR COUGH RELIEF (combined with triprolidine); BENYLIN CHILDREN'S COUGHS AND COLDS (combined with triprolidine); BENYLIN COUGH & CONGESTION (combined with diphenhydramine, menthol, and pseudoephedrine); BENYLIN DRY COUGHS ORIGINAL (combined with diphenhydramine and menthol); BRONALIN DRY COUGH (combined with pseudoephedrine); CABDRIVERS (combined with menthol); COVONIA BRONCHIAL BALSAM (combined with menthol); COVONIA NIGHT TIME FORMULA (combined with diphenhydramine); DAY NURSE (combined with paracetamol and phenylpropanolamine); JUNIOR MELTUS DRY COUGH AND CATARRH (combined with pseudoephedrine); MELTUS DRY COUGH (combined with pseudoephedrine); NIGHT NURSE (combined with paracetamol and promethazine); NIROLEX FOR DRY COUGHS WITH DECONGESTANT (combined with pseudoephedrine); SUDAFED LINCTUS (combined with pseudoephedrine); VICKS COLDCARE (combined with paracetamol and phenylpropanolamine); VICKS MEDINITE (combined with doxylamine, ephedrine, and paracetamol).

dextromoramide An *opioid analgesic used for the treatment of severe pain. It is short acting and causes less sedation than morphine. Dextromoramide is a *controlled drug; it is available as tablets or suppositories.

Side effects and precautions: see MORPHINE. Dextromoramide should not be given to women in labour, since it may cause depression of breathing in the newborn baby.

Interactions with other drugs: see OPIOIDS.

Proprietary preparation: Palfium.

dextropropoxyphene hydrochloride A weak *opioid analgesic

that can be used alone but is more often given in combination with a
non-opioid analgesic, paracetamol (*see* CO-PROXAMOL).
Dextropropoxyphene is available as capsules on *prescription only.
Side effects and precautions: *see* OPIOIDS; CO-PROXAMOL.
Interactions with other drugs:
  Carbamazepine: its effects are enhanced by dextropropoxyphene.
  Ritonavir: should not be given with dextropropoxyphene as it increases
    the plasma concentration of dextropropoxyphene.
  See also OPIOIDS.
Proprietary preparations: Doloxene; Cosalgesic (*see* CO-PROXAMOL);
Distalgesic (*see* CO-PROXAMOL).

DF 118 Forte (Napp Pharmaceuticals) *See* DIHYDROCODEINE TARTRATE.

DHC Continus (Napp Pharmaceuticals) *See* DIHYDROCODEINE TARTRATE.

Diabetamide (Ashbourne Pharmaceuticals) *See* GLIBENCLAMIDE.

diabetes insipidus *See* VASOPRESSIN.

diabetes mellitus A disease in which glucose (sugar) is not adequately
taken up from the bloodstream by the cells of the body and therefore
cannot be metabolized to produce energy or stored in the liver. It is
caused by an abnormality in the synthesis and secretion of the hormone
*insulin. Diabetes mellitus is characterized by high concentrations of
glucose in the blood (**hyperglycaemia**) and in the urine, with symptoms
of thirst, loss of weight, tiredness, and an excessive production of urine.

  People affected with **insulin-dependent** (or **type I**) **diabetes mellitus**
have little or no ability to produce the hormone and depend on daily
injections of insulin. This type of diabetes can also be referred to as
juvenile-onset diabetes because it usually starts during childhood or
adolescence. The dosage of insulin must be carefully controlled and
matched to the dietary intake of glucose. If cells receive insufficient
glucose, fats may be used as an alternative source of energy, which can
lead to alteration of the acidity of the blood, the accumulation of ketones
(formed when fats are metabolized) in the bloodstream (**ketoacidosis**),
and eventually to diabetic coma. **Noninsulin-dependent** (or **type II** or
maturity-onset) **diabetes mellitus** develops in adults, usually over 40
years old, because of a decrease in the production of natural insulin,
although the pancreas still functions to some extent; alternatively, the
body becomes resistant to the effect of insulin. This condition occurs
more often in people who are overweight; it is usually treated by diet,
weight reduction, and *oral hypoglycaemic drugs, but some patients may
need insulin instead.

  All people with diabetes, regardless of which type, must pay attention
to their diet, in which the amount of carbohydrate should be carefully
controlled to suit their body's needs, and be aware of the importance of
monitoring blood glucose concentrations. Very low blood glucose

(*hypoglycaemia) may be caused by excessive dosage of insulin or some oral antidiabetic drugs or by missing a meal. Good control of blood sugar is necessary to prevent such long-term consequences of diabetes as atherosclerosis (giving rise to heart disease), poor circulation in the extremities (causing foot ulcers), impairment of eyesight, and kidney damage.

Diagesil (APS-Berk) *See* DIAMORPHINE HYDROCHLORIDE.

Dialar (Lagap Pharmaceuticals) *See* DIAZEPAM.

Diamicron (Servier Laboratories) *See* GLICLAZIDE.

diamorphine hydrochloride (heroin hydrochloride) An *opioid analgesic that is used to treat acute pain, such as that associated with a heart attack, or long-term chronic pain, such as that caused by advanced cancer. It is also used in the treatment of pulmonary *oedema. Diamorphine is a *controlled drug; it is available as tablets or a form for injection and is usually administered in a hospital.
Side effects and precautions: see MORPHINE.
Interactions with other drugs: see OPIOIDS.
Proprietary preparation: Diagesil.

Diamox, **Diamox SR** (Wyeth Laboratories) *See* ACETAZOLAMIDE.

Dianette (Schering Health Care) A proprietary combination of *ethinyloestradiol <ethinylestradiol> (a synthetic oestrogen) and *cyproterone acetate (an anti-androgen), used for the treatment of severe *acne in women that has not responded to prolonged antibiotic therapy. It is also used to treat hirsutism (abnormal growth of facial and body hair in women). Dianette acts as an *oral contraceptive in women taking it. It is available as tablets on *prescription only.
Side effects: include breast enlargement, fluid retention with a bloated feeling, weight gain, cramps and pains in the legs, headache, nausea, depression, vaginal discharge, skin changes (including brown patches on the face), and breakthrough bleeding. There may be changes in libido, depression, and irritation from contact lenses. The occurrence of a migraine-like headache for the first time, frequent severe headaches, or visual disturbance should be reported immediately to a doctor.
Precautions: Dianette should not be taken by women who are pregnant or have a history of thrombosis. For other precautions, *see* ORAL CONTRACEPTIVES.
Interactions with other drugs: see ORAL CONTRACEPTIVES.

Diarphen (Co-Pharma) *See* CO-PHENOTROPE.

Diarrest (Galen) A proprietary combination of *codeine phosphate (which reduces intestinal motility), *dicyclomine <dicycloverine>

hydrochloride (an antispasmodic), and *potassium chloride, *sodium chloride, and *sodium citrate (all *electrolytes), used for the treatment of diarrhoea (see ANTIDIARRHOEAL DRUGS), vomiting, and abdominal cramp. It is available as a liquid on *prescription only.

Side effects: Diarrest has a sedative effect.

Precautions: Diarrest should not be taken by people with antibiotic-associated inflammation of the colon (bowel) or diverticular disease (a condition of the colon causing colic and altered bowel habits).

Interactions with other drugs:

MAO inhibitors: should not be taken with Diarrest.

diarrhoea *See* ANTIDIARRHOEAL DRUGS.

Diasorb (Norton Healthcare) *See* LOPERAMIDE HYDROCHLORIDE.

Diazemuls (Cox Pharmaceuticals) *See* DIAZEPAM.

diazepam A long-acting *benzodiazepine used for the short-term treatment of anxiety and insomnia. It is also used to relieve the symptoms of alcohol withdrawal and to treat status epilepticus (repeated epileptic seizures), convulsions associated with fever in children, and chronic muscle spasm. Diazepam is also used to relax patients before operations or uncomfortable diagnostic procedures. It is available, on *prescription only, as tablets, an oral solution, an injection, suppositories, or a rectal solution. Some proprietary preparations of diazepam cannot be prescribed on the NHS.

Side effects: include drowsiness, light-headedness, confusion, shaky movements, and unsteady gait (especially in elderly people), amnesia, dependence, and paradoxical overexcitedness (see BENZODIAZEPINES). Rare side effects include headache, vertigo, gastrointestinal upsets (such as nausea or constipation), blurred vision, changes in libido, difficulty in passing urine, rashes, and a fall in blood pressure.

Precautions: diazepam should not be taken by people who have respiratory depression, severe breathing problems, or severe liver disease, and it should not be used for treating depression, chronic psychosis, phobias, or obsessional states. Diazepam should be used with caution in people who have lung disease or a history of alcohol or drug abuse and by women who are pregnant or breastfeeding. *See also* BENZODIAZEPINES.

Interactions with other drugs:

Isoniazid: increases the effects (including sedation) of diazepam.

Rifampicin: reduces the effects of diazepam.

Ritonavir: increases the plasma concentration of diazepam, causing profound sedation; these drugs should therefore not be taken together.

See also BENZODIAZEPINES.

Proprietary preparations: Dialar (oral solution); Diazemuls (injection);

Diazepam Rectubes (rectal solution); Rimapam (tablets); Stesolid (rectal solution); Tensium (tablets); Valium (tablets or injection); Valclair (suppositories).

Diazepam Rectubes (CP Pharmaceuticals) *See* DIAZEPAM.

diazoxide A drug that has two separate actions and uses. When given by intravenous injection it causes *vasodilatation of the small arteries and consequently rapid lowering of blood pressure; it is therefore sometimes used as an emergency treatment of *hypertension. Diazoxide also increases the concentration of glucose in the bloodstream and is taken orally to treat chronic *hypoglycaemia (low blood glucose) resulting from excessive secretion of insulin (for example, by an insulin-secreting tumour in the pancreas). It is not used to treat acute hypoglycaemia resulting from insulin overdosage in people with diabetes. Diazoxide is available as an injection or tablets on *prescription only.

Side effects: include loss of appetite, nausea, vomiting, low blood pressure, a slow heart rate, sweating, abnormal heart rhythms, and *extrapyramidal reactions.

Precautions: diazoxide should be used with caution in people with severe kidney disease. Growth and development of children must be monitored.

Interactions with other drugs:

Anaesthetics: their effects in lowering blood pressure are increased.

Antihypertensive drugs: their effects in lowering blood pressure are enhanced.

Diuretics: their effects in lowering blood pressure are enhanced.

Proprietary preparation: Eudemine.

Dibenyline (Goldshield Pharmaceuticals) *See* PHENOXYBENZAMINE HYDROCHLORIDE.

dichlorobenzyl alcohol An *antiseptic used as an ingredient of lozenges for the treatment of minor infections of the mouth and throat.

Proprietary preparations: STREPSILS (combined with amylmetacresol); STREPSILS DUAL ACTION LOZENGES (combined with amylmetacresol and lignocaine <lidocaine>).

diclofenac sodium An *NSAID used for the treatment of pain and inflammation in rheumatoid arthritis (including arthritis in children) and other disorders of the muscles and joints; it is also used to treat acute gout and postoperative pain. Diclofenac is applied to the skin for the treatment of sprains and strains. It is also applied to the eye to inhibit constriction of the pupil during eye surgery and to reduce inflammation and pain after surgery. It is available, on *prescription only, as tablets, dispersible tablets, *modified-release capsules and tablets, an injection, suppositories, eye drops, and as a gel for topical application.

Side effects: see NSAIDS. Suppositories may cause local irritation.

Precautions: see NSAIDS.

Interactions with other drugs: see NSAIDS. In addition:

   Anticoagulants: should not be used with injections of diclofenac as the risk of bleeding is increased.

   Cyclosporin: increases the plasma concentration of diclofenac, whose dosage will therefore need to be halved.

Proprietary preparations: Acoflam; Acoflam 75 SR (modified-release tablets); Dexomon SR, Dexomon Retard 100 (modified-release tablets); Dicloflex; Dicloflex SR, Dicloflex Retard (modified-release tablets); Diclomax SR, Diclomax Retard (modified-release capsules); Diclotard 75 MR, Diclotard 100 MR (modified-release tablets); Diclovol; Diclovol SR, Diclovol Retard (modified-release tablets); Diclozip; Digenac XL (modified-release tablets); Enzed; Flamatak MR (modified-release tablets); Flamrase; Flamrase SR (modified-release tablets); Flexotard MR 75, Flexotard MR 100 (modified-release tablets); Isclofen; Lofensaid; Lofensaid Retard 75, Lofensaid Retard 100 (modified-release tablets); Motifene 75 mg (modified-release capsules); Rhumalgan CR (modified-release tablets); Slofenac SR (modified-release tablets); Volraman; Volsaid Retard (modified-release tablets); Voltarol; Voltarol Emulgel (gel); Voltarol Ophtha (eye drops); Voltarol 75 mg SR, Voltarol Retard (modified-release tablets); ARTHROTEC (combined with misoprostol).

Dicloflex, Dicloflex Retard, Dicloflex SR (Pharmacia & Upjohn) *See* DICLOFENAC SODIUM.

Diclomax Retard, Diclomax SR (Parke-Davis Medical) *See* DICLOFENAC SODIUM.

Diclotard 75 MR, Diclotard 100 MR (Ashbourne Pharmaceuticals) *See* DICLOFENAC SODIUM.

Diclovol, Dicloval SR, Dicloval Retard (Arun Pharmaceuticals) *See* DICLOFENAC SODIUM.

Diclozip (Ashbourne Pharmaceuticals) *See* DICLOFENAC SODIUM.

dicobalt edetate A drug used for the treatment of poisoning by cyanides. It is given by intravenous injection and is available on *prescription only.

Side effects: include low blood pressure, a fast heart rate, and vomiting.

Precautions: because it is toxic, dicobalt edetate should only be given to patients who are unconscious or about to become unconscious.

Diconal (GlaxoWellcome) A proprietary combination of *cyclizine hydrochloride (an antiemetic antihistamine) and *dipipanone hydrochloride (a strong opioid analgesic), used for the relief of moderate to severe pain; cyclizine is included to prevent the nausea and vomiting associated with opioids. Diconal is available as tablets; it is a *controlled drug.

Side effects: include drowsiness, dry mouth, blurred vision, and dependence (*see* MORPHINE).

Precautions: Diconal is not recommended for children or terminally ill patients. *See also* MORPHINE; OPIOIDS.

Interactions with other drugs: see ANTIHISTAMINES; OPIOIDS.

dicyclomine hydrochloride <dicycloverine hydrochloride> An *antimuscarinic drug used for the treatment of irritable bowel syndrome and other conditions marked by spasms of the gut (*see* ANTISPASMODICS). Dicyclomine is available as tablets or a syrup on *prescription; packs of tablets in which the maximum single dose is 10 mg and the maximum daily dose is 60 mg can be obtained from pharmacies without a prescription.

Side effects and precautions: see ANTIMUSCARINIC DRUGS.

Proprietary preparations: Merbentyl (10 mg); Merbentyl 20 (20 mg); CARBELLON (combined with magnesium hydroxide and charcoal); KOLANTICON GEL (combined with aluminium hydroxide, magnesium hydroxide, and dimethicone <dimeticone>).

dicycloverine hydrochloride *See* DICYCLOMINE HYDROCHLORIDE.

Dicynene (Delandale Laboratories) *See* ETHAMSYLATE <ETAMSYLATE>.

didanosine An *antiviral drug that prevents retrovirus replication: it is a nucleoside analogue that inhibits the action of reverse transcriptase. Didanosine is used, usually in combination with other antiviral agents, to delay the progression of disease in patients with advanced *HIV infection. It is available as tablets on *prescription only.

Side effects: include diarrhoea, nausea, vomiting, damage to peripheral nerves (causing weakness and numbness in the limbs), pancreatitis, blood disorders, and (rarely) liver failure and visual disturbances.

Precautions: didanosine should be used with caution by those with a history of pancreatitis, disease of the peripheral nerves, gout, or impaired kidney or liver function and by women who are pregnant or breastfeeding.

Proprietary preparation: Videx.

Didronel (Procter & Gamble) *See* DISODIUM ETIDRONATE.

Didronel PMO (Procter & Gamble) *See* DISODIUM ETIDRONATE.

dienoestrol <dienestrol> A synthetic *oestrogen that is used mainly as local *hormone replacement therapy to relieve wasting or inflammation of the vagina, shrinkage or itching of the vulva (external genitals), and pain on intercourse in menopausal and postmenopausal women. It is available as a cream on *prescription only.

Side effects, precautions, and interactions with other drugs: see OESTROGENS.

Proprietary preparation: Ortho Dienoestrol.

diethylamine salicylate A *salicylate that is applied to the skin for the relief of muscular aches and pains, including backache, sciatica, lumbago, and sprains. It is available in the form of creams that can be obtained without a prescription; it is also an ingredient of several *rubefacient preparations that are freely available *over the counter.

Side effects and precautions: see RUBEFACIENTS.

Proprietary preparations: Algesal (cream; available only from pharmacies); Lloyds Cream (freely available); FIERY JACK CREAM (combined with capsicum oleoresin, glycol salicylate, and methyl nicotinate); TRANSVASIN HEAT SPRAY (combined with 2-hydroxyethyl salicylate, and methyl nicotinate).

diethylstilbestrol *See* STILBOESTROL.

diethyltoluamide (DEET) A chemical used as an insect repellent. It is an ingredient of various lotions, sprays, and roll-on sticks that are applied to the skin for repelling mosquitoes, midges, and other bloodsucking insects. Preparations containing DEET are effective but their action lasts only a few hours; they are freely available *over the counter.

Side effects and precautions: preparations may occasionally cause skin irritation. They should not be applied to the lips, eyes, or broken skin, and prolonged use in young children should be avoided.

Differin (Galderma) *See* ADAPALENE.

Difflam (3M Health Care) *See* BENZYDAMINE HYDROCHLORIDE.

Diflucan (Pfizer) *See* FLUCONAZOLE.

diflucortolone valerate A potent *topical steroid used for the treatment of a variety of skin disorders. It is available, on *prescription only, as a cream, an oily cream, or an ointment.

Side effects and precautions: see TOPICAL STEROIDS.

Proprietary preparations: Nerisone; Nerisone Forte (a stronger preparation).

diflunisal A *salicylate that is used for the treatment of pain and inflammation in rheumatoid arthritis and other disorders of joints and muscles and for the relief of mild to moderate pain, including period pains. It produces less severe effects on the stomach lining than aspirin. Diflunisal is available as tablets on *prescription only.

Side effects, precautions, and interactions with other drugs: see NSAIDS.

Proprietary preparation: Dolobid.

Digenac XL (Ethical Generics) *See* DICLOFENAC SODIUM.

Digibind (GlaxoWellcome) A proprietary preparation of antibodies to *digoxin, used for the rapid treatment of overdosage of digoxin and other cardiac glycosides. It is given by injection and is available on *prescription only.

digitalis drugs *See* CARDIAC GLYCOSIDES; DIGOXIN.

digitoxin A digitalis drug having the same effects as *digoxin, but with a much longer duration of action. It is available as tablets on *prescription only.
Side effects, precautions, and interactions with other drugs: see DIGOXIN.

digoxin A *cardiac glycoside (digitalis drug). It is used to treat congestive *heart failure and supraventricular *arrhythmias (particularly atrial fibrillation). The effective dose of digoxin can also be the dose at which side effects become common, so treatment must be monitored carefully. Digoxin is available on *prescription only as a solution for infusion, as tablets, or as an elixir.
Side effects: include nausea, vomiting, loss of appetite, diarrhoea, confusion, visual disturbance, and arrhythmias.
Precautions: side effects must be observed and reported to the doctor, since thay can be a sign of too high a dosage.
Interactions with other drugs:
  Amiodarone: increases the plasma concentration of digoxin; the dosage of digoxin should be halved.
  Diuretics: because digoxin is more toxic if potassium is depleted, a potassium-sparing diuretic should be added if patients are taking other diuretics with digoxin.
  Propafenone: increases the plasma concentration of digoxin; the dose of digoxin should be halved.
  Quinidine: increases the plasma concentration of digoxin; the dose of digoxin should be halved.
  Spironolactone: enhances the effect of digoxin.
  Verapamil: increases plasma concentration of digoxin and bradycardia (slow heart rate).
Proprietary preparations: Lanoxin; Lanoxin-PG.

dihydrocodeine tartrate An *opioid analgesic, similar to codeine in its pain-relieving effects, used for the treatment of mild to severe pain (depending on the dosage). It is also used in combination with paracetamol (*see* CO-DYDRAMOL). Dihydrocodeine is available as tablets, *modified-release tablets, or an oral solution on *prescription only; an injection of dihydrocodeine is a *controlled drug.
Side effects and precautions: see MORPHINE.
Interactions with other drugs: see OPIOIDS.

Proprietary preparations: DF 118 Forte (high-strength tablets); DHC Continus (high-strength modified-release tablets); Galake (*see* CO-DYDRAMOL); REMEDEINE (combined with paracetamol).

dihydrotachysterol An *analogue of *vitamin D used for the treatment of tetany, spasm and twitching of the muscles caused by low plasma calcium concentrations due to underworking of the parathyroid glands (*see* PARATHYROID HORMONE). It is available as an oral solution that contains *arachis oil (and should therefore not be used by people who are allergic to peanuts). Dihydrotachysterol can be obtained without a prescription, but only from pharmacies.

Side effects, precautions, and interactions with other drugs: *see* VITAMIN D.

Proprietary preparation: AT 10.

Dijex Suspension (Seton Scholl Healthcare) A proprietary combination of the antacids *aluminium hydroxide and *magnesium hydroxide used for the relief of upset stomach, heartburn, indigestion, and trapped wind (*see* ACID-PEPTIC DISEASES). It is freely available *over the counter.

Side effects and interactions with other drugs: *see* ANTACIDS.

Precautions: this suspension is not recommended for children under six years old.

Dijex Tablets (Seton Scholl Healthcare) A proprietary combination of the antacids *aluminium hydroxide and *magnesium carbonate, used for the relief of upset stomach, heartburn, and indigestion (*see* ACID-PEPTIC DISEASES). It is freely available *over the counter.

Side effects and interactions with other drugs: *see* ANTACIDS.

Precautions: these tablets are not recommended for children.

Dilcardia SR (Generics) *See* DILTIAZEM HYDROCHLORIDE.

dill seed oil An oil distilled from the seeds of the dill plant (*Anethum graveolens*). It is included, either as the oil or as dill water, as an ingredient in preparations to relieve flatulence and wind pains.

Proprietary preparations: NEO GRIPE MIXTURE (combined with ginger tincture and sodium bicarbonate); WOODWARD'S GRIPE WATER (combined with sodium bicarbonate).

diloxanide furoate A drug used for the treatment of chronic infections of the intestine by the amoeba *Entamoeba histolytica*, which causes amoebic dysentry. It is available as tablets on *prescription only.

Side effects: include flatulence and (rarely) vomiting and itching.

Precautions: diloxanide should not be taken by women who are pregnant or breastfeeding.

Proprietary preparation: Furamide.

diltiazem hydrochloride A class III *calcium antagonist used for the treatment of most forms of *angina. Longer-acting formulations are also used for the treatment of *hypertension. A *prescription only medicine, it is available as capsules or tablets in short-acting or *modified-release formulations.

Side effects: see CALCIUM ANTAGONISTS.

Precautions: diltiazem should not be taken by people with severe bradycardia (slow heart rate) or some other forms of heart disease, or by women who are pregnant or breastfeeding. *See also* ANTIHYPERTENSIVE DRUGS.

Interactions with other drugs:

Amiodarone: diltiazem increases the risk of amiodarone having adverse effects on the heart.

Antiepileptic drugs: phenytoin reduces the effects of diltiazem, which itself increases the plasma concentration of phenytoin; diltiazem enhances the effects of carbamazepine; the effects of diltiazem are reduced by phenobarbitone <phenobarbital>.

Beta blockers: the risk of bradycardia (slow heart rate) is increased if beta blockers are taken with diltiazem.

Cyclosporin: its plasma concentration is increased by diltiazem.

Digoxin: its plasma concentration is increased by diltiazem.

Rifampicin: reduces the effect of diltiazem.

Theophylline: its effects are enhanced by diltiazem.

See also CALCIUM ANTAGONISTS.

Proprietary preparations: Adizem-SR (modified-release tablets or capsules); Adizem-XL (modified-release capsules); Angiozem; Angitil SR (modified-release capsules); Calazem; Calcicard CR (modified-release tablets); Dilcardia SR (modified-release capsules); Dilzem SR (modified-release capsules); Dilzem XL (high-strength modified-release capsules); Slozem (modified-release capsules); Tildiem LA (modified-release capsules); Tildiem Retard (low-strength modified-release tablets); Viazem XL (modified-release capsules); Zemtard (modified-release capsules).

Dilzem SR, **Dilzem XL** (Elan Pharma) *See* DILTIAZEM HYDROCHLORIDE.

dimenhydrinate An *antihistamine used for the treatment of nausea, vomiting, vertigo, motion sickness, and disorders of the inner ear affecting balance or hearing (including Ménière's disease). It is available as tablets without a prescription.

Side effects: drowsiness is the most common side effect; *see* ANTIHISTAMINES.

Precautions and interactions with other drugs: see ANTIHISTAMINES.

Proprietary preparation: Dramamine.

dimercaprol (BAL) A drug that is used as an antidote to poisoning by metals, such as antimony, arsenic, bismuth, gold, mercury, and thallium (but not iron, cadmium, or selenium). It is also used as an *adjunct to *sodium calcium edetate for treating lead poisoning. Dimercaprol is available as an injection on *prescription only.

Side effects: include low blood pressure, a fast heart rate, general malaise, nausea, vomiting, increased production of saliva, tears, and sweat, a burning sensation in the mouth, throat, and eyes, a feeling of constriction in the chest and throat, headache, muscle spasms, and (in children) fever.

Precautions: dimercaprol should not be given to people with severely impaired liver function (unless this is caused by arsenic poisoning). It should be used with caution in people with high blood pressure or impaired kidney function, elderly people, and women who are pregnant or breastfeeding.

dimethicone <dimeticone> A water-repellent silicone used in *barrier preparations, for example for the treatment of napkin rash, pressure sores, and eczema. Activated dimethicone (**simethicone**) is used to relieve wind, gripes, and colic in babies and is also included in *antacid preparations to disperse gas in the stomach and gut. Dimethicone is available without a prescription, but some combined preparations can only be obtained from pharmacies.

Proprietary preparations: Dentinox Infant Colic Drops; Infacol (liquid for gripes, colic, and wind); Settlers Wind-Eze; Windcheaters (tablets); Woodward's Colic Drops; ACTONORM GEL (combined with aluminium hydroxide, magnesium hydroxide, and peppermint oil); ALTACITE PLUS (combined with hydrotalcite, aluminium hydroxide, and magnesium hydroxide); ASILONE SUSPENSION (combined with aluminium hydroxide and magnesium hydroxide); BISODOL EXTRA TABLETS (combined with sodium bicarbonate, calcium carbonate, and magnesium carbonate); COBADEX (combined with hydrocortisone); CONOTRANE (combined with benzalkonium chloride); DIOVOL (combined with aluminium hydroxide and magnesium hydroxide); KOLANTICON GEL (combined with dicyclomine hydrochloride, aluminium hydroxide, and magnesium oxide); MAALOX PLUS (combined with aluminium hydroxide and magnesium hydroxide); RENNIE DEFLATINE (combined with calcium carbonate and magnesium carbonate); SIOPEL (combined with cetrimide); SPRILON (combined with zinc oxide); TIMODINE (combined with nystatin, hydrocortisone, and benzalkonium chloride); VASELINE DERMACARE (combined with white soft paraffin); VASOGEN CREAM (combined with zinc oxide and calamine).

dimethyl sulphoxide (<dimethyl sulfoxide>; **DMSO**) A drug that is used to relieve the pain and other symptoms of a form of cystitis that is associated with an ulcer in the wall of the bladder. It is instilled into the bladder and then voided. Dimethyl sulphoxide is available as a solution for instillation on *prescription only. DMSO may also be combined with other drugs in preparations that are applied topically as it improves their absorption.

Side effects: dimethyl sulphoxide may cause bladder spasms and allergic reactions.

Precautions: prolonged use of dimethyl sulphoxide requires six-monthly monitoring of its effects on the eyes, liver, and kidneys.

Proprietary preparations: Rimso-50; Herpid (combined with *idoxuridine).

dimeticone *See* DIMETHICONE.

Dimetriose (Florizel) *See* GESTRINONE.

Dimotane (Wyeth Laboratories) *See* BROMPHENIRAMINE MALEATE.

Dimotane Co (Whitehall Laboratories) A proprietary combination of *brompheniramine (an antihistamine), *codeine (an analgesic and cough suppressant), and *pseudoephedrine (a decongestant), used for the relief of dry coughs and nasal congestion. It is available as a sugar-free liquid; **Dimotane Co Paediatric** is formulated for children under two years old. Both preparations can be bought without a prescription, but only from pharmacies.

Side effects, precautions, and interactions with other drugs: see ANTIHISTAMINES; CODEINE; DECONGESTANTS; EPHEDRINE; OPIOIDS.

Dimotane Expectorant (Whitehall Laboratories) A proprietary combination of *brompheniramine (an antihistamine), *guaiphenesin <guaifenesin> (an expectorant), and *pseudoephedrine (a decongestant), used for the relief of productive coughs and congestion associated with colds. It is available as a liquid without a prescription, but only from pharmacies.

Side effects and interactions with other drugs: see ANTIHISTAMINES; DECONGESTANTS; EPHEDRINE HYDROCHLORIDE; GUAIPHENESIN <GUAIFENESIN>.

Precautions: this medicine is not recommended for children under two years old. *See also* ANTIHISTAMINES; DECONGESTANTS; EPHEDRINE HYDROCHLORIDE; GUAIPHENESIN <GUAIFENESIN>.

Dimotane Plus (Wyeth Laboratories) A proprietary combination of *brompheniramine maleate (an antihistamine) and *pseudoephedrine (a decongestant), used to relieve the symptoms of hay fever and urticaria (nettle rash). It is available as a liquid; **Dimotane Plus Paediatric** is an elixir for children. Both preparations can be bought from pharmacies without a prescription.

Side effects: see ANTIHISTAMINES; EPHEDRINE HYDROCHLORIDE. This medicine may have stimulant effects in children.

Precautions: Dimotane Plus should be used with caution by people with asthma and by pregnant women.

Interactions with other drugs: see ANTIHISTAMINES; EPHEDRINE HYDROCHLORIDE.

Dimotapp (Whitehall Laboratories) A proprietary combination of the antihistamine *brompheniramine and the decongestants *phenylephrine and *phenylpropanolamine, used for the relief of congestion and catarrh associated with colds, sinusitis, and hay fever. It is available as a sugar-free liquid, *modified-release tablets (**Dimotapp LA**), and a children's formulation (**Dimotapp Paediatric**) without a prescription, but only from pharmacies. It cannot be prescribed on the NHS.

Side effects, precautions, and interactions with other drugs: see ANTIHISTAMINES; PHENYLPROPANOLAMINE; PHENYLEPHRINE; EPHEDRINE HYDROCHLORIDE.

Dindevan (Goldshield Pharmaceuticals) *See* PHENINDIONE.

Dinnefords Teejel (Seton Scholl Healthcare) A proprietary combination of *cetalkonium chloride (an antiseptic) and *choline salicylate (an analgesic), used for the relief of pain and discomfort of mouth ulcers, cold sores, denture irritation, and infant teething problems. It is freely available *over the counter.

Precautions: the gel is not recommended for children under four months old. *See also* SALICYLATES.

dinoprost A *prostaglandin, similar to *dinoprostone, that is injected directly into the amniotic sac to induce abortion. It is available on *prescription, but only in hospitals, and is now rarely used.

Side effects, precautions, and interactions with other drugs: see DINOPROSTONE.

Proprietary preparation: Prostin F2 alpha.

dinoprostone A *prostaglandin used to induce labour, to soften the cervix before labour, and to induce abortion. It is available as tablets, a cervical or vaginal gel, pessaries, vaginal tablets, or a solution for intravenous infusion or injection into the amniotic sac. A *prescription only medicine, dinoprostone should only be used under direct medical supervision.

Side effects: include nausea, vomiting, diarrhoea, high body temperature and flushing, and constriction of the airways; less frequently raised blood pressure, breathlessness, chills, headache, and dizziness may occur.

Precautions: dinoprostone should not be given to women with acute pelvic inflammatory disease or heart, kidney, lung, or liver disease. It should be used with caution in women with a history of glaucoma, asthma, high or low blood pressure, anaemia, jaundice, diabetes, or epilepsy.

Proprietary preparations: Prepidil (cervical gel); Propess-RS (pessaries); Prostin E2 Oral, Prostin E2 Vaginal Tablets; Prostin E2 Solution; Prostin E2 Vaginal Gel.

Diocalm Dual Action (Seton Scholl Healthcare) A proprietary combination of *morphine hydrochloride (which reduces gut motility) and *attapulgite (an antidiarrhoeal drug), used for the treatment of occasional diarrhoea and associated discomfort or pain. It is available as tablets and can be obtained without a prescription, but only from pharmacies.

Side effects and interactions with other drugs: *see* MORPHINE; OPIOIDS.

Precautions: this medicine should not be given to children under six years old.

Diocalm Replenish (Seton Scholl Healthcare) A proprietary combination of glucose (a sugar), *sodium chloride, *sodium citrate, and *potassium chloride, used to prevent and treat dehydration, in particular to replace the *electrolytes lost during attacks of acute diarrhoea (*see* ORAL REHYDRATION THERAPY). It is available as a powder to be dissolved in water and can be obtained without a prescription, but only from pharmacies.

Precautions: Diocalm Replenish should not be taken by people with kidney disease or intestinal obstruction.

Diocalm Ultra (SmithKline Beecham Consumer Healthcare) *See* LOPERAMIDE HYDROCHLORIDE.

Diocaps (APS-Berk) *See* LOPERAMIDE HYDROCHLORIDE.

Dioctyl (Schwartz Pharma) *See* DOCUSATE SODIUM.

dioctyl sodium sulphosuccinate *See* DOCUSATE SODIUM.

Dioderm (Dermal Laboratories) *See* HYDROCORTISONE.

Dioralyte Natural (Rhône-Poulenc Rorer) A proprietary combination of glucose, *sodium chloride, *potassium chloride, and *disodium hydrogen citrate, used for the replacement of *electrolytes in people with diarrhoea (*see* ORAL REHYDRATION THERAPY). It is available as a powder to be dissolved in water and can be obtained without a prescription, but only from pharmacies.

Precautions: Dioralyte Natural should not be taken by people with kidney disease or intestinal obstruction.

Dioralyte Relief (Rhône-Poulenc Rorer) A proprietary combination of *sodium chloride, *potassium chloride, *sodium citrate, and precooked rice powder (a carbohydrate), used for the treatment of diarrhoea (*see* ORAL REHYDRATION THERAPY). It is available as a powder to be dissolved in water and can be obtained without a prescription, but only from pharmacies.

Precautions: Dioralyte Relief should not be taken by people with kidney disease or intestinal obstruction.

Dioralyte Tablets (Rhône-Poulenc Rorer) A proprietary combination of *sodium bicarbonate, *citric acid, glucose, *sodium chloride, and *potassium chloride, used for the replacement of electrolytes in infants, children, or adults suffering from diarrhoea (*see* ORAL REHYDRATION THERAPY). The tablets, which are dissolved in water to make an effervescent drink, can be obtained without a prescription, but only from pharmacies.

Precautions: this medicine should not be taken by people with kidney disease or intestinal obstruction.

Diovan (Novartis Pharmaceuticals) *See* VALSARTAN.

Diovol (Pharmax) A proprietary combination of *aluminium hydroxide and *magnesium hydroxide (antacids) and activated *dimethicone <dimeticone> (an antifoaming agent), used for the treatment of peptic ulcers, increased secretion of stomach acid, and flatulence (*see* ACID-PEPTIC DISEASES). It is freely available *over the counter as a sugar-free suspension.

Side effects, precautions, and interactions with other drugs: see ANTACIDS.

Dipentum (Pharmacia & Upjohn) *See* OLSALAZINE SODIUM.

diphenhydramine An *antihistamine used, in the form of the citrate or hydrochloride, mainly as an ingredient in many cough and cold preparations. As it has marked sedative properties, it is also used for the relief of temporary insomnia. Diphenhydramine is also included in preparations for treating irritating skin conditions. It is available as tablets, capsules, syrups, a cream, or a lotion and may be bought from pharmacies without a prescription.

Side effects: sedation is common and *extrapyramidal reactions have been reported. *See also* ANTIHISTAMINES.

Precautions and interactions with other drugs: see ANTIHISTAMINES.

Proprietary preparations: Aller-eze Cream; Bronalin Paediatric (syrup); Medinex (liquid for insomnia); Nytol (tablets for insomnia); BENYLIN CHESTY COUGHS ORIGINAL (combined with ammonium chloride and menthol); BENYLIN CHILDREN'S NIGHT COUGHS (combined with menthol); BENYLIN WITH CODEINE (combined with codeine and menthol); BENYLIN COUGH & CONGESTION (combined with dextromethorphan, pseudoephedrine, and menthol); BENYLIN DAY & NIGHT TABLETS (night tablets; combined with paracetamol); BENYLIN DRY COUGHS ORIGINAL (combined with dextromethorphan and menthol); BENYLIN 4 FLU (combined with paracetamol and phenylephrine); BOOTS CATARRH SYRUP FOR CHILDREN (combined with pseudoephedrine); BOOTS CHILDREN'S 1 YEAR PLUS NIGHT TIME COUGH SYRUP (combined with pholcodine); BOOTS NIGHT COLD COMFORT (combined with paracetamol, pholcodine, and pseudoephedrine); BOOTS NIGHT-TIME COUGH RELIEF (combined with pholcodine); BRONALIN EXPECTORANT (combined with ammonium chloride); CALADRYL (combined with zinc oxide and camphor); COVONIA NIGHT TIME FORMULA (combined with dextromethorphan); ECDYLIN (combined with ammonium chloride); GUANOR EXPECTORANT (combined

with ammonium chloride and menthol); HISTALIX (combined with
ammonium chloride and menthol); PANADOL NIGHT (combined with
paracetamol); PROPAIN (combined with caffeine, codeine, and
paracetamol); TIXYLIX CATARRH SYRUP (combined with menthol); UNIFLU
WITH GREGOVITE C (combined with codeine, paracetamol, and
phenylephrine).

diphenoxylate hydrochloride See CO-PHENOTROPE; OPIOIDS.

diphenylpyraline An *antihistamine that is not used alone but is
included as an ingredient of some proprietary cold or cough remedies
(capsules or syrup). Preparations containing diphenylpyraline are
available without a prescription, but usually only from pharmacies.
Side effects, precautions, and interactions with other drugs: see
ANTIHISTAMINES.
Proprietary preparation: ESKORNADE (combined with
phenylpropanolamine).

dipipanone hydrochloride A strong *opioid analgesic that is used in
combination with an antiemetic drug for the treatment of moderate to
severe pain. Dipipanone is a *controlled drug.
Side effects and precautions: see MORPHINE.
Interactions with other drugs: see OPIOIDS.
Proprietary preparation: DICONAL (combined with cyclizine).

dipivefrin A *sympathomimetic drug used for the treatment of
chronic (open-angle) *glaucoma. It acts in a similar way to *adrenaline
<epinephrine>, to which it is converted in the eye. Dipivefrin is available
as eye drops on *prescription only.
Side effects: there may be transient stinging and allergic reactions.
Precautions: dipivefrin should not be used by people who wear soft
contact lenses and should be used with caution by people with heart
disease and high blood pressure (*hypertension). It should not be used to
treat closed-angle glaucoma.
Proprietary preparation: Propine.

Diprobase (Schering-Plough) A proprietary combination of *liquid
paraffin and *white soft paraffin (both emollients) in the form of a cream
or ointment, used to soothe dry skin conditions. It is freely available
*over the counter .

Diprobath (Schering-Plough) A proprietary combination of light *liquid
paraffin and *isopropyl myristate, used as an emollient to relieve dry
skin conditions. It is available as an emulsion to be added to the bath and
can be obtained without a prescription, but only from pharmacies.

Diprosalic (Schering-Plough) A proprietary combination of
*betamethasone (a corticosteroid) and *salicylic acid (a keratolytic), used

as a potent topical steroid and skin softener for the treatment of *eczema that has not responded to less potent steroids and *psoriasis. A *prescription only medicine, it is available as an ointment and as a lotion for the scalp (**Diprosalic Scalp Application**).

Side effects, precautions, and interactions with other drugs: see TOPICAL STEROIDS; SALICYLIC ACID.

Diprosone (Schering-Plough) *See* BETAMETHASONE.

dipyridamole An *antiplatelet drug that is used as additional therapy (to oral *anticoagulants) for the prevention of thromboembolism (*see* THROMBOSIS). *Modified-release preparations are also used to prevent strokes in people who have already had a stroke. Dipyridamole is available, on *prescription only, as tablets, a suspension, or modified-release capsules.

Side effects: include nausea, indigestion, headache, dizziness, muscle aches, low blood pressure, a fast heart rate, hot flushes, and allergic rashes.

Precautions: dipyridamole should be used with caution by people with severe angina, migraine, or low blood pressure, and by those who have had a recent heart attack.

Interactions with other drugs:

Adenosine: the anti-arrhythmic effects of adenosine are increased and prolonged by dipyridamole.

Antacids: the use of antacids with dipyridamole should be avoided.

Anticoagulants: their effects are enhanced by dipyridamole.

Proprietary preparations: Cerebrovase; Modaplate; Persantin; Persantin Retard (modified-release capsules); ASASANTIN RETARD (combined with aspirin).

Dirythmin SA (AstraZeneca) *See* DISOPYRAMIDE.

disinfectants Agents that destroy or remove bacteria and other microorganisms and are used to cleanse surgical instruments and other objects. Examples are cresol, *hexachlorophane <hexachlorophene>, and *phenol. Dilute solutions of some disinfectants may be used as *antiseptics or as preservatives in solutions of eye drops or injections.

Disipal (Yamanouchi Pharma) *See* ORPHENADRINE.

disodium edetate A compound included in many preparations as an antioxidant and preservative. It is also a chelating agent that binds free calcium, and is included in solutions for washing out urinary catheters.

Proprietary preparations: URIFLEX G (combined with citric acid, sodium bicarbonate, and magnesium oxide); URIFLEX R (combined with citric acid, magnesium carbonate, and gluconolactone); URO-TAINER SUBY G (combined with citric acid, magnesium oxide, and sodium bicarbonate).

disodium etidronate A *bisphosphonate that is used to treat Paget's disease (in which the bones become deformed and fracture easily). Taken with *calcium carbonate, it is also used for the treatment and prevention of postmenopausal osteoporosis of the spine, especially in women for whom *hormone replacement therapy is unsuitable, and corticosteroid-induced osteoporosis. Etidronate is available, on *prescription only, as tablets and a form of infusion.

Side effects: include nausea and diarrhoea, and there may initially be increased bone pain in patients with Paget's disease (this usually disappears as treatment continues); rare side effects are allergic skin reactions (itching or rash), abdominal pain, constipation, headache, and 'pins and needles'.

Precautions: etidronate should not be taken by people with liver or kidney disease or by women who are pregnant or breastfeeding. Food and certain drugs (see below) should be avoided for at least two hours before and after taking the tablets, since they bind to etidronate in the stomach and intestine and prevent its absorption.

Interactions with other drugs:

Aminoglycosides: in combination with etidronate, they may cause abnormally low concentrations of calcium in the plasma.

Antacids: reduce the absorption of etidronate tablets.

Calcium supplements: reduce the absorption of etidronate tablets.

Iron supplements: reduce the absorption of etidronate tablets.

Proprietary preparations: Didronel; Didronel PMO (packaged with effervescent tablets of calcium carbonate).

disodium hydrogen citrate A salt of *sodium that has a clean sharp lemon taste. It is an ingredient of *electrolyte replacement solutions used in *oral rehydration therapy.

Proprietary preparation: DIORALYTE NATURAL (combined with glucose, sodium chloride, and potassium chloride).

disodium pamidronate A *bisphosphonate used to reduce high concentrations of calcium in the blood in the treatment of bone cancer, bone pain due to secondary tumours, and Paget's disease. It is available as an injection on *prescription only.

Side effects: include mild transient fever, influenza-like symptoms, local reactions at the injection site, and transient bone pain or muscle aches.

Precautions: people should not drive or operate machinery immediately after treatment. Pamidronate should not be given to women who are pregnant or breastfeeding and should be used with caution in people with kidney disease.

Interactions with other drugs:

Aminoglycosides: in combination with pamidronate, they may cause abnormally low concentrations of calcium in the plasma.

Proprietary preparation: Aredia.

disodium phosphate dodecahydrate *See* PHOSPHATE LAXATIVES.

disopyramide A class I *anti-arrhythmic drug used to treat superventricular arrhythmias or ventricular arrhythmias after a heart attack (*see* ARRHYTHMIA). It is available, on *prescription only, as capsules, *modified-release tablets, or an injection.

Side effects: include dry mouth, urinary retention, constipation, blurred vision, gastrointestinal upset, and hypotension (low blood pressure).

Precautions: disopyramide should be used with caution during pregnancy and by people with liver or kidney disease, heart failure, enlarged prostate, or glaucoma. *See also* ANTI-ARRHYTHMIC DRUGS.

Interactions with other drugs:

Other anti-arrhythmic drugs: amiodarone increases the risk of ventricular arrhythmias and should not be used with disopyramide; depression of heart function is increased if disopyramide is taken with any other anti-arrhythmic.

Antibiotics: the plasma concentration (and therefore effects) of disopyramide is increased by erythromycin (and possibly clarithromycin) and reduced by rifampicin.

Antihistamines: disopyramide should not be taken with astemizole, terfenadine, or mizolastine as these drugs increase the risk of ventricular arrhythmias.

Antipsychotic drugs: disopyramide should not be taken with pimozide, sertindole, or thioridazine as these drugs increase the risk of ventricular arrhythmias.

Beta blockers: sotalol increases the risk of ventricular arrhythmias and should not be taken with disopyramide; heart function is depressed if other beta blockers are taken with disopyramide.

Cisapride: should not be taken with disopyramide as this combination increases the risk of ventricular arrhythmias.

Diuretics: increase toxicity to the heart through potassium depletion.

Halofantrine: increases the risk of ventricular arrhythmias.

Tricyclic antidepressants: increase the risk of ventricular arrhythmias.

Verapamil: depression of heart function is increased if verapamil is taken with disopyramide.

Proprietary preparations: Dirythmin SA (modifed-release tablets); Rythmodan; Rythmodan Retard (modified-release tablets).

Disprin, **Disprin CV**, **Disprin Direct** (Reckitt & Colman) *See* ASPIRIN.

Disprin Extra (Reckitt & Colman) A proprietary combination of *aspirin and *paracetamol (analgesics and antipyretics), used for the treatment of mild to moderate pain (including headache, neuralgia, toothache, and period pains) and fever and to relieve the symptoms of influenza and colds. It is freely available *over the counter in the form of soluble tablets.

Side effects and interactions with other drugs: see ASPIRIN.

Precautions: Disprin Extra should not be given to children, except on medical advice. *See also* ASPIRIN; PARACETAMOL.

Disprol (Reckitt & Colman) *See* PARACETAMOL.

Distaclor, **Distaclor MR** (Dista) *See* CEFACLOR.

Distalgesic (Dista) *See* CO-PROXAMOL.

Distamine (Dista) *See* PENICILLAMINE.

distigmine bromide An *anticholinesterase drug used for the treatment of myasthenia gravis. It is also used to reverse paralysis of the small intestine and to treat urinary retention, especially after surgery. Distigmine is similar to *pyridostigmine and *neostigmine but has a longer duration of action. It is available as tablets on *prescription only.
Side effects: include nausea and vomiting, sweating, increased salivation, diarrhoea, abdominal cramps, and blurred vision.
Precautions: distigmine should not be taken by people with intestinal or urinary obstruction or by those in postoperative shock. It should be used with caution in people with asthma, low blood pressure, peptic ulcers, epilepsy, Parkinson's disease, or kidney disease.
Interactions with other drugs: see PYRIDOSTIGMINE.
Proprietary preparation: Ubretid.

disulfiram A drug used in the treatment of chronic alcohol dependence, but only under specialist supervision. It causes acetaldehyde, a breakdown product of alcohol, to accumulate in the blood, which results in extremely unpleasant reactions after consuming even a small amount of alcohol; these include flushing, a throbbing headache, palpitation, a fast heart rate, nausea, and vomiting. If large amounts of alcohol are consumed the reaction is severe: an abnormal heart rhythm (*see* ARRHYTHMIA), with low blood pressure and eventually collapse. It is essential for people to abstain from alcohol for at least 24 hours before starting treatment with disulfiram and that they understand the severity and possible dangers of the reaction between disulfiram and alcohol. Disulfiram is available as tablets on *prescription only.
Side effects: include drowsiness and fatigue at the start of the treatment, nausea, vomiting, bad breath, and decreased libido. Rarely, depression, paranoia, mania, allergic skin rashes, liver damage, and damage to peripheral nerves may occur.
Precautions: people taking disulfiram may be advised to carry a warning card, emphasizing the dangerous effects of alcohol taken with disulfiram. Even the small amounts of alcohol in some oral medicines may be sufficient to cause a reaction, and toiletries containing alcohol should be avoided. Disulfiram should not be taken by people who have heart failure, coronary artery disease, a history of stroke, high blood pressure,

psychosis, or personality disorder. It should not be taken by women who are pregnant or breastfeeeding.

Interactions with other drugs:

Anticoagulants: the anticoagulant effects of warfarin and nicoumalone <acenocoumarol> are increased.

Phenytoin: the risk of phenytoin causing adverse effects is increased.

Proprietary preparation: Antabuse.

Ditemic (SmithKline Beecham Pharmaceuticals) A proprietary combination of *ferrous sulphate, *zinc sulphate monohydrate, B vitamins (*see* VITAMIN B COMPLEX), and *vitamin C, used to treat iron-deficiency *anaemia. It is available as *modified-release capsules and can be obtained without a prescription, but only from pharmacies.

Side effects, precautions, and interactions with other drugs: see IRON.

dithranol A drug used in the treatment of mild to moderately severe chronic *psoriasis. Since dithranol is irritant to healthy skin, care must be taken to apply it only to affected areas. Also, as some people are allergic to this drug, a small area of skin should be tested for sensitivity to dithranol before treatment starts. It is usual to start with a low concentration (0.1%), which is gradually built up to higher concentrations (1–3%). Preparations are washed off after each treatment. Dithranol is sometimes used in conjunction with *coal tar and UVB (ultraviolet-B) light. It is available as a cream, ointment, or paste (**Lassar's paste**). Preparations containing more than 1% dithranol are *prescription only medicines, but those with lower concentrations can be obtained from pharmacies without a prescription.

Side effects: dithranol commonly causes local irritation of the skin and a burning sensation; it stains skin, clothing, and other fabrics.

Precautions: dithranol should not be used to treat acute psoriasis. It should not come into contact with the eyes, face, mucous membranes, broken skin, or genitals. It should be used with caution by women who are pregnant or breastfeeding. Soaps or shampoos should not be used to remove the cream.

Proprietary preparations: Dithrocream (0.1–0.25%); Dithrocream Forte (0.5%); Dithrocream HP (1%); Dithrocream 2%; Micanol; PSORIN (combined with coal tar and salicylic acid); PSORIN SCALP GEL (combined with salicylic acid).

Dithrocream (Dermal Laboratories) *See* DITHRANOL.

Ditropan (Lorex Synthélabo) *See* OXYBUTYNIN HYDROCHLORIDE.

Diumide-K Continus (ASTA Medica) A proprietary combination of *frusemide <furosemide> (a loop diuretic) and *potassium chloride. Available on *prescription only, it is taken orally in the form of *modified-release tablets for the treatment of *oedema associated with congestive heart failure, liver disease, or kidney disease.

Side effects, precautions, and interactions with other drugs: see LOOP DIURETICS.

See also DIURETICS.

diuretics A class of drugs that increase the volume of urine (diuresis) by promoting the excretion of salts (especially sodium and potassium) and water via the kidneys. Diuretics are used to reduce the *oedema due to salt and water retention in disorders of the kidneys, heart, or liver. They are also used, alone or in combination with other drugs, in the treatment of high blood pressure (*see* HYPERTENSION). The use of diuretics can result in potassium deficiency; this is corrected by the simultaneous administration of a *potassium supplement or by adding another diuretic with a potassium-sparing effect, such as amiloride or triamterene. (Potassium is essential for the normal functioning of nerves and muscles; low concentrations of potassium cause weakness, confusion, and in severe cases abnormal heart rhythms.) The main classes of diuretics are the *loop diuretics, *thiazide diuretics, and *potassium-sparing diuretics.

Diurexan (ASTA Medica) *See* XIPAMIDE.

Dixarit (Boehringer Ingelheim) *See* CLONIDINE HYDROCHLORIDE.

dobutamine hydrochloride A drug that stimulates beta-adrenoceptors in the heart (*see* SYMPATHOMIMETIC DRUGS). It is used to increase blood pressure in patients who have had a heart attack or open heart surgery or in cases of shock. It may also be used for heart stress testing during diagnostic procedures. Available as an intravenous solution on prescription, it is only used in hospitals.

Side effects and precautions: a fast heart rate and a marked increase in blood pressure may indicate an overdose.

Interactions with other drugs:

 Beta blockers: severe hypertension may result if these drugs are taken with dobutamine.

 Entacapone: may enhance the effects of dobutamine.

Proprietary preparations: Dobutrex; Posiject.

Dobutrex (Eli Lilly & Co) *See* DOBUTAMINE HYDROCHLORIDE.

docetaxel A *taxane used for the treatment of breast *cancer that is resistant to other cytotoxic therapies. Docetaxel can cause fluid retention and (like *paclitaxel) severe allergic reactions: *dexamethasone is usually given before treatment to reduce these side effects. Docetaxel is available as a solution for intravenous infusion on *prescription only.

Side effects: include fluid retention causing swelling of the legs, allergic reactions, *bone marrow suppression, hair loss, and muscle pain. *See also* CYTOTOXIC DRUGS.

Precautions: docetaxel should not be given to women who are pregnant

or breastfeeding and should be used with caution in people with liver disease. *See also* CYTOTOXIC DRUGS.
Proprietary preparation: Taxotere.

docusate sodium (dioctyl sodium sulphosuccinate) A *stimulant laxative and *faecal softener that is used, alone or in combination with other laxatives, in the treatment of constipation and to clear the bowel before X-ray examination. It has a detergent action, which reduces surface tension, and is therefore also used to soften ear wax. Docusate is available as capsules, a solution, enemas, or ear drops and can be obtained without a prescription, but only from pharmacies. *See also* CO-DANTHRUSATE.
Side effects and precautions: see STIMULANT LAXATIVES.
Proprietary preparations: Dioctyl (capsules); Docusol (adult or paediatric solutions); Molcer (ear drops); Norgalax Micro-enema; Waxsol (ear drops); Capsuvac (*see* CO-DANTHRUSATE); FLETCHERS' ENEMETTE (combined with glycerin); Normax (*see* CO-DANTHRUSATE).

Docusol (Typharm) *See* DOCUSATE SODIUM.

Do-Do ChestEze (Novartis Consumer Health) A proprietary combination of *ephedrine (a decongestant), *theophylline (a bronchodilator), and *caffeine, used for the relief of bronchial coughs, wheezing, and breathlessness and to clear the chest of mucus following infections of the upper airways. It is available as tablets without a prescription, but only from pharmacies.
Side effects and interactions with other drugs: see EPHEDRINE HYDROCHLORIDE; DECONGESTANTS; THEOPHYLLINE; XANTHINES.
Precautions: this medicine is not recommended for children under 12 years old except on medical advice. *See also* EPHEDRINE HYDROCHLORIDE; DECONGESTANTS; THEOPHYLLINE; XANTHINES.

Do-Do Expectorant (Novartis Consumer Health) *See* GUAIPHENESIN <GUAIFENESIN>.

Dolmatil (Lorex Synthélabo) *See* SULPIRIDE.

Dolobid (Merck Sharp & Dohme) *See* DIFLUNISAL.

Doloxene (Eli Lilly & Co) *See* DEXTROPROPOXYPHENE HYDROCHLORIDE.

Domical (APS-Berk) *See* AMITRIPTYLINE HYDROCHLORIDE.

domiphen An *antiseptic used in solutions to disinfect the skin and in lozenges for the treatment of minor infections of the mouth and throat.
Proprietary preparation: BRADOSOL PLUS (combined with lignocaine).

Domperamol (Servier Laboratories) A proprietary combination of *paracetamol (an analgesic) and *domperidone (an antiemetic), used for the relief of acute attacks of mild to moderate migraine. It is available as tablets on *prescription only.

Side effects: *see* DOMPERIDONE.

Precautions: Domperamol is not recommended for children. *See also* DOMPERIDONE.

domperidone A drug that antagonizes the action of *dopamine. It is an *antiemetic used to prevent or treat nausea and vomiting, especially that associated with *cytotoxic drug therapy. Domperidone also stimulates gastric motility (*see* PROKINETIC DRUGS) and is used in the treatment of indigestion not due to peptic ulceration. It is available, on *prescription only, as tablets, a suspension, or suppositories; packs of 10 tablets for the relief of indigestion can be obtained from pharmacies without a prescription.

Side effects: include breast enlargement and pain, allergic rashes, and (rarely) *extrapyramidal reactions.

Precautions: domperidone should be used with caution by people with kidney disease and by women who are pregnant or breastfeeding.

Proprietary preparations: Motilium; Motilium 10; DOMPERAMOL (combined with paracetamol).

donepezil hydrochloride An *acetylcholinesterase inhibitor that increases the amounts of acetylcholine in the brain. It is used to treat the symptoms of mild to moderate dementia (including short-term memory loss) that occur in people with Alzheimer's disease and has been shown to have some success in slowing the progress of the disease. Donepezil is not effective in treating other forms of dementia or confusion. It is available as tablets on *prescription only, and treatment should be supervised by a specialist.

Side effects: include nausea, vomiting, diarrhoea, fatigue, insomnia, muscle cramps, and (less commonly) headache, dizziness, fainting, and slowing of the heart rate.

Precautions: donepezil should not be taken by women who are pregnant or breastfeeding and should be used with caution in people who have certain heart conditions, or who are likely to develop a peptic ulcer, or who have asthma or chronic bronchitis.

Interactions with other drugs:

  Muscle relaxants: donepezil may either increase or reduce the effects of muscle relaxants used in surgery to paralyse muscles.

Proprietary preparation: Aricept.

Dopacard (Ipsen) *See* DOPEXAMINE.

dopamine A substance that transmits messages between nerve cells in the brain. Dopamine is also an intermediate product in the biochemical pathway that manufactures other neurotransmitters, noradrenaline <norepinephrine> and adrenaline <epinephrine>. Dopamine also controls the secretion of the hormones prolactin and *growth hormone by exerting an inhibitory effect. Outside the brain, dopamine has effects on the heart and blood vessels and is used in the form of *dopamine hydrochloride to treat circulatory collapse.

Imbalance of dopamine concentrations in the brain causes a variety of conditions that may be treated by drugs that either increase dopamine levels or inhibit the action of dopamine. Drugs that stimulate dopamine receptors (leading to increased production of dopamine) or increase dopamine activity are known as **dopamine receptor agonists**. They include *amantadine, *bromocriptine, *cabergoline, and *quinagolide and are used to treat Parkinson's disease (*see* ANTIPARKINSONIAN DRUGS) and to relieve some hormone disorders.

Drugs that prevent the action of dopamine by competing with it to occupy and block dopamine receptor sites in the brain and elsewhere are called **dopamine receptor antagonists**. It is thought that psychoses may be associated with excessive dopamine activity in the brain, and some *antipsychotic drugs (e.g. the phenothiazines and butyrophenones) are dopamine antagonists. The antiemetic drugs *domperidone and *metoclopramide act partly by blocking the action of dopamine at the vomiting centre in the brain. Antagonism of dopamine action also produces a group of side effects known as *extrapyramidal reactions.

dopamine hydrochloride A preparation of *dopamine used to treat cardiogenic shock (collapse of the circulation) resulting from heart failure, heart attack, or heart surgery; it is thought to stimulate beta-receptors in the heart (*see* SYMPATHOMIMETIC DRUGS) and also dopamine receptors in blood vessels, particularly in the kidney. It is available, on *prescription only, as a solution for injection or infusion.
Side effects: include nausea and vomiting, changes in heart rate and blood pressure, and constriction of the blood vessels in the fingers and toes.
Precautions: dopamine hydrochloride should not be given to patients with phaeochromocytoma (a tumour of the adrenal gland) or abnormal heart rhythms (*see* ARRHYTHMIA).
Interactions with other drugs:
  MAOIs: there is a risk of a dangerous rise in blood pressure; dopamine should not be taken within two weeks of stopping MAOIs.
Proprietary preparations: Dopamine Hydrochloride in Dextrose (Glucose) Injection; Select-a-Jet Dopamine.

dopexamine A beta-adrenoceptor stimulant (*see* SYMPATHOMIMETIC DRUGS) that also has some other pharmacological actions. It increases the output of the heart and increases blood flow to the kidneys and gut. It is used to maintain heart function during heart surgery. Available on *prescription only as an intravenous injection, it is only used in hospitals.
Side effects: include a fast heartbeat; nausea, vomiting, anginal pain, tremor, and headache have also been reported.
Interactions with other drugs:

Adrenaline <epinephrine> and noradrenaline <norepinephrine>: their effects may be increased by dopexamine.

MAOIs: a severe rise in blood pressure may occur if these drugs are taken with dopexamine.

Proprietary preparation: Dopacard.

Dopram (Antigen Pharmaceuticals) *See* DOXAPRAM HYDROCHLORIDE.

Doralese (SmithKline Beecham Pharmaceuticals) *See* INDORAMIN HYDROCHLORIDE.

dornase alfa A *mucolytic drug that breaks down mucus by cleaving DNA; it is a genetically engineered version of a natural human enzyme. Dornase alfa is used for the management of cystic fibrosis patients who accumulate large amounts of tenacious mucus. It is administered by inhalation using a jet nebulizer and is available on *prescription only.

Side effects: include sore throat, hoarseness, laryngitis, chest pain, conjunctivitis, and rash.

Precautions: dornase alfa should not be mixed with other drugs in the nebulizer. It should be used with caution in women who are pregnant or breastfeeding.

Proprietary preparation: Pulmozyme.

dorzolamide A *carbonic anhydrase inhibitor that is used to reduce the pressure inside the eye in the treatment of chronic (open-angle) *glaucoma; it acts by reducing the production of aqueous fluid in the eye. Dorzolamide is used, either alone or in combination with a *beta blocker, to treat patients who have not responded to beta blockers alone or in whom beta blockers should not be used. It is available as eye drops on *prescription only.

Side effects: include burning, stinging, and itching of the eye, a bitter taste in the mouth, blurred vision, increased production of tears, conjunctivitis, inflammation of the eyelid, headache, dizziness, tingling in the fingers, nausea, rash, and allergic reactions.

Precautions: dorzolamide should not be used in people with severe kidney disease or in women who are pregnant or breastfeeding. It should be used with caution in people with liver disease.

Interactions with other drugs:

Phenytoin: there is an increased risk of osteomalacia.

Proprietary preparations: Trusopt; COSOPT (combined with timolol maleate).

Dostinex (Pharmacia & Upjohn) *See* CABERGOLINE.

dosulepin hydrochloride *See* DOTHIEPIN HYDROCHLORIDE.

Dothapax (Ashbourne Pharmaceuticals) *See* DOTHIEPIN <DOSULEPIN> HYDROCHLORIDE.

dothiepin hydrochloride <dosulepin hydrochloride> A *tricyclic antidepressant drug used for the treatment of depressive illness and anxiety with depression, especially when sedation is required. It is available as tablets or capsules on *prescription only.
Side effects, precautions, and interactions with other drugs: see TRICYCLIC ANTIDEPRESSANTS; AMITRIPTYLINE HYDROCHLORIDE.
Proprietary preparations: Dothapax; Prepadine; Prothiaden.

Double Check (Family Planning Sales) *See* NONOXINOL-9.

Dovonex (Leo Pharmaceuticals) *See* CALCIPOTRIOL.

doxapram hydrochloride A drug that stimulates breathing (i.e. it is a respiratory *stimulant). It may be used to reverse the inhibition of breathing (respiratory depression) caused by drugs during surgery. It can also be used to treat acute respiratory failure. Doxapram is available as a form for intravenous injection or infusion on *prescription only.
Side effects: include warmth around the perineum, dizziness, sweating, and increases in blood pressure and heart rate.
Precautions: doxapram should not be used in people with severe asthma or hypertension, coronary artery disease, epilepsy, or an overactive thyroid gland.
Interactions with other drugs:
 MAOIs: may increase the effects of doxapram.
 Sympathomimetic drugs: the risk of high blood pressure is increased if these drugs are given with doxapram.
 Theophylline: stimulation of the central nervous system is increased.
Proprietary preparation: Dopram.

doxazosin An *alpha blocker used to treat *hypertension and to relieve the obstruction of urine flow that can occur in men with an enlarged prostate gland. It is available as tablets on *prescription only.
Side effects, precautions, and interactions with other drugs: see ALPHA BLOCKERS.
Proprietary preparation: Cardura.
See also ANTIHYPERTENSIVE DRUGS; VASODILATORS.

doxepin A *tricyclic antidepressant drug that is taken by mouth for the treatment of depression and is applied to the skin for the relief of itching associated with *eczema. Doxepin is available, on *prescription only, as capsules or a cream.
Side effects: see AMITRIPTYLINE HYDROCHLORIDE. The cream can cause drowsiness and local burning, stinging, irritation, or rash.
Precautions: see TRICYCLIC ANTIDEPRESSANTS. Doxepin capsules should not to be taken by women who are breastfeeding; the cream should not be applied to large areas of skin.

Interactions with other drugs: see TRICYCLIC ANTIDEPRESSANTS.
Proprietary preparations: Sinequan (capsules); Xepin (cream).

doxorubicin One of the most widely used and effective *cytotoxic drugs. A *cytotoxic antibiotic, doxorubicin is administered intravenously for the treatment of acute leukaemias, lymphomas, and a variety of solid tumours (*see* CANCER) and is instilled directly into the bladder to treat bladder cancer. It is also used to treat AIDS-related Kaposi's sarcoma (a tumour of blood vessels in the skin), for which it is available as a lipid formulation for infusion; the lipid enhances its uptake by the tumour cells. Doxorubicin is a *prescription only medicine.

Side effects: include moderate to severe nausea and vomiting, *bone marrow suppression, hair loss, and inflammation of the mouth. High doses can have adverse effects on the heart. Leakage from the infusion tube can damage the surrounding tissue. *See also* CYTOTOXIC DRUGS.

Precautions: doxorubicin should not be given to people with pre-existing heart disease, women who are pregnant or breastfeeding, elderly people, or anyone who has received radiation. Heart function should be closely monitored. Doxorubicin is irritant to the skin and must be handled carefully. *See also* CYTOTOXIC DRUGS.

Interactions with other drugs:

Cyclosporin: the risk of this drug causing nerve damage is increased.

Proprietary preparation: Caelyx (lipid formulation).

doxycycline A tetracycline antibiotic used for the treatment of chronic bronchitis, brucellosis, chlamydial infections, and infections caused by mycoplasmas and rickettsias (*see* TETRACYCLINES). It is also used to treat mouth ulcers, acne, prostatitis, sinusitis, and pelvic inflammatory disease. Although it does not have a *licence for this purpose, doxycycline is also used as a prophylactic protection against malaria, especially in areas, such as southeast Asia, where the malarial parasites are resistant to mefloquine and in people who cannot take chloroquine or mefloquine. Unlike most other tetracyclines, doxycycline does not exacerbate kidney disease and may be taken by those with impaired kidney function. It is available, on *prescription only, as tablets, dispersible tablets, or capsules.

Side effects and precautions: see TETRACYCLINES.

Interactions with other drugs:

Antiepileptics: carbamazepine, phenobarbitone <phenobarbital>, phenytoin, and primidone reduce the plasma concentration of doxycycline.

See also TETRACYCLINES.

Proprietary preparations: Cyclodox (capsules); Demix (capsules); Doxylar (capsules); Ramysis (capsules); Vibramycin (capsules); Vibramycin Acne Pack; Vibramycin-D (dispersible tablets).

doxylamine An *antihistamine that is included as an ingredient of tablets to relieve headaches.

Side effects, precautions, and interactions with other drugs: see
ANTIHISTAMINES.
Proprietary preparation: BOOTS TENSION HEADACHE RELIEF (combined
with paracetamol, caffeine, and codeine).

Doxylar (Lagap Pharmaceuticals) *See* DOXYCYCLINE.

Dozic (Rosemont Pharmaceuticals) *See* HALOPERIDOL.

Dramamine (Searle) *See* DIMENHYDRINATE.

Drapolene Cream (Warner-Lambert Consumer Healthcare) A
proprietary combination of the antiseptics *benzalkonium chloride and
*cetrimide in a base that includes *white soft paraffin and wool fat (*see*
LANOLIN), used as a *barrier preparation for the prevention and
treatment of napkin rash. It is freely available *over the counter.

Driclor (Stiefel Laboratories) *See* ALUMINIUM CHLORIDE.

Dristan Decongestant Tablets (Whitehall Laboratories) A
proprietary combination of *aspirin (an analgesic and antipyretic),
*phenylephrine (a decongestant), *chlorpheniramine <chlorphenamine>
maleate (an antihistamine), and *caffeine (a stimulant), used to relieve
the symptoms of colds and influenza, including congestion, catarrh,
aches and pains, and fever. It can be obtained without a prescription, but
only from pharmacies.
Side effects and interactions with other drugs: see ASPIRIN;
PHENYLEPHRINE; ANTIHISTAMINES.
Precautions: these tablets should not be given to children, except on
medical advice. *See also* ASPIRIN; PHENYLEPHRINE; ANTIHISTAMINES;
CAFFEINE.

Dristan Nasal Spray (Whitehall Laboratories) *See* OXYMETAZOLINE.

Drogenil (Schering-Plough) *See* FLUTAMIDE.

Droleptan (Janssen-Cilag) *See* DROPERIDOL.

droperidol A butyrophenone *antipsychotic drug used for the rapid
calming of manic or agitated patients. It is also used as an *antiemetic for
controlling nausea and vomiting induced by cytotoxic drugs in cancer
patients. Droperidol is available, on *prescription only, as tablets, an oral
liquid, or an injection.
Side effects: as for *chlorpromazine, but droperidol has more
pronounced *extrapyramidal reactions, fewer antimuscarinic effects, and
is less sedating.
Precautions: see CHLORPROMAZINE HYDROCHLORIDE.
Interactions with other drugs:

Anaesthetics: their effect in lowering blood pressure is enhanced.

Antidepressants: there is an increased risk of antimuscarinic effects and arrhythmias (abnormal heartbeats) if droperidol is taken with tricyclic antidepressants.

Antiepileptic drugs: their anticonvulsant effects are antagonized by droperidol.

Antihistamines: there is an increased risk of arrhythmias if droperidol is taken with astemizole or terfenadine.

Halofantrine: there is an increased risk of arrhythmias if this drug is taken with droperidol.

Ritonavir: may increase the effects of droperidol.

Sedatives: the sedative effects of droperidol are increased if it is taken with anxiolytic or hypnotic drugs, or any other drug that causes sedation.

Proprietary preparation: Droleptan.

Dryptal (APS-Berk) *See* FRUSEMIDE <FUROSEMIDE>.

DTIC-Dome (Bayer) *See* DACARBAZINE.

Dubam Cream (Wallace Manufacturing) A proprietary combination of *methyl salicylate, *menthol, and cineole (*see* TURPENTINE OIL), used as a *rubefacient for the relief of aches, pains, and stiffness in muscles, tendons, and joints, including backache, sciatica, lumbago, and fibrositis. It is freely available *over the counter.
Side effects and precautions: *see* RUBEFACIENTS; SALICYLATES.

Dubam Spray (Wallace Manufacturing) A proprietary combination of *methyl salicylate, *ethyl salicylate, *methyl nicotinate, and *glycol salicylate, used as a *rubefacient for the relief of aches, pains, and stiffness in muscles, tendons and joints, including backache, sciatica, lumbago, and fibrositis. It is freely available *over the counter.
Side effects and precautions: *see* RUBEFACIENTS; SALICYLATES.

Dulco-Lax (Boehringer Ingelheim) *See* BISACODYL.

Dulco-Lax Liquid (Boehringer Ingelheim) *See* SODIUM PICOSULPHATE <PICOSULFATE>.

Dumicoat (Cox Pharmaceuticals) *See* MICONAZOLE.

Duofilm (Stiefel Laboratories) A proprietary combination of *salicylic acid and *lactic acid (both keratolytics), used for the treatment of verrucas. It is available as a paint and can be obtained without a prescription, but only from pharmacies.
Side effects and precautions: *see* SALICYLIC ACID.

Duovent (Boehringer Ingelheim) A proprietary combination of the

bronchodilators *fenoterol hydrobromide (a sympathomimetic drug) and *ipratropium bromide (an antimuscarinic drug), used to relieve constriction of the airways associated with chronic bronchitis and emphysema. It is available as a breath-activated metered-dose aerosol *inhaler; **Duovent UDV** is a solution for use in a *nebulizer. Both preparations are *prescription only medicines.
Side effects, precautions, and interactions with other drugs: see SALBUTAMOL; IPRATROPIUM BROMIDE.

Duphalac (Solvay Healthcare) *See* LACTULOSE.

Duphaston (Solvay Healthcare) *See* DYDROGESTERONE.

Duragel (LRC Products) *See* NONOXINOL-9.

Durogesic (Janssen-Cilag) *See* FENTANYL.

Duromine (3M Health Care) *See* PHENTERMINE.

Dutonin (Bristol-Myers Squibb) *See* NEFAZODONE HYDROCHLORIDE.

Dyazide (SmithKline Beecham Pharmaceuticals) A proprietary combination of *triamterene (a potassium-sparing diuretic) and *hydrochlorothiazide (a thiazide diuretic), used for the treatment of *hypertension or *oedema associated with heart failure, liver disease, or kidney disease. It is available as tablets on *prescription only.
Side effects, precautions, and interactions with other drugs: see POTASSIUM-SPARING DIURETICS; THIAZIDE DIURETICS.
See also ANTIHYPERTENSIVE DRUGS; DIURETICS.

dydrogesterone A *progestogen used for the treatment of heavy or painful periods (including those associated with *endometriosis) and other types of irregular vaginal bleeding, premenstrual syndrome, and habitual or threatened abortion. It is also used in conjunction with oestrogens in *hormone replacement therapy (HRT). Dydrogesterone is available as tablets on *prescription only.
Side effects, precautions, and interactions with other drugs: see PROGESTOGENS.
Proprietary preparations: Duphaston; Duphaston HRT; FEMAPAK (packaged with oestradiol <estradiol>); FEMOSTON (combined with oestradiol <estradiol>).

Dynamin (APS-Berk) *See* ISOSORBIDE MONONITRATE.

Dysman 250, **Dysman 500** (Ashbourne Pharmaceuticals) *See* MEFENAMIC ACID.

Dyspamet (SmithKline Beecham Pharmaceuticals) *See* CIMETIDINE.

dyspepsia *See* ACID-PEPTIC DISEASES.

Dysport (Ipsen) *See* BOTULINUM A TOXIN-HAEMAGGLUTININ COMPLEX.

Dytac (Pharmark) *See* TRIAMTERENE.

Dytide (Pharmark) A proprietary combination of *triamterene (a potassium-sparing diuretic) and *benzthiazide (a thiazide diuretic), used for the treatment of *oedema associated with heart failure, liver disease, or kidney disease. It is available as capsules on *prescription only.
Side effects, precautions, and interactions with other drugs: see
POTASSIUM-SPARING DIURETICS; THIAZIDE DIURETICS.
See also DIURETICS.

E

E45 Bath Oil (Crookes Healthcare) A proprietary combination of light *liquid paraffin (an emollient) and cetyl *dimethicone <dimeticone> (a water repellent), used for the relief of *eczema and dry skin conditions. It is freely available *over the counter.

E45 Cream (Crookes Healthcare) A proprietary combination of *white soft paraffin, hypoallergenic *lanolin, and light *liquid paraffin (all emollients), used for the relief of *eczema and dry skin conditions. It is freely available *over the counter.

E45 Wash Cream (Crookes Healthcare) A proprietary combination of *zinc oxide (an astringent) and light *liquid paraffin (an emollient), used as a soap substitute for the relief of *eczema, dermatitis, and dry skin conditions (including ichthyosis and itching in the elderly). It is freely available *over the counter.

Earex Ear Drops (Seton Scholl Healthcare) A proprietary combination of *arachis oil, *almond oil, and *camphor, used for the removal of earwax. It is freely available *over the counter.

Earex Plus Ear Drops (Seton Scholl Healthcare) A proprietary combination of *choline salicylate (an analgesic) and *glycerin, used for the removal of earwax and for the relief of irritation and inflammation of the outer ear. It is available from pharmacies without a prescription.
Precautions: frequent application should be avoided, and the drops should not be used in children under one year old.

Ebufac (DDSA Pharmaceuticals) *See* IBUPROFEN.

Ecdylin (E. C. De Witt & Co) A proprietary combination of *ammonium chloride (an expectorant) and *diphenhydramine (a sedative antihistamine), used to relieve the symptoms of productive coughs. It is available as a syrup without a prescription, but only from pharmacies.
Side effects, precautions, and interactions with other drugs: see ANTIHISTAMINES.

Econacort (Bristol-Myers Squibb) A proprietary combination of *econazole nitrate (an antifungal drug) and *hydrocortisone (a corticosteroid), used for the treatment of fungal and bacterial infections of the skin. It is available as a cream on *prescription only.
Side effects, precautions, and interactions with other drugs: see ECONAZOLE NITRATE; TOPICAL STEROIDS.

econazole nitrate An imidazole *antifungal drug used for the treatment of candidiasis (thrush) of the vagina or penis, napkin rash infected with thrush, and fungal or bacterial skin infections (especially where skin surfaces touch, such as the groin, armpit, or between the toes). Available as *pessaries and as a cream or lotion for topical application, it can be obtained without a prescription, but only from pharmacies (Ecostatin pessaries are available on *prescription only).

Side effects: there may be local mild burning or irritation.

Precautions and interactions with other drugs: the drug should not come in contact with the eyes. Astemizole and terfenadine should not be taken with econazole.

Proprietary preparations: Ecostatin (cream and pessaries); Gyno-Pevaryl 1 (pessaries); Pevaryl (cream and lotion); ECONACORT (combined with hydrocortisone); PEVARYL TC (combined with triamcinolone acetonide).

Ecostatin (Bristol-Myers Squibb) *See* ECONAZOLE NITRATE.

eczema A common itchy skin disease characterized by reddening and vesicle formation, which may lead to weeping and crusting. It is endogenous, i.e. outside agents do not play a primary role, in contrast to **dermatitis**, in which similar symptoms result from contact with irritant substances. However, in some contexts the terms 'dermatitis' and 'eczema' are used interchangeably. There are several types of eczema, the most common of which is **atopic eczema**, which is usually associated with asthma and hay fever. **Seborrhoeic eczema** (or **dermatitis**) involves the scalp, eyelids, nose, and lips, and is associated with the presence of *Pityrosporum* yeasts. **Gravitational** (or **stasis**) **eczema**, incorrectly known as **varicose eczema**, is associated with poor circulation.

Treatment of eczema is with *topical steroids but *emollients are very important, especially in treating mild cases. Other treatments include *coal tar and *ichthammol. *Cyclosporin is reserved for severe atopic eczema that is resistant to other treatments.

Edecrin (Merck Sharp & Dohme) *See* ETHACRYNIC ACID.

Edronax (Pharmacia & Upjohn) *See* REBOXETINE.

Efalith (Searle) A proprietary combination of *zinc sulphate (an astringent) and *lithium succinate (an anti-inflammatory and antifungal drug), used for the treatment of seborrhoeic *eczema. It is available as an ointment on *prescription only.

Side effects: the ointment may irritate the skin.

Precautions: Efalith should not be applied around the eyes or mouth. It may exacerbate psoriasis. It is not recommended for children under 12 years old.

Efamast (Searle) *See* GAMOLENIC ACID.

Efcortelan (GlaxoWellcome) *See* HYDROCORTISONE.

Efcortesol (GlaxoWellcome) *See* HYDROCORTISONE.

Efexor (Wyeth Laboratories) *See* VENLAFAXINE.

Effercitrate (Typharm) *See* POTASSIUM CITRATE.

Effico (Pharmax) A proprietary combination of *caffeine, *nicotinamide and *thiamine hydrochloride (B vitamins), and *compound gentian infusion in the form of a *tonic, used to stimulate the appetite. It is freely available *over the counter and cannot be prescribed on the NHS.

eformoterol fumarate <formoterol fumarate> A *sympathomimetic drug that stimulates beta *adrenoceptors in the airways. It is used as a *bronchodilator mainly to prevent asthma attacks during the night and exercise-induced asthma in people who are taking long-term prophylactic anti-inflammatory drugs (such as corticosteroids). It is not suitable for the treatment of acute attacks of asthma. Eformoterol is available, on *prescription only, as a powder for use in a breath-activated *inhaler.
Side effects: see SALBUTAMOL. In addition, there may be irritation of the mouth, throat, and eyes, altered taste, rash, insomnia, nausea, and itching.
Precautions: eformoterol should not be taken by women who are pregnant or breastfeeding.
Interactions with other drugs: see SALBUTAMOL.
Proprietary preparations: Foradil; Oxis Turbohaler.

Efudix (ICN Pharmaceuticals) *See* FLUOROURACIL.

Elantan, Elantan LA (Schwartz Pharma) *See* ISOSORBIDE MONONITRATE.

Elavil (DDSA Pharmaceuticals) *See* AMITRIPTYLINE HYDROCHLORIDE.

Eldepryl (Orion Pharma) *See* SELEGILINE.

Eldisine (Eli Lilly & Co) *See* VINDESINE SULPHATE.

Electrolade (Eastern Pharmaceuticals) A proprietary combination of *sodium chloride, *potassium chloride, *sodium bicarbonate, and glucose, used to replace fluids and *electrolytes in cases of dehydration (*see* ORAL REHYDRATION THERAPY). It is available as a flavoured powder to be dissolved in water and can be obtained without a prescription, but only from pharmacies.
Precautions: Electrolade should not be taken by people with kidney disease.

electrolyte A solution that produces ions (an ion is an atom or group of atoms that conduct electricity); for example, sodium chloride solution consists of free sodium and free chloride ions. In medical usage electrolyte usually means the ion itself; thus plasma electrolytes are the ions in the circulating blood, which include *sodium, *potassium, *calcium, chloride, bicarbonate, and phosphate. Electrolytes are essential for the normal functioning of cells: imbalances of electrolytes in the body can have serious consequences.

Measurement of plasma electrolytes forms part of a thorough medical examination. Concentrations of various electrolytes can be altered by many diseases in which electrolytes are lost from the body (as in vomiting or diarrhoea) or are not excreted and accumulate (as in kidney failure). Electrolyte depletion or retention can also be caused by drugs (e.g. *diuretics). When electrolyte concentrations are severely reduced they can be corrected by administering the appropriate substance by mouth or intravenously. Severe diarrhoea is also accompanied by dehydration: both fluids and electrolytes can be replaced by *oral rehydration therapy. Excess electrolytes in the blood can be removed by dialysis or by drugs, including special absorbent resins that are taken by mouth or by enema (*see* CALCIUM POLYSTYRENE SULPHONATE; SODIUM POLYSTYRENE SULPHONATE).

elixir A medicinal liquid preparation that is sweetened by the addition of alcohol or glycerin; these mask the taste of bitter or unpleasant drugs.

Elleste Duet (Searle) A proprietary preparation of *oestradiol <estradiol> tablets and *norethisterone tablets, used as sequential combined *hormone replacement therapy for the relief of menopausal symptoms in women who have not had a hysterectomy. The tablets, which are available on *prescription only, must be taken in the prescribed order.
Side effects, precautions, and interactions with other drugs: see HORMONE REPLACEMENT THERAPY.

Elleste Duet Conti (Searle) A proprietary combination of *oestradiol <estradiol> and *norethisterone, used as continuous combined *hormone replacement therapy for the relief of menopausal symptoms and prevention of osteoporosis in women who have not had a hysterectomy and who have not had a period for a year. It is available as tablets on *prescription only.
Side effects, precautions, and interactions with other drugs: see HORMONE REPLACEMENT THERAPY.

Elleste Solo, **Elleste Solo MX** (Searle) *See* OESTRADIOL <ESTRADIOL>; HORMONE REPLACEMENT THERAPY.

Elliman's Universal Embrocation (Seton Scholl Healthcare) A proprietary combination of *acetic acid and *turpentine oil, used as a rubefacient for the relief of aches, pains, and stiffness of muscles, joints,

and tendons, including backache, sciatica, lumbago, and fibrositis. It is freely available *over the counter.
Side effects and precautions: *see* RUBEFACIENTS.

Elocon (Schering-Plough) *See* MOMETASONE FUROATE.

Eltroxin (Goldshield Pharmaceuticals) *See* THYROXINE SODIUM <LEVOTHYROXINE SODIUM>.

Eludril Mouthwash (Chefaro Proprietaries) A proprietary combination of the antiseptics *chlorbutol <chlorobutanol> and *chlorhexidine gluconate, used for the prevention and treatment of gingivitis (inflammation of the gums), mouth ulcers, *Candida* infections (thrush), and minor throat infections and for general oral hygiene. It is freely available *over the counter.
Precautions: this mouthwash is not recommended for children.

Eludril Spray (Chefaro Proprietaries) A proprietary combination of *chlorhexidine gluconate (an antiseptic) and *amethocaine <tetracaine> (a local anaesthetic), used for the treatment of mouth and throat conditions, such as gingivitis (inflammation of the gums), stomatitis (inflammation of the mouth lining), mouth ulcers, tonsillitis, and minor infections. It can be obtained from pharmacies without a prescription.
Precautions: Eludril Spray should not be used immediately before eating and is not suitable for children under 12 years old.

Elyzol (Cox Pharmaceuticals) *See* METRONIDAZOLE.

Emblon (APS-Berk) *See* TAMOXIFEN.

embrocation A lotion that is rubbed onto the body to treat sprains and strains. Embrocations usually include *rubefacients as ingredients.

Emcor, Emcor LS (Merck Pharmaceuticals) *See* BISOPROLOL FUMARATE.

Emeside (Laboratories for Applied Biology) *See* ETHOSUXIMIDE.

emetics Drugs that induce vomiting. *Ipecacuanha is occasionally used to empty the stomach after ingestion of a poisonous substance, although there is little evidence that it significantly reduces absorption of the poison. It should not be used if a corrosive poison or a petroleum distillate has been swallowed (because of the dangers of these if inhaled), and the patient must be fully conscious. Apomorphine, solutions of common salt (sodium chloride), copper sulphate, and mustard are also emetics but should not be used in the treatment of poisoning.

Emfib (APS-Berk) *See* GEMFIBROZIL.

Emflex (Merck Pharmaceuticals) *See* ACEMETACIN.

Eminase (Monmouth Pharmaceuticals) *See* ANISTREPLASE.

Emla (AstraZeneca) A proprietary combination of the local anaesthetics *lignocaine <lidocaine> and *prilocaine, used for surface anaesthesia of the skin (for example, before taking blood samples) and of the genital area preparatory to removing genital warts. It is available as a cream on *prescription only.

Side effects: include transient local pallor, redness, or swelling.

Precautions: Emla should not be applied to wounds or to mucous membranes other than the genital region and should not be used in children under one year old. It should be used with caution in people with anaemia (*see* PRILOCAINE).

Emmolate (Bio-Medical Services) A proprietary combination of wood alcohols and *liquid paraffin in the form of a bath oil, used an an *emollient for the relief of contact dermatitis (an allergic skin condition), dry skin, and itching. It is freely available *over the counter.

emollients Agents that soothe and soften the skin. Emollients are oil-in-water emulsions (*creams) or greasy and insoluble in water (*ointments). They are used alone as moisturizers in the treatment of such conditions as *eczema and *psoriasis to lessen the need for, or complement, active drug therapy (such as corticosteroids) and in skin preparations as a base for a more active drug (such as an antibiotic). They either prevent water loss by forming a greasy layer to stop evaporation from the skin (e.g. *white soft paraffin) or improve the binding of water to the skin, in which case they are called **humectants** (e.g. *urea creams). *Liquid paraffin, *lanolin, and vegetable oils (such as *arachis oil, *almond oil, and *soya oil) are other commonly used emollients. Some emollients are applied directly to the skin; others are added to the bath or used in the shower, in some cases as a substitute for soap.

Emulsiderm (Dermal Laboratories) A proprietary combination of *liquid paraffin and *isopropyl myristate (both emollients) and *benzalkonium chloride (an antiseptic), used for the treatment of dry and itching skin conditions. Available as a liquid to be rubbed into the skin or added to the bath, it can be obtained without a prescription, but only from pharmacies.

emulsion A preparation in which fine droplets of one liquid (such as oil) are dispersed in another liquid (such as water). Medicines are prepared in the form of emulsions to disguise the taste of an oil, which is dispersed in a flavoured liquid.

enalapril hydrochloride An *ACE inhibitor used as an adjunct to *diuretics for the treatment of *heart failure. It is also used to treat all grades of *hypertension. It is available, on *prescription only, as tablets or as wafers to be dissolved on the tongue.

Side effects, precautions, and interactions with other drugs: see ACE INHIBITORS.
Proprietary preparations: Innovace; Innovace Melt (wafers); INNOZIDE (combined with hydrochlorothiazide).
See also ANTIHYPERTENSIVE DRUGS.

Endekay Fluodrops (Stafford-Miller) *See* FLUORIDE.

Endekay Fluotabs (Stafford-Miller) *See* FLUORIDE.

endometriosis The presence of tissue similar to the endometrium (lining of the uterus) at other sites in the pelvis, such as the wall of the uterus, the ovary, Fallopian tubes, or the peritoneum (membrane) lining the pelvis. This tissue undergoes the periodic changes similar to those of the endometrium and causes pelvic pain and painful periods. Drugs used in the treatment of endometriosis include *danazol, *gestrinone, some gonadorelin analogues (*see* LEUPRORELIN; NAFARELIN; TRIPTORELIN), and some progestogens (*see* DYDROGESTERONE; MEDROXYPROGESTERONE).

Endoxana (ASTA Medica) *See* CYCLOPHOSPHAMIDE.

enema A liquid infused into the rectum through a tube passed into the anus. Some drugs are administered in the form of enemas; for example, corticosteroids in the treatment of inflammatory bowel disease.

Eno, **Eno Lemon** (SmithKline Beecham Consumer Healthcare) Proprietary combinations of *sodium bicarbonate, sodium carbonate, and *citric acid used as an antacid for the relief of indigestion, flatulence, and nausea. They are freely available *over the counter in the form of effervescent powders.
Side effects, precautions, and interactions with other drugs: see ANTACIDS.

enoxaparin A *low molecular weight heparin used for the prevention and treatment of deep-vein *thrombosis and in the treatment of unstable *angina. It is also used in patients undergoing kidney dialysis, in order to prevent blood-clot formation. Enoxaparin is available as a solution for subcutaneous injection on *prescription only.
Side effects, precautions, and interactions with other drugs: see HEPARIN.
Proprietary preparation: Clexane.

enoximone A drug that acts on the heart muscles to strengthen the heartbeat and is used for the short-term treatment of congestive *heart failure. It is available as an injection on *prescription only.
Side effects: enoximone may cause abnormal heartbeats or (less commonly) low blood pressure, headache, insomnia, nausea, vomiting, and diarrhoea.
Precautions: enoximone should be used with caution in people with some types of heart disease (in whom heart and blood monitoring will be

required during treatment) and in women who are pregnant or breastfeeding.

Proprietary preparation: Perfan.

entacapone A *dopamine agonist that is used as an *adjunct to *levodopa (with carbidopa or benserazide) for treating Parkinson's disease when levodopa alone has become less effective in controlling symptoms. It is available as tablets on *prescription only.

Side effects: include nausea, vomiting, abdominal pain, constipation, diarrhoea, dry mouth, and abnormal involuntary movements; the urine may become reddish brown.

Precautions: entacapone should not be taken by women who are pregnant or breastfeeding or by people with liver disease or phaeochromocytoma (a tumour of the adrenal gland).

Interactions with other drugs:

Antidepressant drugs: tricyclic antidepressants, MAOIs, maprotiline, and venlafaxine should not be taken with entacapone.

Apomorphine: its effect may be increased by entacapone.

Iron: reduces the absorption of entacapone.

Methyldopa: its effect may be increased by entacapone.

Sympathomimetic drugs: the effects of adrenaline <epinephrine>, noradrenaline <norepinephrine>, dobutamine, dopamine, and isoprenaline may be increased by entacapone.

Proprietary preparation: Comtess.

enteric-coated Describing tablets that are coated with a substance that enables them to pass through the stomach and into the intestine unchanged. Drugs contained in enteric-coated tablets may irritate the stomach, so that it is better for them to be released into the intestine (e.g. aspirin, prednisolone), or they may be destroyed by the acid contents of the stomach (e.g. pancreatin).

Enterocalm (GalPharm International) *See* KAOLIN.

Enterosan (Monmouth Pharmaceuticals) A proprietary combination of *kaolin (an adsorbent), *belladonna extract (an antispasmodic), and *morphine (which reduces gut motility), used for the treatment of diarrhoea and stomach upsets (*see* ANTIDIARRHOEAL DRUGS). It is available as chewable tablets and can be obtained without a prescription, but only from pharmacies.

Side effects, precautions, and interactions with other drugs: see MORPHINE.

Entocort CR, Entocort Enema (AstraZeneca) *See* BUDESONIDE.

Entrotabs (Monmouth Pharmaceuticals) A proprietary combination of *attapulgite (an antidiarrhoeal drug), *aluminium hydroxide (an antacid), and pectin (an adsorbent and bulk-forming agent), used for the treatment of stomach upsets and diarrhoea. It is freely available *over the counter in the form of tablets.

Precautions: this medicine is not recommended for children under six years old.

Enzed (Kent Pharmaceuticals) *See* DICLOFENAC SODIUM.

Epaderm (Dermal Laboratories) A proprietary combination of *yellow soft paraffin, emulsifying wax, and *liquid paraffin in the form of an ointment, used as an *emollient and a soap substitute for the relief of dry skin conditions. It is freely available *over the counter.

Epanutin (Parke-Davis Medical) *See* PHENYTOIN.

ephedrine hydrochloride A *sympathomimetic drug that relaxes smooth muscle and constricts blood vessels. It was formerly widely used as a *bronchodilator in the treatment of such conditions as asthma and chronic bronchitis, but has largely been replaced for treating these conditions by drugs that have fewer adverse effects. Its main use now is as a nasal *decongestant (alone or in combination with other drugs) and it is included as an ingredient in many medicines for treating colds and coughs. It is also used to treat bedwetting in children. Ephedrine hydrochloride is available as tablets or an injection on *prescription only and as an *elixir or nose drops that can be bought from pharmacies without a prescription.

Side effects: with nose drops, side effects are rare; local irritation may occur. When taken by mouth fast heart rate, anxiety, restlessness, insomnia, and palpitation are the most common side effects; tremor, irregular heart rhythms, dry mouth, and cold extremities may also occur.

Precautions: when taken by mouth, ephedrine should be used with caution by the elderly and by people with an overactive thyroid gland, diabetes mellitus, high blood pressure, heart disease, kidney disease, or an enlarged prostate gland.

Interactions with other drugs:

Antihypertensive drugs: ephedrine may antagonize the effects of alpha blockers and possibly other antihypertensive drugs in lowering blood pressure.

MAOIs: may cause a dangerous rise in blood pressure.

Proprietary preparations: CAM (sugar-free mixture); BOOTS INFANT SUGAR FREE COUGH AND CONGESTION SYRUP (combined with ipecacuanha); FRANOL and FRANOL PLUS (combined with theophylline); HAYMINE (combined with chlorpheniramine <chlorphenamine>); VICKS MEDINITE (combined with dextromethorphan, doxylamine, and paracetamol).

Ephynal (Roche Products) *See* VITAMIN E.

epilepsy *See* ANTICONVULSANT DRUGS.

Epilim (Sanofi Winthrop) *See* SODIUM VALPROATE.

Epilim Chrono (Sanofi Winthrop) A proprietary combination of *sodium valproate and valproic acid (anticonvulsants), used for the treatment of epilepsy. A *prescription only medicine, it is available for oral use as *modified-release tablets.
Side effects, precautions, and interactions with other drugs: see SODIUM VALPROATE.

Epimaz (Norton Healthcare) *See* CARBAMAZEPINE.

epinephrine *See* ADRENALINE.

Epipen (ALK) *See* ADRENALINE <EPINEPHRINE>.

epirubicin A *cytotoxic antibiotic similar to *doxorubicin. It is given intravenously for the treatment of breast cancer and is instilled directly into the bladder to treat bladder cancer. Epirubicin is available as an injection on *prescription only.
Side effects and precautions: see DOXORUBICIN; CYTOTOXIC DRUGS.
Proprietary preparation: Pharmorubicin.

Epivir (GlaxoWellcome) *See* LAMIVUDINE.

epoetin *See* ERYTHROPOIETIN.

Epogam (Searle) *See* GAMOLENIC ACID.

epoprostenol An *antiplatelet drug that is used in patients undergoing kidney dialysis to prevent platelets aggregating and forming a blood clot; it may be given alone or with *heparin. Epoprostenol is available as a form for intravenous infusion on *prescription only.
Side effects: epoprostenol has a potent action in dilating blood vessels, causing headache, flushing, and low blood pressure; pallor, sweating, and slowing of the heart rate may occur with higher dosages.
Precautions: if epoprostenol is given with heparin, the clotting time of the patient's blood should be regularly monitored (*see* ANTICOAGULANTS).
Proprietary preparation: Flolan.

Eppy (Chauvin Pharmaceuticals) *See* ADRENALINE <EPINEPHRINE>.

Eprex (Janssen-Cilag) *See* ERYTHROPOIETIN.

Epsom salts *See* MAGNESIUM SULPHATE.

Equagesic (Wyeth Laboratories) A proprietary combination of *aspirin (a non-opioid analgesic), *meprobamate (a muscle relaxant), and ethoheptazine citrate (an *opioid analgesic), used for the short-term treatment of muscle pain. Equagesic is available as tablets; it is a *controlled drug that cannot be prescribed on the NHS.

Side effects: include drowsiness, dizziness, nausea, shaky movements and unsteady gait, rash, blood disorders, low blood pressure, and 'pins and needles'.

Precautions: Equagesic should not be taken by people with severe lung diseases, peptic ulcer, kidney disease, haemophilia, or an allergy to aspirin or NSAIDs, or by women who are pregnant or breastfeeding.

Interactions with other drugs: see ASPIRIN; OPIOIDS.

Equilon (Chefaro Proprietaries) *See* MEBEVERINE HYDROCHLORIDE.

Erecnos (Fournier Pharmaceuticals) *See* THYMOXAMINE <MOXISYLYTE>.

ergocalciferol (vitamin D$_2$) One of the D vitamins (*see* VITAMIN D), which is used for the treatment of simple vitamin D deficiency, such as that caused by lack of sunlight. Ergocalciferol is not available as plain tablets, so is usually given in combination with *calcium lactate and *calcium phosphate as **calcium and ergocalciferol** tablets, which are available without a prescription, but only from pharmacies. A form of ergocalciferol for injection is available on *prescription only (*see* CALCIFEROL).

Side effects, precautions, and interactions with other drugs: see VITAMIN D.

ergometrine maleate An *alkaloid that constricts blood vessels and also stimulates the uterus to contract. It is used in childbirth to bring about delivery of the placenta and, usually in conjunction with oxytocin, to stop bleeding due to an incomplete abortion. Ergometrine is also used to prevent or treat bleeding from the uterus after childbirth. For these purposes it is given by intravenous injection. Oral ergometrine may be used for treating small episodes of bleeding occurring days after delivery. Ergometrine is available, on *prescription only, as a solution for injection or as tablets.

Side effects: include nausea, vomiting, headache, dizziness, tinnitus (the sensation of sounds in the ears), abdominal pain, chest pain, bouts of palpitation, breathlessness, a slow heart rate, and a temporary increase in blood pressure.

Precautions: ergometrine should not be given to women with heart or circulatory disease, impaired kidney or liver function, breathing difficulties, high blood pressure, or infection.

Proprietary preparation: SYNTOMETRINE (combined with oxytocin).

ergotamine tartrate An alkaloid derived from the fungus ergot, used for the treatment of acute attacks of *migraine that have not responded to analgesics; it acts by constricting the arteries in the scalp. Because of the severity of its side effects, *5HT$_1$ agonists are usually preferred.

Ergotamine is available, on *prescription only, as tablets, suppositories, or a metered-dose *inhaler.

Side effects: include nausea, vomiting, abdominal pain, muscle cramps, and (rarely) exacerbation of the headache. Ergotamine can cause vasospasm (constriction of the arteries) of the fingers and toes: if numbness or tingling of the fingers and toes develops, treatment should be stopped and a doctor informed.

Precautions: ergotamine should not be taken by people with heart disease, vascular disease (including Raynaud's syndrome), severe hypertension, liver or kidney disease, or an overactive thyroid gland, or by women who are pregnant or breastfeeding.

Interactions with other drugs:

Antibiotics: erythromycin and possibly azithromycin increase the risk of toxic effects of ergotamine.

Antiviral drugs: nelfinavir and ritonavir increase the risk of ergot toxicity and should not be taken with ergotamine.

5HT$_1$ agonists: should not be taken with ergotamine since they increase the risk of vasospasm.

Proprietary preparations: Cafergot; Lingraine; Medihaler-Ergotamine (metered-dose inhaler); MIGRIL (combined with cyclizine and caffeine).

Erwinase (Ipsen) *See* CRISANTASPASE.

Eryacne (Galderma) *See* ERYTHROMYCIN.

Erycen (APS-Berk) *See* ERYTHROMYCIN.

Erymax (Elan Pharma) *See* ERYTHROMYCIN.

Erythrocin (Abbott Laboratories) *See* ERYTHROMYCIN.

erythromycin The oldest and probably best known of the *macrolide antibiotics. A useful alternative to penicillins for treating patients who are allergic to these drugs, it is used to treat respiratory infections, whooping cough, syphilis, legionnaires' disease, gastrointestinal infections, and *acne. It is also effective against *Chlamydia* bacteria (which cause a variety of diseases, notably sexually transmitted conditions, parrot disease, and eye infections) and mycoplasmas (microorganisms that cause respiratory and genital infections). Erythromycin is also used with *neomycin to sterilize the gut before surgery. It is available, on *prescription only, as tablets, capsules, or a solution for oral use, an alcoholic solution or gel for topical application, or as an *intravenous injection.

Side effects: include nausea, vomiting, abdominal discomfort, diarrhoea, and rashes or other allergic reactions; reversible hearing loss may occur after large doses.

Precautions: erythromycin estolate (in Ilosone) should not be taken by people with liver disease; other forms should be used with caution in those with liver impairment. All forms of erythromycin should be used with caution in those with kidney disease, heart conditions, or porphyria and in women who are pregnant or breastfeeding.

Interactions with other drugs:

Astemizole and terfenadine: erythromycin increases the risk of these drugs causing *arrhythmias and should not be taken with them.

Carbamazepine: plasma concentrations of carbamazepine are increased.

Cisapride: erythromycin increases the risk of this drug causing arrhythmias; the two drugs should not be taken together.

Cyclosporin: plasma concentrations of cyclosporin are increased.

Disopyramide: plasma concentrations of disopyramide are increased, which may cause adverse effects.

Midazolam: plasma concentrations of midazolam are increased, causing sedation.

Theophylline: plasma concentrations of theophylline are increased.

Warfarin and nicoumalone <acenocoumarol>: plasma concentrations of these drugs are increased, which increases the risk of bleeding.

Proprietary preparations: Arpimycin; Eryacne (gel); Erycen; Erymax; Erythrocin; Erythroped; Erythroped A; Ilosone; Rommix Stiemycin (topical solution); Tiloryth; BENZAMYCIN (combined with benzoyl peroxide); ZINERYT (combined with zinc acetate).

Erythroped, Erythroped A (Abbott Laboratories) *See* ERYTHROMYCIN.

erythropoietin A hormone produced naturally by the kidneys that stimulates the production of red blood cells by the bone marrow. A form of erythropoietin (**epoetin**) produced by genetic engineering is used to treat *anaemia associated with chronic kidney failure. Epoetin is also used in patients undergoing chemotherapy with platinum-containing drugs in order to shorten the period of anaemia. It is given by subcutaneous, intravenous, or intramuscular injection and is available on *prescription only.

Side effects: include raised blood pressure, headache, thrombosis, influenza-like symptoms, epileptic seizures, and rashes.

Precautions: erythropoietin should not be given to people with untreated high blood pressure. It should be used with caution in those with vascular disease, cancer, a history of epilepsy, or liver disease and in pregnant or breastfeeding women.

Interactions with other drugs:

ACE inhibitors: there is an increased risk of high concentrations of potassium in the plasma.

Proprietary preparations: Eprex (epoetin alfa); Neorecormon (epoetin beta).

ES Bronchial Mixture (Torbet Laboratories) A proprietary combination of ammonium bicarbonate, *ipecacuanha, and *squill (all

expectorants) and *senna, used for the relief of productive coughs and catarrh. This liquid is freely available *over the counter.
Side effects and precautions: see IPECACUANHA; SQUILL.

Eskamel (Goldshield Pharmaceuticals) A proprietary combination of *sulphur and *resorcinol (both keratolytics), used for the treatment of acne. It is available as a cream and can be obtained without a prescription, but only from pharmacies.
Side effects and precautions: see RESORCINOL.

Eskazol (SmithKline Beecham Pharmaceuticals) *See* ALBENDAZOLE.

Eskornade (Goldshield Pharmaceuticals) A proprietary combination of *phenylpropanolamine (a decongestant) and *diphenylpyraline (an antihistamine), used to relieve the congestive symptoms associated with colds, influenza, and allergies. It is available as *modified-release capsules or a syrup without a prescription, but only from pharmacies.
Side effects, precautions, and interactions with other drugs: see PHENYLPROPANOLAMINE; EPHEDRINE HYDROCHLORIDE; ANTIHISTAMINES.

esmolol hydrochloride A cardioselective *beta blocker used for the treatment and prevention of heart *arrhythmias and the treatment of *hypertension that occurs after surgery. It is available as a solution for intravenous infusion on *prescription only. Since it has a very short duration of action it is usually reserved for diagnostic use in the short term. After stabilization of the heart rate transition is usually made to oral medication.
Side effects, precautions, and interactions with other drugs: see BETA BLOCKERS.
Proprietary preparation: Brevibloc.

Estracombi (Novartis Pharmaceuticals) A proprietary preparation of *oestradiol <estradiol> skin patches (**Estraderm TTS**) and combined oestradiol/*norethisterone skin patches (**Estragest TTS**) used as sequential combined *hormone replacement therapy for the relief of menopausal symptoms and the prevention of osteoporosis in women who have not had a hysterectomy. The patches, which are available on *prescription only, must be applied in the prescribed order.
Side effects, precautions, and interactions with other drugs: see HORMONE REPLACEMENT THERAPY.

Estracyt (Pharmacia & Upjohn) *See* ESTRAMUSTINE.

Estraderm MX (Novartis Pharmaceuticals) *See* OESTRADIOL <ESTRADIOL>; HORMONE REPLACEMENT THERAPY.

Estraderm TTS (Novartis Pharmaceuticals) *See* OESTRADIOL <ESTRADIOL>; HORMONE REPLACEMENT THERAPY; ESTRACOMBI.

estradiol *See* OESTRADIOL.

Estragest TTS (Novartis Pharmaceuticals) *See* ESTRACOMBI.

estramustine An oestrogenic *alkylating drug (a combination of *mustine <chlormethine> and an oestrogen) used for the treatment of prostate *cancer. It is available as capsules on *prescription only.
Side effects: include nausea and vomiting, impairment of liver function, enlargement of the breasts, and (rarely) angina. *See also* CYTOTOXIC DRUGS.
Precautions: estramustine should not be taken by people with peptic ulcers, severe liver disease, or severe heart disease. *See also* CYTOTOXIC DRUGS.
Proprietary preparation: Estracyt.

Estrapak (Novartis Pharmaceuticals) A proprietary preparation of *oestradiol <estradiol> skin patches and *norethisterone tablets used as sequential combined *hormone replacement therapy for the relief of menopausal symptoms and the prevention of osteoporosis in women who have not had a hysterectomy. It is available on *prescription only.
Side effects, precautions, and interactions with other drugs: see HORMONE REPLACEMENT THERAPY.

Estring (Pharmacia & Upjohn) *See* OESTRADIOL <ESTRADIOL>; HORMONE REPLACEMENT THERAPY.

estriol *See* OESTRIOL.

estrone *See* OESTRONE.

estropipate A semisynthetic *oestrogen that is converted to *oestrone <estrone> in the body. It is used as *hormone replacement therapy to relieve menopausal symptoms and to prevent postmenopausal osteoporosis. Women who have not had a hysterectomy may also need to take *progestogen supplements. Estropipate is available as tablets on *prescription only.
Side effects, precautions, and interactions with other drugs: see HORMONE REPLACEMENT THERAPY.
Proprietary preparations: Harmogen; IMPROVERA (packaged with medroxyprogesterone).

etacrynic acid *See* ETHACRYNIC ACID.

etamsylate *See* ETHAMSYLATE.

ethacrynic acid <etacrynic acid> A *loop diuretic that may be given by injection to treat *oedema when rapid fluid loss is urgently required; it is no longer widely used. Ethacrynic acid is available as a form for injection on *prescription only.

Side effects: see LOOP DIURETICS. In addition, there may be nausea and other gastrointestinal upsets, and the injection can be painful.

Precautions: ethacrynic acid should not be given to women who are breastfeeding. *See also* LOOP DIURETICS.

Interactions with other drugs: see LOOP DIURETICS.

Proprietary preparation: Edecrin.

ethambutol hydrochloride An *antibiotic that inhibits the growth of the bacterium that causes *tuberculosis. It is used in combination with other drugs to treat tuberculosis, especially when resistance to the common drugs is suspected, but it may cause visual damage, which limits its use. A *prescription only medicine, it is available as tablets.

Side effects: include inflammation of the optic nerve (causing blurred vision) and red/green colour blindness. Any visual changes should be reported to a doctor immediately.

Precautions: ethambutol should be used with caution in children under six years old, who cannot report visual symptoms reliably, in people with kidney disease, and in women who are pregnant or breastfeeding.

ethamsylate <etamsylate> A *haemostatic drug that reduces bleeding in capillaries (very small blood vessels); it acts by improving the ability of platelets to stick together, which is part of the normal blood-clotting process. Ethamsylate is given by intravenous or intramuscular injection for the prevention and treatment of haemorrhage (excessive bleeding) in low-birth-weight babies. It is taken orally in the short-term treatment of blood loss due to heavy periods. Ethamsylate is available, on *prescription only, as tablets or an injection.

Side effects: include nausea, headache, and rashes.

Precautions: ethamsylate should not be given to people with porphyria.

Proprietary preparation: Dicynene.

ethanolamine oleate An irritant substance that is used in *sclerotherapy to treat varicose veins. It is available, on *prescription only, as a solution for slow injection into the affected vein.

Side effects: ethanolamine oleate may cause allergic reactions, and if it leaks out of the vein it may damage surrounding tissue.

Precautions: ethanolamine oleate should not be used in people who cannot walk, or have obese legs or acutely inflamed veins, or by women taking oral contraceptives.

Ethimil MR (Ethical Generics) *See* VERAPAMIL HYDROCHLORIDE.

ethinyloestradiol <ethinylestradiol> A synthetic *oestrogen that is used mainly in combination with *progestogens in *oral contraceptives and in the so-called 'morning-after pill' (postcoital contraception). Alone, it is occasionally used to treat certain types of breast and prostate cancer. A *prescription only medicine, ethinyloestradiol in nonproprietary form is available as tablets.

Side effects: include nausea, fluid retention, and (in men) impotence and enlargement of the breasts. *See also* OESTROGENS; ORAL CONTRACEPTIVES.

Precautions: ethinyloestradiol should be used with caution by people with cardiovascular disease or jaundice. *See also* OESTROGENS; ORAL CONTRACEPTIVES.

Interactions with other drugs: see OESTROGENS.

Proprietary preparations: BINOVUM (combined with norethisterone); BREVINOR (combined with norethisterone); CILEST (combined with norgestimate); DIANETTE (combined with cyproterone acetate); EUGYNON 30 (combined with levonorgestrel); FEMODENE (combined with gestodene); LOESTRIN 20 and Loestrin 30 (combined with norethisterone); LOGYNON (combined with levonorgestrel); MARVELON (combined with desogestrel); MERCILON (combined with desogestrel); MICROGYNON 30 (combined with levonorgestrel); MINULET (combined with gestodene); NORIMIN (combined with norethisterone); OVRAN (combined with levonorgestrel); OVRANETTE (combined with levonorgestrel); OVYSMEN (combined with norethisterone); SCHERING PC4 (combined with norgestrel); SYNPHASE (combined with norethisterone); TRIADENE (combined with gestodene); TRI-MINULET (combined with gestodene); TRINORDIOL (combined with levonorgestrel); TRINOVUM (combined with norethisterone). See table at *oral contraceptives.

ethoheptazine citrate   *See* EQUAGESIC.

ethosuximide   An *anticonvulsant drug used for the treatment of absence seizures. It is available, on *prescription only, as capsules or a syrup.

Side effects: include gastrointestinal upsets, weight loss, drowsiness, dizziness, shaky movements, hiccups, headache, depression, and skin rashes.

Precautions: ethosuximide should be used with caution in people who have liver or kidney disease and in women who are pregnant or breastfeeding; women who are planning to become pregnant should seek specialist advice.

Interactions with other drugs:

 Anticonvulsants: taking two or more anticonvulsants together may increase their adverse effects.

 Antidepressants: reduce the anticonvulsant effect of ethosuximide.

 Antipsychotics: may reduce the anticonvulsant effect of ethosuximide.

Proprietary preparations: Emeside; Zarontin.

ethyl nicotinate   A drug that is used as a *rubefacient for the relief of muscular aches and pains. It is an ingredient of creams and sprays that are freely available *over the counter.

Side effects and precautions: see RUBEFACIENTS.

Proprietary preparations: BOOTS PAIN RELIEF BALM (combined with glycol salicylate and nonylic acid vanillylamide); BOOTS PAIN RELIEF WARMING

SPRAY (combined with methyl salicylate and camphor); PR HEAT SPRAY (combined with methyl salicylate and camphor); TRANSVASIN HEAT RUB (combined with hexyl nicotinate and tetrahydrofurfuryl salicylate).

ethyl salicylate A *salicylate that is used as an ingredient of several *rubefacient sprays and sticks for the relief of aches, pains, and stiffness in muscles, joints, and tendons. It is freely available *over the counter.
Side effects and precautions: see SALICYLATES.
Proprietary preparations: DEEP HEAT SPRAY (combined with glycol salicylate, methyl salicylate, and methyl nicotinate); DUBAM SPRAY (combined with methyl salicylate, glycol salicylate, and methyl nicotinate); RALGEX STICK (combined with capsicum oleoresin, methyl salicylate, glycol salicylate, and menthol).

ethynodiol diacetate <etynodiol diacetate> A synthetic *progestogen used in progestogen-only *oral contraceptives. It is available as tablets on *prescription only.
Side effects, precautions, and interactions with other drugs: see PROGESTOGENS.
Proprietary preparation: Femulen.

Ethyol (Schering-Plough) *See* AMIFOSTINE.

etidronate disodium *See* DISODIUM ETIDRONATE.

etodolac An *NSAID used for the treatment of pain and inflammation in rheumatoid arthritis and osteoarthritis. It is available as tablets, *modified-release tablets, or capsules on *prescription only.
Side effects, precautions, and interactions with other drugs: see NSAIDS.
Proprietary preparations: Lodine; Lodine SR (modified-release tablets).

Etopophos (Bristol-Myers Squibb) *See* ETOPOSIDE.

etoposide A *cytotoxic drug, derived from an extract of the American mandrake plant, that is similar to the *vinca alkaloids. It acts by causing breaks in DNA so that cell replication cannot take place. Etoposide is used for the treatment of lymphomas, some forms of lung cancer, testicular cancer, acute leukaemias, and brain tumours (*see* CANCER). It is available, on *prescription only, as capsules or a form for intravenous infusion.
Side effects: include hair loss, *bone marrow suppression, nausea, and vomiting; there may be pain and irritation at the injection site. *See also* CYTOTOXIC DRUGS.
Precautions: etoposide should not be taken by women who are pregnant or breastfeeding or by people with severe liver disease.
Proprietary preparations: Etopophos; Vepesid.

etynodiol diacetate *See* ETHYNODIOL DIACETATE.

eucalyptol *See* EUCALYPTUS OIL.

eucalyptus oil An aromatic oil with a cooling effect, distilled from the leaves of various species of eucalyptus tree; its main constituent is **cineole** (or **eucalyptol**). It is used, often in combination with *menthol and/or other volatile substances, in inhalations and other remedies to relieve the congestion associated with colds and catarrh. It is also an ingredient of *rubefacient preparations for the relief of muscular aches and pains. Most preparations containing eucalyptus oil are freely available *over the counter.

Side effects: eucalyptus oil is poisonous in overdose.

Proprietary preparations: CHYMOL EMOLLIENT BALM (combined with terpineol, methyl salicylate, and phenol); DEEP HEAT RUB (combined with methyl salicylate, menthol, and turpentine oil); OLBAS INHALER (combined with menthol, cajuput oil, and peppermint oil); OLBAS OIL (combined with menthol, cajuput oil, clove oil, juniper berry oil, and oil of wintergreen); OLBAS PASTILLES (combined with menthol, peppermint oil, clove oil, juniper berry oil, and oil of wintergreen); TIXYLIX INHALANT (combined with turpentine oil, camphor, and menthol); VICKS VAPORUB (combined with turpentine oil, camphor, and menthol); WOODWARD'S BABY CHEST RUB (combined with turpentine oil and menthol).

Eucardic (Roche Products) *See* CARVEDILOL.

Eucerin (Beiersdorf) *See* UREA.

Eudemine (Medeva) *See* DIAZOXIDE.

Euglucon (Hoechst Marion Roussel) *See* GLIBENCLAMIDE.

Eugynon 30 (Schering Health Care) A proprietary combination of *ethinyloestradiol <ethinylestradiol> (30 micrograms) and *levonorgestrel used as an *oral contraceptive. It is available as tablets on *prescription only.

Side effects, precautions, and interactions with other drugs: see ORAL CONTRACEPTIVES.

Eumovate (GlaxoWellcome) *See* CLOBETASONE BUTYRATE.

Eurax (Novartis Consumer Health) *See* CROTAMITON.

Eurax-Hydrocortisone (Novartis Consumer Health) A proprietary combination of *crotamiton (a soothing agent) and *hydrocortisone (a corticosteroid), used for the treatment of itching skin conditions. It is available as a cream on *prescription only. **Eurax Hc**, which is packaged in a 15-gram tube, is available from pharmacies without a prescription.

Side effects and precautions: see TOPICAL STEROIDS; CROTAMITON.

Evista (Eli Lilly & Co) *See* RALOXIFENE.

Evorel (Janssen-Cilag) *See* OESTRADIOL <ESTRADIOL>; HORMONE REPLACEMENT THERAPY.

Evorel Conti (Janssen-Cilag) A proprietary combination of *oestradiol <estradiol> and *norethisterone used as continuous combined *hormone replacement therapy for the relief of menopausal symptoms and prevention of osteoporosis in women who have not had a hysterectomy and who have not had a period for a year. It is available as skin patches on *prescription only.
Side effects, precautions, and interactions with other drugs: see HORMONE REPLACEMENT THERAPY.

Evorel-Pak (Janssen-Cilag) A proprietary preparation of *oestradiol <estradiol> skin patches and *norethisterone tablets used as sequential combined *hormone replacement therapy for the relief of menopausal symptoms in women who have not had a hysterectomy. It is available on *prescription only.
Side effects, precautions, and interactions with other drugs: see HORMONE REPLACEMENT THERAPY.

Evorel Sequi (Janssen-Cilag) A proprietary preparation of *oestradiol <estradiol> skin patches and combined oestradiol/*norethisterone skin patches used as sequential combined *hormone replacement therapy for the relief of menopausal symptoms in women who have not had a hysterectomy. The patches, which are available on *prescription only, must be applied in the prescribed order.
Side effects, precautions, and interactions with other drugs: see HORMONE REPLACEMENT THERAPY.

excipient A substance that is combined with a drug in order to render it suitable for administration; examples are preservatives included in eye drops and skin preparations. Excipients should have no pharmacological action themselves, but some may cause allergic reactions in sensitive individuals (e.g. parabens (preservatives) and lanolin in creams and ointments).

Exelderm (AstraZeneca) *See* SULCONAZOLE.

Exelon (Novartis Pharmaceuticals) *See* RIVASTIGMINE.

Ex-Lax Senna (Novartis Consumer Health) *See* SENNA.

Exocin (Allergan) *See* OFLOXACIN.

Exorex (Pharmax) *See* COAL TAR.

Exosurf Neonatal (GlaxoWellcome) *See* COLFOSCERIL PALMITATE.

expectorants Drugs that are claimed to decrease the viscosity and increase the volume of mucus in the airways, making it more watery and therefore easier to expel by coughing. Drugs used orally as expectorants irritate the lining of the stomach, which has been said to provide a stimulus for the reflex production of fluid by the glands of the airways. However, there is no evidence that any expectorant works. Expectorants are usually given to relieve chesty productive coughs, but may also be used to increase the secretion of liquid mucus in irritating dry coughs. They include *ammonium chloride, **ammonium acetate**, **ammonium carbonate**, *guaiphenesin <guaifenesin>, **guaiacol**, *ipecacuanha, and *squill, which are incorporated into many proprietary medicines for treating coughs and colds. *Compare* MUCOLYTIC DRUGS.

Expulin (Monmouth Pharmaceuticals) A proprietary combination of *chlorpheniramine <chlorphenamine> (an antihistamine), *pholcodine (a cough suppressant), *pseudoephedrine (a decongestant), and *menthol, used to relieve the dry coughs and congestion associated with colds and influenza. A sugar-free liquid, it is freely available *over the counter.
Side effects, precautions, and interactions with other drugs: see ANTIHISTAMINES; EPHEDRINE HYDROCHLORIDE; PHOLCODINE; OPIOIDS.

Expulin Chesty Cough Linctus (Monmouth Pharmaceuticals) *See* GUAIPHENESIN <GUAIFENESIN>.

Expulin Decongestant for Babies and Children (Monmouth Pharmaceuticals) A proprietary combination of *chlorpheniramine <chlorphenamine> (an antihistamine), *ephedrine (a decongestant), and *menthol, used to relieve the congestion and running nose associated with colds, influenza, and hay fever in children under 12. It is available as a sugar-free liquid without a prescription, but only from pharmacies.
Side effects, precautions, and interactions with other drugs: see ANTIHISTAMINES; EPHEDRINE HYDROCHLORIDE.

Expulin Dry (Monmouth Pharmaceuticals) A proprietary combination of *pholcodine (a cough suppressant) and *menthol, used for the relief of dry persistent coughs. It is available as a liquid without a prescription, but only from pharmacies.
Side effects and interactions with other drugs: see PHOLCODINE; OPIOIDS.
Precautions: this medicine is not recommended for children. *See also* OPIOIDS.

Expulin Paediatric (Monmouth Pharmaceuticals) A proprietary combination of *chlorpheniramine <chlorphenamine> (an antihistamine), *pholcodine (a cough suppressant), and *menthol, used to relieve dry coughs in children under 12. It is available as a sugar-free liquid without a prescription, but only from pharmacies.
Side effects and interactions with other drugs: see ANTIHISTAMINES; PHOLCODINE; OPIOIDS.

Precautions: this medicine is not recommended for children under one year old. *See also* ANTIHISTAMINES; OPIOIDS.

Exterol (Dermal Laboratories) A proprietary combination of *urea hydrogen peroxide and *glycerin, used for the softening and removal of earwax. It is available without a prescription, but only from pharmacies.

Side effects: there may be mild effervescence on application and the drops may cause irritation.

Precautions: Exterol should not be used on perforated eardrums.

extrapyramidal reactions A group of reactions caused by a reduction in the activity of the neurotransmitter *dopamine in the brain. This can result from disease (such as Parkinson's disease) or from taking drugs that antagonize the action of dopamine. Drugs having this effect include *antipsychotic drugs and *metoclopramide (an antiemetic). Extrapyramidal reactions consist of tremor, rigidity, and other symptoms of parkinsonism, abnormal face and body movements (such as twisting of the neck, rolling eyes, and writhing movements of the arms), restlessness, and uncontrolled movements of the jaws, tongue, lips, cheeks, and limbs. Drug-induced extrapyramidal reactions are more common in children and young adults and are dose-related. If alternative drugs that do not cause these reactions cannot be used, the reactions can be prevented or treated with *benztropine <benzatropine>, *benzhexol <trihexyphenidyl>, *biperiden, or *procyclidine.

F

Factor VIIa One of the factors involved in the complex process of blood clotting. Recombinant Factor VIIa, prepared by genetic engineering techniques, is used to control bleeding in people with haemophilia who have developed antibodies to *Factor VIII and *Factor IX. A *prescription only medicine, it is available in a form for injection for use in specialist centres.
Side effects: include skin irritation, nausea, fever, malaise, and changes in blood pressure.
Proprietary preparation: NovoSeven.

Factor VIII (antihaemophilic factor) One of the factors involved in the complex process of blood clotting. Freeze-dried Factor VIII fraction, prepared from human plasma, or recombinant human antihaemophilic factor VIII (**octocog alfa**), prepared by genetic engineering techniques, is used for the prevention and treatment of bleeding in people with classical haemophilia (haemophilia A; *see* HAEMOSTATIC DRUGS). Antihaemophilic factor from pigs is available for treating patients who have developed antibodies to human antihaemophilic factor. All preparations are available in a form for injection on *prescription only.
Side effects: include allergic reactions, such as chills and fever.
Proprietary preparations: Alphanate; Hyate C (porcine antihaemophilic factor); Kogenate (octocog alfa); Liberate; Monoclate-P; Recombinate (octocog alfa); Replenate; 8Y.

Factor IX One of the factors involved in the complex process of blood clotting. Freeze-dried Factor IX fraction, prepared from human plasma, is used for the prevention and treatment of bleeding in people with haemophilia B (*see* HAEMOSTATIC DRUGS). It may also contain other clotting factors. Factor IX preparations are available in a form for injection on *prescription only.
Side effects: there may be allergic reactions, such as chills and fever.
Precautions: Factor IX should not be given to people with disseminated intravascular coagulation (DIC), a rare disorder in which there is generalized blood clotting.
Proprietary preparations: Alpha-Nine; HT Defix; Mononine; Replenine.

faecal softeners *Laxatives that ease straining and are therefore used by people with painful anal or rectal conditions, such as fissures or haemorrhoids. The most commonly used faecal softener is *arachis oil.
See also DOCUSATE SODIUM; GLYCERIN; LIQUID PARAFFIN.

famciclovir An *antiviral drug used for the treatment of herpes zoster infections (shingles) and genital herpes. It is converted in the body to *penciclovir and may be used in preference to *aciclovir as it can be given less often. Famciclovir is available as tablets on *prescription only.

Side effects: include nausea, vomiting, headache, and (less commonly) dizziness and rash.

Precautions: famciclovir should be used with caution in those with impaired kidney function and in women who are pregnant or breastfeeding.

Interactions with other drugs:

Probenecid: increases the plasma concentration of famciclovir.

Proprietary preparation: Famvir.

Famel Expectorant (Seton Scholl Healthcare) *See* GUAIPHENESIN <GUAIFENESIN>.

Famel Linctus (Seton Scholl Healthcare) *See* PHOLCODINE.

Famel Original (Seton Scholl Healthcare) A proprietary combination of *codeine (a cough suppressant) and creosote (an *expectorant), used to relieve the symptoms of dry troublesome coughs. It is available as a syrup without a prescription, but only from pharmacies.

Side effects and interactions with other drugs: see CODEINE; OPIOIDS.

Precautions: this medicine is not recommended for children. *See also* OPIOIDS.

famotidine An *H_2-receptor antagonist used for the treatment of duodenal and gastric ulcers and the Zollinger-Ellison syndrome, and for the prevention of gastro-oesophageal reflux disease (*see* ACID-PEPTIC DISEASES). It is available as tablets or chewable tablets on *prescription only. Packs containing no more than two weeks' supply of tablets, for the relief of indigestion and heartburn in people over 16 years old, can be obtained from pharmacies without a prescription.

Side effects: include headache, dizziness, dry mouth, constipation, diarrhoea, nausea, rash, weakness, and fatigue. Rarely, famotidine may cause reversible breast enlargement in men.

Precautions: famotidine should be used with caution by people with poor kidney function or stomach cancer and by women who are pregnant or breastfeeding.

Proprietary preparations: Boots Excess Acid Control; Pepcid; Pepcid AC; Pepcid AC Chewable.

Famvir (SmithKline Beecham Pharmaceuticals) *See* FAMCICLOVIR.

Fanalgic (Mitchell International Pharmaceuticals) *See* PARACETAMOL.

Fansidar (Roche Products) A proprietary combination of *pyrimethamine (an antimalarial drug) and sulfadoxine (a *sulphonamide), used for the treatment of falciparum *malaria. It is available as tablets on *prescription only.

Side effects, precautions, and interactions with other drugs: see PYRIMETHAMINE; CO-TRIMOXAZOLE.

Fareston (Orion Pharma) *See* TOREMIFENE.

Farlutal (Pharmacia & Upjohn) *See* MEDROXYPROGESTERONE.

Fasigyn (Pfizer) *See* TINIDAZOLE.

Faverin (Solvay Healthcare) *See* FLUVOXAMINE MALEATE.

Fectrim (DDSA Pharmaceuticals) *See* CO-TRIMOXAZOLE.

Fefol (Medeva) A proprietary combination of *ferrous sulphate and *folic acid, used to prevent deficiencies of iron and folic acid during pregnancy. It is available as *modified-release capsules and can be obtained without a prescription, but only from pharmacies. It cannot be prescribed on the NHS.
Side effects, precautions, and interactions with other drugs: see IRON.

felbinac An *NSAID that is one of the active agents produced by the metabolism of *fenbufen. Felbinac is applied to the skin to relieve the pain and inflammation of sprains, strains, and similar injuries. It is available as a gel or foam on *prescription only; a gel with a lower concentration of felbinac can be obtained from pharmacies without a prescription.
Side effects and precautions: see NSAIDS.
Proprietary preparations: Traxam (gel or foam); Traxam Pain Relief (lower-strength gel).

Feldene, **Feldene Melt** (Pfizer) *See* PIROXICAM.

Feldene P Gel (Pfizer) *See* PIROXICAM.

felodipine A class II *calcium antagonist used for the treatment of all grades of *hypertension. It is available as *modified-release capsules on *prescription only.
Side effects: see CALCIUM ANTAGONISTS.
Precautions: felodipine should not be used to treat unstable angina or to treat patients who have had a heart attack during the previous month. It should not be taken during pregnancy. *See also* CALCIUM ANTAGONISTS; ANTIHYPERTENSIVE DRUGS.
Interactions with other drugs:
  Antiepileptic drugs: the effects of felodipine are reduced by phenytoin, carbamazepine, phenobarbitone <phenobarbital>, and primidone.
  Erythromycin: increases the plasma concentration of felodipine.

Itraconazole: increases the plasma concentration of felodipine.
See also CALCIUM ANTAGONISTS.
Proprietary preparation: Plendil.

Femapak 40 (Solvay Healthcare) A proprietary preparation of
*oestradiol <estradiol> (40-microgram) patches and *dydrogesterone
tablets used as sequential combined *hormone replacement therapy for
the relief of menopausal symptoms in women who have not had a
hysterectomy. **Femapak 80**, containing 80-microgram oestradiol
<estradiol> patches, is used in addition for the prevention of
postmenopausal osteoporosis. Both preparations are available on
*prescription only.
Side effects, precautions, and interactions with other drugs: *see* HORMONE
REPLACEMENT THERAPY.

Femara (Novartis Pharmaceuticals) *See* LETROZOLE.

Fematrix (Solvay Healthcare) *See* OESTRADIOL <ESTRADIOL>; HORMONE
REPLACEMENT THERAPY.

Femeron (Janssen-Cilag) *See* MICONAZOLE.

Femigraine (Roche Products) A proprietary combination of *aspirin (an
analgesic) and *cyclizine (an antiemetic antihistamine), used to relieve
the headache and nausea associated with migraine. It is available as
effervescent tablets and can be obtained from pharmacies without a
prescription.
Side effects: include drowsiness and stomach upsets (*see* ASPIRIN;
CYCLIZINE; ANTIHISTAMINES).
Precautions and interactions with other drugs: *see* ASPIRIN;
ANTIHISTAMINES.

Feminax (Roche Products) A proprietary combination of *paracetamol
(a non-opioid analgesic), *codeine (an opioid analgesic), *caffeine (a
stimulant), and *hyoscine hydrobromide (an antispasmodic), used for the
relief of period pains. It is available as tablets and can be obtained
without a prescription, but only from pharmacies.
Side effects and precautions: *see* PARACETAMOL; CODEINE; OPIOIDS;
ANTIMUSCARINIC DRUGS.
Interactions with other drugs: *see* OPIOIDS.

Femodene (Schering Health Care) A proprietary combination of
*ethinyloestradiol <ethinylestradiol> and *gestodene used as an *oral
contraceptive. **Femodene ED** contains both active and dummy tablets so
that a tablet is taken each day of a 28-day cycle. Both preparations are
available as tablets on *prescription only.
Side effects and interactions with other drugs: *see* ORAL CONTRACEPTIVES.
Precautions: these preparations should not be used by women who are at

risk of developing thromboembolism, for example because they are very overweight or have varicose veins or a history of thrombosis. They should therefore only be taken by women who cannot tolerate other brands and who are prepared to accept the increased risk. *See also* ORAL CONTRACEPTIVES.

Femoston 2/10 (Solvay Healthcare) A proprietary preparation of *oestradiol <estradiol> (2-milligram tablets) and combined oestradiol (2 mg)/*dydrogesterone (10 mg) tablets used as sequential combined *hormone replacement therapy for the relief of menopausal symptoms and the prevention of osteoporosis in women who have not had a hysterectomy. **Femoston 2/20** (in which the tablets contain 20 mg dydrogesterone) is given if breakthrough bleeding occurs with Femoston 2/10. **Femoston 1/10** (in which the tablets contain 1 mg oestradiol <estradiol>) are used only for the relief of menopausal symptoms. All preparations are available on *prescription only.
Side effects, precautions, and interactions with other drugs: see HORMONE REPLACEMENT THERAPY.

FemSeven (Merck Pharmaceuticals) *See* OESTRADIOL <ESTRADIOL>; HORMONE REPLACEMENT THERAPY.

Femulen (Searle) *See* ETHYNODIOL DIACETATE <ETYNODIOL DIACETATE>; ORAL CONTRACEPTIVES.

Fenbid Gel, **Fenbid Spansule** (Goldshield Pharmaceuticals) *See* IBUPROFEN.

fenbufen An *NSAID used for the treatment of pain and inflammation in rheumatoid arthritis and other disorders of the joints or muscles. It is available as tablets or capsules on *prescription only. *See also* FELBINAC.
Side effects: see NSAIDS. In addition, fenbufen is more likely than some other NSAIDs to cause rashes, in which case a doctor should be informed as the treatment may need to be discontinued immediately; allergic lung disorders may follow the rash.
Precautions and interactions with other drugs: see NSAIDS.
Proprietary preparations: Fenbuzip; Lederfen.

Fenbuzip (Ashbourne Pharmaceuticals) *See* FENBUFEN.

Fennings Children's Cooling Powders (Anglian Pharma) *See* PARACETAMOL.

Fennings Little Healers (Anglian Pharma) *See* IPECACUANHA.

fenofibrate A *fibrate used for the treatment of a wide variety of *hyperlipidaemias that have not responded to dietary intervention and other appropriate measures. It is available as capsules on *prescription only.

Side effects and precautions: see FIBRATES.
Interactions with other drugs: see BEZAFIBRATE.
Proprietary preparation: Lipantil Micro (in two strengths of tablets).

Fenoket (Opus) *See* KETOPROFEN.

fenoprofen An *NSAID used for the treatment of pain and inflammation in rheumatoid arthritis and other disorders of the joints or muscles. It is also used to relieve mild or moderate pain caused by other conditions. Fenoprofen is available as tablets on *prescription only.
Side effects: see NSAIDS. Additional side effects may include infections of the upper airways and cystitis.
Precautions and interactions with other drugs: see NSAIDS.
Proprietary preparation: Fenopron.

Fenopron (Novex Pharma) *See* FENOPROFEN.

fenoterol hydrobromide A *sympathomimetic drug that stimulates beta *adrenoceptors. It is used as a *bronchodilator in the treatment of asthma, bronchitis, and emphysema. Fenoterol is available as a metered-dose aerosol *inhaler on *prescription only.
Side effects, precautions, and interactions with other drugs: see SALBUTAMOL.
Proprietary preparations: Berotec 100; DUOVENT (combined with ipratropium bromide).

Fenox (Seton Scholl Healthcare) *See* PHENYLEPHRINE.

Fentamox (Opus) *See* TAMOXIFEN.

fentanyl A strong *opioid used for the treatment of severe pain, such as that due to cancer. It is also used for pain relief during surgical operations and to depress breathing in patients on ventilators. Fentanyl is a *controlled drug; it is available as *transdermal (skin) patches (for use during surgery or for people on ventilators) and as an injection.
Side effects and precautions: see MORPHINE.
Interactions with other drugs: see OPIOIDS.
Proprietary preparations: Durogesic (skin patches); Sublimaze (injection).

Fentazin (Goldshield Pharmaceuticals) *See* PERPHENAZINE.

fenticonazole An imidazole *antifungal drug used for the treatment of vaginal candidiasis (thrush). It is available as pessaries on *prescription only.
Side effects: there may be local mild irritation.
Precautions: fenticonazole is not suitable for use with barrier

contraceptives. It should not be used by women who are pregnant or breastfeeding.

Proprietary preparation: Lomexin.

Feospan (Medeva) *See* FERROUS SULPHATE.

Ferfolic SV (Sinclair Pharmaceuticals) A proprietary combination of *ferrous gluconate, *folic acid, and vitamin C, used during pregnancy to prevent deficiencies of iron and folic acid in the mother and spina bifida and other neural-tube defects in the baby. It is available as tablets on *prescription only.

Side effects, precautions, and interactions with other drugs: see IRON.

ferric ammonium citrate *See* LEXPEC WITH IRON-M.

ferric hydroxide sucrose A complex of *iron (in the form of ferric hydroxide) and sucrose, used in the treatment of iron-deficiency anaemia. It is given by slow intravenous injection or infusion and is available on *prescription only.

Side effects: include nausea, vomiting, changes in taste, headache, low blood pressure, and (less commonly) 'pins and needles', abdominal disorders, muscle pain, fever, flushing, and nettle rash.

Precautions: oral iron should not be taken until five days after the last injection. Injections should not be given to pregnant women or to people with liver disease, infection, or a history of asthma or other allergic disorders.

Interactions with other drugs: see IRON.

Proprietary preparation: Venofer.

Ferrograd (Abbott Laboratories) *See* FERROUS SULPHATE.

Ferrograd C (Abbott Laboratories) A proprietary combination of *ferrous sulphate and ascorbic acid (vitamin C), used for the treatment of iron-deficiency anaemia. It is available as tablets and may be obtained without a prescription, but only from pharmacies.

Side effects, precautions, and interactions with other drugs: see IRON.

Ferrograd Folic (Abbott Laboratories) A proprietary combination of *ferrous sulphate and *folic acid, used to prevent deficiencies of iron and folic acid during pregnancy. It is available as tablets and can be obtained without a prescription, but only from pharmacies.

Side effects, precautions, and interactions with other drugs: see IRON.

ferrous fumarate An *iron supplement used for the treatment of iron-deficiency anaemia. It is available, as tablets or capsules, without a prescription: some preparations are freely available *over the counter; others can be bought only from pharmacies. Ferrous fumarate is also included in many preparations combined with *folic acid.

Side effects, precautions, and interactions with other drugs: see IRON.
Proprietary preparations: Fersaday (tablets); Fersamal (tablets); Galfer (capsules); Galfer Syrup; GALFER FA (combined with folic acid); GIVITOL (combined with B group vitamins and vitamin C); IRON JELLOIDS (combined with B group vitamins and vitamin C); PHYLLOSAN (combined with B group vitamins and vitamin C); PREGADAY (combined with folic acid).

ferrous gluconate An *iron supplement used for the treatment and prevention of iron-deficiency anaemia. It is available as tablets that can be obtained without a prescription, but only from pharmacies.
Side effects, precautions, and interactions with other drugs: see IRON.
Proprietary preparation: FERFOLIC SV (combined with ferrous fumarate and folic acid).

ferrous glycine sulphate An *iron supplement used to treat iron-deficiency anaemia. It is available as tablets and can be obtained without a prescription, but only from pharmacies.
Side effects, precautions, and interactions with other drugs: see IRON.
Proprietary preparation: Plesmet.

ferrous sulphate An *iron supplement used for the treatment of iron-deficiency anaemia. It is available as tablets, a solution for children, and as *modified-release preparations and can be obtained without a prescription, but only from pharmacies.
Side effects, precautions, and interactions with other drugs: see IRON.
Proprietary preparations: Feospan (modified-release capsules); Ferrograd (tablets); Slow-Fe (modified-release tablets); DENCYL (combined with folic acid and zinc sulphate monohydrate); DITEMIC (combined with B vitamins and zinc sulphate monohydrate); FEFOL (combined with folic acid); FERROGRAD C (combined with ascorbic acid); FERROGRAD FOLIC (combined with folic acid); FESOVIT Z (combined with vitamins B and C and zinc sulphate monohydrate); FORTESPAN (combined with folic acid); SLOW-FE FOLIC (combined with folic acid).

Fersaday (Goldshield Pharmaceuticals) *See* FERROUS FUMARATE.

Fersamal (Goldshield Pharmaceuticals) *See* FERROUS FUMARATE.

Fertiral (Hoechst Marion Roussel) *See* GONADORELIN.

Fesovit Z (Medeva) A proprietary combination of *ferrous sulphate, *zinc sulphate monohydrate, B vitamins (*see* VITAMIN B COMPLEX), and *vitamin C, used to treat iron-deficiency *anaemia. It is available as *modified-release capsules on *prescription only.
Side effects, precautions, and interactions with other drugs: see IRON.

fexofenadine hydrochloride One of the newer (non-sedating) *antihistamines, used for the relief of symptoms of such allergic conditions as hay fever and urticaria. It is available as tablets on *prescription only.

Side effects, precautions, and interactions with other drugs: see ANTIHISTAMINES.

Proprietary preparations: Telfast 120; Telfast 180.

fibrates A group of *lipid-lowering drugs that lower plasma *triglycerides and increase the breakdown of LDL-*cholesterol (*see* LIPOPROTEINS), thereby reducing plasma LDL-cholesterol by up to 18%. They also tend to raise plasma HDL-cholesterol (which has a beneficial effect). Fibrates are used to treat a variety of *hyperlipidaemias. *See* BEZAFIBRATE; CIPROFIBRATE; CLOFIBRATE; FENOFIBRATE; GEMFIBROZIL.

Side effects: fribrates can cause gastrointestinal upset (nausea and/or vomiting), rash, and muscle pain. Less often itching, impotence, headache, dizziness, drowsiness, and hair loss may occur.

Precautions and interactions with other drugs: fibrates can cause rhabdomyolysis (inflammation and destruction of muscle tissue). Muscle pain, tenderness, or weakness must therefore be reported to a doctor promptly and investigated. Rhabdomyolysis can be a serious condition and is more likely to occur in people who are also taking *statins or *cyclosporin. People with kidney disease or hypothyroidism are at a higher risk of developing this condition. Fibrates should not be taken by women who are pregnant or breastfeeding. See also entries for individual drugs.

fibrinolytic drugs A class of drugs that are used to dissolve blood clots. They act by stimulating production of the body's own enzymes that break down fibrin, the protein that forms the basis of blood clots (thrombi), i.e. they are **thrombolytic drugs**. The common fibrinolytic drugs are *streptokinase, *alteplase, *reteplase, *anistreplase, and *urokinase. Most of them are used to dissolve blood clots in the coronary arteries (which supply the heart) in people who have had a heart attack; some of them have other uses in addition to or instead of this. Fibrinolytic drugs are available as solutions for injection or infusion on *prescription only.

Side effects: include nausea, vomiting, and bleeding (which is usually limited to the injection site). Back pain has been reported, and low blood pressure can occur after a heart attack.

Precautions and interactions with other drugs: fibrinolytic drugs should not be given to people who have an active peptic ulcer, a bleeding disorder, active lung disease, severe liver disease, or acute pancreatitis, or to those who have recently had a stroke, haemorrhage, or injury, or who have recently undergone surgery (including tooth extraction). They should be used with caution in pregnant women. The risk of bleeding is increased if fibrinolytic drugs are used with anticoagulants or antiplatelet drugs.

Fibro-Vein (STD Pharmaceutical Products) *See* SODIUM TETRADECYL SULPHATE.

Fiery Jack Cream (J. Pickles & Sons) A proprietary combination of *capsicum oleoresin, *diethylamine salicylate, *glycol salicylate, and *methyl nicotinate, used as a *rubefacient for the relief of muscular aches and pains, including backache, sciatica, lumbago, and strains. It is freely available *over the counter.
Side effects and precautions: see RUBEFACIENTS; SALICYLATES.

Fiery Jack Ointment (J. Pickles & Sons) *See* CAPSICUM OLEORESIN.

Filair (3M Health Care) *See* BECLOMETHASONE <BECLOMETASONE> DIPROPIONATE.

filgrastim Recombinant human granulocyte-colony stimulating factor, a form of *granulocyte-colony stimulating factor produced by genetic engineering. It is used for the treatment of neutropenia (a decrease in the number of neutrophils, a type of white blood cell) induced by *cytotoxic drug treatment for *cancer or resulting from destruction of the bone marrow prior to bone marrow transplantation. It may be given to cancer patients who are about to undergo blood collection before aggressive treatment; neutrophil production will thus be boosted in this collected blood, which is used to replace the white cells destroyed by the treatment. Filgrastim is also used for treating some other forms of neutropenia (such as that present at birth) when this causes recurrent serious infections. It is available as a form for injection on *prescription only; its use is restricted to specialist units.
Side effects: include pain in muscles or bones, transient low blood pressure, difficult or painful urination, allergic reactions, headache, diarrhoea, anaemia, nose bleeds, hair loss, osteoporosis, and rash.
Precautions: white blood cell counts should be carefully monitored during treatment. Filgrastim should be used with caution in women who are pregnant or breastfeeding.
Proprietary preparation: Neupogen.

finasteride An *anti-androgen that acts by inhibiting the enzyme that metabolizes *testosterone to the more active dihydrotestosterone. It is used in the treatment of benign enlargement of the prostate. It is available as tablets on *prescription only.
Side effects: include impotence, decreased libido, a reduced volume of semen on ejaculation, breast tenderness and enlargement, and allergic reactions (including lip swelling and rash).
Precautions: finasteride should be used with caution in men with urinary obstruction and prostate cancer. The use of barrier contraception is recommended if the patient's sexual partner is pregnant or capable of

becoming pregnant; women who are pregnant or capable of becoming so should avoid handling crushed or broken tablets.
Proprietary preparation: Proscar.

first-line treatment Drug therapy that is the first choice for treating a particular condition; other drugs are only used if first-line therapy has failed.

fish oils *See* OMEGA-3 MARINE TRIGLYCERIDES.

Flagyl (Rhône-Poulenc Rorer) *See* METRONIDAZOLE.

Flagyl Compak (Rhône-Poulenc Rorer) A proprietary preparation of *metronidazole tablets packaged with *nystatin pessaries, used for the treatment of vaginal infections. It is available on *prescription only.
Side effects, precautions, and interactions with other drugs: see METRONIDAZOLE; NYSTATIN.

Flamatak MR (Cox Pharmaceuticals) *See* DICLOFENAC SODIUM.

Flamatrol (APS-Berk) *See* PIROXICAM.

Flamazine (Smith & Nephew Healthcare) *See* SILVER SULPHADIAZINE <SULFADIAZINE>.

Flamrase, **Flamrase SR** (APS-Berk) *See* DICLOFENAC SODIUM.

flavoxate hydrochloride An *antimuscarinic drug used to treat urinary incontinence, abnormal frequency or urgency in passing urine, and bladder spasms due to the presence of a catheter. It acts in the same way as *oxybutynin but is less effective, although it may be preferred to this drug as its side effects are less severe. Flavoxate is available as tablets on *prescription only.
Side effects: include dry mouth, constipation, blurred vision, nausea, and headache.
Precautions: flavoxate is not recommended for children under 12 years old. *See also* OXYBUTYNIN.
Interactions with other drugs: see ANTIMUSCARINIC DRUGS.
Proprietary preparation: Urispas 200.

flecainide acetate A class I *anti-arrhythmic drug used for the treatment of a variety of *arrhythmias. It is available as an injection or tablets on *prescription only.
Side effects: include dizziness, visual disturbances, and less commonly nausea and vomiting.
Precautions: therapy with flecainide acetate should be initiated under hospital supervision. It should not usually be taken during pregnancy,

because of the lack of data on its effects on the baby, or after a heart attack. *See also* ANTI-ARRHYTHMIC DRUGS.

Interactions with other drugs:

Other anti-arrhythmic drugs: amiodarone increases the risk of arrhythmias and should not be taken with flecainide; depression of heart function is increased if flecainide is taken with any other anti-arrhythmic.

Antidepressants: tricyclic antidepressants increase the risk of arrhythmias; fluoxetine increases the plasma concentration of flecainide.

Antihistamines: the risk of arrhythmias is increased if astemizole or terfenadine are taken with flecainide.

Antimalarial drugs: quinine increases the plasma concentration of flecainide; halofantrine increases the risk of arrhythmias.

Beta blockers: depression of heart function is increased if these drugs are taken with flecainide.

Diuretics: increase adverse effects on the heart through potassium loss.

Ritonavir: increases the plasma concentration of flecainide and should therefore not be taken with flecainide.

Verapamil: depression of heart function is increased if verapamil is taken with flecainide.

Proprietary preparation: Tambocor.

Fleet Micro-enema (E. C. De Witt & Co) A proprietary combination of *sodium citrate (an osmotic laxative) and *sodium lauryl sulphoacetate (a wetting agent), used for the treatment of constipation. It can be obtained without a prescription, but only from pharmacies.

Precautions: *see* SODIUM CITRATE.

Fleet Phospho-soda (E. C. De Witt & Co) A proprietary combination of sodium dihydrogen phosphate dihydrate and disodium phosphate dodecahydrate (both *phosphate laxatives), used to evacuate the bowel before investigative procedures or surgery. It is available as an oral solution and can be obtained without a prescription, but only from pharmacies.

Side effects: *see* BOWEL-CLEANSING SOLUTIONS.

Precautions: this solution is not recommended for children. *See also* BOWEL-CLEANSING SOLUTIONS.

Fleet Ready-to-Use Enema (E. C. De Witt & Co) A proprietary combination of the osmotic laxatives *sodium acid phosphate and sodium phosphate (*see* PHOSPHATE LAXATIVES), used for the treatment of constipation or to evacuate the bowel before investigative procedures or surgery. It is available from pharmacies without a prescription.

Precautions: this enema is not recommended for children under three years old and should be used with caution in elderly people. *See also* PHOSPHATE LAXATIVES.

Fletchers' Arachis Oil Retention Enema (Pharmax) *See* ARACHIS OIL.

Fletchers' Enemette (Pharmax) A proprietary combination of
*docusate sodium and *glycerin, used as a stimulant laxative and faecal
softener in the treatment of constipation and to clear the bowel before
surgery, childbirth, or X-ray examination. It is available as an enema and
can be obtained from pharmacies without a prescription.
Side effects and precautions: see STIMULANT LAXATIVES.

Fletchers' Phosphate Enema (Pharmax) A proprietary combination
of the osmotic laxatives *sodium acid phosphate and sodium phosphate
(*see* PHOSPHATE LAXATIVES), used for the treatment of constipation or to
evacuate the bowel before investigative procedures or surgery. It is
available from pharmacies without a prescription.
Precautions: this enema is not recommended for children under three
years old and should be used with caution in elderly people. *See also*
PHOSPHATE LAXATIVES.

Flexin Continus (Napp Pharmaceuticals) *See* INDOMETHACIN
<INDOMETACIN>.

Flexotard MR (Pharmacia & Upjohn) *See* DICLOFENAC SODIUM.

Flixonase (Allen & Hanburys) *See* FLUTICASONE PROPIONATE.

Flixotide (Allen & Hanburys) *See* FLUTICASONE PROPIONATE.

Flolan (GlaxoWellcome) *See* EPOPROSTENOL.

Flomax MR (Yamanouchi Pharma) *See* TAMSULOSIN HYDROCHLORIDE.

Florinef (Bristol-Myers Squibb) *See* FLUDROCORTISONE ACETATE.

Floxapen (SmithKline Beecham Pharmaceuticals) *See* FLUCLOXACILLIN.

Flu-Amp (Generics) *See* CO-FLUAMPICIL.

Fluanxol (Lundbeck) *See* FLUPENTHIXOL <FLUPENTIXOL>.

Fluclomix (Ashbourne Pharmaceuticals) *See* FLUCLOXACILLIN.

flucloxacillin A *penicillin that is resistant to beta-lactamase (*see*
PENICILLINS). It is used for the treatment of infections due to
penicillinase-producing bacteria, including ear infections, pneumonia,
impetigo, cellulitis (an infection of the deep layers of the skin), and
infections of the lining of the heart cavity or valves. It is available, on
*prescription only, as capsules or a syrup for oral use and as an injection.
Side effects: include diarrhoea and allergic reactions (*see*
BENZYLPENICILLIN). In addition, hepatitis and jaundice may occur (the
jaundice may develop up to several weeks after treatment has stopped).
Precautions: see BENZYLPENICILLIN; PENICILLINS.

Interactions with other drugs: see BENZYLPENICILLIN.

Proprietary preparations: Floxapen; Fluclomix; Galfloxin; Ladropen; Zoxin; Flu-Amp (*see* CO-FLUAMPICIL); Magnapen (*see* CO-FLUAMPICIL).

fluconazole A triazole *antifungal drug used for the treatment of many fungal infections, especially candidiasis (of the mouth, vagina, or throat), athlete's foot, and cryptococcal meningitis (a form of meningitis that can occur as an opportunistic infection in AIDS patients). Available on *prescription, fluconazole can be taken orally, as capsules or a suspension, or it can be given by intravenous infusion. Capsules for treating vaginal candidiasis (maximum dose 150 mg) can be bought from pharmacies without a prescription.

Side effects: include abdominal discomfort, diarrhoea, and flatulence. Rarely, allergic reactions may occur; if a rash develops, the treatment should be stopped and a doctor consulted.

Precautions: fluconazole should be used with caution by people with impaired kidney function and by women who are pregnant or breastfeeding.

Interactions with other drugs:

Antacids: reduce the absorption of fluconazole.

Anticoagulants: the anticoagulant effects of warfarin and nicoumalone <acenocoumarol> are enhanced by fluconazole.

Antidiabetic drugs: the plasma concentrations of the sulphonylureas are increased.

Astemizole: should not be taken with fluconazole because of the risk of abnormal heart rhythms.

Cisapride: should not be taken with fluconazole.

Hydrochlorothiazide: increases the plasma concentration of fluconazole.

Phenytoin: its effect is enhanced.

Rifampicin: reduces the plasma concentration of fluconazole.

Terfenadine: should not be taken with fluconazole because of the risk of abnormal heart rhythms.

Theophylline: fluconazole increases the plasma concentration of theophylline, which may increase its side effects in patients receiving high doses of this drug.

Proprietary preparations: Diflucan; Diflucan One (available without a prescription).

flucytosine An *antifungal drug used for the treatment of systemic (generalized) yeast infections, such as candidiasis. It enhances the effects of *amphotericin, and is therefore used with this drug for treating severe or longstanding fungal infections, including cryptococcal meningitis and severe *Candida* infections. Flucytosine is available as a solution for intravenous infusion on *prescription only; tablets may be obtained for named patients.

Side effects: include nausea, vomiting, diarrhoea, rashes, and (more rarely) confusion, hallucinations, convulsions, headache, sedation, vertigo, and blood disorders (including bone marrow suppression).

Precautions: flucytosine should be used with caution in the elderly, in people with impaired kidney function or blood disorders, and in women who are pregnant or breastfeeding. Regular blood counts and tests for liver and kidney function should be carried out during treatment.

Interactions with other drugs:

  Amphotericin: may enhance the adverse effects of flucytosine.

  Cytarabine: may reduce the plasma concentration of flucytosine.

Proprietary preparation: Alcobon.

Fludara (Schering Health Care) *See* FLUDARABINE.

fludarabine An *antimetabolite that is used for the treatment of chronic lymphocytic leukaemia (*see* CANCER) after treatment with an *alkylating drug has failed. It is available as a form for injection or infusion on *prescription only.

Side effects: see CYTOTOXIC DRUGS. Very rarely, fludarabine may have adverse effects on the nervous system and lungs.

Precautions: fludarabine should not be given to pregnant women or people with severe kidney disease. The dosage may need to be reduced for those with moderate kidney disease. *See also* CYTOTOXIC DRUGS.

Interactions with other drugs:

  Pentostatin: increases the adverse effects of fludarabine on the lungs.

Proprietary preparation: Fludara.

fludrocortisone acetate A mineralocorticoid (*see* CORTICOSTEROIDS) used as replacement therapy in people with a deficiency of the natural hormone (aldosterone), as in Addison's disease or following surgical removal of the adrenal glands. It is also used to treat a certain kind of low blood pressure (orthostatic hypotension). Fludrocortisone is available as tablets on *prescription only.

Side effects: include high blood pressure, sodium and water retention, and potassium loss.

Precautions and interactions with other drugs: see CORTICOSTEROIDS.

Proprietary preparation: Florinef.

fludroxycortide *See* FLURANDRENOLONE.

flumazenil A drug that is used to reverse the sedative effects of *benzodiazepines that have been given during anaesthesia, in intensive care, or in diagnostic procedures. It is available as an injection on *prescription only.

Side effects: include nausea, vomiting, and flushing; agitation, anxiety, and fear can occur if sedation is reversed too rapidly. Patients in intensive care may have a transient increase in heart rate and blood pressure.

Precautions: flumazenil may cause withdrawal symptoms in people who are dependent on benzodiazepines; it should not be used in people who are receiving long-term treatment with benzodiazepines for epilepsy. Flumazenil should be used with caution in people with liver disease or a severe head injury, the elderly, children, and women who are pregnant or breastfeeding.

Proprietary preparation: Anexate.

flumethasone pivalate <flumetasone pivalate> A *corticosteroid used in combination with an antibacterial drug for the treatment of inflammation of the outer ear in which eczema is present. It is available as ear drops on *prescription only.

Side effects: flumethasone may cause local allergic reactions. *See* TOPICAL STEROIDS.

Precautions: prolonged use of flumethasone should be avoided. *See* TOPICAL STEROIDS.

Proprietary preparation: LOCORTEN-VIOFORM (combined with clioquinol).

flunisolide A *corticosteroid used for the treatment of allergic rhinitis (including hay fever). It is available as a metered-dose nasal spray on *prescription only; a nasal spray specifically for hay fever can be bought from pharmacies without a prescription.

Side effects: include transient local irritation.

Precautions: flunisolide should not be used when infection is present and should be used with caution by pregnant women and by people suffering from ulceration of the nose or who have recently suffered trauma to the nose or undergone nasal surgery.

Proprietary preparations: Syntaris; Syntaris Hayfever Nasal Spray.

flunitrazepam A long-acting *benzodiazepine used for the short-term treatment of insomnia. Flunitrazepam is a *controlled drug; it is available as tablets but cannot be prescribed on the NHS.

Side effects and precautions: see BENZODIAZEPINES; DIAZEPAM.

Interactions with other drugs: see BENZODIAZEPINES.

Proprietary preparation: Rohypnol.

fluocinolone acetonide A potent *topical steroid used for the treatment of a variety of skin disorders. It is available, on *prescription only, as a cream or ointment of varying strengths or as a gel.

Side effects and precautions: see TOPICAL STEROIDS.

Proprietary preparations: Synalar; Synalar 1:4 (diluted preparation), Synalar Cream 1:10 (weaker preparation), Synalar Gel; SYNALAR C (combined with clioquinol); SYNALAR N (combined with neomycin sulphate).

fluocinonide A potent *topical steroid used for the treatment of a variety of skin disorders. It is available, on *prescription only, as a cream, ointment, or scalp lotion.

Side effects and precautions: see TOPICAL STEROIDS.
Proprietary preparations: Metosyn; Metosyn Scalp Lotion.

fluocortolone A moderately potent *topical steroid, consisting of fluocortolone pivalate and fluocortolone hexanoate, used for the treatment of a variety of skin disorders. These compounds are combined in a cream and an ointment that are available on *prescription only. Fluocortolone combined with a local anaesthetic is used for relieving the symptoms of *haemorrhoids.
Side effects and precautions: see TOPICAL STEROIDS.
Proprietary preparations: Ultralanum; ULTRAPROCT (combined with cinchocaine hydrochloride).

Fluor-a-Day (Dental Health Products) *See* FLUORIDE.

fluorescein sodium A dye that is applied to the eye for diagnostic purposes: to highlight damaged areas of the cornea and locate foreign bodies. It is sometimes used in combination with a *local anaesthetic. Fluorescein sodium is available as eye drops and can be obtained without a prescription, but only from pharmacies.
Proprietary preparations: Minims Fluorescein Sodium; MINIMS LIGNOCAINE AND FLUORESCEIN (combined with lignocaine <lidocaine>).

fluoride A salt of fluorine, which in solution produces fluoride ions (*see* ELECTROLYTE). The incorporation of fluoride ions into the enamel of developing teeth strengthens the enamel and makes the teeth more resistant to dental caries (tooth decay). An adequate fluoride intake is provided by drinking water with a fluoride content of 1 part per million (ppm). When the natural fluoride content is significantly less than this, fluoride can be added to the public water supplies by the water authorities. In areas where tap water is not fluoridated, **sodium fluoride** supplements may be given to children. Sodium fluoride is available as tablets, drops, mouthwashes, and gels and can be obtained without a prescription, but only from pharmacies. **Monofluorophosphate**, which is added to some toothpastes or used in gels, is another source of fluoride.
Side effects: there may be occasional white flecks on the teeth; overdosage may produce yellowish-brown discoloration of the teeth.
Precautions: fluoride supplements should not be used if the fluoride content of drinking water exceeds 0.7 ppm.
Proprietary preparations: En-De-Kay (mouthwash); En-De-Kay Fluodrops (drops for children up to two years old); En-De-Kay Fluotabs (tablets for children over two years old); Fluor-a-Day (tablets); FluoriGard (tablets, drops, mouthwash, or gel).

FluoriGard (Colgate-Palmolive) *See* FLUORIDE.

fluorometholone A *corticosteroid used for the short-term treatment of inflammatory eye conditions that are not infected. It is available as eye drops on *prescription only.

Side effects: include an increase in pressure in the eye after a few weeks' treatment, thinning of the cornea, and fungal infections.

Precautions: fluorometholone should not be used by people with viral, fungal, tuberculous, or weeping infections or by those who wear soft contact lenses; it should be used with caution by people with glaucoma. Prolonged use by pregnant women and infants should be avoided. *See also* TOPICAL STEROIDS.

Proprietary preparations: FML; FML-NEO (combined with neomycin sulphate).

fluorouracil (5-fluorouracil; 5-FU) An *antimetabolite used for the treatment of solid tumours (*see* CANCER), especially those of the gastrointestinal tract (such as cancers of the colon and rectum) and breast cancer. It is usually administered intravenously, sometimes in conjunction with *folinic acid, which increases its effectiveness. It is usually given as intensive courses of several days' treatment every 3–4 weeks. Fluorouracil can also be used topically to treat certain malignant skin tumours. A *prescription only medicine, it is available as a solution for injection, capsules, or a cream.

Side effects: injections or capsules may cause *bone marrow suppression, inflammation of the mucous membranes lining the mouth, stomach, and intestine, and nausea and vomiting. *See* CYTOTOXIC DRUGS.

Precautions: see CYTOTOXIC DRUGS.

Proprietary preparation: Efudix (cream).

fluoxetine An *antidepressant drug of the *SSRI group. It is used for the treatment of depressive illness, obsessive-compulsive disorder, and bulimia nervosa. Fluoxetine is available as capsules or liquid on *prescription only.

Side effects and precautions: see SSRIS.

Interactions with other drugs:

Antiepileptics: the plasma concentrations of carbamazepine and phenytoin are increased by fluoxetine.

Antipsychotics: plasma concentrations of clozapine, haloperidol, and sertindole are increased by fluoxetine.

Selegiline: there is an increased risk of hypertension and adverse effects on the central nervous system.

Terfenadine: there is an increased risk of *arrhythmias and fluoxetine should not be taken with terfenadine.

For other interactions, *see* SSRIS.

Proprietary preparation: Prozac.

flupenthixol <flupentixol> A thioxanthene *antipsychotic drug used for the treatment of schizophrenia and other psychoses, particularly in patients who are apathetic and withdrawn. It is also used for the short-term treatment of depression. Flupenthixol is available, on *prescription only, as tablets or as a *depot injection.

Side effects: as for *chlorpromazine, but flupenthixol is less sedating and more likely to produce *extrapyramidal reactions.

Precautions: flupenthixol should not be used to treat senile confused patients or those who are hyperactive or excitable. *See also* CHLORPROMAZINE HYDROCHLORIDE.

Interactions with other drugs:

 Anaesthetics: their effect in lowering blood pressure is enhanced.

 Antidepressants: there is an increased risk of antimuscarinic effects and arrhythmias if flupenthixol is taken with tricyclic antidepressants.

 Antiepileptic drugs: their anticonvulsant effects are antagonized by flupenthixol.

 Antihistamines: there is an increased risk of arrhythmias if flupenthixol is taken with astemizole or terfenadine.

 Halofantrine: there is an increased risk of arrhythmias if this drug is taken with flupenthixol.

 Ritonavir: may increase the effects of flupenthixol.

 Sedatives: the sedative effects of flupenthixol are increased if it is taken with anxiolytic or hypnotic drugs, or any other drug that causes sedation.

Proprietary preparations: Depixol; Depixol Conc. (depot injection); Depixol Low Volume (depot injection); Fluanxol.

fluphenazine hydrochloride A phenothiazine *antipsychotic drug used for the treatment of schizophrenia and other psychoses and mania. It is also used as an *adjunct in the treatment of severe anxiety, agitation, and behavioural disorders. Fluphenazine is available, on *prescription only, as tablets or a *depot injection.

Side effects: as for *chlorpromazine but fluphenazine has more *extrapyramidal reactions, fewer antimuscarinic effects, and is less sedating.

Precautions: fluphenazine should not be used to treat patients who are severely depressed. *See also* CHLORPROMAZINE HYDROCHLORIDE.

Interactions with other drugs: *see* CHLORPROMAZINE HYDROCHLORIDE.

Proprietary preparations: Modecate, Modicate Concentrate (depot injections); Moditen; MOTIPRESS (combined with nortriptyline); MOTIVAL (combined with nortriptyline).

flurandrenolone <fludroxycortide> A moderately potent *topical steroid used for the treatment of a variety of skin conditions. It is available, on *prescription only, as a cream, ointment, or impregnated tape.

Side effects and precautions: *see* TOPICAL STEROIDS.

Proprietary preparations: Haelan.

flurazepam A long-acting *benzodiazepine used for the short-term treatment of insomnia. It is available as tablets on *prescription only, but cannot be prescribed on the NHS.

Side effects and precautions: see BENZODIAZEPINES; DIAZEPAM.

Interactions with other drugs:

Ritonavir: increases the plasma concentration of flurazepam, causing profound sedation; these two drugs should therefore not be taken together.

See also BENZODIAZEPINES.

Proprietary preparation: Dalmane.

flurbiprofen An *NSAID used for the treatment of pain and inflammation in rheumatoid arthritis and other disorders of the muscles or joints. It is also used to treat mild to moderate pain (such as period pains) and to relieve postoperative pain. Flurbiprofen (as the sodium salt) is applied to the eye to prevent constriction of the pupil during eye surgery and to reduce inflammation after surgery or laser treatment. It is available, on *prescription only, as tablets, modified-release capsules, suppositories, or eye drops.

Side effects: see NSAIDS. Suppositories may cause local irritation.

Precautions and interactions with other drugs: see NSAIDS.

Proprietary preparations: Froben; Froben SR (modified-release capsules); Ocufen (eye drops).

flutamide An *anti-androgen used for the treatment of advanced *cancer of the prostate gland. It is available as tablets on *prescription only.

Side effects: include breast enlargement and tenderness (sometimes with milk production), nausea, vomiting, diarrhoea, increased appetite, insomnia, and tiredness.

Precautions: liver function tests will need to be performed regularly during treatment. People with heart disease may suffer from fluid retention.

Interactions with other drugs:

Warfarin: the anticoagulant effect of warfarin is increased.

Proprietary preparations: Chimax; Drogenil.

fluticasone propionate A *corticosteroid most often used as an anti-inflammatory drug for treating skin disorders, such as dermatitis and eczema, and for the prevention of *asthma attacks and the prevention and treatment of allergic rhinitis, including hay fever. When used topically it is classed as a potent steroid. It is available, on *prescription only, as a cream, an ointment, a metered-dose nasal spray, a metered-dose *inhaler, a breath-activated inhaler, disks of powder to be used in a breath-activated delivery system, or as single-dose units for use in a *nebulizer.

Side effects: see CORTICOSTEROIDS. The nasal spray may cause irritation, nosebleeds, and disturbances in smell and taste.

Precautions: fluticasone should be used with caution by women who are pregnant or breastfeeding.

Proprietary preparations: Cultivate (cream); Flixonase (nasal spray); Flixotide (inhaler); Flixotide Accuhaler; Flixotide Diskhaler; Flixotide Nebules.

fluvastatin A *statin used for the treatment of primary hypercholesterolaemia (see HYPERLIPIDAEMIA) that has not responded to dietary measures. It is available as capsules on *prescription only.

Side effects, precautions, and interactions with other drugs: see STATINS.

Proprietary preparation: Lescol.

fluvoxamine maleate An *antidepressant drug of the *SSRI group. It is used for the treatment of depressive illness and obsessive-compulsive disorder. Fluvoxamine is available as tablets on *prescription only.

Side effects: see SSRIS.

Precautions: see SSRIS. In addition, dosage of this drug should be reduced gradually at the end of treatment.

Interactions with other drugs:

Antiepileptics: the plasma concentrations of carbamazepine and phenytoin are increased by fluvoxamine.

Clozapine: its plasma concentration may be increased by fluvoxamine.

Terfenadine: there is an increased risk of *arrhythmias and fluvoxamine should not be taken with terfenadine.

Theophylline and aminophylline: plasma concentrations of these drugs are increased to toxic values by fluvoxamine, which should therefore not be used in combination with them; if this is unavoidable, the dosage of theophylline or aminophylline must be reduced.

See also SSRIS.

Proprietary preparation: Faverin.

FML (Allergan) *See* FLUOROMETHOLONE.

FML-Neo (Allergan) A proprietary combination of *neomycin sulphate (an antibiotic) and *fluorometholone (a corticosteroid), used for the short-term treatment of inflammatory conditions of the eye that are infected. It is available as eye drops on *prescription only.

Side effects and precautions: see FLUOROMETHOLONE.

folic acid A vitamin of the B group (see VITAMIN B COMPLEX) that has an important role in DNA and RNA synthesis. Good dietary sources of folic acid are liver, yeast, and green vegetables. The proper functioning of folic acid depends on that of another B vitamin, B_{12}, and deficiency of one vitamin may lead to deficiency of the other. Deficiency of folic acid causes certain types of *anaemia (including megaloblastic anaemia), in which the cells that give rise to red blood cells do not develop normally. These can be treated with folic acid. A good intake of folic acid is particularly necessary during pregnancy. Folic acid supplements taken before and during pregnancy help to prevent spina bifida and other neural-tube defects (in which the spinal cord or brain fail to develop normally) in the fetus. It is recommended that women should take 400 micrograms of folic acid daily while trying to conceive and for the first three months of pregnancy. This dosage should be increased to 400–500 milligrams for women who have previously given birth to a baby with a neural-tube defect. Folic acid is also combined with *iron supplements in preparations used to prevent deficiencies of folic acid and iron during pregnancy. Folic acid is available as tablets, a syrup, or a solution and can be obtained from pharmacies without a prescription, but preparations in which the daily dose exceeds 500 micrograms are *prescription only medicines.

Side effects: there may be mottling of the teeth.

Proprietary preparations: Folicare (solution); Lexpec (syrup); Preconceive (tablets); DENCYL (combined with ferrous sulphate and zinc sulphate monohydrate); FEFOL (combined with ferrous fumarate); FERFOLIC SV (combined with ferrous gluconate and vitamin C); FERROGRAD FOLIC (combined with ferrous sulphate); GALFER FA (combined with ferrous fumarate); LEXPEC WITH IRON-M (combined with ferric ammonium citrate); PREGADAY (combined with ferrous fumarate): PREGNACARE (combined with vitamins and minerals); SLOW-FE FOLIC (combined with ferrous sulphate).

Folicare (Rosemont Pharmaceuticals) *See* FOLIC ACID.

folinic acid An agent that counteracts the side effects of *methotrexate and is given as 'rescue' treatment, usually 24 hours after administration of methotrexate, when inflammation of the lining of the mouth and other mucous membranes or *bone marrow suppression are causing problems. It also enhances the activity of *fluorouracil and is used as part of the combination treatment for cancers of the colon and rectum. Folinic acid is given in the form of **calcium folinate** (or **calcium leucovorin**), available as tablets or a solution for injection, or **calcium levofolinate** (**calcium levoleucovorin**), which is available as an injection. Both these drugs are *prescription only medicines.

Side effects: fever occasionally occurs after injection.

Proprietary preparations: Isovorin (calcium levofolinate); Lederfolin (calcium folinate); Refolinon (calcium folinate).

follitropin A synthetic preparation of follicle-stimulating hormone (a *gonadotrophin) used for the treatment of infertility in men and women that is due to underactivity of the pituitary gland (resulting in insufficient production of gonadotrophins). It is also used to induce superovulation (production of a large number of eggs) in women undergoing fertility treatment, such as *in vitro* fertilization. Follitropin is given by subcutaneous or intramuscular injection and is available on *prescription only.

Side effects: include ovarian hyperstimulation (the uncontrolled production of large numbers of follicles in the ovaries) and multiple pregnancy; allergic reactions may occur in both sexes.

Precautions: follitropin should be used with caution in women with ovarian cysts and in people with thyroid or adrenal disorders or pituitary tumours.

Proprietary preparations: Gonal-F (follitropin alpha); Puregon (follitropin beta).

Fomac (APS-Berk) *See* MEBEVERINE HYDROCHLORIDE.

Foradil (Novartis Pharmaceuticals) *See* EFORMOTEROL <FORMOTEROL> FUMARATE.

Forceval (Unigreg) A proprietary combination of *vitamin A, vitamins of the B group (*see* VITAMIN B COMPLEX), ascorbic acid (*see* VITAMIN C), vitamin D_2 (*see* ERGOCALCIFEROL), *vitamin E, and various minerals and trace elements, used as a multivitamin and mineral supplement for treating vitamin and mineral deficiency and for people on special diets that lack these substances. It is available as capsules or junior capsules (which also contain *vitamin K) and can be obtained without a prescription, but only from pharmacies.

formaldehyde A caustic liquid that is used to remove verrucas and warts (*see* KERATOLYTICS). It is available as a lotion or gel that can be obtained without a prescription, but only from pharmacies.

Side effects: formaldehyde may cause irritation of the treated skin.

Precautions: formaldehyde should not be used on facial or genital warts or on warts around the anus. It should not be applied to healthy skin around the wart or to broken skin.

Proprietary preparation: Veracur.

formestane An *aromatase inhibitor used for the treatment of breast *cancer in women who have undergone a natural menopause or in whom the menopause has been induced (for example, by removal of the ovaries). It is available as an injection for deep intramuscular use on *prescription only.

Side effects: include pain and irritation at the injection site, rash, itching, hot flushes, nausea and vomiting, and (rarely) growth of facial hair, baldness, vaginal bleeding, pelvic and muscle cramps, joint pain, headache, dizziness, drowsiness, and sore throat.

Precautions: formestane should not be given to women who have not reached the menopause or who are pregnant or breastfeeding.

Proprietary preparation: Lentaron.

formoterol fumarate *See* EFORMOTEROL FUMARATE.

formulation The form in which a drug is presented. Tablets, a syrup, and an injection are examples.

Fortagesic (Sanofi Winthrop) A proprietary combination of *pentazocine (an opioid analgesic) and *paracetamol (a non-opioid analgesic), used for the treatment of moderate pain of muscle and joint disorders. Fortagesic is available as tablets; it is a *controlled drug and cannot be prescribed on the NHS.
Side effects and precautions: see MORPHINE; PARACETAMOL.
Interactions with other drugs: see OPIOIDS.

Fortespan (SmithKline Beecham Pharmaceuticals) A proprietary combination of *ferrous sulphate and *folic acid, used to prevent deficiencies of iron and folic acid during pregnancy. It is available as *modified-release capsules and can be obtained without a prescription, but only from pharmacies.
Side effects, precautions, and interactions with other drugs: see IRON.

Fortipine LA 40 (Nycomed Amersham) *See* NIFEDIPINE.

Fortral (Sanofi Winthrop) *See* PENTAZOCINE.

Fortum (GlaxoWellcome) *See* CEFTAZIDIME.

Fosamax (Merck Sharp & Dohme) *See* ALENDRONIC ACID.

foscarnet An *antiviral drug used for the treatment of cytomegalovirus retinitis, a serious eye infection, occurring mainly in AIDS patients, that can lead to blindness. It is also used for treating herpes simplex infections, such as cold sores and genital herpes, in people whose immune systems are compromised and who have not responded to *aciclovir. However, it does not deplete white blood cells to the same extent as ganciclovir. Foscarnet is available as an intravenous infusion on *prescription only.
Side effects: include nausea, vomiting, diarrhoea, abdominal pains, headache, fatigue, impairment of kidney function, reduced concentrations of calcium and haemoglobin in the blood, rash, fever, and genital irritation or ulcers.
Precautions: foscarnet should be used with caution in people with kidney disease and it should not be given to women who are pregnant or breastfeeding. Plenty of fluids should be taken during treatment.
Proprietary preparation: Foscavir.

Foscavir (AstraZeneca) *See* FOSCARNET.

fosfestrol tetrasodium A synthetic *oestrogen used for the treatment of *cancer of the prostate gland; it is broken down in the body to produce *stilboestrol <diethylstilbestrol> (another synthetic oestrogen). Fosfestrol is available, on *prescription only, as tablets or as a solution for intravenous injection.

Side effects: include nausea and vomiting, fluid retention, thrombosis, breast enlargement, impotence, and (after intravenous injection) pain behind the testicles.

Precautions and interactions with other drugs: see OESTROGENS.

Proprietary preparation: Honvan.

fosinopril An *ACE inhibitor used as an adjunct to *diuretics for the treatment of *heart failure. It is available as tablets on *prescription only.

Side effects, precautions, and interactions with other drugs: see ACE INHIBITORS.

Proprietary preparation: Staril.

Frador (Fenton) A proprietary combination of *chlorbutol <chlorobutanol> (an antiseptic), *menthol, *styrax, and balsamic benzoin (an antiseptic and astringent) in the form of a *tincture, used to relieve the pain of mouth ulcers. It is freely available *over the counter.

Fragmin (Pharmacia & Upjohn) *See* DALTEPARIN SODIUM.

framycetin sulphate An *aminoglycoside antibiotic used for the treatment of bacterial infections of the eyes (such as conjunctivitis), the outer ear, or the skin. It is available as eye drops, ointment, or ear drops on *prescription only.

Side effects: there is a small risk of ear damage, especially if the eardrum is perforated; local allergic reactions may occur.

Precautions: ear drops containing framycetin should not be used in people with a perforated eardrum. Contact lenses should not be worn by people taking eye drops containing framycetin. The ointment should not be applied to large areas of damaged skin.

Proprietary preparations: Soframycin (eye drops or ointment); SOFRADEX (combined with dexamethasone and gramicidin); SOFRAMYCIN (skin ointment; combined with gramicidin).

frangula *See* NORMACOL PLUS.

Franol (Sanofi Winthrop) A proprietary combination of *ephedrine hydrochloride (a sympathomimetic drug) and *theophylline (a bronchodilator), used for the treatment of bronchitis and asthma. **Franol Plus** is a stronger preparation containing a higher concentration of ephedrine. Both preparations are available as tablets on *prescription only.

Side effects: include palpitation, nausea, stomach upset, headache, insomnia, arrhythmias (irregular heart rhythms), anxiety, flushing, and tremor.

Precautions: Franol and Franol Plus should not be taken by people with unstable angina, porphyria, arrhythmias, severe high blood pressure, or coronary disease or by pregnant women. They should be used with caution in people with poor kidney function, heart or liver disease, peptic ulcers, an overactive thyroid gland, or glaucoma and in women who are breastfeeding.

Interactions with other drugs: see EPHEDRINE HYDROCHLORIDE; XANTHINES.

friar's balsam *See* BENZOIN TINCTURE COMPOUND.

Frisium (Hoechst Marion Roussel) *See* CLOBAZAM.

Froben, Froben SR (Knoll) *See* FLURBIPROFEN.

Froop (APS-Berk; Ashbourne Pharmaceuticals) *See* FRUSEMIDE <FUROSEMIDE>.

Froop-Co (Ashbourne Pharmaceuticals) *See* CO-AMILOFRUSE.

Fru-Co (Norton Healthcare) *See* CO-AMILOFRUSE.

Frumil, Frumil Forte, Frumil LS (Rhône-Poulenc Rorer) *See* CO-AMILOFRUSE.

frusemide <furosemide> A *loop diuretic used for the treatment of *oedema associated with heart failure, liver disease with ascites (accumulation of fluid in the abdominal cavity), or kidney disease. It is available, on *prescription only, as tablets, a suspension, or a solution for intravenous injection. *See also* CO-AMILOFRUSE.

Side effects, precautions, and interactions with other drugs: see LOOP DIURETICS.

Proprietary preparations: Dryptal; Froop; Lasix; Rusyde; Aridil (*see* CO-AMILOFRUSE); DIUMIDE-K CONTINUS (combined with potassium chloride); Froop-Co (*see* CO-AMILOFRUSE); Fru-Co (*see* CO-AMILOFRUSE); Frumil (*see* CO-AMILOFRUSE); FRUSENE (combined with triamterene); LASIKAL (combined with potassium chloride); LASILACTONE (combined with spironolactone); Lasoride (*see* CO-AMILOFRUSE).

See also DIURETICS.

Frusene (Orion Pharma) A proprietary combination of *frusemide <furosemide> (a loop diuretic) and *triamterene (a potassium-sparing diuretic), used for the treatment of *oedema associated with congestive heart failure, liver disease, or kidney disease. It is available as tablets on *prescription only.

Side effects, precautions, and interactions with other drugs: see LOOP DIURETICS; POTASSIUM-SPARING DIURETICS.

See also DIURETICS.

5-FU *See* FLUOROURACIL.

Fucibet (Leo Pharmaceuticals) A proprietary combination of *fusidic acid (an antibiotic) and *betamethasone (a potent steroid), used for the treatment of eczema occurring with bacterial infection. It is available as a cream on *prescription only.
Side effects, precautions, and interactions with other drugs: see CORTICOSTEROIDS.

Fucidin (Leo Pharmaceuticals) *See* FUSIDIC ACID.

Fucidin H (Leo Pharmaceuticals) A proprietary combination of *fusidic acid (an antibiotic) and *hydrocortisone (a moderately potent steroid), used for the treatment of eczema and dermatitis occurring with bacterial infection. It is available, on *prescription only, as an ointment, gel, or cream.
Side effects, precautions, and interactions with other drugs: see CORTICOSTEROIDS.

Fucithalmic (Leo Pharmaceuticals) *See* FUSIDIC ACID.

Fulcin (AstraZeneca) *See* GRISEOFULVIN.

Full Marks (Seton Scholl Healthcare) *See* PHENOTHRIN.

Fungilin (Bristol-Myers Squibb) *See* AMPHOTERICIN.

Fungizone (Bristol-Myers Squibb) *See* AMPHOTERICIN.

Furadantin (Procter & Gamble) *See* NITROFURANTOIN.

Furamide (Knoll) *See* DILOXANIDE FUROATE.

furosemide *See* FRUSEMIDE.

fusafungine An *antibiotic that also reduces inflammation. It is used for the treatment of infections and inflammation in the nose and throat. Fusafungine is available as a metered-dose aerosol spray on *prescription only.
Proprietary preparation: Locabiotal.

fusidic acid A narrow-spectrum *antibiotic used, often in the form of its salt, sodium fusidate, for the treatment of infections caused by penicillin-resistant staphylococci, especially bone and skin infections and abscesses. It is available, on *prescription only, as a gel, cream, or ointment for topical use, as tablets or a solution for oral use, or as an *intravenous infusion.
Side effects: include nausea, vomiting, rashes, and reversible jaundice, especially after high doses.

Precautions: regular monitoring of liver function during treatment is desirable.

Proprietary preparations: Fucidin; Fucithalmic (eye drops); FUCIBET (combined with betamethasone); FUCIDIN H (combined with hydrocortisone).

Fybogel (Reckitt & Colman) *See* ISPAGHULA HUSK.

Fybogel Mebeverine (Reckitt & Colman) A proprietary combination of *mebeverine hydrochloride (an antispasmodic) and *ispaghula husk (a bulking agent), used for the treatment of irritable bowel syndrome. It is available as effervescent granules on *prescription only.

Precautions: Fybogel Mebeverine should not be taken by people with intestinal obstruction. This medicine should be taken with a full glass of water and should not be taken immediately before going to bed.

Fybozest Orange (Reckitt & Colman) *See* ISPAGHULA HUSK.

Fynnon Calcium Aspirin (Seton Scholl Healthcare) *See* ASPIRIN.

Fynnon Salts (Seton Scholl Healthcare) *See* SODIUM SULPHATE.

G

gabapentin An *anticonvulsant drug used as an *adjunct in the treatment of partial epilepsy. It is available as tablets on *prescription only.

Side effects: include somnolence, dizziness, shaky movements, fatigue, headache, nausea and vomiting, rhinitis, weight gain, and nervousness.

Precautions: dosages should be reduced gradually when stopping medication. The dosage may need to be reduced in the elderly. Women who are planning to become pregnant, or who are already pregnant, should seek specialist advice. Gabapentin is not recommended for women who are breastfeeding.

Interactions with other drugs:

Anatacids: reduce the absorption of gabapentin.

Proprietary preparation: Neurontin.

Gabitril (Sanofi Winthrop) *See* TIAGABINE.

Galake (Galen) *See* CO-DYDRAMOL.

Galcodine, **Galcodine Paediatric** (Galen) *See* CODEINE.

Galenamet (Galen) *See* CIMETIDINE.

Galenamox (Galen) *See* AMOXYCILLIN <AMOXICILLIN>.

Galenphol, **Galenphol Paediatric**, **Galenphol Strong** (Galen) *See* PHOLCODINE.

Galfer (Galen) *See* FERROUS FUMARATE.

Galfer FA (Galen) A proprietary combination of *ferrous fumarate and *folic acid, used to prevent deficiencies of iron and folic acid during pregnancy. It is available as tablets and can be obtained without a prescription, but only from pharmacies.

Side effects, precautions, and interactions with other drugs: see IRON.

Galfloxin (Galen) *See* FLUCLOXACILLIN.

Galloways Cough Syrup (Pfizer Consumer Healthcare) A proprietary combination of *ipecacuanha and *squill (both expectorants), used for the relief of coughs and hoarseness. It may be bought freely *over the counter.

Side effects and precautions: see IPECACUANHA; SQUILL.

Galprofen (GalPharm International) *See* IBUPROFEN.

Galpseud (Galen) *See* PSEUDOEPHEDRINE.

Galpseud Plus (Galen) A proprietary combination of
*chlorpheniramine <chlorphenamine> maleate (an antihistamine) and
*pseudoephedrine (a sympathomimetic drug), used as a *decongestant
for the treatment of hay fever and colds. It is available as tablets and may
be bought from pharmacies without a prescription.
Side effects and interactions with other drugs: see ANTIHISTAMINES;
EPHEDRINE HYDROCHLORIDE.
Precautions: Galpseud Plus should not be taken by people with epilepsy
or high blood pressure. *See also* ANTIHISTAMINES; EPHEDRINE
HYDROCHLORIDE.

Gamanil (Merck Pharmaceuticals) *See* LOFEPRAMINE.

gamolenic acid A fatty acid that is a constituent of evening primrose
oil and borage oil. It is used to relieve the symptoms of *eczema and to
treat breast pain (including that associated with menstrual periods), in
which it is thought to reduce the responses of the breasts to the
hormones that cause breast tenderness during periods: it works slowly
and may not have a beneficial effect until it has been taken for 2–3
months. Gamolenic acid is available as capsules on *prescription only.
Side effects: include nausea and headache.
Precautions: gamolenic acid should not be taken by people with epilepsy.
Proprietary preparations: Efamast (for breast pain); Epogam (for eczema).

ganciclovir An *antiviral drug used for the treatment of
cytomegalovirus (CMV) infections. These occur mainly in AIDS patients
and in the recipients of transplants. The most serious CMV infection in
AIDS patients is retinitis (which may lead to blindness); in transplant
patients it is CMV pneumonia. Ganciclovir is available, on *prescription
only, as an intravenous infusion or capsules.
Side effects: the most serious side effect is *bone marrow suppression,
resulting in susceptibility to infection and bleeding; other side effects
include anaemia, fever, and rash may occur. Less frequently, chills, fever,
malaise, nausea, vomiting, abdominal pain, mouth ulcers, diarrhoea, loss
of appetite, headache, and itching may occur.
Precautions: ganciclovir should not be given to women who are pregnant
or breastfeeding; pregnancy during treatment should be avoided by using
adequate contraceptive measures. Blood counts must be monitored
during treatment.
Interactions with other drugs:
  Primaxin: ganciclovir increases the side effects of this antibiotic.
  Zidovudine: causes profound reduction of white-blood-cell production by
    the bone marrow and should not be used with ganciclovir.
Proprietary preparation: Cymevene.

Ganda (Chauvin Pharmaceuticals) A proprietary combination of *adrenaline <epinephrine> (a sympathomimetic drug) and *guanethidine monosulphate (which prolongs and enhances its effects), used in the treatment of *glaucoma to reduce the production of aqueous fluid in the eye and to increase its drainage from the eye. It is available as eye drops on *prescription only.

Side effects: see ADRENALINE <EPINEPHRINE>.

Precautions: prolonged use may damage the conjunctiva and cornea, which should therefore be examined every six months.

Garamycin (Schering-Plough) *See* GENTAMICIN.

Gastrobid Continus (Napp Pharmaceuticals) *See* METOCLOPRAMIDE.

Gastrocote (Seton Scholl Healthcare) A proprietary combination of *alginic acid, *aluminium hydroxide, *magnesium trisilicate, and *sodium bicarbonate, used as an *antacid in the treatment of indigestion, oesophagitis, and heartburn due to reflux (see ACID-PEPTIC DISEASES). It is freely available *over the counter as chewable tablets or a sugar-free liquid.

Side effects and interactions with other drugs: see ANTACIDS.

Precautions: the tablets are not recommended for children under six years old and should be used with caution by people with diabetes, since they have a high sugar content.

Gastroflux (Ashbourne Pharmaceuticals) *See* METOCLOPRAMIDE.

Gastromax (Pfizer) *See* METOCLOPRAMIDE.

gastro-oesophageal reflux *See* ACID-PEPTIC DISEASES.

Gaviscon Advance (Reckitt & Colman) A proprietary combination of sodium alginate (*see* ALGINIC ACID) and *potassium bicarbonate, used for the treatment of heartburn, oesophagitis, and indigestion due to reflux (*see* ACID-PEPTIC DISEASES). It is available as a sugar-free suspension and can be obtained without a prescription, but only from pharmacies.

Precautions: Gaviscon Advance has a high sodium content and should therefore be avoided by people following salt-restricted diets and by those who have heart failure or impaired liver or kidney function.

Gaviscon Infant (Reckitt & Colman) *See* ALGINIC ACID.

Gaviscon Liquid (Reckitt & Colman) A proprietary combination of sodium alginate (*see* ALGINIC ACID), *sodium bicarbonate, and *calcium carbonate, used as an *antacid for the treatment of heartburn, oesophagitis, and indigestion due to reflux (*see* ACID-PEPTIC DISEASES). It can be obtained without a prescription, but only from pharmacies.

Side effects and interactions with other drugs: see ANTACIDS.

Precautions: Gaviscon Liquid has a high sodium content and should therefore be avoided by people following salt-restricted diets and by those who have heart failure or impaired liver or kidney function.

Gaviscon Tablets (Reckitt & Colman) A proprietary combination of *alginic acid, *aluminium hydroxide, *magnesium trisilicate, and *sodium bicarbonate, used as an *antacid for the treatment of heartburn, oesophagitis, and indigestion due to reflux (*see* ACID-PEPTIC DISEASES). It can be obtained without a prescription, but only from pharmacies. **Gaviscon 500** is a similar formulation; **Gaviscon 250** (half-strength tablets) cannot be prescribed on the NHS.

Side effects and interactions with other drugs: see ANTACIDS.

Precautions: Gaviscon Tablets have a high sodium content and should therefore be avoided by people following salt-restricted diets and by those who have heart failure or impaired liver or kidney function.

gel A jelly-like substance consisting of a colloid in which a liquid is dispersed in a solid. Some drugs are formulated as gels for *topical application. The bases may be soluble or insoluble in water.

Gelcosal (Quinoderm) A proprietary combination of strong *coal tar solution, pine *tar, and *salicylic acid (all keratolytics), used for the treatment of *psoriasis and flaking *eczema. It is available as a gel and can be obtained without a prescription, but only from pharmacies.

Side effects and precautions: see COAL TAR; SALICYLIC ACID.

Gelcotar (Quinoderm) A proprietary combination of strong *coal tar solution and pine *tar (both keratolytics), used for the treatment of *psoriasis and flaking *eczema. It is available as a gel, which can be obtained without a prescription, but only from pharmacies. A shampoo formulation, which contains strong coal tar solution and *cade oil, is freely available *over the counter.

Side effects and precautions: see COAL TAR.

Geltears (Chauvin Pharmaceuticals) *See* CARBOMER.

gemcitabine An *antimetabolite used intravenously for the palliative treatment of some forms of advanced lung *cancer and of pancreatic cancer (*see* CYTOTOXIC DRUGS). It is available as an injection on *prescription only.

Side effects: include mild nausea and vomiting and rashes; influenza-like symptoms and kidney impairment may also occur. *See* CYTOTOXIC DRUGS.

Precautions: gemcitabine should not be given with radiotherapy or to pregnant women. *See* CYTOTOXIC DRUGS.

Proprietary preparation: Gemzar.

gemeprost A *prostaglandin that is used to soften and dilate the cervix (neck of the uterus) to allow operations to be carried out on the uterus or fetus during the first three months of pregnancy. It is also given to induce abortion (*see also* MIFEPRISTONE) or to cause expulsion of a fetus that has died in the uterus. Gemeprost is available, on *prescription only, as pessaries to be inserted into the vagina.

Side effects: include vaginal bleeding, pain in the uterus, nausea, vomiting, diarrhoea, headache, muscle weakness, dizziness, flushing, chills, backache, breathlessness, chest pain, bouts of palpitation, and mild fever.

Precautions: gemeprost should be used with caution in women with obstructive airways disease (e.g. asthma), certain heart conditions, glaucoma, or inflammation of the cervix or vagina.

gemfibrozil A *fibrate used for the treatment of a wide variety of *hyperlipidaemias and to prevent coronary heart disease in middle-aged people who have not responded to dietary modification and other appropriate measures. It is available as capsules or tablets on *prescription only.

Side effects and precautions: see FIBRATES. Gemfibrozil can also cause blurred vision, jaundice, atrial fibrillation (*see* ARRHYTHMIA), and painful extremities. It should not be taken by people with alcoholism, liver disease, or gallstones.

Interactions with other drugs: see BEZAFIBRATE.

Proprietary preparations: Emfib; Lopid.

Gemzar (Eli Lilly & Co) *See* GEMCITABINE.

generic name The nonproprietary name of a drug or chemical, which is not protected by a trademark. *Compare* PROPRIETARY NAME.

Genotropin (Pharmacia & Upjohn) *See* SOMATROPIN.

gentamicin The most important of the *aminoglycoside antibiotics. It is widely used for the treatment of serious infections, when it may be given with a *penicillin and/or *metronidazole. It is used for the treatment of septicaemia, septicaemia in the newborn, meningitis and other infections of the central nervous system, infections of the bile ducts, kidney infections, infections of the prostate, infections of the membranes or valves of the heart, and pneumonia. It is also used to treat ear and eye infections. Gentamicin is available on *prescription only. For *systemic infections it is given by injection; for ear and eye infections as drops.

Side effects: damage to the ears and kidneys may occur if concentrations in the blood become high.

Precautions: gentamicin should not be taken by pregnant women or by people with myasthenia gravis. It should be used with caution in those with kidney disease, in children, and in the elderly, and should not be used for prolonged periods. Blood and urine tests are required to monitor concentrations of gentamicin and kidney function.

Interactions with other drugs (with injections only):

Amphotericin: increases the risk of kidney toxicity.

Antibacterials: there is an increased risk of ear and kidney toxicity with colistin, capreomycin, and vancomycin.

Cisplatin: increases the risk of kidney toxicity.

Cyclosporin: increases the risk of kidney toxicity.

Loop diuretics: increase the risk of ear toxicity.

Muscle relaxants: the effects of some muscle relaxants used during surgery is increased.

Neostigmine and pyridostigmine: the effects of these drugs are antagonized.

Proprietary preparations: Cidomycin (injection, ear and eye drops); Garamycin (ear and eye drops); Genticin (injection, ear and eye drops); Isotonic Gentamicin Injection; Minims Gentamicin (single-dose eye drops); GENTISONE HC (combined with hydrocortisone).

gentian mixture A combination of *compound gentian infusion and either hydrochloric acid (**compound gentian mixture, acid**) or sodium bicarbonate (**compound gentian mixture, alkaline**), used as a *tonic to stimulate the appetite. Both mixtures can be obtained without a prescription, but only from pharmacies.

gentian violet *See* CRYSTAL VIOLET.

Genticin (Roche Products) *See* GENTAMICIN.

Gentisone HC (Roche Products) A proprietary combination of *gentamicin (an antibiotic) and *hydrocortisone (a corticosteroid), used for the treatment of infections of the outer ear. It is available as ear drops on *prescription only.

Side effects, precautions, and interactions with other drugs: see GENTAMICIN; TOPICAL STEROIDS.

Geref 50 (Serono Laboratories) *See* SERMORELIN.

Germolene Cream (SmithKline Beecham Consumer Healthcare) A proprietary combination of the antiseptics *chlorhexidine and *phenol, used for the treatment of minor cuts and grazes, minor burns, scalds, blisters, insect bites, stings, and spots. It is freely available *over the counter.

Germolene Ointment (SmithKline Beecham Consumer Healthcare) A proprietary combination of *zinc oxide, *methyl salicylate, *phenol, *white soft paraffin, *liquid paraffin, light anhydrous *lanolin, *yellow soft paraffin, and *octaphonium <octafonium> chloride, used as an emollient antiseptic treatment for minor cuts and grazes, burns, scalds, blisters, sore or rough skin, sunburn, muscular pain, and stiffness. It is freely available *over the counter.

Germoloids (SmithKline Beecham Consumer Healthcare) A proprietary combination of *zinc oxide (an astringent) and *lignocaine <lidocaine> (a local anaesthetic), used to relieve the pain and discomfort of *haemorrhoids and anal itching. It is freely available *over the counter in the form of a cream, ointment, or suppositories.

gestodene A synthetic *progestogen used as an ingredient in combined *oral contraceptives. There is a higher risk of thromboembolism with this progestogen than with certain others. Gestodene is available on *prescription only.

Side effects and interactions with other drugs: see ORAL CONTRACEPTIVES.

Precautions: gestodene should not be used by women who are at risk of developing thromboembolism, for example because they are very overweight or have varicose veins or a history of thrombosis. It should therefore only be taken by women who cannot tolerate other oral contraceptives and who are prepared to accept the increased risk. *See also* ORAL CONTRACEPTIVES.

Proprietary preparations: FEMODENE and FEMODENE ED (combined with ethinyloestradiol <ethinylestradiol>); MINULET (combined with ethinyloestradiol <ethinylestradiol>); TRIADENE (combined with ethinyloestradiol <ethinylestradiol>); TRI-MINULET (combined with ethinyloestradiol <ethinylestradiol>).

Gestone (Ferring Pharmaceuticals) *See* PROGESTERONE.

gestonorone hexanoate *See* GESTRONOL HEXANOATE.

gestrinone A drug that inhibits the release of *gonadotrophins from the pituitary gland and therefore reduces the secretion of oestrogen and progesterone by the ovaries. It is used for the treatment of *endometriosis. Gestrinone is available as capsules on *prescription only.

Side effects: include spotting (vaginal bleeding), acne, fluid retention, weight gain, headache, stomach and bowel upsets, cramp, depression, and (rarely) growth of body hair, voice changes, and changes in appetite.

Precautions: gestrinone should not be taken by women who are pregnant (it must be stopped if pregnancy occurs) or breastfeeding or by women who have severe liver, kidney, or heart disease.

Interactions with other drugs:

Antiepileptic drugs: carbamazepine, phenobarbitone <phenobarbital>, phenytoin, and primidone reduce the plasma concentrations (and therefore effectiveness) of gestrinone.

Rifampicin: reduces the plasma concentrations (and therefore effectiveness) of gestrinone.

Proprietary preparation: Dimetriose.

gestronol hexanoate <gestonorone hexanoate> A *progestogen used in the treatment of breast cancer, endometrial cancer (cancer of the lining of the womb), and enlargement of the prostate gland. It is available as an injection on *prescription only.

Side effects and precautions: see MEDROXYPROGESTERONE.

Interactions with other drugs: see PROGESTOGENS.

Proprietary preparation: Depostat.

ginger tincture An extract from the root of the ginger plant (*Zingiber officinale*). It is used as a flavouring agent and is included as an ingredient in preparations to relieve flatulence and wind pain.

Proprietary preparation: NEO GRIPE MIXTURE (combined with sodium bicarbonate and dill seed oil).

Givitol (Galen) A proprietary combination of *ferrous fumarate, B group vitamins (see VITAMIN B COMPLEX), and vitamin C (ascorbic acid), used as a supplement during pregnancy. It is available as capsules and can be obtained without a prescription, but only from pharmacies. Givitol cannot be prescribed on the NHS.

Side effects, precautions, and interactions with other drugs: see IRON.

Glandosane (Fresenius) A proprietary combination of carboxymethylcellulose (a protective agent; see CARMELLOSE), salts of potassium, sodium, magnesium, and calcium (see ELECTROLYTE), and sorbitol (a sugar), used as an artificial saliva to relieve dry mouth, which occurs, for example, after radiotherapy. It is freely available *over the counter in the form of an aerosol spray.

glaucoma A condition in which loss of vision occurs because of damage to the optic nerve, which in most cases is caused by an abnormally high pressure in the eye. This is known as **primary glaucoma** and there are two distinct types. In **acute** (or **closed-angle**) **glaucoma**, there is an abrupt rise in pressure due to sudden closure of the angle between the cornea and iris where aqueous fluid usually drains from the eye. This is accompanied by pain and marked blurring of vision. In the more common **chronic simple** (or **open-angle**) **glaucoma**, the pressure increases gradually, usually without producing pain, and the visual loss is insidious. The same type of visual loss may rarely occur in eyes with a normal pressure: this is called **low-tension glaucoma**. Primary glaucoma occurs increasingly with age and is an important cause of blindness. **Secondary glaucoma** may occur when some other eye disease impairs the normal circulation of the aqueous fluid and causes the pressure inside the eye to rise.

In all types of glaucoma treatment is focused on reducing the pressure inside the eye. Drops are instilled into the eye at regular intervals to improve the outflow of aqueous fluid from the eye and/or to reduce the production of aqueous fluid. Drugs used include some *beta blockers (see BETAXOLOL HYDROCHLORIDE; CARTEOLOL HYDROCHLORIDE; LEVOBUNOLOL HYDROCHLORIDE; TIMOLOL MALEATE); *miotics, such as *pilocarpine and *carbachol; *adrenaline <epinephrine> and drugs with similar effects to adrenaline (*see* DIPIVEFRIN); the sympathomimetic drugs *apraclonidine and *brimonidine; and the prostaglandin analogue *latanoprost. Carbonic anhydrase inhibitors, in the form of tablets or eye drops, are also used (*see* ACETAZOLAMIDE; DORZOLAMIDE).

glibenclamide   A long-acting *sulphonylurea used for the treatment of noninsulin-dependent (type II) *diabetes mellitus. It is available as tablets on *prescription only.
Side effects and interactions with other drugs: see SULPHONYLUREAS.
Precautions: glibenclamide should not be used in the elderly. *See also* SULPHONYLUREAS.
Proprietary preparations: Calabren; Daonil; Diabetamide; Euglucon; Gliken; Libanil; Malix; Semi-Daonil.

Glibenese (Pfizer) *See* GLIPIZIDE.

gliclazide   A *sulphonylurea used for the treatment of noninsulin-dependent (type II) *diabetes mellitus. It is available as tablets on *prescription only.
Side effects, precautions, and interactions with other drugs: see SULPHONYLUREAS.
Proprietary preparation: Diamicron.

Gliken (Kent Pharmaceuticals) *See* GLIBENCLAMIDE.

glimepiride   A *sulphonylurea used for the treatment of noninsulin-dependent (type II) *diabetes mellitus. It is available as tablets on *prescription only.
Side effects: include jaundice and hepatitis, severe allergic reactions, and a decrease in plasma *sodium concentration. *See also* SULPHONYLUREAS.
Precautions: blood tests and monitoring of liver function should be carried out regularly during treatment. Glimepiride should not be taken by those with severely impaired liver or kidney function or by pregnant women (*see also* SULPHONYLUREAS).
Interactions with other drugs: see SULPHONYLUREAS.
Proprietary preparation: Amaryl.

glipizide   A *sulphonylurea used for the treatment of noninsulin-dependent (type II) *diabetes mellitus. It is available as tablets on *prescription only.
Side effects, precautions, and interactions with other drugs: see SULPHONYLUREAS.
Proprietary preparations: Glibenese; Minodiab.

gliquidone   A *sulphonylurea used for the treatment noninsulin-dependent (type II) *diabetes mellitus. It is available as tablets on *prescription only.

Side effects, precautions, and interactions with other drugs: see
SULPHONYLUREAS.
Proprietary preparation: Glurenorm.

GlucaGen (Novo Nordisk Pharmaceutical) *See* GLUCAGON.

glucagon A protein hormone secreted by the alpha cells of the islets of
Langerhans in the pancreas. It acts in opposition to *insulin and
increases blood glucose by stimulating the breakdown of glycogen to
glucose in the liver. Glucagon is used to counteract *hypoglycaemia
resulting from insulin overdosage in the treatment of *diabetes mellitus.
It is given by intramuscular, subcutaneous, or intravenous injection and
is available on *prescription only.
Side effects: include nausea, vomiting, diarrhoea, and low concentrations
of *potassium in the blood; rarely, allergic reactions may occur.
Precautions: glucagon must not be given to people with tumours of the
insulin- or glucagon-producing cells of the islets of Langerhans in the
pancreas or to those with phaeochromocytoma (a tumour of the adrenal
gland).
Proprietary preparation: GlucaGen.

Glucamet (Opus) *See* METFORMIN HYDROCHLORIDE.

Glucobay (Bayer) *See* ACARBOSE.

glucocorticoids *See* CORTICOSTEROIDS.

gluconolactone A compound that can bind free calcium and is
included in solutions for washing out catheters.
Proprietary preparation: URIFLEX R (combined with disodium edetate,
citric acid, and magnesium carbonate).

Glucophage (Merck Pharmaceuticals) *See* METFORMIN HYDROCHLORIDE.

Glurenorm (Sanofi Winthrop) *See* GLIQUIDONE.

glutaraldehyde A caustic liquid that is used to destroy warts and
verrucas (*see* KERATOLYTICS). The process is slow and the wart may need to
be pared down and repainted several times. Glutaraldehyde is available as
a liquid and can be obtained without a prescription, but only from
pharmacies.
Side effects: glutaraldehyde stains the skin brown and may cause local
irritation.
Precautions: glutaraldehyde should not be used on facial or genital warts
or on warts around the anus. It should not be applied to healthy skin
around the wart or to broken skin or come into contact with the eyes,
mouth, or other mucous membranes.
Proprietary preparation: Glutarol.

Glutarol (Dermal Laboratories) *See* GLUTARALDEHYDE.

glycerin (glycerol) A clear viscous liquid obtained by hydrolysis of fats and mixed oils. It is used as an *emollient in many skin preparations, as an earwax softener, as a *stimulant laxative and faecal softener (particularly in the form of suppositories and enemas), as a *demulcent and sweetening agent in linctuses and pastilles, and in combination with *thymol in a mouthwash.

Proprietary preparations: AUDAX (combined with choline salicylate); EAREX PLUS EAR DROPS (combined with choline salicylate); EXTEROL (combined with urea hydrogen peroxide); FLETCHERS' ENEMETTE (combined with docusate sodium); LEMSIP COUGH + COLD DRY COUGH MEDICINE (combined with honey); MICOLETTE MICRO-ENEMA (combined with sodium lauryl sulphoacetate and sodium citrate).

glycerol *See* GLYCERIN.

glyceryl trinitrate A *nitrate drug used in treatment of *angina, to prevent or shorten attacks. It is short acting and rapidly absorbed across the lining of the mouth. Therefore to abort attacks it is usually taken as

Proprietary preparations of glyceryl trinitrate

Preparation	Formulation	Availability
Coro-Nitro Pump Spray	metered-dose sublingual aerosol spray	*P
Deponit	24-hour skin patches	P
Glytrin Spray	metered-dose sublingual aerosol spray	P
GTN 300 mcg	sublingual tablets	P
Minitran	24-skin patches	P
Nitrocine	injection	†POM
Nitro-Dur	24-hour skin patches	P
Nitrolingual Pumpspray	metered-dose sublingual aerosol spray	P
Nitromin	metered-dose sublingual aerosol spray	P
Nitronal	injection	POM
Percutol	ointment	P
Suscard	modified-release buccal tablets	P
Sustac	modified-release tablets	P
Transiderm-Nitro	24-hour skin patches	P

* P = pharmacy medicine

† POM = prescription only medicine

tablets to be dissolved in the mouth – often under the tongue (sublingual) or between the upper lip and the gum (buccal) – or as a sublingual spray. Relief of pain is rapid. Glyceryl trinitrate can be taken before exercise to prevent an angina attack. Prevention of symptoms is achieved by means of *modified-release tablets or by ointment or skin patches applied to the chest. Glyceryl trinitrate is also available for injection. Some preparations are *prescription only medicines; others can be obtained from pharmacies without a prescription. Glyceryl trinitrate tablets are unstable; they must be stored in light-proof, containers, without cotton wool wadding, and discarded after eight weeks. Glyceryl trinitrate spray can be stored for a long time.

Side effects, precautions, and interactions with other drugs: see NITRATES.
Proprietary preparations: see table.

glycol monosalicylate   *See* GLYCOL SALICYLATE.

glycol salicylate (glycol monosalicylate) A *salicylate that is an ingredient of many *rubefacient creams and sprays for the relief of aches, pains, and stiffness in muscles, joints, and tendons. It is also included in preparations for soothing *haemorrhoids. These preparations are freely available *over the counter.

Side effects and precautions: see SALICYLATES.
Proprietary preparations: ALGIPAN RUB (combined with capsicum oleoresin and methyl nicotinate); BOOTS PAIN RELIEF BALM (combined with ethyl nicotinate and nonylic acid vanillylamide); BOOTS SUPPOSITORIES FOR HAEMORRHOIDS (combined with benzyl alcohol, methyl salicylate, and zinc oxide); CREMALGIN (combined with capsicum oleoresin and methyl nicotinate); DEEP HEAT SPRAY (combined with methyl salicylate, methyl nicotinate, and ethyl salicylate); DUBAM SPRAY (combined with ethyl salicylate, methyl salicylate, and methyl nicotinate); FIERY JACK CREAM (combined with capsicum oleoresin, diethylamine salicylate, and methyl nicotinate); RALGEX CREAM (combined with capsicum oleoresin and methyl nicotinate); RALGEX FREEZE SPRAY (combined with methoxymethane and isopentane); RALGEX HEAT SPRAY (combined with methyl nicotinate); RALGEX STICK (combined with capsicum oleoresin, ethyl salicylate, methyl salicylate, and menthol); SALONAIR (combined with benzyl nicotinate, camphor, menthol, methyl salicylate, and squalane); SALONPAS PLASTERS (combined with methyl salicylate, camphor, and menthol).

glycopyrronium bromide An *antimuscarinic drug that is used before surgery to reduce the secretion of saliva and of mucus in the airways (which are increased when a tube is inserted into the air passage and anaesthetics are inhaled). It is also used, combined with *neostigmine, after surgery to prevent the adverse effects of neostigmine. Glycopyrronium is available as an injection on *prescription only.

Side effects, precautions, and interactions with other drugs: see ANTIMUSCARINIC DRUGS.

Proprietary preparations: Robinul; ROBINUL-NEOSTIGMINE (combined with neostigmine).

Glypressin (Ferring Pharmaceuticals) *See* TERLIPRESSIN.

Glytrin Spray (Sanofi Winthrop) *See* GLYCERYL TRINITRATE.

Goddard's White Oil Embrocation (LRC Products) A proprietary combination of dilute *acetic acid, *turpentine oil, and dilute *ammonia solution, used as a *rubefacient for the relief of pain and stiffness in muscles, joints, and tendons, including backache, sciatica, lumbago, and fibrositis. It is freely available *over the counter.
Side effects and precautions: see RUBEFACIENTS.

goitre *See* IODINE; THYROID HORMONES.

Golden Eye (Typharm) *See* PROPAMIDINE ISETHIONATE <ISETIONATE>.

gold salts *See* AURANOFIN; SODIUM AUROTHIOMALATE.

gonadorelin *Gonadotrophin-releasing hormone, which is used to treat amenorrhoea (absence of periods) and certain types of infertility in women. It acts by increasing the concentrations of pituitary *gonadotrophins in the blood, which promote the production of oestrogens and egg cells. Gonadorelin is given by *subcutaneous infusion in short pulses every 90 minutes, delivered by means of a portable pump connected to a tube inserted beneath the skin, and is available on *prescription only.
   *Analogues of gonadorelin are more powerful than the natural hormone, initially increasing the secretion of gonadotrophins by the pituitary gland (and hence of oestrogen by the ovaries or testosterone by the testes). However, continued use acts to inhibit the further release of gonadotrophins, resulting in decreased secretion of oestrogen or testosterone. Gonadorelin analogues are used to treat *endometriosis, infertility, breast cancer, and prostate cancer. *See* BUSERELIN; GOSERELIN; LEUPRORELIN; NAFARELIN; TRIPTORELIN.
Side effects: include nausea, headache, abdominal pain, and increased menstrual bleeding; there may be local reactions at the site of injection.
Precautions: gonadorelin should not be used by women with cysts in the ovaries or womb or amenorrhoea due to excessive weight loss. It should not be used for longer than six months and treatment should be stopped if pregnancy occurs.
Proprietary preparations: Fertiral; HRF; Relefact LH-RH.

gonadotrophin-releasing hormone (GnRH) A hormone that is produced by the hypothalamus and acts on the pituitary gland to promote the release of *gonadotrophins; since it stimulates the production of luteinizing hormone (LH) and follicle-stimulating hormone (FSH), it is also called **LH-RH** or **LH-FSH-RH**. *See* GONADORELIN.

gonadotrophins Hormones produced by the pituitary gland that act on the ovaries in women and on the testes in men to promote the production of sex hormones and either ova (eggs) or sperm. In pregnancy another gonadotrophin, *human chorionic gonadotrophin (HCG), is produced by the placenta. Its presence in the urine is the basis of pregnancy tests. Gonadotrophins are used mainly in the treatment of female infertility that is caused by underactivity of the pituitary gland, which results in poor ovulation. They are also used to induce superovulation (the production of large numbers of eggs) in women undergoing assisted conception (such as *in vitro* fertilization). The gonadotrophins for therapeutic use are natural and synthetic forms of follicle-stimulating hormone (FSH), which stimulates the growth of the egg-producing follicles in the ovaries (*see* UROFOLLITROPHIN <UROFOLLITROPIN>; FOLLITROPIN), and luteinizing hormone (LH), which stimulates the release of the egg from the ovary. These hormones are available in combination as *human menopausal gonadotrophin (HMG or menotrophin).

Gonal-F (Serono Laboratories) *See* FOLLITROPIN.

Gopten (Knoll) *See* TRANDOLAPRIL.

goserelin An analogue of *gonadorelin that is used to treat *endometriosis and to reduce the thickness of the endometrium (lining of the uterus) before a surgical 'scrape' to treat excessively heavy periods. It is also used to suppress the release of gonadotrophins by the pituitary gland before stimulating ovulation in women undergoing fertility treatment, such as *in vitro* fertilization. Goserelin initially causes increased secretion of gonadotrophins by the pituitary gland, which stimulates secretion of oestrogen by the ovaries, but this acts on the pituitary gland to suppress further release of gonadotrophins and therefore production of oestrogen. In men goserelin is used to treat prostate cancer, having an action similar to that of *leuprorelin. It is available as a solution for *depot subcutaneous injection on *prescription only.

Side effects: in women these include hot flushes, changes in libido, vaginal dryness, mood changes and other symptoms similar to those of the menopause. There may be weight gain, reduction in bone density (which can exacerbate osteoporosis), and (rarely) nausea, headache, and abdominal pain. Side effects in men include hot flushes, decreased libido, impotence, a temporary increase in bone pain from secondary tumours in the bones, allergic reactions at the injection site, and a temporary increase in blood pressure. Rarely there may be enlargement of the breasts, nausea, vomiting, and dizziness.

Precautions: goserelin should not be taken by women with undiagnosed vaginal bleeding or by those who are pregnant or breastfeeding; a nonhormonal method of contraception should be used during treatment. The drug should be used with caution by women at risk of developing osteoporosis. Treatment should not be continued to longer than six months. In men there is a risk of compression of the spinal cord and of kidney stones blocking the ureters leading from the kidneys; patients should be monitored carefully during the first month of treatment.

Proprietary preparation: Zoladex.

gramicidin An *antibiotic that is only used topically, to treat skin, eye, and ear infections, since it is too toxic to be given systemically (i.e. by mouth or injection). It is usually combined with other antimicrobial agents, such as *neomycin and *polymyxin B, or with a *corticosteroid. Preparations containing gramicidin are available on *prescription only.

Side effects: gramicidin may cause allergic reactions (rash or itching).

Proprietary preparations: ADCORTYL WITH GRANEODIN (combined with triamcinolone acetonide and neomycin); GRANEODIN (combined with neomycin); NEOSPORIN (combined with neomycin and polymyxin B); SOFRADEX (combined with dexamethasone and framycetin sulphate); SOFRAMYCIN (combined with framycetin sulphate); TRI-ADCORTYL and TRI-ADCORTYL OTIC (combined with triamcinolone acetonide, nystatin, and neomycin).

Graneodin (Bristol-Myers Squibb) A proprietary combination of the antibiotics *neomycin sulphate and *gramicidin, used to treat bacterial skin infections. It is available as an ointment on *prescription only.

Side effects: use of this ointment may lead to impaired hearing and cause allergic reactions.

Precautions: Graneodin should not be used for treating viral, fungal, or deep-seated infections. It should not be used with dressings or be applied to large areas of damaged skin or perforated eardrums.

granisetron An *antiemetic used for the prevention or treatment of nausea and vomiting associated with *cytotoxic chemotherapy or radiotherapy or occurring after surgery. It acts by opposing the action of the neurotransmitter 5-hydroxytryptamine (*serotonin) at receptors in the central nervous system and in the gut. It is available, on *prescription only, as tablets, liquid, or an intravenous injection.

Side effects: include headache, constipation, and rash.

Precautions: granisetron should be used with caution in women who are pregnant or breastfeeding.

Proprietary preparation: Kytril.

Granocyte (Chugai Pharma) *See* LENOGRASTIM.

granulocyte-colony stimulating factor (G-CSF) A protein that stimulates the cells of the bone marrow that produce granulocytes (a type of white blood cell with granular cytoplasm), including neutrophils, which have an important role in the body's defence against infection by destroying bacteria. **Recombinant human granulocyte-colony stimulating factor** is manufactured in the laboratory by genetic engineering techniques. It is used to boost neutrophil production in people whose natural production is poor or in those who have received drugs, especially *cytotoxic drugs, that suppress their natural white cell production (*see* FILGRASTIM; LENOGRASTIM). **Granulocyte macrophage-colony stimulating factor (GM-CSF)** stimulates the production of both granulocytes and macrophages, which develop from white blood cells called monocytes and engulf invading bacteria. A genetically engineered form is available (*see* MOLGRAMOSTIM); its uses are similar to those of filograstim and lenograstim.

Graves' disease *See* THYROID HORMONES.

Gregoderm (Unigreg) A proprietary combination of the antibiotics *neomycin sulphate, *nystatin, and *polymyxin B sulphate and the corticosteroid *hydrocortisone, used for the treatment of infected inflammatory skin conditions and anal itching. It is available as an ointment on *prescription only.
Side effects and precautions: see TOPICAL STEROIDS.

griseofulvin An *antifungal drug that is used for treating fungal infections of the skin, scalp, hair, and nails. Treatment may need to be continued for weeks or even months, but side effects are uncommon. Griseofulvin is available as tablets on *prescription only.
Side effects: include headache, nausea, vomiting, and less commonly rashes, dizziness, fatigue, and sensitivity to light; blood disorders have also been reported.
Precautions: griseofulvin should not be taken by people with liver failure, lupus erythematosus, or porphyria or by pregnant women. Women should avoid becoming pregnant for one month after treatment has ceased, and men should not father a child within six months of treatment. Griseofulvin enhances the effects of alcohol and may impair the ability to drive and operate machinery.
Interactions with other drugs:
  Anticoagulants: the effects of warfarin and nicoumalone
    <acenocoumarol> are reduced.
  Oral contraceptives: their effects are reduced by griseofulvin; additional
    contraceptive measures should be taken during treatment and for one
    month after treatment has ceased.
  Phenobarbitone <phenobarbital>: reduces the effect of griseofulvin.
Proprietary preparations: Fulcin; Grisovin.

Grisovin (GlaxoWellcome) *See* GRISEOFULVIN.

growth hormone A hormone, secreted by the pituitary gland, that promotes growth of the long bones in the limbs and increases protein synthesis. Its release is controlled by the opposing actions of two hormones: **growth hormone releasing hormone** (or **somatorelin**), which stimulates its release, and **somatostatin**, which inhibits this. Excessive production of growth hormone results in gigantism before puberty and acromegaly in adults. Lack of growth hormone in children causes dwarfism. Acromegaly can be treated by injections of somatostatin analogues (*see* OCTREOTIDE; LANREOTIDE); dwarfism is treated with a genetically engineered form of human growth hormone (*see* SOMATROPIN).

GSL (general sales list) *See* OVER THE COUNTER.

GTN 300 mcg (Martindale Pharmaceuticals) *See* GLYCERYL TRINITRATE.

guaifenesin *See* GUAIPHENESIN.

guaiphenesin <guaifenesin> A drug that is reported to reduce the viscosity of sputum and is included as an *expectorant in many cough preparations. However, there is no good evidence that it is effective. Guaiphenesin is available without a prescription, but preparations containing other ingredients can usually only be bought from pharmacies.
Side effects: gastrointestinal discomfort has occasionally been reported; very large doses cause nausea and vomiting.
Precautions: guaiphenesin should not be taken by people with porphyria.
Proprietary preparations: Beechams Veno's Expectorant; Benylin Children's Chesty Coughs; Do-Do Expectorant; Expulin Chesty Cough Linctus; Famel Expectorant; Hill's Balsam Chesty Cough Liquid; Jackson's All Fours; Lemsip Cough + Cold Chesty Cough Medicine; Liquifruta Garlic Cough Medicine; Meltus Expectorant; Meltus Honey and Lemon; Nirolex Chesty Cough Linctus; Nurse Sykes Bronchial Balsam; Robitussin Chesty Cough; Tixylix Chesty Cough; Vicks Vaposyrup Chesty Cough; ACTIFED EXPECTORANT (combined with pseudoephedrine and triprolidine); ADULT MELTUS EXPECTORANT WITH DECONGESTANT (combined with pseudoephedrine and menthol); BEECHAMS ALL-IN-ONE (combined with paracetamol and phenylephrine); BENYLIN CHESTY COUGHS NON DROWSY (combined with menthol); BOOTS BRONCHIAL COUGH MIXTURE (combined with ammonium carbonate and ammonium chloride); DIMOTANE EXPECTORANT (combined with brompheniramine and pseudoephedrine); JUNIOR MELTUS EXPECTORANT (combined with cetylpyridinium); NIROLEX FOR CHESTY COUGHS WITH DECONGESTANT (combined with pseudoephedrine); ROBITUSSIN CHESTY COUGH WITH CONGESTION (combined with pseudoephedrine); SUDAFED EXPECTORANT (combined with pseudoephedrine).

guanethidine A drug that prevents the release of noradrenaline <norepinephrine> from nerve endings in the *sympathetic nervous system and may be used, in combination with other antihypertensive drugs, in the treatment of resistant *hypertension. It is available as tablets on *prescription only. Guanethidine is also combined with *adrenaline <epinephrine> in eye drops for the treatment of *glaucoma.

Side effects: include low blood pressure, and therefore dizziness, on standing up (orthostatic hypotension), fluid retention, slow heart rate, failure of ejaculation, and diarrhoea.

Precautions: guanethidine should not be taken by people with phaeochromocytoma (a tumour of the adrenal gland), kidney disease, or heart failure.

Interactions with other drugs:

Anaesthetics: their effect in lowering blood pressure is increased.

Sympathomimetic drugs: methylphenidate and some drugs used in cough and cold remedies (e.g. ephedrine) antagonize the effect of guanethidine in lowering blood pressure.

Proprietary preparations: Ismelin; GANDA (combined with adrenaline <epinephrine>).

Guanor Expectorant (Rosemont Pharmaceuticals) A proprietary combination of *ammonium chloride (an expectorant), *diphenhydramine (a sedative antihistamine), and *menthol, used for the relief of coughs and congestion. It is available as a linctus without a prescription, but only from pharmacies.

Side effects, precautions, and interactions with other drugs: see ANTIHISTAMINES.

Guarem (Shire Pharmaceuticals) See GUAR GUM.

guar gum A soluble fibre extracted from the seeds of an Indian plant, Cyamopsis psoraloides. Used as an *oral hypoglycaemic drug, it reduces the rise in blood-sugar concentrations that occur after a meal: it is thought to act by delaying the absorption of carbohydrate from the intestine. Guar gum is used as an *adjunct to other antidiabetic drugs in the treatment of *diabetes mellitus. It is also used to treat dumping syndrome, in which the stomach empties very rapidly after a meal (especially one rich in carbohydrate), causing a drop in blood sugar and drawing fluid from the bloodstream into the intestine. Guar gum is available as granules, which can be dispersed in water or sprinkled onto food and taken with fluid, and can be obtained without a prescription, but only from pharmacies.

Side effects: include flatulence, distension of the abdomen, and intestinal obstruction.

Precautions: adequate fluid intake must be maintained since the gum swells and absorbs liquid. Granules should always be taken with plenty of water and not immediately before going to bed.

Proprietary preparation: Guarem.

Gyno-Daktarin (Janssen-Cilag) See MICONAZOLE.

Gynol-II (Janssen-Cilag) See NONOXINOL-9

Gyno-Pevaryl 1 (Janssen-Cilag) See ECONAZOLE NITRATE.

H₂-receptor antagonists (histamine H₂-receptor antagonists) A class of drugs that block a type of *histamine receptor in the stomach (called H₂ receptors) and thereby reduce the secretion of gastric (stomach) acid. They reduce both the volume and the acidity of gastric juice and are used in the treatment of gastric and duodenal ulcers. *See* CIMETIDINE; FAMOTIDINE; NIZATIDINE; RANITIDINE; RANITIDINE BISMUTH CITRATE.

Side effects: side effects are generally rare and minor. Dizziness, drowsiness or fatigue, and rash have been reported with all H₂-receptor antagonists; more rarely headache, changes in liver function, and blood disorders may occur. More information is provided in the entries for individual H₂-receptor antagonists.

Precautions and interactions with other drugs: see entries for individual H₂-receptor antagonists.

Haelan (Novex Pharma) *See* FLURANDRENOLONE <FLUDROXYCORTIDE>.

haemophilia *See* HAEMOSTATIC DRUGS.

haemorrhoids (piles) Swelling of the spongy blood-filled cushions in the wall of the anus, usually a consequence of prolonged constipation or, occasionally, diarrhoea. Haemorrhoids may protrude beyond the anus. They bleed and may cause pain after defaecation due to an **anal fissure** (a break in the skin lining the anal canal). Soothing preparations available for relief of the symptoms of haemorrhoids contain *local anaesthetics (such as *lignocaine <lidocaine> or *pramoxine <pramocaine> hydrochloride), mild astringents (such as *zinc oxide, *bismuth subgallate, or *hamamelis), and often lubricants, mild antiseptics, and *vasoconstrictor drugs. Some preparations also contain *corticosteroids to relieve inflammation. If bleeding persists, an irritant fluid (such as *phenol) may be injected around the haemorrhoids to make them shrivel up (*see* SCLEROTHERAPY).

Soothing preparations containing local anaesthetics and/or corticosteroids can be absorbed and may cause *systemic effects; local anaesthetics may irritate the skin around the anus. For these reasons such preparations should not be used for prolonged periods; treatment should be directed towards avoiding precipitating factors for haemorrhoids, such as constipation.

haemostatic drugs Drugs that are used to stop or prevent haemorrhage (excessive bleeding). **Antifibrinolytic drugs** inhibit or prevent the activation of enzymes that digest blood clots in the circulation; they include *tranexamic acid and *aprotinin. *Ethamsylate <etamsylate> acts by encouraging platelets (specialized blood cells) to stick together, which is part of the blood-clotting process. **Haemophilia**

is an inherited bleeding disorder in which blood does not clot naturally, or does so only very slowly. The clotting process is a complex reaction involving several clotting factors, some of which are missing in haemophiliacs. The most important of these are *Factor VIII, lack of which results in classical haemophilia (haemophilia A) and von Willebrand's disease; and *Factor IX, lack of which causes Christmas disease (haemophilia B). Blood products containing these factors are used in the treatment of these disorders. *See also* PHYTOMENADIONE; VITAMIN K.

Halciderm (Bristol-Myers Squibb) *See* HALCINONIDE.

halcinonide A very potent *topical steroid used for the treatment of eczema, psoriasis, and a variety of other skin conditions. It is available as a cream on *prescription only.
Side effects and precautions: see TOPICAL STEROIDS.
Proprietary preparation: Halciderm.

Haldol, Haldol Decanoate (Janssen-Cilag) *See* HALOPERIDOL.

Halfan (SmithKline Beecham Pharmaceuticals) *See* HALOFANTRINE HYDROCHLORIDE.

Half-Beta Prograne (Tillomed Laboratories) *See* PROPRANOLOL HYDROCHLORIDE.

Half-Inderal LA (AstraZeneca) *See* PROPRANOLOL HYDROCHLORIDE.

Half Securon SR (Knoll) *See* VERAPAMIL HYDROCHLORIDE.

Half Sinemet CR (Du Pont Pharmaceuticals) *See* CO-CARELDOPA.

halibut-liver oil A combination of *vitamin A and *vitamin D used as a vitamin supplement. It is freely available *over the counter in the form of capsules.
Side effects, precautions, and interactions with other drugs: see VITAMIN A.

halofantrine hydrochloride A drug used for the treatment of falciparum *malaria, although its use is declining. It is not suitable for prevention of the disease. Halofantrine is available as tablets on *prescription only.
Side effects: include gastrointestinal disturbance, abdominal pain, and abnormal heart rhythms.
Precautions and interactions with other drugs: halofantrine should not be taken by people with certain heart conditions or by women who are pregnant or breastfeeding. It should be used with caution in women who are pregnant or are capable of becoming pregnant and it should not be taken with food. Halofantrine should not be taken with any drug that can

have an effect on a certain phase of the heartbeat (the QT interval); such drugs include anti-arrhythmic drugs, chloroquine, mefloquine, quinine, tricyclic antidepressants, antipsychotics, and certain antihistamines (such as astemizole and terfenadine).

Proprietary preparation: Halfan.

haloperidol A butyrophenone *antipsychotic drug used for the treatment of schizophrenia and other psychoses and mania. In the short term it is used to calm severely agitated or violent patients and to relieve severe anxiety. Haloperidol is also used to treat intractable hiccups, tics, and severe nausea. It is available, on *prescription only, as tablets, capsules, an oral solution, an injection, and a *depot injection.

Side effects: as for *chlorpromazine, but haloperidol has more pronounced *extrapyramidal reactions, fewer antimuscarinic effects, and is less sedating.

Precautions: see CHLORPROMAZINE HYDROCHLORIDE.

Interactions with other drugs:

Amiodarone: should not be taken with haloperidol as this combination increases the risk of abnormal heart rhythms.

Anaesthetics: their effect in lowering blood pressure is enhanced.

Antidepressants: there is an increased risk of antimuscarinic effects and arrhythmias if haloperidol is taken with tricyclic antidepressants; fluoxetine increases the plasma concentration of haloperidol.

Antiepileptic drugs: their anticonvulsant effects are antagonized by haloperidol; carbamazepine reduces the effects of haloperidol.

Antihistamines: there is an increased risk of arrhythmias if haloperidol is taken with astemizole or terfenadine.

Cisapride: should not be taken with haloperidol as this combination increases the risk of arrhythmias.

Halofantrine: there is an increased risk of arrhythmias if this drug is taken with haloperidol.

Rifampicin: reduces the effects of haloperidol.

Ritonavir: may increase the effects of haloperidol.

Sedatives: the sedative effects of haloperidol are increased if it is taken with anxiolytic or hypnotic drugs, or any other drug that causes sedation.

Proprietary preparations: Dozic; Haldol; Haldol Decanoate (depot injection); Serenace.

Halycitrol (Laboratories for Applied Biology) A proprietary combination of *vitamin A and *vitamin D, used as a vitamin supplement. It is freely available *over the counter in the form of a syrup.

Side effects, precautions, and interactions with other drugs: see VITAMIN A.

hamamelis (witch hazel) An extract of the shrub *Hamamelis virginiana*, which has mild *astringent properties. It is used in lotions to soothe and cool bruises, sprains, or tired sore eyes. It is also included in preparations for soothing *haemorrhoids.

Proprietary preparation: Optrex (eye drops and eye lotion).

Harmogen (Pharmacia & Upjohn) *See* ESTROPIPATE.

Hay-Crom (Norton Healthcare) *See* SODIUM CROMOGLYCATE <CROMOGLICATE>.

Haymine (Pharmax) A proprietary combination of *chlorpheniramine <chlorphenamine> maleate (an antihistamine) and *ephedrine (a decongestant), used for the treatment of hay fever, urticaria, and other allergic conditions. It is available as tablets and may be bought from pharmacies without a prescription.

Side effects and interactions with other drugs: *see* ANTIHISTAMINES; EPHEDRINE HYDROCHLORIDE.

Precautions: Haymine should not be taken by people who have suffered from coronary thrombosis, high blood pressure, or thyroid problems. *See also* ANTIHISTAMINES; EPHEDRINE HYDROCHLORIDE.

Hc45 (Crookes Healthcare) *See* HYDROCORTISONE.

HDL (high-density lipoproteins) *See* LIPOPROTEINS.

heart block *See* ARRHYTHMIA.

heartburn *See* ACID-PEPTIC DISEASES.

heart failure (congestive heart failure) A condition produced by inadequate output of blood from the heart. Because the tissues of the body do not receive enough blood, and therefore enough oxygen, the body takes actions to compensate for this deficiency, which include: constricting the peripheral blood vessels (so that the overall volume of the blood vessels is smaller), retaining sodium and thus water (so that blood volume increases), and making the heart pump faster. These effects occur because a hormonal system called the **renin-angiotensin** system is stimulated. The symptoms of heart failure are *oedema, fatigue, breathlessness, reduced ability to exercise, and attacks of shortness of breath on exercise or during the night. Heart failure is treated with a variety of drugs, including *ACE inhibitors (which prevent the activation of the renin-angiotensin system), *cardiac glycosides (which improve the force of contraction and therefore the output of the heart), *nitrates, and *diuretics.

Hedex Caplets (SmithKline Beecham Consumer Healthcare) *See* PARACETAMOL.

Hedex Extra (SmithKline Beecham Consumer Healthcare) A proprietary combination of *paracetamol (an analgesic) and *caffeine (a stimulant), used to relieve headache (including migraine), toothache, neuralgia, rheumatic pains, and period pains. It is freely available *over the counter in the form of tablets.

Precautions: Hedex Extra should not be given to children, except on medical advice. *See also* PARACETAMOL; CAFFEINE.

Hedex Ibuprofen (SmithKline Beecham Consumer Healthcare) *See* IBUPROFEN.

Helicobacter *See* ACID-PEPTIC DISEASES.

Hemabate (Pharmacia & Upjohn) *See* CARBOPROST.

Heminevrin (AstraZeneca) *See* CHLORMETHIAZOLE <CLOMETHIAZOLE>.

Hemocane (Eastern Pharmaceuticals) A proprietary combination of *lignocaine <lidocaine> (a local anaesthetic), *benzoic acid and cinnamic acid (which have antiseptic properties), and *zinc oxide and *bismuth oxide (astringents), used to relieve the pain and itching of *haemorrhoids. It is freely available *over the counter in the form of a cream.

heparin A naturally occurring *anticoagulant that consists of several molecules of different sizes. **Standard heparin** is used to treat deep-vein *thrombosis and pulmonary embolism, and is given before and after surgery to prevent these conditions. People undergoing kidney dialysis may be given heparin to prevent clots forming. Heparin may also be given to people who have had a heart attack if there is a risk of further blood clots. Solutions of heparin are used to wash out cannulas (tubes inserted into veins for *infusion of substances) to stop blood clots forming. A *prescription only medicine, heparin (in the form of heparin calcium or heparin sodium) is available as a solution for intravenous or subcutaneous injection. *See also* LOW MOLECULAR WEIGHT HEPARINS; DANAPAROID SODIUM.

Side effects: excessive bleeding is the most serious side effect (*see* ANTICOAGULANTS); if this occurs, treatment should be stopped and *protamine sulphate may need to be given. Other side effects include destruction of the skin surrounding the injection site and thrombocytopenia (loss of platelets, blood cells that are involved in the clotting process, resulting in bruising and prolonged bleeding after injury). Long-term use of heparin can cause osteoporosis.

Precautions: the anticoagulant effect of heparin should be monitored with regular blood tests, particularly if it is given intravenously. Heparins should be used with caution in people with haemophilia or other bleeding disorders. They should not be given to people with active peptic ulcer, recent cerebral haemorrhage, severe *hypertension, severe liver disease, or kidney failure, or after major trauma or recent surgery.

Interactions with other drugs:

Aspirin: increases the anticoagulant effect of heparin and the risk of excessive bleeding.

Dipyridamole: increases the anticoagulant effect of heparin and the risk of excessive bleeding.

Glyceryl trinitrate: infusion of glyceryl trinitrate reduces the anticoagulant effect of heparin.

NSAIDs: there is an increased risk of gastric bleeding with diclofenac and ketorolac.

Proprietary preparations: Calciparine; Canusal; Hep-Flush; Heplok; Hepsal; Minihep; Minihep Calcium; Monoparin; Monoparin Calcium; Multiparin; Pump-Hep; Unihep; Uniparin Calcium; Uniparin Forte.

heparinoids Derivatives of *heparin that have the anticoagulant properties of heparin. They are used in creams, ointments, and gels to improve the circulation in such conditions as bruising, superficial thrombophlebitis (inflammation of a vein with the formation of small blood clots), chilblains, varicose veins, and haemorrhoids. They are not thought to be very effective. Heparinoids can be obtained without a prescription, but only from pharmacies. *Danaparoid sodium is a heparinoid that is injected before and after surgery to prevent deep vein thrombosis and pulmonary embolism.

Proprietary preparations: Hirudoid (cream or ointment); ANACAL (combined with lauromacrogols); LASONIL (combined with hyaluronidase); MOVELAT (combined with salicyclic acid).

Hep-Flush (Leo Pharmaceuticals) *See* HEPARIN.

Heplok (Leo Pharmaceuticals) *See* HEPARIN.

Hepsal (CP Pharmaceuticals) *See* HEPARIN.

heroin hydrochloride *See* DIAMORPHINE HYDROCHLORIDE.

Herpetad (Boehringer Ingelheim) *See* ACICLOVIR.

Herpid (Yamanouchi Pharma) *See* IDOXURIDINE.

Hewletts Cream (Kestrel Healthcare) A proprietary combination of *zinc oxide and *white soft paraffin, used as an *emollient to soothe dry skin. It is freely available *over the counter.

hexachlorophane <hexachlorophene> An *antiseptic that is active against a wide range of bacteria. It is used for disinfecting the hands before performing surgery, disinfecting the skin, especially pre-operatively, and (in the form of a powder) for preventing staphylococcal infections in newborn babies. Hexachlorophane is available as a cream on *prescription only or as a dusting powder or solution, which can be obtained without a prescription but only from pharmacies.

Precautions: the cream should not be used on children under two years old; the powder should not be used on damaged skin.
Proprietary preparations: Ster-Zac DC (cream); Ster-Zac Powder; DERMALEX (combined with allantoin and squalane).

Hexalen (Ipsen) *See* ALTRETAMINE.

hexamine hippurate <**methenamine hippurate**> An *antiseptic used for the treatment of recurrent infections of the urinary tract; it acts by being transformed to *formaldehyde. It is available as tablets without a *prescription.
Side effects: include gastrointestinal disturbances, bladder irritation, and rash.
Precautions: hexamine should not be taken by people who are severely dehydrated or by those with severe kidney disease.
Proprietary preparation: Hiprex.

hexetidine An *antiseptic with activity against bacteria and fungi that is used in mouthwashes for minor mouth and throat conditions, such as oral thrush, gingivitis (inflammation of the gums), sore throat, recurrent mouth ulcers, and halitosis. It is also used before and after dental surgery. Hexetidine, in the form of a solution, is freely available *over the counter.
Side effects: there may be local irritation; alterations in taste and smell have occasionally been reported.
Proprietary preparation: Oraldene.

Hexopal (Sanofi Winthrop) *See* INOSITOL NICOTINATE.

hexyl nicotinate A *rubefacient similar to *methyl nicotinate. It is an ingredient of a cream that is freely available *over the counter.
Side effects and precautions: see RUBEFACIENTS.
Proprietary preparation: TRANSVASIN HEAT RUB (combined with ethyl nicotinate and tetrahydrofurfuryl salicylate).

hexylresorcinol An *antiseptic used in solutions for cleansing wounds and in mouthwashes and throat lozenges for the relief of minor infections of the mouth and throat. Preparations containing hexylresorcinol are freely available *over the counter.
Proprietary preparations: Lemsip Sore Throat Antibacterial Lozenges; TCP Sore Throat Lozenges; BEECHAMS THROAT-PLUS LOZENGES (combined with benzalkonium chloride).

hiatus hernia *See* ACID-PEPTIC DISEASES.

Hibicet (AstraZeneca) *See* CHLORHEXIDINE.

Hibicet Hospital Concentrate (AstraZeneca) A proprietary combination of the antiseptics *chlorhexidine gluconate and *cetrimide, used to cleanse and disinfect the skin. It is freely available *over the counter in the form of a solution.

Hibiscrub (AstraZeneca) *See* CHLORHEXIDINE.

Hibisol (AstraZeneca) *See* CHLORHEXIDINE.

Hibitane (AstraZeneca) *See* CHLORHEXIDINE.

Hill's Balsam Chesty Cough Liquid (Boehringer Ingelheim) *See* GUAIPHENESIN <GUAIFENESIN>.

Hill's Balsam Chesty Cough Liquid for Children (Boehringer Ingelheim) *See* IPECACUANHA.

Hill's Balsam Chesty Cough Pastilles (Boehringer Ingelheim) A proprietary combination of *ipecacuanha (an expectorant), *benzoin tincture, *menthol, and *peppermint oil, used for the relief of coughs, colds, and catarrh. **Hill's Balsam Extra Strong '2 in 1' Pastilles** contains a higher concentration of menthol. Both preparations are freely available *over the counter.
Side effects: see IPECACUANHA.
Precautions: this medicine is not recommended for children. *See also* IPECACUANHA.

Hill's Balsam Dry Cough Liquid (Boehringer Ingelheim) *See* PHOLCODINE.

Hill's Balsam Nasal Congestion Pastilles (Boehringer Ingelheim) *See* MENTHOL.

Hioxyl (Quinoderm) *See* HYDROGEN PEROXIDE.

Hiprex (3M Health Care) *See* HEXAMINE <METHENAMINE> HIPPURATE.

Hirudoid (Sankyo Pharma) *See* HEPARINOIDS.

Hismanal (Janssen-Cilag) *See* ASTEMIZOLE.

Histafen (APS-Berk) *See* TERFENADINE.

Histalix (Wallace Manufacturing) A proprietary combination of *ammonium chloride (an expectorant), *diphenhydramine (a sedative antihistamine), and *menthol, used to relieve the symptoms of coughs and colds. It is available as a syrup without a prescription, but only from pharmacies. It cannot be prescribed on the NHS.
Side effects and interactions with other drugs: see ANTIHISTAMINES.

Precautions: this medicine should not be given to children under one year old. *See also* ANTIHISTAMINES.

histamine A compound found in nearly all tissues of the body, with high concentrations in the skin, lungs, and intestines. Histamine causes dilatation of blood vessels and contraction of smooth muscle (for example in the airways) and regulates the secretion of gastric (stomach) acid. It plays an important role in inflammation and is released in large amounts after skin damage (such as that due to animal venoms). It is also released in anaphylactic reactions (*see* ANAPHYLAXIS) and allergic conditions, giving rise to some of the symptoms of these conditions. Histamine acts at specific sites (receptors) in the tissues, of which there are two main types, H_1 receptors and H_2 receptors. *Antihistamines (H_1-receptor antagonists) block H_1 receptors in the skin, nose, and airways and are used for treating such allergic reactions as urticaria (nettle rash) and hay fever. *H_2-receptor antagonists block H_2 receptors, which are found mainly in the stomach; they are used for treating peptic ulcers and other types of *acid-peptic diseases.

HIV The human immunodeficiency virus, which destroys a subgroup of white blood cells (the helper T-cells, or CD4 lymphocytes), resulting in suppression of the body's immune response. HIV infection is essentially sexually transmitted; the two other main routes of spread are via infected blood or blood products and from an infected woman to her fetus (it may also be acquired from maternal blood during childbirth or be transmitted in breast milk). Acute infection following exposure to the virus results in the production of antibodies, their presence indicating that infection has taken place. Some people who are HIV-positive progress to chronic infection. This can include the **AIDS-related complex** – persistent generalized involvement of the lymph nodes marked by intermittent fever, weight loss, diarrhoea, fatigue, and night sweats – and **AIDS** itself, in which the individual is susceptible to opportunistic infections – especially pneumonia caused by the protozoan *Pneumocystis carinii*, cytomegalovirus (CMV) infections, generalized candidiasis or other fungal infections, and tuberculosis – and/or tumours, such as **Kaposi's sarcoma**.

   Although there is currently no cure for HIV infection, a combination of two nucleoside reverse transcriptase inhibitors and either a protease inhibitor or a non-nucleoside reverse transcriptase inhibitor (*see* ANTIVIRAL DRUGS) has been shown to be effective in delaying the progress of the disease.

Hivid (Roche Products) *See* ZALCITABINE.

homatropine hydrobromide An *antimuscarinic drug that is very similar to *atropine sulphate. Like atropine, it is used to dilate the pupils and paralyse the ciliary muscle during examination of the interior of the eye. Homatropine hydrobromide is available as eye drops on *prescription only.

Side effects, precautions, and interactions with other drugs: see ATROPINE SULPHATE; ANTIMUSCARINIC DRUGS.

Proprietary preparation: Minims Homatropine Hydrobromide (single-dose eye drops).

Honvan (ASTA Medica) *See* FOSFESTROL TETRASODIUM.

hormone replacement therapy (HRT) The use of female hormones to relieve the symptoms that occur when the ovaries cease to function, either naturally (the menopause) or following surgical removal of the ovaries ('surgical menopause'). HRT controls such symptoms as hot flushes and vaginal dryness, and there is often an improvement in psychological wellbeing. It also has beneficial effects on bone density, preventing osteoporosis, and on plasma lipids (fats), which may decrease the incidence of coronary heart disease. HRT may, however, increase the incidence of endometrial cancer and possibly of breast cancer.

Replacement is usually with natural *oestrogens (*see* OESTRADIOL <ESTRADIOL>; OESTRIOL <ESTRIOL>; OESTRONE <ESTRONE>) or conjugated oestrogens (a mixture of natural oestrogens obtained from the urine of pregnant mares). In women who have had a hysterectomy oestrogens alone may be given, in the form of tablets, skin patches, a gel for topical application, or a vaginal cream, ring, or tablets. For women who still have a uterus a *progestogen must also be taken to protect against overgrowth of the endometrium (lining of the uterus), which is stimulated by oestrogens and may give rise to cancer. In **sequential combined therapy** a progestogen is added for 10–14 days at the end of each monthly (or for some preparations three-monthly) cycle. The combination of an oestrogen and a progestogen on a cyclical basis may give episodes of monthly or three-monthly bleeding. In **continuous combined therapy** an oestrogen and a progestogen are given every day. With this therapy, which is suitable for women who have not had a natural period for at least a year, most women stop having episodes of bleeding after an initial 2–3 month period of adjustment. Sequential and continuous combined preparations are available as tablets and/or skin patches; in sequential therapy these must be taken (or applied) in the prescribed order as the dosage of oestrogens may vary or the progestogen may be added on specific days. Progestogens may alternatively be taken in the form of tablets or a vaginal gel as an *adjunct to oestrogen-only therapy. Synthetic and semisynthetic oestrogens are also used in HRT (*see* DIENOESTROL <DIENESTROL>; ESTROPIPATE; STILBOESTROL <DIETHYLSTILBESTROL>; TIBOLONE). All HRT preparations are *prescription only medicines.

Side effects: include nausea, vomiting, weight gain, breast tenderness and enlargement, breakthrough bleeding, headache, dizziness, migraine, and increased blood pressure. The occurrence of migraine-type headaches for the first time, frequent severe headaches, or acute visual disturbances should be reported to a doctor immediately.

Precautions: HRT should not be used by women who have cancer of the breast, uterus, or genital tract, thrombosis, or severe heart, liver, or kidney disease or by those who are pregnant or breastfeeding. It should be used with caution by women who have had thrombosis or thromboembolism, migraine, diabetes, epilepsy, porphyria, fibroids, or tetanus. If pregnancy occurs HRT should be stopped immediately. HRT may need to be discontinued before surgery.

Interactions with other drugs: as for *oestrogen, but interactions are much less likely to occur as the doses of oestrogen are relatively low.

Proprietary preparations: see table.

Hormone replacement therapy

Proprietary preparation	Oestrogen	Progestogen (alone or combined with an oestrogen)
Sequential combined therapy		
Climagest	oestradiol tablets	norethisterone tablets
Cyclo-Progynova	oestradiol tablets	levonorgestrel/oestradiol tablets
Elleste Duet	oestradiol tablets	norethisterone tablets
Estracombi	oestradiol patches	norethisterone/oestradiol patches
Estrapak	oestradiol patches	norethisterone tablets
Evorel-Pak	oestradiol patches	norethisterone tablets
Evorel Sequi	oestradiol patches	norethisterone/oestradiol patches
Femapak	oestradiol patches	dydrogesterone tablets
Femoston	oestradiol tablets	dydrogesterone/oestradiol tablets
Improvera	estropipate tablets	medroxyprogesterone tablets
Menophase	mestranol tablets	norethisterone/mestranol tablets
Nuvelle	oestradiol tablets	levonorgestrel/oestradiol tablets
Nuvelle TS	oestradiol patches	levonorgestrel/oestradiol patches
Premique Cycle	conjugated oestrogen tablets	medroxyprogesterone tablets
Prempak-C	conjugated oestrogen tablets	norgestrel tablets
Tridestra	oestradiol tablets	medroxyprogesterone/oestradiol tablets
Trisequens	oestradiol/oestriol tablets	norethisterone/oestradiol/oestriol tablets
Trisequens Forte	oestradiol/oestriol tablets	norethisterone/oestradiol/oestriol tablets

Proprietary preparation	Oestrogen	Progestogen	Formulation
Continuous combined therapy			
Climesse	oestradiol	norethisterone	tablets
Elleste Duet Conti	oestradiol	norethisterone	tablets
Evorel Conti	oestradiol	norethisterone	patches
Kliofem	oestradiol	norethisterone	tablets
Kliovance	oestradiol	norethisterone	tablets
Premique	conjugated oestrogens	medroxyprogesterone	tablets
Oestrogen-only therapy			
Climaval	oestradiol		tablets
Dermestril	oestradiol		patches
Elleste Solo	oestradiol		tablets
Elleste Solo MX	oestradiol		patches
Estraderm TTS	oestradiol		patches
Estraderm MX	oestradiol		patches
Estring	oestradiol		vaginal ring
Evorel	oestradiol		patches
Fematrix	oestradiol		patches
Femseven	oestradiol		patches
Harmogen	estropipate		tablets
Hormonin	oestriol/oestradiol/oestrone		tablets
Menorest	oestradiol		patches
Oestrogel	oestradiol		gel
Ortho Dienoestrol	dienoestrol		vaginal cream
Ortho-Gynest	oestriol		pessary or vaginal cream
Ovestin	oestriol		vaginal cream
Premarin	conjugated oestrogens		tablets or vaginal cream
Progynova	oestradiol		tablets
Progynova TS	oestradiol		patches
Sandrena	oestradiol		gel
Tampovagan	stilboestrol		pessary
Vagifem	oestradiol		vaginal tablets
Zumenon	oestradiol		tablets
Adjunctive progestogen therapy			
Crinone		progesterone	vaginal gel
Duphaston HRT		dydrogesterone	tablets
Micronor HRT		norethisterone	tablets

Hormonin (Shire Pharmaceuticals) A proprietary combination of
*oestriol <estriol>, *oestrone <estrone>, and *oestradiol <estradiol> used
as *hormone replacement therapy to relieve menopausal symptoms and
to prevent postmenopausal osteoporosis. Women who have not had a
hysterectomy may also need to take *progestogen supplements.
Hormonin is available as tablets on *prescription only.
Side effects, precautions, and interactions with other drugs: see HORMONE
REPLACEMENT THERAPY

HRF (Monmouth Pharmaceuticals) *See* GONADORELIN.

HRT *See* HORMONE REPLACEMENT THERAPY.

HT Defix (Scottish National Blood Transfusion Service) *See* FACTOR IX.

5HT₁ agonists Drugs that stimulate receptors for the neurotransmitter
*serotonin (5-hydrotryptamine; 5HT) and are used in the treatment of
*migraine. They have effects similar to serotonin, rapidly reversing the
dilatation of the blood vessels in the brain that is thought to cause a
migraine attack. $5HT_1$ agonists are used to treat acute attacks of
migraine; they should not be taken with other drugs used for this
purpose. *See* NARATRIPTAN; RIZATRIPTAN; SUMATRIPTAN; ZOLMITRIPTAN.
Side effects, precautions, and interactions with other drugs: see entries
for individual $5HT_1$ agonists.

Humalog (Eli Lilly & Co) *See* INSULIN.

Humalog Mix25 (Eli Lilly & Co) *See* INSULIN.

Human Actrapid (Novo Nordisk Pharmaceutical) *See* INSULIN.

human chorionic gonadotrophin (HCG) A *gonadotrophin
produced during pregnancy by the placenta. Therapeutically, it is used in
males for the treatment of undescended testicles, delayed puberty, and
poor sperm production. In women it is used for the treatment of
infertility due to failure of the ovary to release mature eggs. It is used in
conjunction with *human menopausal gonadotrophin to promote
superovulation (the production of large numbers of eggs) in women
undergoing fertility treatment. It is given by subcutaneous or
intramuscular *injection and is available on *prescription only.
Side effects: include oedema (fluid retention), particularly in men,
headache, tiredness, mood changes, and allergic reactions; high doses
result in increased sexuality.
Precautions: HCG should be used with caution by people with asthma,
epilepsy, migraine, or disorders of the heart or kidneys.
Proprietary preparations: Choragon; Pregnyl; Profasi.

Human Insulatard (Novo Nordisk Pharmaceutical) *See* INSULIN.

human menopausal gonadotrophin (menotrophin) A combination of follicle-stimulating hormone and luteinizing hormone (*see* GONADOTROPHINS), extracted from the urine of postmenopausal women. It is used for the treatment of infertility in women and men caused by underactivity of the pituitary gland (resulting in insufficient production of gonadotrophins). It is also used to stimulate the ovaries in women undergoing fertility treatment. Human menopausal gonadotrophin is given by subcutaneous or intramuscular injection and is available on *prescription only.

Side effects: include ovarian hyperstimulation (the uncontrolled production of large numbers of follicles in the ovaries) and multiple pregnancy; in both sexes there may be allergic reactions.

Precautions: the drug should be used with caution in women with ovarian cysts and in people with thyroid or adrenal disorders or pituitary tumours.

Proprietary preparations: Humegon; Menogon; Normegon; Pergonal.

Human Mixtard 10, **20**, **30**, **40**, **50** (Novo Nordisk Pharmaceutical) *See* INSULIN.

Human Monotard (Novo Nordisk Pharmaceutical) *See* INSULIN.

Human Ultratard (Novo Nordisk Pharmaceutical) *See* INSULIN.

Human Velosulin (Novo Nordisk Pharmaceutical) *See* INSULIN.

Humatrope (Eli Lilly & Co) *See* SOMATROPIN.

humectants *See* EMOLLIENTS.

Humegon (Organon Laboratories) *See* HUMAN MENOPAUSAL GONADOTROPHIN.

Humiderm (ConvaTec) *See* SODIUM PYRROLIDONE CARBOXYLATE.

Humulin I (Eli Lilly & Co) *See* INSULIN.

Humulin Lente (Eli Lilly & Co) *See* INSULIN.

Humulin M1, **M2**, **M3**, **M4**, **M5** (Eli Lilly & Co) *See* INSULIN.

Humulin S (Eli Lilly & Co) *See* INSULIN.

Humulin Zn (Eli Lilly & Co) *See* INSULIN.

Hyalase (CP Pharmaceuticals) *See* HYALURONIDASE.

hyaluronidase An enzyme that increases the permeability of connective tissue and is given in conjunction with injections of other drugs (such as local anaesthetics) to enhance the penetration of the drug into the tissues. It is available, on *prescription only, as a form for injection. Hyaluronidase is also included as an ingredient in creams to encourage the resorption of blood and other fluids in inflamed tissues.

Side effects: hyaluronidase may occasionally cause a severe allergic reaction.

Precautions: hyaluronidase should not be used to reduce the swelling of bites or stings and must not be given intravenously. It should not be applied to the eyes or to infected or cancerous tissues.

Proprietary preparations: Hyalase; LASONIL (combined with heparinoids).

Hyate C (Speywood) *See* FACTOR VIII.

Hycamtin (SmithKline Beecham Pharmaceuticals) *See* TOPOTECAN.

Hydergine (Novartis Pharmaceuticals) *See* CO-DERGOCRINE MESYLATE <MESILATE>.

hydralazine hydrochloride A *vasodilator drug used as an adjunct to *diuretics and *cardiac glycosides for the treatment of moderate to severe *heart failure and, in conjunction with beta blockers, moderate to severe *hypertension. Its use is declining, especially for treatment of hypertension, due to its side effects. It is available, on *prescription only, as tablets or as a solution for injection.

Side effects: include a rapid heart rate, dizziness, headache, nausea, vomiting, fluid retention, and (less commonly) diarrhoea, constipation, rashes, and numbness or tingling in the hands or feet.

Precautions: hydralazine should not be taken by people with systemic lupus erythematosus or some types of heart disease. It should be used with caution in people with kidney disease or a history of stroke and in women who are pregnant or breastfeeding. *See also* ANTIHYPERTENSIVE DRUGS.

Interactions with other drugs:

  Anaesthetics: their effects in lowering blood pressure are enhanced.

Proprietary preparation: Apresoline.

Hydrea (Bristol-Myers Squibb) *See* HYDROXYUREA <HYDROXCARBAMIDE>.

hydrochlorothiazide A *thiazide diuretic used for the treatment of *hypertension and *oedema associated with *heart failure, liver disease, or kidney disease. Because it reduces the amount of calcium in the urine it is sometimes used to prevent the recurrence of kidney stones. It is available as tablets on *prescription only. *See also* CO-AMILOZIDE.

Side effects, precautions, and interactions with other drugs: see THIAZIDE DIURETICS; ANTIHYPERTENSIVE DRUGS.

Proprietary preparations: Hydrosaluric; ACCURETIC (combined with quinapril); ACEZIDE (combined with captopril); Amil-Co (*see* CO-AMILOZIDE); Amilmaxco 5/50 (*see* CO-AMILOZIDE); CAPOZIDE (combined with captopril);

CARACE PLUS (combined with lisinopril); CO-BETALOC (combined with metoprolol); COZAAR-COMP (combined with losartan); Delvas (see CO-AMILOZIDE); DYAZIDE (combined with triamterene); INNOZIDE (combined with enalapril); KALTEN (combined with atenolol and amiloride hydrochloride); MODUCREN (combined with amiloride hydrochloride and timolol maleate); Moduret 25 (see CO-AMILOZIDE); MONOZIDE 10 (combined with bisoprolol fumarate); SECADREX (combined with acebutolol); TRIAM-CO (combined with triamterene); ZESTORETIC (combined with lisinopril); Zida-Co (see CO-AMILOZIDE).

See also DIURETICS.

hydrocortisone (cortisol; 17-hydroxycorticosterone) A moderately potent *corticosteroid with both mineralocorticoid and glucocorticoid activity, used for the treatment of poorly functioning adrenal glands, anaphylactic shock (see ANAPHYLAXIS), inflammatory bowel disease, *haemorrhoids, rheumatic disease, and inflammatory conditions of the eyes or skin. It is available as tablets, a solution for injection, eye drops or ointment, ear drops, a cream or ointment for skin conditions, and a rectal foam, usually on *prescription only. A few preparations, containing low doses of hydrocortisone, are available without a prescription.

Side effects: see CORTICOSTEROIDS; TOPICAL STEROIDS. In addition, perineal or scrotal warmth, irritation, and pain can occur if intravenous injections are given too rapidly.

Precautions and interactions with other drugs: see CORTICOSTEROIDS; TOPICAL STEROIDS.

Proprietary preparations: Colifoam (rectal foam); Corlan (lozenges); Dermacort (cream); Dioderm (cream); Efcortelan (cream); Efcortesol (injection); Hc45 (cream); Hydrocortistab (injection); Hydrocortisyl (cream); Hydrocortone (tablets); Lanacort (cream and ointment); Mildison Lipocream; Solu-Cortef (injection); Zenoxone (cream); ACTINAC (combined with chloramphenicol, butoxyethyl nicotinate, allantoin, and sulphur); ALPHADERM (combined with urea); ALPHOSYL HC (combined with coal tar and allantoin); ANUGESIC-HC (combined with pramoxine <pramocaine> hydrochloride, zinc oxide, Peru balsam, benzyl benzoate, and bismuth oxide); ANUGESIC-HC SUPPOSITORIES (combined with zinc oxide, bismuth oxide, bismuth subgallate, pramoxine <pramocaine> hydrochloride, and Peru balsam); ANUSOL-HC (combined with benzyl benzoate, bismuth subgallate, Peru balsam, and zinc oxide); CALMURID HC (combined with lactic acid); CANESTEN HC (combined with clotrimazole); COBADEX (combined with dimethicone <dimeticone>); DAKTACORT (combined with miconazole nitrate); ECONACORT (combined with econazole nitrate); EURAX-HYDROCORTISONE (combined with crotamiton); FUCIDIN H (combined with fusidic acid); GENTISONE HC (combined with gentamicin); GREGODERM (combined with neomycin sulphate, polymyxin B sulphate, and nystatin); NEO-CORTEF (combined with neomycin sulphate); NYSTAFORM-HC (combined with nystatin and chlorhexidine); OTOSPORIN (combined with polymyxin B sulphate and neomycin sulphate); PERINAL (combined with lignocaine <lidocaine> hydrochloride); PROCTOFOAM HC (combined with pramoxine <pramocaine> hydrochloride); PROCTOSEDYL (combined with cinchocaine hydrochloride); QUINOCORT (combined with potassium hydroxyquinoline sulphate); TARCORTIN (combined with coal tar); TERRA-CORTRIL (combined with oxytetracycline); TERRA-CORTRIL NYSTATIN (combined with nystatin and oxytetracycline); TIMODINE (combined with nystatin, benzalkonium chloride, and dimethicone <dimeticone>); UNIROID-HC (combined with cinchocaine hydrochloride); VIOFORM-HYDROCORTISONE (combined with clioquinol); XYLOPROCT (combined with zinc oxide, lignocaine <lidocaine>, and aluminium acetate).

hydrocortisone butyrate   A potent *topical steroid used for the treatment of eczema, psoriasis, and other inflammatory skin diseases and also seborrhoea of the scalp. It is available, on *prescription only, as a cream, ointment, emulsion, or scalp lotion.
Side effects and precautions: see TOPICAL STEROIDS.
Proprietary preparations: Locoid; Locoid Crelo; Locoid Lipocream; Locoid Scalp Lotion; LOCOID C (combined with chlorquinaldol).

Hydrocortistab (Knoll)   See HYDROCORTISONE.

Hydrocortisyl (Hoechst Marion Roussel)   See HYDROCORTISONE.

Hydrocortone (Merck Sharp & Dohme)   See HYDROCORTISONE.

hydroflumethiazide   A *thiazide diuretic used for the treatment of *hypertension or *oedema associated with heart failure, liver disease, or kidney disease. It is available, in combination with spironolactone, as tablets on *prescription only (see CO-FLUMACTONE).
Side effects, precautions, and interactions with other drugs: see THIAZIDE DIURETICS; ANTIHYPERTENSIVE DRUGS.
Proprietary preparations: Aldactide 25; Aldactide 50 (see CO-FLUMACTONE).
See also DIURETICS.

hydrogen peroxide   An oxidizing agent that has *antiseptic, disinfectant, and deodorizing properties. It is a weak antibacterial agent. Diluted hydrogen peroxide has been used in preparations for cleansing, disinfecting, and removing dead tissue from wounds, ulcers, and pressure sores and to release dressings compacted with dried blood, but it may cause more harm than good. A solution is used for disinfecting contact lenses. Hydrogen peroxide is available as a solution, mouthwash, or cream and may be bought without a *prescription, but only from pharmacies.
Precautions: preparations should not be allowed to come into contact with the eyes. Stronger solutions can be irritating and bleaching.
Proprietary preparations: Crystacide (solution); Hioxyl (cream); Peroxyl (mouthwash).
See also UREA HYDROGEN PEROXIDE.

Hydromol Cream (Quinoderm)   A proprietary combination of *arachis oil and *liquid paraffin (both emollients), *isopropyl myristate, sodium lactate, and *sodium pyrrolidone carboxylate (a humectant), used for the relief of dry skin conditions. It is freely available *over the counter.

Hydromol Emollient (Quinoderm) A proprietary combination of light *liquid paraffin (an emollient) and an *isopropyl myristate, used to relieve dry skin conditions. It is available as an emulsion to be added to the bath and can be obtained without a prescription, but only from pharmacies.

hydromorphone hydrochloride An *opioid analgesic that is a derivative of *morphine. It is used for the treatment of severe pain in people terminally ill with cancer. Hydromorphone is available as capsules or *modified-release capsules; it is a *controlled drug.
Side effects and precautions: see MORPHINE; OPIOIDS.
Interactions with other drugs: see OPIOIDS.
Proprietary preparations: Palladone; Palladone SR (modified-release capsules).

Hydrosaluric (Merck Sharp & Dohme) *See* HYDROCHLOROTHIAZIDE.

hydrotalcite A compound preparation of aluminium magnesium carbonate hydroxide hydrate, used as an *antacid for the treatment of indigestion. It is available as tablets or a suspension and can be obtained without a prescription, but only from pharmacies.
Side effects, precautions, and interactions with other drugs: see ANTACIDS.
Proprietary preparation: ALTACITE PLUS (combined with dimethicone <dimeticone>).

hydroxocobalamin A form of vitamin B_{12} (*see* VITAMIN B COMPLEX) used to treat pernicious *anaemia, which is caused by lack of intrinsic factor, a substance that is produced in the intestines and allows vitamin B_{12} to be absorbed. Hydroxocobalamin has replaced *cyanocobalamin for treating this condition since it remains in the body for a longer period; it is available as an injection on *prescription only.
Side effects: include itching, rash, fever, chills, hot flushes, nausea, and dizziness.
Proprietary preparations: Cobalin-H; Neo-Cytamen.

hydroxyapatite A natural mineral that is a component of bones and teeth; for therapeutic use it is usually prepared from cow bones. Hydroxyapatite consists of a complex form of calcium phosphate with small amounts of protein. It is used to supplement *calcium and phosphate in the treatment of osteoporosis, osteomalacia, and rickets. Hydroxyapatite is freely available *over the counter in the form of tablets or granules.
Precautions: hydroxyapatite should not be taken by people with high concentrations of calcium in the blood or urine and it should be used

with caution by people with kidney stones or kidney disease and by those who are immobilized for prolonged periods.

Proprietary preparations: Ossopan 800 (tablets); Ossopan Granules.

hydroxycarbamide *See* HYDROXYUREA.

hydroxychloroquine sulphate A drug similar to *chloroquine, used for the treatment of rheumatoid arthritis, juvenile arthritis, and lupus erythematosus (a chronic inflammatory condition of connective tissue). It is also used to treat skin conditions that are aggravated by sunlight. Available as tablets on *prescription only, it should be administered under specialist supervision.

Side effects, precautions, and interactions with other drugs: see CHLOROQUINE.

Proprietary preparation: Plaquenil.

17-hydroxycorticosterone *See* HYDROCORTISONE.

hydroxyethylcellulose An agent used in the treatment of dry eyes due to deficient production of natural tears. It is available as single-dose eye drops and can be obtained without a prescription, but only from pharmacies.

Proprietary preparation: MINIMS ARTIFICIAL TEARS (combined with sodium chloride).

hydroxyprogesterone hexanoate <hydroxyprogesterone caproate> A *progestogen that has been used to prevent miscarriage in women who have had recurrent miscarriages, although it is not recommended for this. Hydroxyprogesterone is given by intramuscular injection during the first half of pregnancy. It is available on *prescription only.

Side effects and precautions: see MEDROXYPROGESTERONE.

Interactions with other drugs: see PROGESTOGENS.

Proprietary preparation: Proluton Depot.

2-hydroxyethyl salicylate A *salicylate that is included in *rubefacients for the relief of muscular and rheumatic aches and pains. It is an ingredient of preparations that are freely available *over the counter.

Side effects and precautions: see SALICYLATES.

Proprietary preparation: TRANSVASIN HEAT SPRAY (combined with diethylamine salicylate and methyl nicotinate).

5-hydroxytryptamine *See* SEROTONIN.

hydroxyurea <hydroxycarbamide> A *cytotoxic drug used to treat chronic myeloid leukaemia (*see* CANCER). It may occasionally be used to

treat the blood disease polycythaemia. Hydroxyurea is available as capsules on *prescription only, and is likely to be used only in specialist units.

Side effects: include nausea (and possibly vomiting), *bone marrow suppression, and skin reactions (*see* CYTOTOXIC DRUGS).

Precautions: see CYTOTOXIC DRUGS.

Proprietary preparation: Hydrea.

hydroxyzine hydrochloride One of the original (sedating) *antihistamines, used to relieve the symptoms of such allergic conditions as hay fever and urticaria. It is also used for the short-term treatment of anxiety. Hydroxyzine is available as tablets or a syrup on *prescription only.

Side effects, precautions, and interactions with other drugs: see ANTIHISTAMINES.

Proprietary preparations: Atarax; Ucerax.

Hygroton (Novartis Pharmaceuticals) *See* CHLORTHALIDONE <CHLORTALIDONE>.

hyoscine butylbromide An *antimuscarinic drug (known as **scopolamine** in the USA) that is used for the relief of gut spasms; for example, those associated with irritable bowel syndrome (*see* ANTISPASMODICS). It is available as tablets or an injection on *prescription only, but packs containing limited quantities of tablets can be obtained from pharmacies without a prescription.

Side effects and precautions: see ANTIMUSCARINIC DRUGS.

Proprietary preparation: Buscopan.

hyoscine hydrobromide An *antimuscarinic drug (known as **scopolamine** in the USA) that is used to prevent or treat motion sickness and is given before surgery to reduce secretions and prevent vomiting. It is also used as an *antispasmodic for the relief of period pains. Hyoscine is available as tablets (for motion sickness) that can be obtained from pharmacies without a prescription, and as skin patches (for motion sickness) and an injection, which are available on *prescription only.

Side effects: include drowsiness and dizziness. *See also* ANTIMUSCARINIC DRUGS.

Precautions: drowsiness may affect driving and the performance of other skilled tasks and is enhanced by alcohol. *See also* ANTIMUSCARINIC DRUGS.

Proprietary preparations: Joy-rides; Kwells; Scopoderm TTS (patches); FEMINAX (combined with paracetamol, codeine, and caffeine).

hypercholesterolaemia The presence of high concentrations of *cholesterol in the blood. *See* HYPERLIPIDAEMIA.

hyperlipidaemia (hyperlipoproteinaemia) A condition in which the plasma concentration of *lipoproteins carrying *cholesterol and/or *triglycerides is increased. There are different classes of hyperlipidaemia, depending on which lipids are present in excess and the underlying cause of the condition. In **primary hypercholesterolaemia** the main lipid to be elevated is cholesterol; in **hypertriglyceridaemia** triglycerides are present in excess. **Mixed** (or **combined**) **hyperlipidaemias** are conditions in which both cholesterol and triglycerides are increased. Different *lipid-lowering drugs can be used to treat the various types of hyperlipidaemia.

hypertension High blood pressure, i.e. an elevation of arterial blood pressure above the normal range expected for a person of a particular age and sex. It may result from a variety of disorders, such as kidney or endocrine (glandular) disease. However, more often the cause is not known; in these cases it is called **essential hypertension**. Hypertension is initially symptomless, although severely raised blood pressure may cause headaches and palpitations. It usually requires long-term drug treatment to prevent such complications as damage to arteries (*atherosclerosis), heart attack, *heart failure, stroke, and kidney failure. Certain individuals are more at risk of hypertension, including people with *diabetes mellitus, smokers, and those whose blood lipids (fats) are high (*see* HYPERLIPIDAEMIA). Weight loss, a low salt diet, avoidance of excess alcohol, and regular exercise are important measures to reduce high blood pressure, but for more severe cases drug therapy may be necessary. Drugs used in the treatment of hypertension are known as *antihypertensive drugs, of which there are several groups (*see* ACE INHIBITORS; ALPHA BLOCKERS; BETA BLOCKERS; CALCIUM ANTAGONISTS; DIURETICS; VASODILATORS).

hyperthyroidism *See* THYROID HORMONES.

hypertriglyceridaemia The presence of high concentrations of *triglycerides in the blood. *See* HYPERLIPIDAEMIA.

hypnotic drugs Drugs that produce sleep by depressing brain function. They are used to treat insomnia, but should only be taken for short periods – no more than three weeks and preferably only one week. Hypnotics should be avoided in elderly people, who are at risk of becoming unsteady on their feet and confused, and therefore likely to fall and injure themselves. They should not be given to children unless there are exceptional reasons for doing so (such as night terrors). Hypnotics may impair judgment and increase reaction time, affecting the ability to drive or operate machinery. They increase the effects of alcohol, and the hangover effects of a dose may impair driving the following day. The commonly used hypnotics are the *benzodiazepines and some sedative *antihistamines; *zopiclone and *zolpidem tartrate are newer hypnotics. *Barbiturates were formerly used as hypnotics but can now only be prescribed for patients who are already taking them. *See also* CHLORAL HYDRATE; CHLORMETHIAZOLE <CLOMETHIAZOLE>; TRICLOFOS SODIUM.

Hypnovel (Roche Products) *See* MIDAZOLAM.

hypoglycaemia A deficiency of glucose in the bloodstream, which can cause muscular weakness and incoordination, mental confusion, and sweating. If severe it can lead to convulsions, unconsciousness, and coma. Low blood sugar most commonly occurs with overdosage of *insulin or *sulphonylureas in the treatment of *diabetes mellitus. Mild hypoglycaemia can be treated by giving glucose or sugar, usually in a readily absorbable form, such as dextrose tablets, sweet tea, fruit juice, or jam, but if the individual is unconscious an injection of *glucagon or glucose (50%) is necessary. Chronic hypoglycaemia due to excessive secretion of insulin by a tumour is treated with *diazoxide.

hypoglycaemic drugs See ORAL HYPOGLYCAEMIC DRUGS.

Hypolar Retard 20 (Lagap Pharmaceuticals) See NIFEDIPINE.

hypolipidaemic drugs See LIPID-LOWERING DRUGS.

Hypotears (CIBA Vision Ophthalmics) See POLYVINYL ALCOHOL.

hypothyroidism See THYROID HORMONES.

Hypovase (Pfizer) See PRAZOSIN.

hypromellose A drug used for the treatment of dry eyes when the watery component of natural tears is absent or reduced. It is available as eye drops and can be obtained from pharmacies without a prescription.
Precautions: hypromellose should not be used with soft contact lenses.
Proprietary preparations: Isopto Alkaline; Isopto Plain; Moisture-Eyes; ISOPTO CARPINE (combined with pilocarpine); ISOPTO FRIN (combined with phenylephrine hydrochloride); ILUBE (combined with acetylcysteine); MAXITROL (combined with dexamethasone, neomycin sulphate, and polymyxin B sulphate); TEARS NATURALE (combined with dextran).

Hypurin Bovine Isophane (CP Pharmaceuticals) See INSULIN.

Hypurin Bovine Lente (CP Pharmaceuticals) See INSULIN.

Hypurin Bovine Neutral (CP Pharmaceuticals) See INSULIN.

Hypurin Bovine Protamine Zinc Insulin (CP Pharmaceuticals) See INSULIN.

Hypurin Porcine Biphasic Isophane 30/70 (CP Pharmaceuticals) See INSULIN.

Hypurin Porcine Isophane (CP Pharmaceuticals) See INSULIN.

Hypurin Porcine Neutral (CP Pharmaceuticals) See INSULIN.

Hytrin (Abbott Laboratories) See TERAZOSIN.

Ibufem (GalPharm International) *See* IBUPROFEN.

Ibugel (Dermal Laboratories) *See* IBUPROFEN.

Ibuleve, **Ibuleve Sports** (DDD) *See* IBUPROFEN.

Ibumousse (Dermal Laboratories) *See* IBUPROFEN.

ibuprofen An *NSAID used for the treatment of pain and inflammation in rheumatoid arthritis (including arthritis in children) and other disorders of the muscles or joints. It is also used to treat period pains, pain after surgery, and fever and pain in children. Ibuprofen is applied to the skin to relieve the pain of sprains, strains, bruises, and rheumatic and muscular pain. Ibuprofen has the lowest incidence of gastrointestinal side effects of all the NSAIDs, but its anti-inflammatory effects are weaker. It is available as tablets, effervescent granules, *modified-release tablets and capsules, a syrup, and a gel for topical application. Some preparations are *prescription only medicines. Some non-prescription preparations are freely available *over the counter, but higher dosages and large pack sizes must be bought from pharmacies.
Side effects, precautions, and interactions with other drugs: see NSAIDS.
Proprietary preparations: Advil; Advil Extra Strength; Anadin Ultra; Arthrofen; Brufen; Brufen Retard (modified-release tablets); Cuprofen; Cuprofen Ibutop Gel; Cuprofen Maximum Strength; Ebufac; Fenbid Gel; Fenbid Spansule (modified-release capsules); Galprofen; Hedex Ibuprofen; Ibrufhalal; Ibufem; Ibugel (gel); Ibuleve (gel and spray); Ibuleve Sports (gel); Ibumousse (foam); Ibuspray; Inoven; Isisfen; Junifen (sugar-free suspension for children); Librofem; Lidifen; Migrafen; Motrin; Novaprin; Nurofen; Nurofen for Children (suspension); Pacifene; Pacifene Maximum Strength; PhorPain; Proflex (tablets and cream); Radian B Ibuprofen Gel; Ralgex Ibutop Gel; Relcofen; Rimafen; CODAFEN CONTINUS (combined with codeine); DEEP RELIEF (combined with menthol); LEMSIP PHARMACY POWERCAPS (combined with pseudoephedrine); NUROFEN COLDS & FLU (combined with pseudoephedrine); NUROFEN PLUS (combined with codeine); SOLPAFLEX (combined with codeine); VICKS ACTION (combined with pseudoephedrine).

Ibuspray (Dermal Laboratories) *See* IBUPROFEN.

ichthammol A *keratolytic that is milder than *coal tar; it is used for the treatment of chronic *eczema in which the skin has become thick and hard. It is available as an ointment and – combined with *zinc oxide – as a cream or medicated bandage that can be obtained without a prescription, but only from pharmacies.

Side effects: ichthammol may cause local irritation of the skin.

Proprietary preparations: ICHTHOPASTE (combined with zinc oxide); ICTHABAND (combined with zinc oxide).

Ichthopaste (Smith & Nephew Healthcare) A proprietary preparation consisting of a bandage impregnated with a paste containing *zinc oxide (an astringent protective agent) and *ichthammol (a mild keratolytic). It is used in the treatment of chronic *eczema in which the skin has become thick and hard. Icthopaste can be obtained from pharmacies without a prescription.

Icthaband (Smith & Nephew Healthcare) A proprietary preparation consisting of a bandage impregnated with a paste containing *zinc oxide (an astringent protective agent) and *ichthammol (a mild keratolytic). It is used in the treatment of chronic *eczema in which the skin has become thick and hard. Icthaband can be obtained from pharmacies without a prescription.

idarubicin A *cytotoxic antibiotic used for the treatment of advanced breast cancer that has not responded to other chemotherapy. It is also used to treat acute leukaemias, myeloma (cancer of the plasma cells of the bone marrow), and non-Hodgkin's lymphoma (*see* CANCER). Idarubicin is available as capsules or an injection on *prescription only.

Side effects: see DOXORUBICIN; CYTOTOXIC DRUGS.

Precautions: idarubicin should not be given to pregnant women and should be used with caution in people with liver or kidney disease. *See also* DOXORUBICIN; CYTOTOXIC DRUGS.

Proprietary preparation: Zavedos.

idoxuridine A nucleoside analogue (*see* ANTIVIRAL DRUGS) used for the treatment of herpes zoster (shingles) and herpes simplex infections (such as cold sores and genital herpes). A *prescription only medicine, it is available as a solution for topical application with *dimethyl sulphoxide <sulfoxide> to aid its absorption.

Side effects: include skin irritation and allergic reactions; there may be a strange taste when applied near the mouth.

Precautions: idoxuridine should not be used by women who are pregnant or breastfeeding. It may damage or stain clothing.

Proprietary preparation: Herpid (combined with dimethyl sulphoxide <sulfoxide>).

ifosfamide An *alkylating drug, similar to *cyclophosphamide, that is used for the treatment of a wide variety of *cancers. Like cyclophosphamide, it releases acrolein in the body, which can cause irritation and bleeding in the bladder. It is therefore given with *mesna to prevent this effect. Ifosfamide is available as an injection on *prescription only.

Side effects: include nausea and vomiting, blood in the urine, *bone marrow suppression, lack of periods in women, and decreased fertility in men. In high doses ifosfamide can cause drowsiness, confusion, and fits. *See also* CYTOTOXIC DRUGS.

Precautions: ifosfamide should not be given to people who are already passing blood in their urine, those who have a urinary-tract infection, or to women who are pregnant or breastfeeding. *See also* CYTOTOXIC DRUGS.

Interactions with other drugs:
  Warfarin: ifosfamide enhances the anticoagulant effect of warfarin.

Proprietary preparation: Mitoxana.

Ikorel (Rhône-Poulenc Rorer) *See* NICORANDIL.

Ilosone (Novex Pharma) *See* ERYTHROMYCIN.

Ilube (Alcon Laboratories) A proprietary combination of *acetylcysteine (a mucolytic drug) and *hypromellose (a lubricant), used for the treatment of dry eyes associated with excessive production of mucus in the eyes. It is available as eye drops on *prescription only.

Precautions: Ilube should not be used with soft contact lenses.

Imbrilon (APS-Berk) *See* INDOMETHACIN <INDOMETACIN>.

Imdur Durules (AstraZeneca) *See* ISOSORBIDE MONONITRATE.

imidazoles A group of chemically related drugs that are active against fungi and are also effective against a wide range of bacteria. The group includes the *antifungal drugs *econazole nitrate, *clotrimazole, *fenticonazole, *isoconazole nitrate, *ketoconazole, *miconazole *sulconazole, and *tioconazole. Some imidazoles, such as *thiabendazole <tiabendazole> and *mebendazole, have marked activity against parasitic worms and are used chiefly as (*anthelmintics).

imiglucerase An enzyme preparation produced by genetic engineering techniques that is used to replace an enzyme whose deficiency results in Gaucher's disease, an inherited disorder in which lipids accumulate in the bone marrow, liver, spleen, lymph nodes, and other tissues. Imiglucerase is available, on *prescription only, as a form for intravenous infusion; its use is restricted to specialists.

Side effects: include itching, pain or swelling at the injection site, and allergic reactions; nausea, vomiting, and diarrhoea have also been reported.

Precautions: imiglucerase should be used with caution in women who are pregnant or breastfeeding.

Proprietary preparation: Cerezyme.

Imigran (GlaxoWellcome) *See* SUMATRIPTAN.

imipenem A broad-spectrum beta-lactam *antibiotic, similar to the

*penicillins, that is used for the treatment of intra-abdominal, genitourinary, and gynaecological infections and for infections of the lower respiratory tract, bones, joints, skin, and soft tissues. It is also used to treat septicaemia and to prevent infections after surgery. Imipenem is given in combination with **cilastatin**, an agent that inhibits its breakdown in the kidneys and therefore prolongs its action. It is administered by intravenous infusion or intramuscular injection and is available on *prescription only.

Side effects: include nausea, vomiting, diarrhoea, taste disturbances, blood disorders, allergic reactions, convulsions, confusion, and mental disturbances.

Precautions: imipenem should not be given to women who are breastfeeding or to anyone who is allergic to it. It should be used with caution in patients allergic to other beta-lactam antibiotics, in those with kidney disease or any disease of the central nervous system (such as epilepsy), and in pregnant women.

Interactions with other drugs:

Ganciclovir: the adverse effects of ganciclovir are increased if it is administered with imipenem.

Proprietary preparation: Primaxin (combined with cilastatin).

imipramine hydrochloride A *tricyclic antidepressant drug used for the treatment of depressive illness and also bedwetting in children; it is less sedative than *amitriptyline. It is available as tablets or syrup on *prescription only.

Side effects, precautions, and interactions with other drugs: see AMITRIPTYLINE HYDROCHLORIDE; TRICYCLIC ANTIDEPRESSANTS.

Proprietary preparation: Tofranil.

immunoglobulins A group of proteins that act as antibodies as part of the immune response to help the body fight infection. They belong to a class of proteins called **gammaglobulins** and are produced by certain white blood cells in response to the presence of antigens, substances that the body regards as foreign or potentially dangerous, which occur, for example, on the surface of bacteria or viruses.

Normal immunoglobulin, which is prepared from human plasma and contains antibodies to a number of viruses, is used to treat immunoglobulin deficiency that occurs in congenital agammaglobulinaemia and hypogammaglobulinaemia, conditions that are present at birth and result in extreme susceptibility to infections. It is also used to prevent damage to the coronary arteries in Kawasaki syndrome, in which inflammation of the blood vessels is associated with fever and rash, and in the treatment of idiopathic thrombocytopenic purpura, in which platelets (blood cells involved in blood clotting) are destroyed by the body's own antibodies. In addition, normal immunoglobulin is given to prevent infections developing in patients who have received a bone marrow transplant, which is preceded by treatment to destroy the patient's own bone marrow (*see* BONE MARROW

SUPPRESSION). For all these purposes immunoglobulin is given by intravenous injection. Intramuscular injections of normal immunoglobulin may be used to provide temporary immunity against hepatitis A, measles, and rubella in people at risk. Normal immunoglobulin is available as a solution for injection on *prescription only.

Side effects: include malaise, chills, and fever.

Precautions: normal immunoglobulin should not be given within three weeks of vaccination as it may interfere with the immune response to vaccines that contain live viruses.

Proprietary preparations (for intravenous injection): Alphaglobin; Octagam; Sandoglobulin; Vigam.

Immunoprin (Ashbourne Pharmaceuticals) *See* AZATHIOPRINE.

immunosuppressants Drugs that suppress the activity of the immune system. They are given after organ transplantation to prevent the body's immune system causing tissue rejection. Some are also used in the treatment of autoimmune diseases (in which the body's immune system attacks the body's own tissues), including rheumatoid arthritis and myasthenia gravis. The immunosuppressants used to prevent transplant rejection include *azathioprine, *cyclosporin, *mycophenolate mofetil, *corticosteroids (such as prednisolone), and *tacrolimus.

   Because immunity is lowered during treatment with immunosuppressants, there is an increased susceptibility to infection (*see* BONE MARROW SUPPRESSION), and regular blood counts may need to be carried out. Some drugs, especially the *cytotoxic drugs used to treat cancer, cause immunosuppression as a side effect.

Imodium (Janssen-Cilag) *See* LOPERAMIDE HYDROCHLORIDE.

implant A medicinal preparation that is inserted into the patient's tissues, usually beneath the skin. This enables slow and steady release of the active ingredient over a period of weeks or months. Some hormonal contraceptives can be administered in this way.

Improvera (Pharmacia & Upjohn) A proprietary preparation of *estropipate tablets and *medroxyprogesterone tablets used as sequential combined as *hormone replacement therapy for the relief of menopausal symptoms and the prevention of osteoporosis in women who have not had a hysterectomy. It is available on *prescription only.

Side effects, precautions, and interactions with other drugs: see HORMONE REPLACEMENT THERAPY.

Imuderm Therapeutic Oil (Goldshield Pharmaceuticals) A proprietary combination of *almond oil and *liquid paraffin (both emollients), which is added to the bath or applied directly to the skin for the treatment of *eczema, *psoriasis, and other skin conditions associated with dry, itching, scaly, or cracked skin. It is freely available *over the counter.

Imunovir (Nycomed Amersham) *See* INOSINE PRANOBEX.

Imuran (GlaxoWellcome) *See* AZATHIOPRINE.

indapamide hemihydrate A thiazide-like diuretic (*see* THIAZIDE DIURETICS) used for the treatment of *hypertension. It is available as tablets or *modified-release tablets on *prescription only.
Side effects: include headache, dizziness, fatigue, and muscle cramps due to loss of potassium.
Precautions: indapamide should be discontinued if there are signs of deteriorating kidney function, and it should not be taken by people who have recently had a stroke or by those with severe liver disease.
Proprietary preparations: Natramid; Natrilix; Natrilex SR (modified-release tablets); Nindaxa 2.5; Opumide.

Inderal, **Inderal LA** (AstraZeneca) *See* PROPRANOLOL HYDROCHLORIDE.

Inderetic (AstraZeneca) A proprietary combination of *propranolol hydrochloride (a non-cardioselective beta blocker) and *bendrofluazide <bendroflumethiazide> (a thiazide diuretic), used in the treatment of *hypertension. It is available as capsules on *prescription only. **Inderex** is a similar preparation twice the strength of Inderetic.
Side effects, precautions, and interactions with other drugs: see BETA BLOCKERS; THIAZIDE DIURETICS.

Inderex (AstraZeneca) *See* INDERETIC.

indigestion *See* ACID-PEPTIC DISEASES.

indinavir A protease inhibitor (*see* ANTIVIRAL DRUGS) that is used in combination with other antiviral drugs for the treatment of *HIV infection. Indinavir is available as tablets on *prescription only.
Side effects: include stomach and bowel upsets, headache, fatigue, dizziness, insomnia, dry mouth, disturbances of taste, rash, tingling in the extremities, and aching muscles.
Precautions: indinavir should not be taken by women who are breastfeeding. It should be used with caution in people with liver disease and in pregnant women.
Interactions with other drugs:
  Itraconazole: the dose of indinavir may need to be reduced.
  Ketoconazole: the dose of indinavir may need to be reduced.
  Rifabutin: the dosage of rifabutin may need to be reduced and that of indinavir increased.
  Rifampicin: reduces the plasma concentration of indinavir.
Proprietary preparation: Crixivan.

Indocid, Indocid-R (Merck Sharp & Dohme) *See* INDOMETHACIN
<INDOMETACIN>.

Indolar SR (Lagap Pharmaceuticals) *See* INDOMETHACIN <INDOMETACIN>.

Indomax, Indomax 75 SR (Ashbourne Pharmaceuticals) *See*
INDOMETHACIN <INDOMETACIN>.

indomethacin <indometacin> An *NSAID used for the treatment of
the pain and inflammation in rheumatoid arthritis and other disorders of
muscles or joints. It is also used to relieve the pain of acute gout and
period pains. Indomethacin is available, on *prescription only, as
capsules, *modified-release capsules or tablets, a suspension, and
suppositories.
Side effects: indomethacin commonly causes indigestion, nausea,
vomiting, and diarrhoea, gastrointestinal ulceration and bleeding,
dizziness, headache, and light-headedness. It may rarely cause
drowsiness, confusion, insomnia, psychiatric disturbances, blood
disorders, and blurred vision. Suppositories can cause local irritation and
occasionally bleeding.
Precautions: see NSAIDS. In addition, indomethacin should be used with
caution in people with epilepsy, parkinsonism, or psychiatric illness;
suppositories should not be used in people with haemorrhoids. Eye and
blood tests are advisable for those taking indomethacin on a long-term
basis.
Interactions with other drugs: see NSAIDS.
Proprietary preparations: Flexin Continus (modified-release tablets);
Imbrilon; Indocid (capsules, sugar-free suspension for children, and
suppositories); Indocid-R (modified-release capsules); Indolar SR (modified-
release capsules); Indomax; Indomax 75 SR (modified-release capsules);
Indomod; Indotard (modified-release capsules); Pardelprin (modified-
release capsules); Rheumacin LA (modified-release capsules); Rimacid; Slo-
Indo (modified-release capsules).

Indomod (Pharmacia & Upjohn) *See* INDOMETHACIN <INDOMETACIN>.

indoramin hydrochloride An *alpha blocker used to treat all grades
of *hypertension and to relieve the obstruction of urine flow that can
occur in men with an enlarged prostate gland. It is available as tablets on
*prescription only.
Side effects and interactions with other drugs: see ALPHA BLOCKERS.
Precautions: people with heart failure should be treated appropriately
before taking indoramin. Indoramin should be used with caution in
people with liver or kidney disease, epilepsy, Parkinson's disease, or
depression. *See also* ANTIHYPERTENSIVE DRUGS.
Proprietary preparations: Baratol; Doralese.
See also VASODILATORS.

Indotard (Ashbourne Pharmaceuticals) *See* INDOMETHACIN
<INDOMETACIN>.

Infacol (Pharmax) *See* DIMETHICONE <DIMETICONE>.

Infaderm Therapeutic Oil (Goldshield Pharmaceuticals) A
proprietary combination of *almond oil and *liquid paraffin (both
emollients), which is added to the bath or applied directly to the skin for
the treatment of *eczema, *psoriasis, and other skin conditions
associated with dry, itching, scaly, or cracked skin. It is freely available
*over the counter.

Infadrops (Goldshield Pharmaceuticals) *See* PARACETAMOL.

Infestat (Opus) *See* NYSTATIN.

infusion The slow injection of a substance, usually into a vein
(**intravenous infusion**; *see* INTRAVENOUS INJECTION), enabling large
volumes to be administered over a period of minutes, hours, or even
days. This is a common method for replacing water, electrolytes, and
blood products and is also used for the continuous administration of
drugs (e.g. antibiotics, painkillers) or *parenteral nutrition. The infused
substance flows under gravity from a suspended bottle through a tube
ending in a hollow needle inserted into the patient's vein. Many
infusions are controlled by electronically regulated infusion pumps to
ensure an accurate rate of flow.

inhaler A device for breathing in a drug in order to deliver it to the
airways or lungs. Inhalers are most commonly used for administering
bronchodilators or corticosteroids in the treatment of *asthma. **Aerosol**
(or **metered-dose**) **inhalers** deliver a measured dose of the drug in the
form of a suspension of extremely small liquid or solid particles, which is
dispensed from the inhaler by a propellant under pressure. Such inhalers
are placed into the mouth and depressed (activated) to release drug as the
individual takes a breath. This requires a certain amount of coordination
and may therefore be unsuitable for children. **Spacers** (or **spacing
devices**), which are available for use with some aerosol inhalers, extend
the space between the inhaler and the mouth. This reduces the speed at
which the aerosol travels to the back of the mouth, allowing more time
for the propellant to evaporate and therefore reducing the impact of the
propellant on the back of the mouth (which can cause irritation) and
enabling a higher proportion of the particles of the drug to be inhaled.
There is also less need to coordinate breathing in with activation of the
inhaler. **Breath-activated** (or **breath-actuated**) **inhalers** deliver the drug,
in the form of an aerosol or a dry powder, only when the user places his
(or her) mouth over the outlet and breathes in. This obviates the need to
coordinate breathing in with depressing the dispenser. The dose of drug
will still be measured (metered) and is not dependent on the size of
breath taken. **Dry-powder inhalers** are loaded with capsules of the drug

in powder form; as the inhaler is activated (by taking a breath), the capsule is punctured and a type of fan mechanism disperses the powder so that it can be inhaled (these inhalers are called 'Spinhalers' or 'Rotahalers'). 'Turbohalers' are fitted with canisters that deliver measured doses of the drug in powder form. *See also* NEBULIZER.

injection The introduction into the body of drugs in liquid form by means of a syringe, usually drugs that would be destroyed by the digestive processes if taken by mouth. Common routes for injection are below the skin (*subcutaneous), e.g. for insulin; into a muscle (*intramuscular), for drugs that are slowly absorbed; and into a vein (*intravenous), for drugs to be rapidly absorbed. *Enemas are also regarded as injections.

Innohep (Leo Pharmaceuticals) *See* TINZAPARIN SODIUM.

Innovace, Innovace Melt (Merck Sharp & Dohme) *See* ENALAPRIL HYDROCHLORIDE.

Innozide (Merck Sharp & Dohme) A proprietary preparation consisting of *enalapril (an ACE inhibitor) and *hydrochlorothiazide (a thiazide diuretic), used in the treatment of mild to moderate *hypertension. It is available as tablets on *prescription only.
Side effects, precautions, and interactions with other drugs: see ACE INHIBITORS; THIAZIDE DIURETICS.
See also ANTIHYPERTENSIVE DRUGS; DIURETICS.

inosine pranobex An *antiviral drug used for the treatment of herpes simplex infections in mucous membranes and adjacent skin, such as cold sores and genital herpes, and genital warts. It is available as tablets on *prescription only.
Side effects: there may be reversible increases in the concentrations of uric acid in the blood and urine.
Precautions: inosine pranobex should be not be taken by people with kidney disease, gout, or raised plasma concentrations of uric acid.
Proprietary preparation: Imunovir.

inositol *See* VITAMIN B COMPLEX.

inositol nicotinate A *nicotinic acid derivative used for the treatment of Raynaud's syndrome (poor circulation of hands and feet) or intermittent claudication (cramping pain in the legs on walking due to insufficient blood to the muscles). It is available as tablets or a suspension and can be obtained from pharmacies without a prescription.
Side effects: as for *nicotinic acid, but side effects are less severe and occur less frequently.
Precautions: inositol nicotinate should not be taken during pregnancy.
Proprietary preparation: Hexopal.

Inoven (Janssen-Cilag) *See* IBUPROFEN.

Instillagel (Clinimed) A proprietary combination of *lignocaine <lidocaine> hydrochloride (a local anaesthetic) and *chlorhexidine gluconate (an antiseptic), used for the disinfection, lubrication, and local anaesthesia of the urethra preparatory to passing a catheter or a cystoscope (a fibre-optic viewing device) through the urethra to the bladder. It is instilled into the urethra before the procedure and is available as a gel in a disposable syringe without a prescription.

instillation The application of liquid medication drop by drop, as into the eye or the bladder.

insulin A protein hormone, secreted by the beta cells of the islets of Langerhans in the pancreas, that controls the concentration of glucose in the blood. It is secreted in response to a rise in blood glucose, which occurs after a meal; its secretion is inhibited by low blood glucose and its action is opposed by some other hormones, mainly *glucagon and *adrenaline <epinephrine>. Insulin's actions are to promote the uptake of glucose from the blood by the body's cells, mainly in muscles, where it is used as energy, and in the liver, where it is converted to glycogen for storage. It also stops fat being broken down in the body and increases protein synthesis. A lack of insulin causes *diabetes mellitus. People with type I (insulin-dependent) diabetes usually require injections of insulin once or twice a day; those with type II (noninsulin-dependent) diabetes may require insulin rather than *oral hypoglycaemic drugs. Insulin cannot be taken orally (it is broken down in the gut) and must therefore always be injected; after instruction, patients can inject themselves subcutaneously (beneath the skin) in the thigh, buttocks, upper arm, or abdomen. In emergencies soluble insulin can be injected intramuscularly or intravenously; this should only be done in hospital.

Preparations of insulin for therapeutic use are derived from animal sources; they are **highly purified insulins**, which have been treated to remove impurities that would cause allergic reactions. Pork (or porcine) insulin (from pigs) is closer chemically to human insulin and causes fewer local reactions than beef (or bovine) insulin (from cows), but most preparations are synthetic **human insulins**. These are manufactured by altering the structure of pork insulin, either by enzymatic modification or by genetic engineering (to produce recombinant insulin), using bacteria or yeasts. They are labelled according to their method of manufacture: **emp** (enzyme-modified pork), **prb** (pork recombinant, using bacteria), or **pyr** (pork recombinant, using yeasts).

Insulin is available in formulations that are short-acting, intermediate-acting, or long-acting. **Short-acting insulins** are solutions of highly purified soluble insulin that, when given subcutaneously, act rapidly (within 30–60 minutes) and are effective for up to eight hours; blood concentrations have a peak between two and four hours. Administration of short-acting insulins should usually be followed by a meal within 15–30 minutes. They are used for diabetic emergencies since they can be injected intravenously as well as subcutaneously or intramuscularly. The effect of intravenous insulin disappears within 30 minutes. **Insulin lispro** is an *analogue of human insulin that acts very rapidly (15 minutes after injection) and has a short duration of action (2–3 hours), which allows doses to be timed more accurately to coincide with meals. The duration of action of soluble insulin can be prolonged by the addition of zinc, producing **insulin zinc suspensions (IZS)**, or by zinc and protamine (a protein), producing **protamine zinc insulin (PZI)**. Zinc and protamine combine with insulin to delay its release in the body. **Intermediate-acting insulins** include **amorphous IZS** and **isophane insulin** (neutral protamine Hagedorn, or NPH insulin). When injected subcutaneously, they start to act at around 1 hour after injection, with maximum effects at 2–8 hours; activity lasts 18–20 hours. Some intermediate-acting insulins are given twice daily in conjunction with short-acting insulin; others are given once a day. **Long-acting insulins** include amorphous IZS and **crystalline IZS (ultralente)**, or a mixture of these (**lente**), and protamine zinc insulin. They start to act 2–3 hours after subcutaneous injection, with peak activity at 4–16 hours, and can have a duration of action up to 36 hours. Often combinations of short-, intermediate-, and long-acting insulins are prescribed. **Biphasic insulins** are stable mixtures of a short-acting and an intermediate-acting insulin in fixed proportions, which give a two-stage action. The speed of onset of action will vary with the proportion of short-acting insulin (the higher the proportion, the more rapid the onset). Generally, peak activity is at 1–9 hours and duration of action is around 18–20 hours.

Insulin is supplied either as a solution in vials to be drawn up into a syringe for injection or in dispensing **insulin pens** designed to inject measured doses. These pens are available as prefilled disposable devices or as reusable devices that can be fitted with cartridges of insulin and disposable needles. When taking insulin it is usually necessary to measure glucose concentrations in the blood or urine to ensure that the dose is correct. Most diabetic people can make these measurements themselves at home. Insulin is available from pharmacies without a prescription, but the preparations listed in the table are *prescription only medicines and several formulations of insulin, reusable pens, and needles cannot be prescribed on the NHS.

Side effects: the most common side effect is *hypoglycaemia (low blood sugar), which occurs when the patient receives too much insulin or misses a meal and can cause loss of consciousness if untreated (e.g. by taking a glucose sweet). However, most individuals learn to recognize the warning signs of a 'hypo' attack, which include sweating, irritability, muscular weakness, and confusion. Local reactions (e.g. irritation, rash) may occur at the injection site. Hyperglycaemia (high blood sugar; *see* DIABETES MELLITUS) can result when the patient takes too little insulin for the food consumed; changes to the dosing regime are necessary to avoid this problem.

Precautions: expert counselling, training, and dosage adjustment are needed when an individual first starts taking insulin. People using insulin should drive or operate machinery only if they are aware of the nature

Proprietary preparations of insulin

Proprietary preparation	Type of insulin (highly purified)	Packaged as
Short-acting		
Humalog	insulin lispro	vials or cartridges for reusable pens
Human Actrapid	human neutral insulin (pyr)	vials, prefilled pens, cartridges for reusable pens
Human Velosulin	human neutral insulin (emp)	vials
Humulin S	human neutral insulin (prb)	vials, prefilled pens, cartridges for reusable pens
Hypurin Bovine Neutral	beef neutral insulin	vials, cartridges for reusable pens
Hypurin Porcine Neutral	pork neutral insulin	vials, cartridges for reusable pens
Pork Velosulin	pork neutral insulin	vials
Intermediate-acting		
Human Insulatard	human isophane insulin (pyr)	vials, prefilled pens, cartridges for reusable pens
Human Monotard	human insulin zinc suspension (pyr)	vials
Humulin I	human isophane insulin (prb)	vials, prefilled pens, cartridges for reusable pens
Hypurin Bovine Isophane	beef isophane insulin	vials, cartridges for reusable pens
Hypurin Porcine Isophane	pork isophane insulin	vials, cartridges for reusable pens
Pork Insulatard	pork isophane insulin	vials
Long-acting		
Human Ultratard	human insulin zinc suspension (pyr)	vials
Humulin Lente	30% human amorphous insulin + 70% human crystalline insulin (prb)	vials
Humulin Zn	human insulin zinc suspension (prb)	vials
Hypurin Bovine Lente	long-acting beef insulin	vials
Hypurin Bovine Protamine Zinc Insulin	beef protamine zinc insulin	vials
Lentard MC	70% beef insulin zinc suspension + 30% pork insulin zinc suspension	vials

Proprietary preparations of insulin (cont)

Proprietary preparation	Type of insulin (highly purified)	Packaged as
Biphasic		
Humalog Mix25	25% insulin lispro + 75% insulin lispro protamine	prefilled pens, cartridges for reusable pens
Human Mixtard 10– Human Mixtard 50	mixtures of human neutral insulin (pyr; 10–50%) + human isophane insulin (prb; 90–50%)	prefilled pens, cartridges for reusable pens
Humulin M1– Humulin M5	mixtures of human neutral insulin (prb; 10–50%) + human isophane insulin (prb; 90–50%)	vials, prefilled pens, cartridges for reusable pens
Hypurin Porcine Biphasic Isophane 30/70	30% pork neutral insulin + 70% pork isophane insulin	vials, cartridges for reusable pens
Pork Mixtard 30	30% pork neutral insulin + 70% pork isophane insulin	vials

and risks of hypoglycaemia; alcohol enhances the effect of insulin in lowering blood sugar. Insulin requirements usually fall during the first three months of pregnancy and rise during the last six months; close monitoring of insulin requirements is necessary during pregnancy. Any diabetic woman should consult a doctor if she suspects that she is pregnant.

Interactions with other drugs:
   ACE inhibitors: possibly enhance the effect of insulin in lowering blood glucose.
   Anabolic steroids: possibly enhance the effect of insulin in lowering blood glucose.
   Beta blockers: enhance the effect of insulin in lowering blood glucose and mask many of the symptoms of hypoglycaemia.
   Corticosteroids: reduce the effect of insulin in lowering blood glucose.
   Diuretics: loop and thiazide diuretics reduce the effect of insulin in lowering blood glucose.
   MAOIs: enhance the effect of insulin in lowering blood glucose.
   Oral contraceptives: reduce the effect of insulin in lowering blood glucose.
Proprietary preparations: see table.

insulin lispro *See* INSULIN.

Intal (Pantheon Healthcare) *See* SODIUM CROMOGLYCATE <CROMOGLICATE>.

interferon-alfa (INF-α) A type of *interferon used for the treatment of certain cancers: it has some activity against lymphomas, leukaemias, and

Kaposi's sarcoma (a skin cancer prevalent in AIDS patients) and is capable of reducing certain solid tumours (*see* CANCER). Its use is usually restricted to specialist cancer centres since it has many side effects. INF-α is also used in the treatment of genital warts, genital herpes, hepatitis B, and hepatitis C. It is available, on *prescription only, as forms for injection.

Side effects: include influenza-like symptoms (chills, fever, fatigue, aching muscles and joints), loss of appetite, weight loss, and (less commonly) dizziness, vertigo, forgetfulness, depression, drowsiness, confusion, nervousness, sleep disturbance, and depressed production of blood cells by the bone marrow. Changes in blood pressure, abnormal heart rhythms, and allergic reactions have also been reported.

Precautions: INF-α should not be given to people with severe kidney or liver disease, epilepsy or other neurological disorders, or severe heart disease. It should only be given by a specialist and should be used with caution in people who have diabetes. It may impair the ability to drive and operate machinery.

Interactions with other drugs: INF-α enhances the effects of theophylline, warfarin, phenytoin, opioids, and sedatives.

Proprietary preparations: Intron A; Roferon-A; Wellferon; Viraferon.

interferon-beta A type of *interferon used for reducing the frequency and degree of severity of relapses in patients with relapsing remitting multiple sclerosis. It is usually given only to those individuals who have had at least two attacks in the last 2–3 years and in whom the disease has not progressed between relapses; it is not usually given to those who are wheelchair bound. Interferon-beta is available as an injection on *prescription only.

Side effects: include reactions at the injection site, influenza-like symptoms, menstrual disturbances, depression, allergic reactions, insomnia, mood swings, anxiety, confusion, sometimes nausea and vomiting, and rarely hair loss.

Precautions and interactions with other drugs: interferon-beta should not be given to women who are pregnant or breastfeeding. It should be used with caution in people with severe depression, suicidal tendencies, or uncontrolled epilepsy and in those taking certain antiepileptic drugs, warfarin, theophylline, and some antidepressants.

Proprietary preparations: Avonex; Betaferon; Rebif.

interferons Proteins that are produced by cells infected with a virus and have the ability to enhance the resistance of other cells to attack by other viruses. Interferons are active against many different viruses, but particular interferons are effective only in the species that produces them. There are three types of human interferon: alpha (from white blood cells), beta (from fibroblasts), and gamma (from lymphocytes). Human interferon can now be produced by genetic engineering for clinical use in treating hepatitis B and C, hairy-cell leukaemia, Kaposi's sarcoma, and certain other forms of *cancer, and multiple sclerosis. Side effects, including influenza-like symptoms, lethargy, and depression, may be severe. *See* INTERFERON-ALFA; INTERFERON-BETA.

interleukins A family of proteins that control some aspects of the immune response by conveying signals between white blood cells. Different interleukins are designated by numbers. For example, **interleukin-2** (IL-2) stimulates activity in certain T-lymphocytes that results in the destruction of virus-infected cells. A genetically engineered form of IL-2 is used in the treatment of certain cancers (*see* ALDESLEUKIN).

Intralgin (3M Health Care) A proprietary combination of salicylamide (a *salicylate) and *benzocaine (a local anaesthetic), used to relieve the pain of muscle strains and sprains. It is available as a gel and can be obtained from pharmacies without a prescription.
Side effects and precautions: see SALICYLATES; LOCAL ANAESTHETICS.

intramuscular injection The *injection of a drug into the body of a muscle. Usually a larger volume of liquid is injected than for *subcutaneous injections (more than 2 mL) and a slightly wider needle is used. Common sites for intramuscular injections are the deltoid muscle on the outer side of the shoulder and the gluteal muscles of the buttocks.

intravenous injection *Injection of a drug directly into a vein. A small or large volume can be injected; large volumes can be injected over a long period: this is known as intravenous *infusion. Because the drug mixes rapidly with the bloodstream, intravenous injection is the fastest way of introducing a drug into the body.

Intron A (Schering-Plough) *See* INTERFERON ALFA.

Invirase (Roche Products) *See* SAQUINAVIR.

Iocare (CIBA Vision Ophthalmics) *See* BALANCED SALT SOLUTION.

iodine An element required in small amounts for healthy growth and development. Iodine accumulates in the thyroid gland, where it is required for the production of *thyroid hormones. A deficiency of iodine leads to **goitre** (swelling of the neck due to enlargement of the thyroid gland). Aqueous iodine oral solution (**Lugol's solution**) is given to patients with thyrotoxicosis (overproduction of thyroid hormones) in order to reduce the size of the thyroid gland before surgery. It acts as a signal to turn off production of thyroid hormones by the gland. This solution is available from pharmacies without a prescription.
 Iodine is also an *antiseptic and is used to disinfect the skin (*see* POVIDONE–IODINE).
Side effects: Lugol's solution can cause allergic reactions, headache, tear production, conjunctivitis, pain in the salivary glands, laryngitis, bronchitis, and rashes. Prolonged use results in depression, insomnia, and impotence.

Precautions: Lugol's solution should not be used for long-term treatment. It should not be taken by women who are breastfeeding and should be used with caution in pregnant women and in children.

Iodoflex (Smith & Nephew Healthcare) *See* CADEXOMER IODINE.

Iodosorb (Smith & Nephew Healthcare) *See* CADEXOMER IODINE.

Ionamin (Torbet Laboratories) *See* PHENTERMINE.

Ionax Scrub (Galderma) A proprietary combination of polyethylene granules (an abrasive) and *benzalkonium chloride (an antiseptic), used for the treatment of acne. It is available in the form of a foaming face gel and can be obtained without a prescription, but only from pharmacies. It cannot be prescribed on the NHS.
Precautions: Ionax Scrub should not be used by people with telangiectasia (in which spidery red spots of distended blood vessels can be seen beneath the skin). It should not come into contact with the eyes. It should be discontinued if the skin becomes irritated.

Ionil T (Galderma) A proprietary combination of *salicylic acid and *coal tar (both keratolytics) and *benzalkonium chloride (an antiseptic), used for the treatment of *psoriasis and seborrhoeic *eczema of the scalp and dandruff. It is available as a shampoo and can be obtained without a prescription, but only from pharmacies.
Side effects and precautions: see SALICYLIC ACID; COAL TAR.

Iopidine (Alcon Laboratories) *See* APRACLONIDINE.

ipecacuanha (ipecac) A plant extract that contains two alkaloids, emetine and cephaeline, that irritate the lining of the stomach and intestines and act as *emetics. Ipecacuanha has been used to induce vomiting in people (especially children) who have swallowed a non-corrosive poison. In very small doses it can act as an *expectorant, being available as syrups and tablets and included in many cough medicines. Ipecacuanha is freely available *over the counter.
Side effects: large doses produce excessive vomiting, bleeding from the stomach and intestines, and damage to the heart.
Precautions: overdosage can be fatal in children.
Proprietary preparations: Buttercup Infant Cough Syrup; Fennings Little Healers (tablets); Hill's Balsam Chesty Cough Liquid for Children; Melo (syrup); Throaties Family Cough Linctus; BOOTS INFANT SUGAR FREE COUGH AND CONGESTION SYRUP (combined with ephedrine); ES BRONCHIAL MIXTURE (combined with ammonium bicarbonate, senna, and squill); GALLOWAYS COUGH SYRUP (combined with squill); HILL'S BALSAM CHESTY COUGH PASTILLES (combined with benzoin tincture, menthol, and peppermint oil).

ipratropium bromide An *antimuscarinic drug used as a *bronchodilator to relieve the wheezing and breathlessness associated with chronic bronchitis, especially in people who fail to respond to beta-adrenoceptor stimulants (such as salbutamol or terbutaline). It is also used to treat perennial allergic rhinitis. Ipratropium has its maximum effect 30–60 minutes after use; its duration of action is 3–6 hours. It is available, on *prescription only, as an aerosol or powder for inhalation, a nasal spray, and a solution for use in a *nebulizer.

Side effects: these are rare – a dry mouth and dryness and irritation of the nose may occur; difficulties in urinating and constipation are less likely.

Precautions: ipratropium should be used with caution by people with glaucoma, men with an enlarged prostate, and pregnant women.

Proprietary preparations: Atrovent (metered-dose aerosol inhaler); Atrovent Aerocaps (powder for inhalation); Atrovent Autohaler (breath-activated aerosol inhaler); Atrovent Forte (a stronger preparation); Atrovent UDV (solution for use in a nebulizer); Respontin (solution for use in a nebulizer); Rinatec (nasal spray); Steri-Neb Ipratropium (solution for use in a nebulizer); COMBIVENT (combined with salbutamol); DUOVENT (combined with fenoterol hydrobromide).

irbesartan An *angiotensin II inhibitor used in the treatment of *hypertension. It is available as tablets on *prescription only.

Side effects: include headache, dizziness, and muscle and bone pain.

Precautions: irbesartan should not be taken by women who are pregnant or breastfeeding. It should be used with caution by people with kidney disease, severe liver disease, heart failure, and some types of heart disease.

Interactions with other drugs: see ACE INHIBITORS.

Proprietary preparation: Aprovel.

irinotecan A *topoisomerase inhibitor used for the treatment of *cancers of the colon and rectum that have failed to respond to treatment with *fluorouracil. It is available as a solution for intravenous infusion on *prescription only.

Side effects: include diarrhoea occurring more than 24 hours after treatment (which should be reported to a doctor immediately), early diarrhoea (i.e. less than 24 hours after treatment), nausea, vomiting (which can be severe), loss of appetite, *bone marrow suppression, hair loss, weakness, fatigue, breathlessness, cramps, and tingling in fingers or toes. *See also* CYTOTOXIC DRUGS.

Precautions: irinotecan should not be given to people with chronic inflammatory bowel disease, bowel obstruction, liver or kidney disease, or bone marrow suppression or to women who are pregnant or breastfeeding. *See also* CYTOTOXIC DRUGS.

Proprietary preparation: Campto.

iron A metallic element essential to life: most importantly, it is a constituent of haemoglobin, the oxygen-carrying pigment of red blood cells. The main dietary sources of iron are meat and liver. Iron deficiency, which results in iron-deficiency *anaemia, can be caused by blood loss (for example due to heavy menstrual periods or a bleeding peptic ulcer or occurring after childbirth), pregnancy, low dietary intake, or illnesses in which absorption of iron from the gut is affected. It can also occur in premature babies, babies born by Caesarean section, and in patients after surgical removal of the stomach.

Iron supplements are used for the treatment and prevention of iron-deficiency anaemia. They contain soluble iron in the form of iron salts (*see* FERROUS SULPHATE; FERROUS FUMARATE; FERROUS GLUCONATE; FERROUS GLYCINE SULPHATE; POLYSACCHARIDE–IRON COMPLEX; SODIUM IRON EDETATE). Iron salts are sometimes combined with *folic acid; this combination is used mainly during pregnancy to prevent deficiencies of iron and folic acid. Preparations for use during pregnancy often contain other supplemental vitamins and minerals. Some preparations include *vitamin C (ascorbic acid) to help absorption. Iron is best absorbed on an empty stomach, but this can result in gastrointestinal upsets. These can be largely avoided by using *modified-release preparations (although iron from these is sometimes poorly absorbed), by gradually increasing the dose, or by taking the supplements after meals. Iron supplements are usually taken orally – as tablets, modified-release capsules, or syrup; they may occasionally need to be given by injection (*see* IRON SORBITOL–CITRIC ACID COMPLEX; FERRIC HYDROXIDE SUCROSE). Most iron supplements are available without a prescription.

Side effects: include nausea, stomach pain, diarrhoea and constipation (which may cause problems in the elderly). Iron salts colour the stools black.

Precautions: iron supplements should be used with caution by people with gastrointestinal obstruction (since they may worsen constipation) or inflammatory bowel disease (because the iron may not be absorbed).

Interactions with other drugs:

Antacids: reduce the absorption of iron.

Levodopa: its absorption is reduced by iron.

Penicillamine: its absorption is reduced by iron.

Tetracycline antibiotics: the absorption of both tetracyclines and iron is reduced.

Zinc salts: the absorption of both zinc and iron salts is reduced.

Iron Jelloids (Seton Scholl Healthcare) A proprietary combination of *ferrous fumarate, B vitamins (*see* VITAMIN B COMPLEX), and vitamin C, used for the prevention of deficiencies of iron, B vitamins, and vitamin C. It is available as tablets that can be obtained without a prescription, but only from pharmacies. Iron Jelloids are not recommended for children.

Side effects, precautions, and interactions with other drugs: see IRON.

iron sorbitol–citric acid complex A combination of *iron, sorbitol, and citric acid, used to treat iron-deficiency anaemia. It is available as an intramuscular injection on *prescription only.

Side effects: include nausea, vomiting, changes in taste, dizziness, flushing, and occasionally severe disturbances in heart rhythm (*see* ARRHYTHMIA); the urine may darken on standing.

Precautions: oral iron should be stopped 24 hours before injection; other injectable iron preparations should be stopped a week before. Iron injections should not be given during early pregnancy or to people with liver or kidney disease, untreated urinary-tract infections, or heart conditions.

Interactions with other drugs: see IRON.

Proprietary preparation: Jectofer.

Irriclens (ConvaTec) *See* SODIUM CHLORIDE.

irrigation The process of washing out a wound or a hollow organ (such as the bladder) with a continuous flow of water or medicated solution. For example, an infected bladder may be irrigated with an antibiotic or antiseptic solution.

Isclofen (ISIS Products) *See* DICLOFENAC SODIUM.

Isib, **Isib 60XL** (Ashbourne Pharmaceuticals) *See* ISOSORBIDE MONONITRATE.

Isisfen (ISIS Products) *See* IBUPROFEN.

Ismelin (Alliance Pharmaceuticals) *See* GUANETHIDINE.

Ismo, **Ismo Retard** (Roche Products) *See* ISOSORBIDE MONONITRATE.

isocarboxazid A *monoamine oxidase inhibitor used for the treatment of depressive illness. It is available as tablets on *prescription only.

Side effects, precautions, and interactions with other drugs: see MONOAMINE OXIDASE INHIBITORS.

Isocard (Eastern Pharmaceuticals) *See* ISOSORBIDE DINITRATE.

isoconazole nitrate An imidazole *antifungal drug used for the treatment of vaginal candidiasis (thrush) and bacterial infections of the vagina. It is available as pessaries on *prescription only.

Side effects: there may be transient local irritation and burning.

Proprietary preparation: Travogyn.

Isogel (Pfizer) *See* ISPAGHULA HUSK.

Isoket, **Isoket Retard** (Schwartz Pharma) *See* ISOSORBIDE DINITRATE.

isometheptene mucate A *sympathomimetic drug that acts as a *vasoconstrictor; it is used in combination with *paracetamol (an analgesic) for the relief of *migraine attacks. Isometheptene is available as capsules with or without a prescription (depending on the dosage).

Side effects: include dizziness and (more rarely) disorders of blood circulation and rashes.

Precautions: isometheptene should not be taken by people with glaucoma, severe heart disease or hypertension, severe liver or kidney disease, or by women who are pregnant or breastfeeding. It should be used with caution in people with diabetes or an overactive thyroid gland.

Interactions with other drugs:

Bromocriptine: there is an increased risk of adverse effects if isometheptene is taken with bromocriptine.

MAOIs: a severe rise in blood pressure can occur if MAOIs are taken with isometheptene.

Proprietary preparation: MIDRID (combined with paracetamol).

isoniazid A bactericidal *antibiotic used for the treatment of *tuberculosis; it is usually given in combination with other antituberculosis agents, such as *rifampicin and *pyrazinamide. A *prescription only medicine, it is available as tablets, an elixir, or as a solution for injection.

Side effects: include nausea, vomiting, insomnia, and restlessness. Nerve damage, producing weakness, numbness, and 'pins and needles', may occur; this can be prevented by taking isoniazid with *pyridoxine (vitamin B_6). More serious (but rare) are psychiatric disturbances and hepatitis.

Precautions: isoniazid should be used with caution in patients with liver or kidney disease or a history of psychosis or alcoholism and in women who are pregnant or breastfeeding.

Interactions with other drugs:

Antacids: reduce the absorption of isoniazid.

Antiepileptics: the effects of carbamazepine, ethosuximide, and phenytoin are enhanced.

Cycloserine: the toxic effects of this drug may be increased.

Diazepam: the effects of this drug are enhanced.

Proprietary preparations: RIMACTAZID (combined with rifampicin); RIFATER (combined with rifampicin and pyrazinamide); RIFINAH (combined with rifampicin).

isoprenaline hydrochloride A *sympathomimetic drug, similar to *adrenaline <epinephrine>, that stimulates beta *adrenoceptors in the heart. It is used to produce an increase in the rate and force of contraction of the heart as emergency treatment for severe bradycardia (slowing of the heart rate) and heart block (in which the pumping action of the heart is reduced). Isoprenaline hydrochloride is available as a form for intravenous infusion on *prescription only. (The sulphate was formerly used as a bronchodilator in the treatment of asthma, but has been superseded by drugs that act more selectively on the beta-adrenoceptors of the airways and are therefore less likely to have adverse effects on the heart.)

Side effects: include a fast heart rate, abnormal heart rhythms, low blood pressure, sweating, tremor, and headache.

Precautions: isoprenaline should be used with caution in people with heart disease, diabetes, or an overactive thyroid gland.

Interactions with other drugs:

Anaesthetics: the risk of abnormal heart rhythms is increased if isoprenaline is given with halothane or similar volatile liquid anaesthetics.

Entacapone: may increase the effects of isoprenaline.

Proprietary preparation: Saventrine IV.

isopropyl myristate An oily liquid that is readily absorbed by the skin and is used as a base for relatively nongreasy creams and ointments. It also acts as a solvent for many medications that need to be applied to the skin. Isopropyl myristate is an ingredient or base of several *emollient skin preparations used for treating dry skin conditions.

Proprietary preparations: DERMOL (combined with liquid paraffin); DIPROBATH (combined with light liquid paraffin); EMULSIDERM (combined with benzalkonium chloride); HYDROMOL EMOLLIENT (combined with light liquid paraffin).

Isopto Alkaline (Alcon Laboratories) *See* HYPROMELLOSE.

Isopto Atropine (Alcon Laboratories) *See* ATROPINE SULPHATE.

Isopto Carbachol (Alcon Laboratories) A proprietary combination of *carbachol (a cholinergic drug) and *hypromellose (a lubricant), used for the treatment of *glaucoma. It is available as eye drops on *prescription only.

Side effects: include blurred vision, stinging, and headache.

Precautions: see CARBACHOL.

Isopto Carpine (Alcon Laboratories) A proprietary combination of *pilocarpine (a cholinergic drug) and *hypromellose (a lubricant), used for the treatment of *glaucoma. It is available as eye drops on *prescription only.

Side effects, precautions, and interactions with other drugs: see PILOCARPINE.

Isopto Frin (Alcon Laboratories) A proprietary combination of *phenylephrine (a sympathomimetic drug) and *hypromellose (a lubricant), used for the relief of red eyes due to minor irritations. It is available as eye drops and can be obtained without a prescription, but only from pharmacies.

Precautions: the drops should not be used with soft contact lenses or by people with acute glaucoma.

Isopto Plain (Alcon Laboratories) *See* HYPROMELLOSE.

Isordil (Monmouth Pharmaceuticals) *See* ISOSORBIDE DINITRATE.

Isordil Tembids (Monmouth Pharmaceuticals) *See* ISOSORBIDE DINITRATE.

Proprietary preparations of isosorbide dinitrate

Preparation	Formulation	Availability
Cedocard Retard 20, 40	modified-release tablets (20 or 40 mg)	*P
Isocard	metered-dose transdermal spray	P
Isoket	injection	†POM
Isoket Retard 20, 40	modified-release tablets (20 or 40 mg)	P
Isordil	tablets or sublingual tablets	P
Isordil Tembids	modified-release capsules	P
Jeridin	tablets	P
Sorbichew	chewable tablets	P
Sorbid SA 20, 40	modified-release capsules (20 or 40 mg)	P
Sorbitrate	tablets	P

* P = pharmacy medicine

† POM = prescription only medicine

isosorbide dinitrate A *nitrate drug used in treatment of *angina and also as an adjunct to *cardiac glycosides and *diuretics in the treatment of congestive *heart failure. Isosorbide dinitrate is converted in the body to *isosorbide mononitrate, which is the active form of the drug. It is available as tablets to be swallowed, chewed, or dissolved sublingually (under the tongue), as *modified-release tablets or capsules, as a sublingual spray, as a transdermal spray (to be applied to the chest wall), and as an intravenous injection. Some preparations are *prescription only medicines; others can be obtained from pharmacies without a prescription. Oral preparations (unlike those of *glyceryl trinitrate) are stable and can be stored for a long time.

Side effects, precautions, and interactions with other drugs: see NITRATES.

Proprietary preparations: see table.

Proprietary preparations of isosorbide mononitrate

Preparation	Formulation	Availability
Angeze	tablets	*P
Angeze SR	modified-release tablets	P
Dynamin	tablets	P
Elantan 10	tablets (10 mg)	P
Elantan 20	tablets (20 mg)	†POM
Elantan 40	tablets (40 mg)	POM
Elantan LA	modified-release capsules	P
Imdur Durules	modified-release tablets	†POM
Isib	tablets	P
Isib 60 XL	modified-release tablets	P
Ismo	tablets	P
Ismo Retard	modified-release tablets	P
Isotard 25 XL, 40 XL, 50 XL, or 60 XL	modified-release tablets (25, 40, 50, or 60 mg)	P
MCR-50	modified-release capsules	P
Modisal XL	modified-release tablets	P
Monit	tablets	P
Monit SR	modified-release tablets	P
Mono Cedocard 10, 20, or 40	tablets (10, 20 or 40 mg)	P
Monomax SR	modified-release capsules	P
Monosorb XL 60	modified-release tablets	P

* P = pharmacy medicine

† POM = prescription only medicine

isosorbide mononitrate A *nitrate drug used in the treatment of *angina and also as an adjunct to *cardiac glycosides and *diuretics in the treatment of congestive *heart failure. It is available as tablets or capsules, in either short-acting or *modified-release formulations. Some preparations are *prescription only medicines; others can be obtained from pharmacies without a prescription. Unlike some oral preparations of *glyceryl trinitrate, isosorbide mononitrate is stable and can be stored for a long time.

Side effects, precautions, and interactions with other drugs: see NITRATES.
Proprietary preparations: see table.

Isotard (Ashbourne Pharmaceuticals) *See* ISOSORBIDE MONONITRATE.

Isotonic Gentamicin Injection (Baxter Healthcare) *See* GENTAMICIN.

isotretinoin A *retinoid used topically for the treatment of *acne. It may also be given by mouth, under the supervision of a hospital specialist, for severe cases of acne that are unresponsive to antibiotics. Isotretinoin is available, on *prescription only, as a gel or capsules.

Side effects: the gel may cause redness, local irritation, and peeling of the skin at the start of treatment, but this should not last; it may cause changes in skin pigmentation and make the skin more sensitive to light. The capsules commonly cause dryness, flaking, and thinning of the skin, dryness of the nose (with nosebleeds), throat, and eyes, and pain in the joints and muscles. Other side effects may include visual impairment (which should be reported to a doctor immediately), hair loss, nausea, headache, drowsiness, sweating, mood changes, and menstrual irregularities.

Precautions: the gel should not be used on damaged or sunburnt skin, by people with eczema or a personal or family history of skin cancer, or by pregnant women. It should not come into contact with the eyes, nostrils, or mouth, and exposure of treated skin to ultraviolet light (including excessive sunlight) should be avoided. The gel should not be used with other topical preparations (e.g. *keratolytics) that may irritate the skin. The capsules should not be taken by women who are pregnant or breastfeeding, and contraception must be used for one month before and during treatment and for at least one month after treatment (*see* RETINOIDS). They should not be taken by people with liver or kidney disease. Tests to monitor liver function and to measure concentrations of fats in the blood should be performed before and during treatment. Donation of blood should be avoided during treatment and for at least one month after stopping treatment.

Interactions with other drugs:
   Vitamin A: the risk of vitamin A poisoning is increased if supplements are taken with isotretinoin capsules.

Proprietary preparations: Isotrex (gel); Roaccutane (capsules); ISOTREXIN (combined with erythromycin).

Isotrex (Stiefel Laboratories) *See* ISOTRETINOIN.

Isotrexin (Stiefel Laboratories) A proprietary combination of *isotretinoin (a retinoid) and *erythromycin (an antibiotic), used for the treatment of mild to moderate acne. A *prescription only medicine, it is available as a gel to be applied to the skin.

Side effects, precautions, and interactions with other drugs: see ISOTRETINOIN.

Isovorin (Wyeth Laboratories) *See* FOLINIC ACID.

ispaghula husk A natural fibre used as a *bulk-forming laxative. It is also used to lower plasma *cholesterol concentrations in the treatment of primary hypercholesterolaemia (*see* HYPERLIPIDAEMIA). Ispaghula is

available as powder or granules and can be obtained without a
prescription, but only from pharmacies.

Side effects: include flatulence and abdominal distension.

Precautions: ispaghula should not be taken by people who have difficulty
in swallowing, intestinal obstruction, impacted faeces, or colonic atony (a
poorly functioning large bowel). Preparations containing ispaghula
should always be taken with plenty of fluid and should not be taken
immediately before going to bed.

Proprietary preparations: Fybogel; Fybozest Orange (for
hypercholesterolaemia); Konsyl; Isogel; Regulan; FYBOGEL MEBEVERINE
(combined with mebeverine hydrochloride).

isradipine A class II *calcium antagonist used for the treatment of
*hypertension. It is available as tablets on *prescription only.

Side effects and precautions: see CALCIUM ANTAGONISTS;
ANTIHYPERTENSIVE DRUGS.

Interactions with other drugs:

  Antiepileptic drugs: the effects of isradipine are reduced by phenytoin,
    carbamazepine, phenobarbitone <phenobarbital>, and primidone.

  See also CALCIUM ANTAGONISTS.

Proprietary preparation: Prescal.

Istin (Pfizer) *See* AMLODIPINE.

itraconazole A triazole *antifungal drug that is used to treat a wide
variety of fungal infections, including tinea (ringworm) of the skin,
scalp, and nails, and candidiasis (thrush), and to prevent fungal
infections in people whose immune systems are functioning poorly,
such as AIDS patients and the recipients of transplants. Itraconazole is
taken by mouth, as capsules or a liquid, and is available on *prescription
only.

Side effects: include nausea, abdominal pain, indigestion, constipation
(people taking the liquid may have diarrhoea), headache, dizziness,
menstrual disorders, and allergic reactions.

Precautions: itraconazole should not be taken by people with a history of
liver disease or kidney disease or by women who are pregnant or
breastfeeding.

Interactions with other drugs:

  Antacids: reduce the absorption of itraconazole.

  Anticoagulants: the effects of warfarin and nicoumalone
    <acenocoumarol> are enhanced.

  Astemizole: should not be taken with itraconazole because of the risk of
    irregular heart rhythms.

  Cisapride: should not be taken with itraconazole because of the risk of
    irregular heart rhythms.

  Cyclosporin: its plasma concentration (and therefore side effects) is
    increased by itraconazole.

Digoxin: its plasma concentration (and therefore side effects) is increased by itraconazole.

H₂-receptor antagonists: reduce the absorption of itraconazole.

Midazolam: its plasma concentration (and therefore side effects) is increased by itraconazole.

Phenytoin: reduces the plasma concentration of itraconazole.

Simvastatin: there is an increased risk of myopathy (muscle disease) and therefore simvastatin should not be used with itraconazole.

Terfenadine: should not be taken with itraconazole because of the risk of irregular heart rhythms.

Proprietary preparations: Sporanox; Sporanox Liquid; Sporanox Pulse.

Jackson's All Fours (Anglian Pharma) *See* GUAIPHENESIN
<GUAIFENESIN>.

Japp's Health Salts (Roche Products) A proprietary combination of
*sodium bicarbonate, sodium potassium tartrate, and *tartaric acid, used
as an *antacid for the relief of indigestion and heartburn and as a mild
*laxative. It is freely available *over the counter as a powder to be
dissolved to make an effervescent drink.
Precautions and interactions with other drugs: see ANTACIDS.

J Collis Browne's Mixture (Seton Scholl Healthcare) A proprietary
combination of *morphine (which reduces gut motility) and
*peppermint oil (an antispasmodic), used to treat diarrhoea and stomach
upsets (*see* ANTIDIARRHOEAL DRUGS). It can be obtained from pharmacies
without a prescription.
Side effects and interactions with other drugs: see MORPHINE; OPIOIDS.
Precautions: the mixture should not be given to children under six years
old. *See also* MORPHINE.

J Collis Browne's Tablets (Seton Scholl Healthcare) A proprietary
combination of *calcium carbonate (an antacid), *kaolin (an adsorbent),
and *morphine (which reduces gut motility), used for the treatment of
diarrhoea and stomach upsets (*see* ANTIDIARRHOEAL DRUGS). It can be
obtained without a prescription, but only from pharmacies.
Side effects and interactions with other drugs: see MORPHINE.
Precautions: these tablets should not be taken by children under six
years old. *See* KAOLIN; MORPHINE.

Jectofer (AstraZeneca) *See* IRON SORBITOL–CITRIC ACID COMPLEX.

Jeridin (APS-Berk) *See* ISOSORBIDE DINITRATE.

Jomethid XL (Cox Pharmaceuticals) *See* KETOPROFEN.

Joy-rides (Stafford-Miller) *See* HYOSCINE HYDROBROMIDE.

Junifen (Crookes Healthcare) *See* IBUPROFEN.

Junior Meltus Dry Cough and Catarrh (Seton Scholl Healthcare) A
proprietary combination of *dextromethorphan (a cough suppressant)
and *pseudoephedrine (a decongestant), used for the relief of dry coughs
accompanied by congestion of the upper airways. It is available as a
liquid without a prescription, but only from pharmacies.

Junior Meltus Expectorant

338

Side effects, and interactions with other drugs: *see* DEXTROMETHORPHAN; OPIOIDS; EPHEDRINE HYDROCHLORIDE; DECONGESTANTS.

Precautions: this medicine should not be taken by children under two years old. *See also* OPIOIDS; EPHEDRINE HYDROCHLORIDE; DECONGESTANTS.

Junior Meltus Expectorant (Seton Scholl Healthcare) A proprietary combination of *guaiphenesin <guaifenesin> (an expectorant) and *cetylpyridinium (an antiseptic), used to relieve coughs and catarrh associated with colds, influenza, and throat infections in children. **Junior Meltus Sugar and Colour Free Expectorant** is a similar formulation. Both are available as liquids and may be bought freely *over the counter.

Side effects and precautions: *see* GUAIPHENESIN <GUAIFENESIN>. Neither medicine is recommended for children under one year old, except on medical advice.

juniper berry oil An oil extracted from juniper berries. It relieves flatulence, has a *diuretic action, and has antiseptic and anti-inflammatory properties. Juniper berry oil is an ingredient of remedies for treating infections of the urinary tract and of topical preparations for the relief of muscle and joint pain. Combined with other aromatic oils, it is included in inhalations and pastilles to relieve congestion due to colds and catarrh.

Side effects and precautions: prolonged use can irritate the stomach and high doses can damage the kidneys.

Proprietary preparations: JUNO JUNIPAH SALTS (combined with sodium sulphate, sodium phosphate, and sodium bicarbonate); OLBAS OIL (combined with eucalyptus oil, menthol, cajuput oil, clove oil, and oil of wintergreen); OLBAS PASTILLES (combined with eucalyptus oil, menthol, peppermint oil, clove oil, and oil of wintergreen).

juniper tar *See* CADE OIL.

Juno Junipah Salts (Torbet Laboratories) A proprietary combination of *sodium sulphate (an osmotic laxative), sodium phosphate (a *phosphate laxative), *sodium bicarbonate, and *juniper berry oil (which relieves flatulence), used for the treatment of constipation. It is freely available *over the counter in the form of an effervescent powder.

Side effects and precautions: *see* OSMOTIC LAXATIVES; JUNIPER BERRY OIL.

JW Cetrimide Cream (Quinoderm) *See* CETRIMIDE.

Kabikinase (Pharmacia & Upjohn) *See* STREPTOKINASE.

Kalspare (Dominion Pharma) A proprietary combination of
*chlorthalidone <chlortalidone> (a thiazide-like diuretic) and
*triamterene (a potassium-sparing diuretic), used for the treatment of
*hypertension or *oedema associated with heart failure, liver disease, or
kidney disease. It is available as tablets on *prescription only.
Side effects, precautions, and interactions with other drugs: see THIAZIDE
DIURETICS; POTASSIUM-SPARING DIURETICS.
See also ANTIHYPERTENSIVE DRUGS; DIURETICS.

Kalten (AstraZeneca) A proprietary combination of
*hydrochlorothiazide (a thiazide diuretic), *amiloride hydrochloride (a
potassium-sparing diuretic), and *atenolol (a cardioselective beta blocker),
used for the treatment of mild to moderate *hypertension. It is available
as tablets on *prescription only.
Side effects, precautions, and interactions with other drugs: see THIAZIDE
DIURETICS; POTASSIUM-SPARING DIURETICS; BETA BLOCKERS.
See also ANTIHYPERTENSIVE DRUGS; DIURETICS.

Kamillosan (Norgine) A proprietary preparation consisting of extracts
of chamomile (camomile) in a base containing purified *lanolin and
*yellow soft paraffin, used as an *emollient for the relief of sore nipples,
napkin rash, and chapped hands. It is freely available *over the counter
in the form of an ointment.

kanamycin An *aminoglycoside antibiotic whose use has declined
since it has been superseded by other aminoglycosides. It is given as an
*intramuscular or *intravenous injection and is available on
*prescription only.
Side effects, precautions, and interactions with other drugs: see
GENTAMICIN.
Proprietary preparation: Kannasyn.

Kannasyn (Sanofi Winthrop) *See* KANAMYCIN.

Kao-C (Torbet Laboratories) A proprietary combination of *calcium
carbonate (an antacid) and *kaolin (an adsorbent), used for the treatment
of diarrhoea in children (*see* ANTIDIARRHOEAL DRUGS). It is freely available
*over the counter in the form of a sugar-free suspension.
Precautions: Kao-C is not recommended for treating acute diarrhoea and
should not be given to children under one year old. *See also* KAOLIN.

Kaodene (Knoll) A proprietary combination of *codeine phosphate (which reduces gut motility) and light *kaolin (an adsorbent), used for the treatment of diarrhoea. It is freely available *over the counter as a suspension.

Side effects and interactions with other drugs: see CODEINE; OPIOIDS.

Precautions: this medicine is not recommended for treating acute diarrhoea and should not be given to children under five years old. *See also* CODEINE; KAOLIN.

kaolin A purified and powdered adsorbent white clay. It adsorbs fluid and irritants from the gut and is used in the treatment of diarrhoea, but is not recommended for acute diarrhoea. It is used alone (as an oral suspension) or in combination with other ingredients, including morphine, in a variety of *antidiarrhoeal preparations. Kaolin is also used in dusting powders to adsorb moisture and as an ingredient in poultices. It is available as a suspension or an ingredient in tablets, pastes, and powders, and can be obtained without a prescription.

Precautions: kaolin should not be taken by people with gastrointestinal obstruction.

Proprietary preparations: Enterocalm; DE WITT'S ANTACID POWDER (combined with sodium bicarbonate, magnesium carbonate, magnesium trisilicate, calcium carbonate, and peppermint oil); ENTEROSAN (combined with belladonna extract and morphine); J COLLIS BROWNE'S TABLETS (combined with calcium carbonate and morphine); KAO-C (combined with calcium carbonate); KAODENE (combined with codeine phosphate); MOORLAND (combined with aluminium hydroxide, bismuth, magnesium trisilicate, magnesium carbonate, and calcium carbonate); OPAZIMES (combined with aluminium hydroxide, belladonna extract, and morphine).

Kapake, **Kapake Insts** (Galen) *See* CO-CODAMOL.

Kaplon (APS-Berk) *See* CAPTOPRIL.

Karvol (Crookes Healthcare) A proprietary combination of levomenthol (*see* MENTHOL), *chlorbutol <chlorobutanol> (an antiseptic), *terpineol, *thymol, *pumilio pine oil, and pine oil sylvestris in the form of capsules or drops, used for the relief of nasal congestion. The contents of the capsules or the drops are placed on a handkerchief or added to hot water, and the vapour is inhaled. Karvol preparations are freely available *over the counter.

Kay-Cee-L (Geistlich Sons) *See* POTASSIUM CHLORIDE.

Kefadim (Eli Lilly & Co) *See* CEFTAZIDIME.

Kefadol (Dista) *See* CEPHAMANDOLE <CEFAMANDOLE>.

Keflex (Eli Lilly & Co) *See* CEPHALEXIN <CEFALEXIN>.

Kefzol (Eli Lilly & Co) *See* CEPHAZOLIN <CEFAZOLIN>.

Kelfizine W (Pharmacia & Upjohn) *See* SULFAMETOPYRAZINE.

Kemadrin (GlaxoWellcome) *See* PROCYCLIDINE.

Kemicetine (Pharmacia & Upjohn) *See* CHLORAMPHENICOL.

Kenalog (Bristol-Myers Squibb) *See* TRIAMCINOLONE ACETONIDE.

Kentene (Kent Pharmaceuticals) *See* PIROXICAM.

keratolytics Drugs that cause softening and swelling of the cells at the surface of the skin, so that the outer layer of the skin peels off or can easily be removed. Keratolytics are used to remove thickened and horny patches of skin or scaly areas produced by *eczema or *psoriasis. They are also used in the treatment of acne, warts, and corns. Keratolytics include *salicylic acid, *benzoic acid, *benzoyl peroxide, *coal tar, *tar, *resorcinol, and *sulphur. **Caustics** are drugs that are applied to the skin to destroy tissue. Used for treating warts and corns, they include *silver nitrate, *podophyllum, *podophyllotoxin, *formaldehyde, and *glutaraldehyde.

Keri (Bristol-Myers Squibb) *See* LIQUID PARAFFIN.

Kerlone (Lorex Synthélabo) *See* BETAXOLOL HYDROCHLORIDE.

Ketil CR (Tillomed Laboratories) *See* KETOPROFEN.

Ketocid (Trinity Pharmaceuticals) *See* KETOPROFEN.

ketoconazole A powerful imidazole *antifungal drug used for the treatment of fungal infections and to prevent fungal infections in those whose immune systems are functioning poorly (such as AIDS patients and the recipients of transplants). Ketoconazole is particularly useful for treating resistant candidiasis (thrush), gastrointestinal infections, and infections of the skin, nails, and scalp. It is available on *prescription only as tablets and a suspension for oral use and as a cream or shampoo for topical application; shampoos for the prevention and treatment of dandruff can be bought without a prescription.
Side effects: when taken by mouth, side effects include nausea, vomiting, abdominal pain, headache, rashes, itching, and (more rarely) tingling sensations, dizziness, hair loss, breast enlargement in men, and liver damage. When applied topically it can irritate the skin.
Precautions: ketoconazole tablets or suspension should not be taken by people with liver disease or by women who are pregnant or

breastfeeding. Liver function may need to be monitored during treatment.

Interactions with other drugs:

Antacids: reduce the absorption of ketoconazole.

Anticoagulants: the effects of warfarin and nicoumalone <acenocoumarol> are enhanced.

Antimuscarinics: reduce the absorption of ketoconazole.

Astemizole: should not be taken with ketoconazole because of the risk of irregular heart rhythms.

Cisapride: should not be taken with ketoconazole because of the risk of irregular heart rhythms.

Indinavir: the dosage of this drug should be reduced.

Midazolam: its sedative effect is increased.

Oral contraceptives: their effect may be reduced.

Phenytoin: reduces the plasma concentration of ketoconazole.

Rifampicin: the plasma concentrations of both drugs are reduced.

Terfenadine: should not be taken with ketoconazole because of the risk of irregular heart rhythms.

Proprietary preparations: Neutrogena Long Lasting Dandruff Control Shampoo; Nizoral; Nizoral Suspension; Nizoral Dandruff Shampoo; Nizoral Shampoo.

ketoprofen An *NSAID used for the treatment of pain and mild inflammation in rheumatoid arthritis and other disorders of muscles or joints. It is also used to relieve period pains, acute gout, sciatica, and pain occurring after orthopaedic surgery. It is available, on *prescription only, as capsules, *modified-release capsules, suppositories, an injection, and a gel for topical application (some gel formulations are also available without a prescription).

Side effects: *see* NSAIDS. Suppositories may cause local irritation; there may be pain at the site of the injection.

Precautions and interactions with other drugs: *see* NSAIDS.

Proprietary preparations: Boots Muscular Pain Relief Gel; Fenoket (modified-release capsules); Jomethid XL (modified-release capsules); Ketil CR (modified-release capsules); Ketocid (modified-release capsules); Ketoprofen CR (modified-release capsules); Ketotard 200 XL (modified-release capsules); Ketovail (modified-release capsules); Ketozip XL (modified-release capsules); Larafen CR (modified-release capsules); Orudis (capsules and suppositories); Oruvail (modified-release capsules, gel, and injection); Powergel (gel); Solpaflex Gel.

Ketoprofen CR (Du Pont Pharmaceuticals) *See* KETOPROFEN.

ketorolac trometamol An *NSAID used for the treatment of moderate to severe postoperative pain. It is applied to the eye to prevent or reduce inflammation following eye surgery. Ketorolac is available, on *prescription only, as tablets, an injection, or eye drops.

Side effects: severe allergic reactions have been reported when ketorolac is given by mouth or injection; these include rash, constriction of the airways, and swelling of the larynx (*see* ANAPHYLAXIS). *See also* NSAIDS.

Precautions: see NSAIDS.

Interactions with other drugs: see NSAIDS. In addition:

Anticoagulants: should not be used with injections of ketorolac as the risk of bleeding is increased.

Lithium: should not be used with ketorolac tablets or injection, which reduce its excretion and therefore increase the risk of it having adverse effects.

Oxpentifylline <pentoxifylline>: should not be used with ketorolac tablets or injection since it increases the risk of ketorolac causing bleeding.

Probenecid: should not be used with ketorolac tablets or injection, which delay its excretion and therefore increase the risk of it having adverse effects.

Proprietary preparations: Acular (eye drops); Toradol (tablets and injection).

Ketotard 200 XL (Ashbourne Pharmaceuticals) *See* KETOPROFEN.

ketotifen A drug that is thought to prevent the release of *histamine, an important mediator of allergic responses (*see* ANTIHISTAMINES). It is used for the treatment of hay fever and allergic conjunctivitis. Ketotifen is available, on *prescription only, as capsules, tablets, or an elixir.

Side effects: include drowsiness, impaired reactions, dry mouth, and occasionally excitement and weight gain.

Precautions: alcohol enhances its sedative effect. Ketotifen should not be taken by women who are pregnant or breastfeeding. Dosage should be reduced gradually over 2–4 weeks at the end of treatment.

Interactions with other drugs:

Metformin: there is a risk of blood disorders.

Proprietary preparation: Zaditen.

Ketovail (APS-Berk) *See* KETOPROFEN.

Ketovite (Paines & Byrne) A proprietary combination of vitamins used to prevent vitamin deficiency in people with metabolic disorders. It is available as tablets or a liquid; these can be taken together as a vitamin supplement by people on special diets that lack vitamins. The tablets, which are available on *prescription only, contain ascorbic acid (*see* VITAMIN C), members of the *vitamin B complex (including inositol, riboflavin, and thiamine), and alpha tocopheryl acetate (*see* VITAMIN E). The liquid contains *vitamin A, *ergocalciferol (vitamin D_2), and the B vitamins choline chloride and cyanocobalamin; it can be obtained from pharmacies without a prescription.

Ketozip XL (Ashbourne Pharmaceuticals) *See* KETOPROFEN.

Kiflone (APS-Berk) *See* CEPHALEXIN <CEFALEXIN>.

Kinidin Durules (AstraZeneca) *See* QUINIDINE BISULPHATE.

Klaricid, **Klaricid XL** (Abbott Laboratories) *See* CLARITHROMYCIN.

Klean-Prep (Norgine) A proprietary combination of macrogol '3350' (*see* POLYETHYLENE GLYCOLS), anhydrous *sodium sulphate, *sodium bicarbonate, *sodium chloride, and *potassium chloride, used to evacuate the bowel before investigative procedures or surgery. It is available as an oral powder to be mixed with water and can be obtained without a prescription, but only from pharmacies.
Side effects and precautions: see BOWEL-CLEANSING SOLUTIONS; POLYETHYLENE GLYCOLS.

Kliofem (Novo Nordisk Pharmaceutical) A proprietary combination of *oestradiol <estradiol> and *norethisterone, used as continuous combined *hormone replacement therapy for the relief of menopausal symptoms and prevention of osteoporosis in women who have not had a hysterectomy and who have not had a period for a year. It is available as tablets on *prescription only.
Side effects, precautions, and interactions with other drugs: see HORMONE REPLACEMENT THERAPY.

Kliovance (Novo Nordisk Pharmaceutical) A proprietary combination of *oestradiol <estradiol> and *norethisterone, used as continuous combined *hormone replacement therapy for the relief of menopausal symptoms in women who have not had a hysterectomy and who have not had a period for a year. It is available as tablets on *prescription only.
Side effects, precautions, and interactions with other drugs: see HORMONE REPLACEMENT THERAPY.

Kloref (Cox Pharmaceuticals) A proprietary combination of *potassium chloride, *betaine hydrochloride, *potassium benzoate, and *potassium bicarbonate, in the form of tablets that dissolve in water to produce an effervescent drink. **Kloref-S** is a similar preparation in the form of soluble granules. Both are used as *potassium supplements and can be obtained without a prescription, but only from pharmacies.
Side effects, precautions, and interactions with other drugs: see POTASSIUM.

Kogenate (Bayer) *See* FACTOR VIII.

Kolanticon Gel (Hoechst Marion Roussel) A proprietary combination of *dicyclomine <dicycloverine> hydrochloride (an antispasmodic), *aluminium hydroxide and light *magnesium oxide (antacids), and activated *dimethicone <dimeticone> (an antifoaming agent), used for the treatment of gut spasm, excess stomach acid, flatulence, and peptic ulceration. It is available as a sugar-free gel and can be obtained without a prescription, but only from pharmacies.

Side effects: *see* ANTIMUSCARINIC DRUGS.

Precautions: Kolanticon should not be taken by people with gastrointestinal obstruction, severe ulcerative colitis, or myasthenia gravis. It should be used with caution by people with glaucoma or an enlarged prostate gland.

Konakion, Konakion MM (Roche Products) *See* PHYTOMENADIONE.

Konsyl (Eastern Pharmaceuticals) *See* ISPAGHULA HUSK.

Kwells (Roche Products) *See* HYOSCINE HYDROBROMIDE.

Kytril (SmithKline Beecham Pharmaceuticals) *See* GRANISETRON.

L

labetalol hydrochloride A combined *alpha and *beta blocker used in the treatment of *hypertension. It is commonly used for the treatment of hypertension during late pregnancy, although it does not have a *licence for this. It is available on *prescription only as tablets or as a solution for injection.

Side effects: include low blood pressure on standing, tiredness, weakness, headache, rash, tingling of the scalp, difficulty in passing urine, stomach pain, nausea, vomiting, and liver damage (in which case treatment may need to be stopped).

Precautions: labetalol should not be given to people with certain liver disorders as it has the potential for causing liver damage. *See also* ANTIHYPERTENSIVE DRUGS.

Interactions with other drugs: see BETA BLOCKERS.

Proprietary preparation: Trandate.

Labiton (Laboratories for Applied Biology) A proprietary combination of *caffeine, kola nut dried extract, and *thiamine hydrochloride (vitamin B_1) in the form of a *tonic, used to stimulate the appetite. It is freely available *over the counter and cannot be prescribed on the NHS.

Labosept (Laboratories for Applied Biology) *See* DEQUALINIUM CHLORIDE.

lacidipine A class II *calcium antagonist used in the treatment of *hypertension. It is available as tablets on *prescription only.

Side effects and interactions with other drugs: see CALCIUM ANTAGONISTS.

Precautions: lacidipine should not be taken by people who have had a heart attack within the previous month or by women who are pregnant or breastfeeding. *See also* CALCIUM ANTAGONISTS; ANTIHYPERTENSIVE DRUGS.

Proprietary preparation: Motens.

Lacri-Lube (Allergan) A proprietary combination of *white soft paraffin, *liquid paraffin, and wool fat (anhydrous *lanolin), used for the lubrication of dry eyes. It is available as an eye ointment and can be obtained without a prescription, but only from pharmacies.

lactic acid A weak acid that has mild *antibiotic properties and is also a *keratolytic. It is used, usually in combination with *salicylic acid, for the removal of warts. It is also included as an ingredient in preparations for the treatment of skin conditions.

Proprietary preparations: CALMURID (combined with urea); CALMURID HC (combined with hydrocortisone and urea); CUPLEX (combined with salicylic acid); DUOFILM (combined with salicylic acid); LACTICARE (combined with sodium pyrrolidone carboxylate); SALACTOL (combined with salicylic acid); SALATAC (combined with salicylic acid).

Lacticare (Stiefel Laboratories) A proprietary combination of *lactic acid and *sodium pyrrolidone carboxylate, used as an *emollient lotion for the relief of chronic dry skin conditions. It is freely available *over the counter.

lactitol An *osmotic laxative, similar to *lactulose, used for treating constipation. It has a delayed action and the laxative response may not occur until 2–3 days after administration. Lactitol is available as a powder to be sprinkled on to food or mixed in a drink and can be obtained without a prescription, but only from pharmacies.
Side effects and precautions: see LACTULOSE.

Lactugal (Galen) *See* LACTULOSE.

lactulose An *osmotic laxative used for the treatment of constipation. Lactulose is a semisynthetic derivative of sugar that is not absorbed from the gut; it may take up to 48 hours to work. It is available as a solution or powder and can be obtained without a prescription, but only from pharmacies. Some preparations cannot be prescribed on the NHS.
Side effects: lactulose may cause flatulence, cramps, and abdominal discomfort.
Precautions: lactulose should not be taken by people with intestinal obstruction or galactosaemia (a congenital inability to metabolize certain sugars).
Proprietary preparations: Duphalac; Duphalac Dry (powder); Lactugal; Laxose; Osmolax; Regulose.
See also LACTITOL.

Ladropen (APS-Berk) *See* FLUCLOXACILLIN.

Lamictal (GlaxoWellcome) *See* LAMOTRIGINE.

Lamisil, **Lamisil Cream** (Novartis Pharmaceuticals) *See* TERBINAFINE.

lamivudine An *antiviral drug that prevents retrovirus replication: it is a reverse transcriptase inhibitor. Lamivudine is used, usually in combination with other antiviral drugs, to delay the progression of disease in *HIV-infected patients. It is available, on *prescription only, as tablets or a solution.
Side effects: include nausea, vomiting, diarrhoea, abdominal pain, cough, headache, insomnia, malaise, muscle and joint pain, fatigue, and (rarely) pancreatitis.
Precautions: lamivudine should be used with caution in people with impaired kidney function (the dosage is usually reduced). It should not be

taken by women who are breastfeeding and is generally not recommended in the first three months of pregnancy.

Interactions with other drugs:
   Trimethoprim: increases the plasma concentration (and therefore side effects) of lamivudine.

Proprietary preparations: Epivir; COMBIVIR (combined with zidovudine).

lamotrigine An *anticonvulsant drug used for the treatment of partial seizures and generalized tonic-clonic seizures. It is available, on *prescription only, as tablets or dispersible tablets.

Side effects: include rashes, fever, malaise, influenza-like symptoms, drowsiness, and (rarely) liver disorders.

Precautions: people taking lamotrigine should be closely monitored initially: liver, kidney, and blood-clotting functions should be assessed. If rashes, influenza-like symptoms, or drowsiness occur, or if the drug becomes less effective in controlling seizures, treatment may need to be stopped. When stopping medication, lamotrigine should be withdrawn gradually over a two-week period.

Interactions with other drugs:
   Other anticonvulsants: taking two or more anticonvulsants together may enhance their toxicity.

Proprietary preparation: Lamictal.

Lamprene (Novartis Pharmaceuticals) *See* CLOFAZIMINE.

Lanacane Creme (Combe International) *See* BENZOCAINE.

Lanacort (Combe International) *See* HYDROCORTISONE.

lanolin (hydrous wool fat) A mixture of **wool fat** (obtained from the wool of sheep) and 25–30% water. Wool fat itself is also called **anhydrous lanolin**. Lanolin and wool fat are used as a base for creams and as *emollients: when mixed with vegetable oil or soft paraffin (*see* YELLOW SOFT PARAFFIN) they form creams that are readily absorbed.

Side effects: lanolin and wool fat may cause allergic reactions. Highly purified lanolin causes fewer allergic reactions.

Lanoxin, Lanoxin-PG (GlaxoWellcome) *See* DIGOXIN.

lanreotide A long-acting *analogue of **somatostatin**, a hormone that is produced in the brain, gastrointestinal tract, and pancreas and inhibits the release of *growth hormone. It is used for the short-term treatment of patients awaiting surgery for acromegaly (a condition due to excessive secretion of growth hormone by a tumour of the pituitary gland) and for the long-term treatment of acromegaly that does not respond to surgery, *dopamine receptor antagonists, or radiotherapy. It can also be used as an interim treatment until radiotherapy has been effective in reducing concentrations of growth hormone. Lanreotide is also used to inhibit the secretions (and thus relieve the symptoms) of hormone-secreting tumours of the gastrointestinal tract. It is available as an injection on *prescription only.

Side effects: include pain, stinging, and swelling at the injection site, loss of appetite, nausea, vomiting, and abdominal pain; gallstones may develop with long-term treatment.

Precautions: lanreotide should not be given to women who are pregnant or breastfeeding. Diabetic patients may need to reduce their dosage of insulin or oral antidiabetic drugs. Gall-bladder function should be monitored. Lanreotide should be withdrawn gradually at the end of treatment.

Interactions with other drugs:

Antidiabetic drugs: doses of these may need to be reduced (see precautions).

Cyclosporin: lanreotide reduces the absorption of cyclosporin.

Proprietary preparation: Somatuline LA.

lansoprazole A *proton pump inhibitor used for the treatment of reflux oesophagitis, gastric and duodenal ulcers (including those associated with *Helicobacter pylori* infection and the use of *NSAIDs), Zollinger-Ellison syndrome, and other kinds of *acid-peptic disease. It is available as capsules or a suspension on *prescription only.

Side effects: include headache, dizziness, fatigue, malaise, diarrhoea, constipation, sore throat, rashes, and muscle aches.

Precautions: *see* PROTON PUMP INHIBITORS.

Interactions with other drugs:

Antifungal drugs: the absorption of ketoconazole and itraconazole may be reduced by lansoprazole.

Oral contraceptives: their metabolism may be accelerated (and therefore their effects reduced) by lansoprazole.

Phenytoin: lansoprazole should be used with caution in people taking phenytoin.

Warfarin: lansoprazole should be used with caution in people taking warfarin.

Proprietary preparation: Zoton.

Lanvis (GlaxoWellcome) *See* THIOGUANINE <TIOGUANINE>.

Laractone (Lagap Pharmaceuticals) *See* SPIRONOLACTONE.

Larafen CR (Lagap Pharmaceuticals) *See* KETOPROFEN.

Larapam (Lagap Pharmaceuticals) *See* PIROXICAM.

Largactil (Hawgreen) *See* CHLORPROMAZINE HYDROCHLORIDE.

Lariam (Roche Products) *See* MEFLOQUINE.

Lasikal (Hoechst Marion Roussel) A proprietary combination of
*frusemide <furosemide> (a loop diuretic) and *potassium chloride in the
form of *modified-release tablets, used for the treatment of *oedema
associated with congestive *heart failure, liver disease, or kidney disease.
It is available on *prescription only.
Side effects, precautions, and interactions with other drugs: see LOOP
DIURETICS.
See also DIURETICS.

Lasilactone (Hoechst Marion Roussel) A proprietary combination of
*frusemide <furosemide> (a loop diuretic) and *spironolactone (a
potassium-sparing diuretic), used for the treatment of *oedema
associated with congestive *heart failure, liver disease, or kidney disease.
It is available as capsules on *prescription only.
Side effects, precautions, and interactions with other drugs: see LOOP
DIURETICS; POTASSIUM-SPARING DIURETICS.
See also DIURETICS.

Lasix (Borg Medicare) *See* FRUSEMIDE <FUROSEMIDE>.

Lasma (Pharmax) *See* THEOPHYLLINE.

Lasonil (Bayer) A proprietary combination of *heparinoids and
*hyaluronidase, used to improve the circulation and reduce the swelling
and inflammation of bruises, sprains and similar injuries, chilblains, and
varicose veins. It is available as an ointment and can be obtained without
a prescription, but only from pharmacies.
Side effects and precautions: see HYALURONIDASE.

Lasoride (Borg Medicare) *See* CO-AMILOFRUSE.

Lassar's paste *See* DITHRANOL.

latanoprost A *prostaglandin analogue that is used to reduce the
pressure inside the eye in the treatment of open-angle (chronic)
*glaucoma and raised blood pressure in the eye. It acts by increasing the
outflow of aqueous fluid from the eye. Latanoprost is used for treating
people who have not responded to or cannot tolerate other drugs. It is
available as eye drops on *prescription only.
Side effects: latanoprost may increase the brown pigment in the iris, and
people should be warned to notice any changes in eye colour. The eyes
may become irritated or bloodshot, and the eyelashes may become
darker, longer, and thicker.
Precautions: latanoprost should be used with caution by people with
asthma and is not recommended for women who are pregnant or
breastfeeding.
Proprietary preparation: Xalatan.

lauromacrogols A group of compounds that are used as *surfactants. They also have some local *antipruritic activity and are included in preparations to treat dry skin conditions or haemorrhoids.
Side effects: lauromacrogols occasionally cause allergic skin reactions.
Proprietary preparations: ANACAL (combined with heparinoid); BALNEUM PLUS CREAM (combined with urea); BALNEUM PLUS OIL (combined with soya oil).

laxatives Drugs that stimulate, or increase the frequency of, bowel evacuation (these laxatives are also called **cathartics** or **purgatives**) or that encourage the passage of a softer or bulkier stool. Laxatives should not be used for prolonged periods. Excessive use can lead to low plasma concentrations of *potassium and colonic atony (a nonfunctioning large bowel). A balanced diet with adequate fibre and fluid intake and the development of a regular bowel habit should obviate the need for laxatives in most people. However, laxatives are required when drugs are causing constipation or if bowel evacuation is necessary, for example before childbirth or surgery (*see also* BOWEL-CLEANSING SOLUTIONS). The main types of laxatives are *bulk-forming laxatives, *faecal softeners, *osmotic laxatives, and *stimulant laxatives.

Laxoberal (Boehringer Ingelheim) *See* SODIUM PICOSULPHATE <PICOSULFATE>.

Laxose (APS-Berk) *See* LACTULOSE.

LDL (low-density lipoproteins) *See* LIPOPROTEINS; CHOLESTEROL.

Ledclair (Sinclair Pharmaceuticals) *See* SODIUM CALCIUM EDETATE.

Lederfen (Wyeth Laboratories) *See* FENBUFEN.

Lederfolin (Wyeth Laboratories) *See* FOLINIC ACID.

Ledermycin (Wyeth Laboratories) *See* DEMECLOCYCLINE HYDROCHLORIDE.

Lederspan (Wyeth Laboratories) *See* TRIAMCINOLONE ACETONIDE.

Lemsip Cold + Flu Combined Relief Capsules (Reckitt & Colman) A proprietary combination of *paracetamol (an analgesic and antipyretic), *caffeine (a stimulant), and *phenylephrine (a decongestant), used to relieve the symptoms of colds and influenza, including aches and pains, nasal congestion, and fever. **Lemsip Cold + Flu Max Strength Capsules** contains higher doses of the active ingredients. Both preparations are freely available *over the counter.
Side effects and interactions with other drugs: see PHENYLEPHRINE.
Precautions: this medicine should not be given to children, except on medical advice. *See also* PARACETAMOL; CAFFEINE; PHENYLEPHRINE.

Lemsip Cold + Flu Original Lemon (Reckitt & Colman) A
proprietary combination of *paracetamol (an analgesic and antipyretic),
*phenylephrine (a decongestant), and *vitamin C, used to relieve the
symptoms of colds and influenza, including aches, pains, fevers, and
nasal congestion. Similar preparations are **Lemsip Cold + Flu Breathe
Easy** and **Lemsip Cold + Flu Blackcurrant**; **Lemsip Cold + Flu Max
Strength** contains higher doses of the active ingredients. All these
preparations are freely available *over the counter in the form of
powders.

Side effects and interactions with other drugs: see PHENYLEPHRINE.

Precautions: these medicines should not be given to children except on
medical advice. *See also* PARACETAMOL; PHENYLEPHRINE.

Lemsip Cough + Cold Chesty Cough Medicine (Reckitt &
Colman) *See* GUAIPHENESIN <GUAIFENESIN>.

Lemsip Cough + Cold Dry Cough Medicine (Reckitt & Colman) A
proprietary combination of honey and *glycerin, used as a *demulcent
for the relief of dry irritating coughs. It is freely available *over the
counter in the form of a liquid.

Lemsip Pharmacy Powercaps (Reckitt & Colman) A proprietary
combination of *ibuprofen (an NSAID) and *pseudoephedrine (a
decongestant), used to relieve the symptoms of colds and influenza,
including nasal congestion, aches and pains, headaches, sore throat, and
fever. It is available as *modified-release capsules and can be obtained
without a prescription, but only from pharmacies.

Side effects and interactions with other drugs: see NSAIDS;
DECONGESTANTS; EPHEDRINE HYDROCHLORIDE.

Precautions: these preparations should not be taken by children. *See also*
NSAIDS; DECONGESTANTS.

Lemsip Pharmacy Power + Paracetamol (Reckitt & Colman) A
proprietary combination of *paracetamol (an analgesic and antipyretic)
and *pseudoephedrine (a decongestant), used to relieve the symptoms of
colds and influenza, including nasal congestion, fever, and aches and
pains. It is available in the form of powders and can be obtained without
a prescription, but only from pharmacies.

Side effects and interactions with other drugs: see EPHEDRINE
HYDROCHLORIDE; DECONGESTANTS.

Precautions: this medicine should not be given to children, except on
medical advice. *See also* PARACETAMOL; DECONGESTANTS; EPHEDRINE
HYDROCHLORIDE.

Lemsip Sore Throat Antibacterial Lozenges (Reckitt &
Colman) *See* HEXYLRESORCINOL.

Lenium (Janssen-Cilag) *See* SELENIUM SULPHIDE.

lenograstim Recombinant human granulocyte-colony stimulating factor, a form of *granulocyte-colony stimulating factor produced by genetic engineering. It is used for the treatment of neutropenia (a decrease in the number of neutrophils, a type of white blood cell) induced by *cytotoxic drug treatment for *cancer or resulting from destruction of the bone marrow prior to bone marrow transplantation. It may be given to cancer patients who are about to undergo blood collection before aggressive treatment; neutrophil production will thus be boosted in this collected blood, which is used to replace the white cells destroyed by the treatment. Lenograstim is available as a form for injection on *prescription only; its use is restricted to specialist units.

Side effects and precautions: see FILGRASTIM.

Proprietary preparation: Granocyte.

Lentard MC (Novo Nordisk Pharmaceutical) *See* INSULIN.

Lentaron (Novartis Pharmaceuticals) *See* FORMESTANE.

Lentizol (Parke-Davis Medical) *See* AMITRIPTYLINE HYDROCHLORIDE.

lepirudin An *anticoagulant used for the prevention and treatment of *thrombosis and thromboembolism in people who have developed thrombocytopenia with *heparin therapy. It is available in a form for injection or infusion on *prescription only.

Side effects: include bleeding (*see* ANTICOAGULANTS), anaemia, fever, and allergic reactions (such as rashes).

Precautions and interactions with other drugs: lepirudin should not be given to women who are pregnant or breastfeeding and should be used with caution in people with liver or kidney disease and in people who have recently undergone major surgery. The risk of bleeding is increased if lepirudin is used with other anticoagulants, antiplatelet drugs, or fibrinolytic drugs.

Proprietary preparation: Refludan.

lercanidipine A class II *calcium antagonist used for the treatment of mild to moderate *hypertension. It is available as tablets on *prescription only.

Side effects: see CALCIUM ANTAGONISTS.

Precautions: lercanidipine should not be taken by people with unstable angina or uncontrolled heart failure, or by those who have had a heart attack within the previous month, or by women who are pregnant or breastfeeding. *See also* CALCIUM ANTAGONISTS.

Interactions with other drugs:

 Beta blockers: lercanidipine may increase the effects of propranolol and metoprolol in lowering blood pressure. *See also* CALCIUM ANTAGONISTS.

Proprietary preparation: Zanidip.

Lescol (Novartis Pharmaceuticals) *See* FLUVASTATIN.

letrozole An *aromatase inhibitor used for the treatment of advanced breast *cancer in postmenopausal women when treatment with *tamoxifen has failed. It is available as tablets on *prescription only.
Side effects: include pain in muscles or bones, headache, fatigue, indigestion, constipation, abdominal pain, diarrhoea, breathlessness, cough, chest pain, and hot flushes.
Precautions: letrozole should not be taken by women who have not reached the menopause, who are pregnant or breastfeeding, or who have liver disease. It should be used with caution in those with kidney disease.
Proprietary preparation: Femara.

Leucomax (Novartis Pharmaceuticals; Schering-Plough) *See* MOLGRAMOSTIM.

leukaemia *See* CANCER.

Leukeran (GlaxoWellcome) *See* CHLORAMBUCIL.

leukotriene receptor antagonists A class of drugs that block leukotriene receptors in the body. Leukotrienes are a group of compounds that are released from cells and cause actions that result in inflammation. They are responsible for the swelling, redness, and warmth of inflamed tissue and constriction of the airways in people with *asthma and severe hay fever. Leukotriene receptor antagonists thus prevent the inflammatory response produced by leukotrienes; the drugs of this class in current use are *montelukast and *zafirlukast, which are used in the treatment of asthma.

leuprorelin An analogue of *gonadorelin that is used for the treatment of *endometriosis. It is also used to treat advanced prostate cancer that depends on the male sex hormone testosterone for growth. Here leuprorelin acts by causing an initial rise in plasma concentrations of testosterone, followed by a reduction to the same low concentrations achieved by castration. It is given by intramuscular or subcutaneous injection and is available on *prescription only.
Side effects: in women, *see* GOSERELIN. In men side effects include impotence, decreased libido, and (rarely) fatigue, nausea, and irritation at the injection site; there may be bone pain and difficulty in passing urine at the start of treatment, when testosterone concentrations are high.
Precautions: *see* GOSERELIN. In men an *anti-androgen may need to be given at the start of treatment, when high concentrations of testosterone may cause adverse effects.
Proprietary preparations: Prostap SR; Prostap 3.

Leustat (Janssen-Cilag) *See* CLADRIBINE.

levobunolol hydrochloride A *beta blocker used for the treatment of chronic (open-angle) *glaucoma. It is available, on *prescription only, as eye drops – either as a solution or in single-dose preservative-free units.

Side effects: include irritation of the eyes, headache, and dizziness. The drops can trickle into the back of the nose and be swallowed, causing *systemic effects and possibly interactions with other drugs (*see* BETA BLOCKERS).

Precautions: levobunolol should be used with caution by people with diabetes, asthma or breathing problems, or heart failure and by women who are pregnant or breastfeeding.

Proprietary preparations: Betagan; Betagan Unit Dose.

levocabastine An *antihistamine used to relieve the symptoms of hay fever. It is available, on *prescription only, as a nasal spray or eye drops.

Side effects: include local irritation, blurred vision (with eye drops), headache, fatigue, and somnolence.

Precautions: levocabastine should not be used by people with severe kidney disease and should be used with caution by pregnant women. Eye drops should be used with caution by wearers of soft contact lenses.

Interactions with other drugs: *see* ANTIHISTAMINES.

Proprietary preparation: Livostin.

levodopa An *antiparkinsonian drug used to increase concentrations of *dopamine in the brain in people with idiopathic parkinsonism (i.e. parkinsonism of unknown origin). Levodopa is converted to dopamine in the body, but to be effective it must cross into the brain before conversion. However, a large proportion of levodopa is transformed to dopamine in peripheral tissues (those outside the brain), which can cause the side effects of vomiting and low blood pressure. To prevent this effect levodopa is often given in combination with *carbidopa or *benserazide. After several years of levodopa therapy patients may deteriorate, as the effectiveness of the treatment wanes, and unpredictable fluctuations in mobility can occur (the 'on-off' effect). Symptoms can usually be improved by increasing the dosage or dividing the existing daily dose into smaller and more frequent quantities. Alternatively, *modified-release preparations may be of benefit. In some cases a low protein diet may increase the absorption of levodopa. (*See also* APOMORPHINE HYDROCHLORIDE.) Levodopa is available as tablets on *prescription only.

Side effects: include nausea and vomiting, loss of appetite, involuntary abnormal movements of the limbs and face, insomnia, agitation, postural hypotension (a sudden drop in blood pressure on standing), dizziness, fast heart rate, and a reddish discoloration of the urine (which is harmless). Rarely, allergic reactions may occur.

Precautions: levodopa should be used with caution in people with lung disease, peptic ulcers, diabetes, or psychiatric illness. Those who do benefit from therapy should resume normal activities slowly. Dosage should be reduced gradually at the end of treatment. Levodopa should not be taken by pregnant women or by people who have acute glaucoma.

Interactions with other drugs:

  MAOIs: a dangerous rise in blood pressure can occur; levodopa should be avoided for at least two weeks after stopping MAOIs.

  Metoclopramide: increases the plasma concentration of levodopa.

Proprietary preparations: Madopar and Madopar CR (*see* CO-BENELDOPA); Sinemet (*see* CO-CARELDOPA).

levofloxacin A *quinolone antibiotic used for the treatment of pneumonia, acute sinusitis, chronic bronchitis, infections of the urinary tract, and skin and soft tissue infections. It is available, on *prescription only, as tablets or a solution for intravenous infusion.

Side effects and interactions with other drugs: see QUINOLONES.

Precautions: levofloxacin should be used with caution in people with kidney disease. *See also* QUINOLONES.

Proprietary preparation: Tavanic.

levomenthol *See* MENTHOL.

levomepromazine *See* METHOTRIMEPRAZINE.

levonorgestrel A synthetic *progestogen used mainly in *oral contraceptives, either in combination with an *oestrogen or as a progestogen-only preparation. It is also used in *depot contraceptives in the form of implants or an intrauterine system. The implants are flexible rods that are inserted in a fan-shaped pattern under the skin of the upper arm and release levonorgestrel for a period of up to five years. They should be fitted by a trained practitioner under local anaesthetic. The intrauterine formulation consists of an intrauterine contraceptive device (IUCD) that releases levonorgestrel for up to three years; it can be removed at any time within this period. This formulation is a more effective contraceptive than an IUCD alone and is associated with a lower incidence of pelvic inflammatory disease, a potential risk for IUCD users. Levonorgestrel is also used in *hormone replacement therapy (HRT). It is available on *prescription only.

Side effects: see ORAL CONTRACEPTIVES; PROGESTOGENS. The implants may in addition cause prolonged menstrual bleeding, an increase in body hair, and loss of hair on the scalp; there may be local reactions around the implants. The IUCD may cause pain in the lower abdomen or back and skin problems.

Precautions (with oral contraceptives and HRT): *see* ORAL CONTRACEPTIVES; PROGESTOGENS. The implants should not be used during pregnancy or by women with a history of heart or arterial disease, liver disease, undiagnosed vaginal bleeding, or breast or genital cancer. The IUCD should not be used during pregnancy or by women with undiagnosed vaginal bleeding, genital infections, arterial disease, leukaemia, or liver tumours; it should be used with caution by women with hormone-dependent cancer, heart disease, or diabetes, who are on long-term steroid therapy, or who have had an ectopic pregnancy.

Interactions with other drugs: see PROGESTOGENS.

Proprietary preparations: Microval (contraceptive pill); Mirena (IUCD); Norgeston (contraceptive pill); Norplant (implants); CYCLO-PROGYNOVA (combined with oestradiol <estradiol>); EUGYNON 30 (combined with ethinyloestradiol <ethinylestradiol>); LOGYNON and LOGYNON ED (combined with ethinyloestradiol <ethinylestradiol>); MICROGYNON 30 and MICROGYNON 30 ED (combined with ethinyloestradiol <ethinylestradiol>); NUVELLE and NUVELLE TS (combined with oestradiol <estradiol>); OVRAN and OVRAN 30 (combined with oestradiol <estradiol>); OVRANETTE (combined with oestradiol <estradiol>); TRINORDIOL (combined with ethinyloestradiol <ethinylestradiol>).

Levophed, Levophed Special (Sanofi Winthrop) *See* NORADRENALINE <NOREPINEPHRINE>.

levothyroxine sodium *See* THYROXINE SODIUM.

Lexotan (Roche Products) *See* BROMAZEPAM.

Lexpec (Rosemont Pharmaceuticals) *See* FOLIC ACID.

Lexpec with Iron-M (Rosemont Pharmaceuticals) A proprietary combination of *folic acid and ferric ammonium citrate (an *iron supplement), used to prevent deficiencies of iron and folic acid during pregnancy. It is available as a syrup on *prescription only.

Side effects, precautions, and interactions with other drugs: see IRON.

Libanil (APS-Berk) *See* GLIBENCLAMIDE.

Liberate (Scottish National Blood Transfusion Service) *See* FACTOR VIII.

Librium (Roche Products) *See* CHLORDIAZEPOXIDE.

Librofem (Novartis Consumer Health) *See* IBUPROFEN.

lice Small wingless insects that live as parasites on the skin. Lice infestations cause intense itching; scratching to relieve this may result in secondary infection. Head lice are common in schoolchildren and do not indicate poor hygiene. They can be treated with *malathion, *permethrin, *carbaryl, or *phenothrin, which kill the lice (i.e. they are **pediculicides**); some health authorities suggest that malathion should be alternated with carbaryl to prevent the development of resistance. Crab (or pubic) lice adhere to body hair (in the pubic region and armpits); they may also infest the eyelashes. Carbaryl and malathion provide effective treatment.

licence A document given to a pharmaceutical company that allows that company to market a particular drug. The company must apply for a licence to the regulatory body that issues them: in the UK this is the Medicines Control Agency (MCA); in the USA it is the Food and Drug Administration (FDA). The regulatory body issues the licence only for defined uses (called indications), which should be adhered to by the doctor prescribing the drug. However, some drugs may be given for an 'unlicensed indication'; in these circumstances the doctor not adhering to the licence may be vulnerable to litigation if anything untoward occurs due to use of the drug.

Lidifen (APS-Berk) *See* IBUPROFEN.

lidocaine *See* LIGNOCAINE.

lignocaine <lidocaine> A *local anaesthetic that is applied to parts of the body where pain relief is required or given by local injection for infiltration anaesthesia. It is a component of preparations used to treat *haemorrhoids and other causes of anal pain and itching. It is used for relieving sore throats, teething discomfort in babies, and mouth discomfort due to ulcers in adults, to numb areas of skin before injections, and to numb regions of the body before such procedures as insertion of urinary catheters, vaginal examinations, and ophthalmic procedures. It is combined with a *corticosteroid for local use in inflammatory or rheumatic conditions. Lignocaine is also a class I *anti-arrhythmic drug administered by injection for the treatment of ventricular *arrhythmias. It is available as solutions for injection (for local anaesthesia lignocaine may be combined with *adrenaline <epinephrine>) and is included in a variety of ointments, gels, creams, and other preparations for topical application. Solutions for injection are *prescription only medicines; topical preparations are usually available without a prescription.

Side effects: injections of lignocaine may cause dizziness, 'pins and needles', or drowsiness. Less often confusion and hypotension (low blood pressure) may occur.

Precautions: lignocaine injections should not be given to patients with heart block or certain other heart conditions and should be used with caution in people with liver disease, breathing difficulties, or epilepsy.

Proprietary preparations: Strepsils Pain Relief Spray; Vagisil Medicated Creme; Xylocaine (injection with or without adrenaline <epinephrine>, ointment, or spray); Xylocard (injection); ANODESYN (combined with allantoin); BETNOVATE RECTAL (combined with betamethasone and phenylephrine); BOOTS HAEMORRHOID OINTMENT (combined with zinc oxide); BRADOSOL PLUS (combined with domiphen); CALGEL (combined with cetylpyridinium); DENTINOX TEETHING GEL (combined with cetylpyridinium); DEPO-MEDRONE WITH LIDOCAINE (combined with methylprednisolone); DETTOL ANTISEPTIC PAIN RELIEF SPRAY (combined with benzalkonium chloride); EMLA (combined with prilocaine); GERMOLOIDS (combined with zinc oxide); INSTILLAGEL (combined with chlorhexidine); MEDIJEL (combined with aminacrine <aminoacridine>);

MINIMS LIGNOCAINE AND FLUORESCEIN (combined with fluorescein); PERINAL (combined with hydrocortisone); RINSTEAD TEETHING GEL (combined with cetylpyridium); STREPSILS DUAL ACTION LOZENGES (combined with dichlorobenzyl alcohol and amylmetacresol); WOODWARD'S TEETHING GEL (combined with cetylpyridinium); XYLOCAINE ANTISEPTIC GEL (combined with chlorhexidine); XYLOPROCT (combined with aluminium acetate, zinc oxide, and hydrocortisone).

Li-Liquid (Rosemont Pharmaceuticals) *See* LITHIUM CITRATE.

Limclair (Sinclair Pharmaceuticals) *See* TRISODIUM EDETATE.

linctus A syrupy liquid medicine, particularly one used in the treatment of irritating coughs.

Lingraine (Sanofi Winthrop) *See* ERGOTAMINE TARTRATE.

liniment A medicinal preparation that is rubbed onto the skin or applied on a surgical dressing. Liniments often contain camphor.

Lioresal (Novartis Pharmaceuticals) *See* BACLOFEN.

liothyronine sodium (L-triiodothyronine) A preparation of the *thyroid hormone triiodothyronine that is given to replace a lack of natural thyroid hormone and is also used for the treatment of goitre and thyroid cancer. Liothyronine has a more rapid onset and shorter duration of action than *thyroxine sodium <levothyroxine sodium>. It is available as tablets on *prescription only.
Side effects, precautions, and interactions with other drugs: see THYROXINE SODIUM <LEVOTHYROXINE SODIUM>.
Proprietary preparation: Tertroxin.

Lipantil Micro (Fournier Pharmaceuticals) *See* FENOFIBRATE.

lipid-lowering drugs (hypolipidaemic drugs) Drugs that lower the concentrations of *lipoproteins, the agents that transport *cholesterol and *triglycerides, in blood. It is advised that these drugs are given when other risk factors for coronary heart disease have been controlled or eliminated. The most important risk factors are smoking, alcohol consumption, *obesity, *diabetes, *hypertension, and inactivity. Dietary intervention is the first-line treatment of raised lipid concentrations, and adherence to a low-fat/high-fibre diet should accompany the use of lipid-lowering drugs, along with maintenance of near-ideal body weight, reduction of blood pressure, and cessation of smoking. The lipid-lowering drugs include *statins, *fibrates, *bile-acid sequestrants, *nicotinic acid and *acipimox, *omega-3 marine triglycerides, and *ispaghula.

Lipitor (Parke-Davis Medical) *See* ATORVASTATIN.

Lipobase (Yamanouchi Pharma) A proprietary combination of cetostearyl alcohol, cetomacrogol, *liquid paraffin, and *white soft paraffin, used as an *emollient for the relief of dry and itching skin conditions. It is freely available *over the counter.

Lipobay (Bayer) See CERIVASTATIN.

lipoproteins Complex molecules that transport lipids, especially *cholesterol and *triglycerides, in the blood. Lipids do not mix with water (the blood is largely water), and in order to circulate and be taken up by tissues these fatty compounds need to be 'tucked' inside larger molecules, the lipoproteins, which do mix with blood. Lipoproteins are classified according to their density; the most important lipoproteins in terms of heart disease are the **high-density lipoproteins** (**HDL**) and **low-density lipoproteins** (**LDL**). High concentrations of LDL-cholesterol in the blood increase the risk for coronary heart disease; HDL-cholesterol has a protective effect. See LIPID-LOWERING DRUGS.

Lipostat (Bristol-Myers Squibb) See PRAVASTATIN.

Liqui-Char (Oxford Pharmaceuticals) See ACTIVATED CHARCOAL.

liquid paraffin A mineral oil used as an *emollient and as an ingredient in lubricants to treat dry eyes. It was formerly widely used as a *faecal softener to lubricate the passage of faeces in the treatment of constipation, but is no longer recommended for this purpose. It can be obtained without a prescription, but some preparations containing liquid paraffin are available only from pharmacies.

Side effects: when used as a faecal softener, anal seepage of paraffin and anal irritation occur after long-term use, absorption of fat-soluble vitamins may be affected, and life-threatening pneumonia can develop if it is accidentally taken into the lungs.

Proprietary preparations: Alcoderm (emollient cream or lotion); Keri (lotion); Oilatum Bath Formula and Junior Bath Formula; Oilatum Emollient (bath additive); Oilatum Hand Aquagel; ALPHA KERI BATH (combined with lanolin); DERMAMIST (combined with white soft paraffin); DERMOL (combined with benzalkonium chloride, isopropyl myristate, and chlorhexidine hydrochloride); DIPROBASE (combined with white soft paraffin); E45 BATH OIL (combined with dimethicone <dimeticone>); E45 CREAM (combined with lanolin and white soft paraffin); E45 WASH CREAM (combined with zinc oxide); EMULSIDERM (combined with benzalkonium chloride and isopropyl myristate); EMMOLATE (combined with wood alcohols); EPADERM (combined with yellow soft paraffin and wax); GERMOLENE OINTMENT (combined with zinc oxide, methyl salicylate, lanolin, phenol, white soft paraffin, yellow soft paraffin and octaphonium <octafonium> chloride); HYDROMOL CREAM (combined with isopropyl myristate, arachis oil, sodium lactate, and sodium pyrrolidone carboxylate); HYDROMOL EMOLLIENT (combined with isopropyl myristate); INFADERM THERAPEUTIC OIL (combined with almond oil); LACRI-LUBE (combined with white soft paraffin and wool fat); LIPOBASE (combined with white soft paraffin); LUBRI-TEARS (combined with white soft paraffin and wool fat); MIL-PAR (combined with magnesium hydroxide); OILATUM PLUS (combined with benzalkonium chloride and triclosan); ULTRABASE (combined with white soft paraffin); UNGUENTUM M (combined with white soft paraffin and other emollients).

Liquifilm Tears (Allergan) *See* POLYVINYL ALCOHOL.

Liquifruta Garlic Cough Medicine (Pfizer Consumer Healthcare) *See* GUAIPHENESIN <GUAIFENESIN>.

lisinopril An *ACE inhibitor used as an adjunct to *diuretics for the treatment of *heart failure. It is also taken after myocardial infarction (heart attack) to reduce recurrence and is used to treat all grades of *hypertension. Available as tablets on *prescription only, it is usually taken once a day.

Side effects, precautions, and interactions with other drugs: see ACE INHIBITORS.

Proprietary preparations: Carace; Zestril; CARACE PLUS (combined with hydrochlorothiazide); ZESTORETIC (combined with hydrochlorothiazide).

See also ANTIHYPERTENSIVE DRUGS.

Liskonum (SmithKline Beecham Pharmaceuticals) *See* LITHIUM CARBONATE.

lisuride maleate *See* LYSURIDE MALEATE.

Litarex (Cox Pharmaceuticals) *See* LITHIUM CITRATE.

lithium A drug used in the form of its salts for the prevention and treatment of manic-depressive illness (bipolar depression) and in the prevention of recurrent depression (unipolar depression). Its mechanism of action is unclear, but it inhibits the action of an important enzyme involved in the transmission of signals in the brain. Lithium may be added to *tricyclic antidepressants to increase their effectiveness. The concentrations of lithium in the blood that are therapeutically effective may be close to those that produce toxic effects. Plasma concentrations of lithium should therefore be monitored carefully and the dosage adjusted as necessary. Overdosage can be fatal. Lithium is available as *lithium carbonate and *lithium citrate. Different products have different absorption characteristics, therefore it is not advisable to change brands of medication unless specifically instructed to do so.

Side effects: these are dose-related and develop as concentrations of lithium in the blood increase. They include nausea, vomiting, and diarrhoea, fine tremor, increased urine production, weight gain, and oedema. Signs of lithium intoxication include blurred vision, increasing gastrointestinal disturbances, drowsiness and lethargy, giddiness, coarse tremor, and lack of coordination. Treatment may need to be stopped.

Precautions: lithium salts should not be used to treat children, people with kidney or heart disease, or those with *sodium imbalance (lithium toxicity is exacerbated by sodium depletion). They should be used with caution in elderly people and in women who are pregnant or breastfeeding.

Interactions with other drugs: lithium interacts with a wide variety of drugs including:

ACE inhibitors: increase concentrations of lithium in the blood.

Antibiotics: metronidazole and spectinomycin increase concentrations of lithium in the blood.

Anticonvulsants: carbamazepine and phenytoin may increase lithium toxicity without increasing plasma concentrations of lithium.

Antiemetics: there is an increased risk of *extrapyramidal reactions with domperidone and metoclopramide.

Calcium antagonists: diltiazem and verapamil may increase lithium toxicity without increasing plasma concentrations of lithium.

Diuretics: increase concentrations of lithium in the blood. As lithium toxicity is exacerbated by sodium depletion, the use of diuretics, especially thiazides, with lithium is hazardous.

Haloperidol: increases concentrations of lithium in the blood.

Methyldopa: may increase toxicity of lithium without increasing plasma lithium concentrations.

NSAIDs: increase concentrations of lithium in the blood and their use with lithium should be avoided.

SSRIs: increase concentrations of lithium in the blood.

Sumatriptan: increases the adverse effects of lithium on the nervous system.

Theophylline: may reduce concentrations of lithium in the blood.

lithium carbonate A *lithium salt used for the treatment and prevention of mania, manic-depressive illness, and recurrent depression. It is also used to treat aggressive and self-mutilating behaviour. It is available as tablets and *modified-release tablets on *prescription only.
Side effects, precautions, and interactions with other drugs: see LITHIUM.
Proprietary preparations: Camcolit; Liskonum; Lithonate; Priadel.

lithium citrate A *lithium salt used for the treatment and prevention of mania, manic-depressive illness, and recurrent depression. It is also used to treat aggressive and self-mutilating behaviour. It is available as *modified-release tablets or a liquid on *prescription only.
Side effects, precautions, and interactions with other drugs: see LITHIUM.
Proprietary preparations: Li-Liquid; Litarex; Priadel.

lithium succinate A salt of lithium that has anti-inflammatory and antifungal activity and is used for the treatment of seborrhoeic *eczema.

In combination with *zinc sulphate, it is available as an ointment on *prescription only.
Proprietary preparation: EFALITH (combined with zinc sulphate).

Lithonate (APS-Berk) *See* LITHIUM CARBONATE.

Livial (Organon Laboratories) *See* TIBOLONE.

Livostin (CIBA Vision Ophthalmics) *See* LEVOCABASTINE.

Lloyds Cream (Seton Scholl Healthcare) *See* DIETHYLAMINE SALICYLATE.

Locabiotal (Servier Laboratories) *See* FUSAFUNGINE.

local anaesthetics Drugs that inhibit the conduction of impulses in sensory nerves in the region where they are applied and therefore reduce or abolish sensations in that area of the body. Local anaesthetics are used for local pain relief, including that required before painful procedures, such as venepuncture (taking a blood sample) or injections. They are usually applied topically, to the skin or mucous membranes, for **surface anaesthesia**, but some (e.g. **bupivacaine**, *lignocaine <lidocaine>, and *prilocaine) can be injected for **infiltration** (or **local**) **anaesthesia**. Although local anaesthetics are used for their local analgesic effects, most of them also cause dilatation of blood vessels, so that they are quickly absorbed into the bloodstream and removed from their intended site of action. For this reason they are often administered with a *vasoconstrictor drug, such as *adrenaline <epinephrine> or *phenylephrine. Local anaesthetics absorbed into the bloodstream can cause unwanted *systemic effects (see side effects below).
  Local anaesthetics that are ingredients of creams, sprays, or gels for the skin, to relieve the pain of stings or minor cuts, abrasions, and burns, include *amethocaine <tetracaine>, *benzocaine, and lignocaine <lidocaine>. These anaesthetics are also included in sprays and lozenges for painful conditions of the mouth, gums, and throat, and lignocaine <lidocaine> is used in teething gels. Local anaesthetics applied in eye drops include amethocaine <tetracaine>, **oxybuprocaine**, **proxymetacaine**, and lignocaine <lidocaine>. Soothing preparations for the relief of haemorrhoids often contain local anaesthetics, such as lignocaine <lidocaine>, benzocaine, *pramoxine <pramocaine> hydrochloride, or *cinchocaine hydrochloride.
Side effects: rapid and extensive absorption of local anaesthetics causes light-headedness followed by sedation. Some local anaesthetics cause allergic reactions. For specific side effects, see entries for individual drugs.

Loceryl, Loceryl Lacquer (Roche Products) *See* AMOROLFINE.

Locoid, Locoid Crelo, Locoid Lipocream, Locoid Scalp Lotion (Yamanouchi Pharma) *See* HYDROCORTISONE BUTYRATE.

Locoid C (Yamanouchi Pharma) A proprietary combination of *hydrocortisone butyrate (a corticosteroid) and chlorquinaldol (an *antifungal drug), used for the treatment of eczema, psoriasis, and other skin conditions in which infection is present or suspected. It is available as a cream or ointment on *prescription only.
Side effects and precautions: see TOPICAL STEROIDS.

Locorten-Vioform (Novartis Pharmaceuticals) A proprietary combination of *clioquinol (an antibiotic) and *flumethasone <flumetasone> pivalate (a topical steroid), used for the treatment of inflammatory conditions of the outer ear in which secondary infection is suspected. It is available as ear drops on *prescription only.
Side effects: this preparation may irritate the skin and discolour the hair.
Precautions: this medicine should not be used on perforated eardrums or for treating primary infections of the outer ear. It should be used with caution by women who are pregnant or breastfeeding. It is not recommended for children under two years old.

Lodiar (Ashbourne Pharmaceuticals) *See* LOPERAMIDE HYDROCHLORIDE.

Lodine, **Lodine SR** (Wyeth Laboratories) *See* ETODOLAC.

lodoxamide A drug used for the treatment of allergic conjunctivitis. It is available as eye drops on *prescription only.
Side effects: include mild transient stinging, burning, itching, and tear production.
Precautions: lodoxamide should not be used by wearers of soft contact lenses, and should be used with caution by women who are pregnant or breastfeeding.
Proprietary preparation: Alomide.

Loestrin 20 (Parke-Davis Medical) A proprietary combination of *ethinyloestradiol <ethinylestradiol> (20 micrograms) and *norethisterone acetate used as an *oral contraceptive. **Loestrin 30** contains 30 micrograms of ethinyloestradiol <ethinylestradiol>. Both preparations are available as tablets on *prescription only.
Side effects, precautions, and interactions with other drugs: see ORAL CONTRACEPTIVES.

Lofensaid, **Lofensaid Retard** (Opus) *See* DICLOFENAC SODIUM.

lofepramine A *tricyclic antidepressant drug used for the treatment of depressive illness; it is less sedating than *amitriptyline hydrochloride. Lofepramine is available as tablets on *prescription only.
Side effects: similar to those of *amitriptyline hydrochloride, but lofepramine has fewer antimuscarinic effects (e.g. dry mouth, blurred vision, difficulty in urinating) than amitriptyline; it can have adverse effects on the liver.

Precautions and interactions with other drugs: see TRICYCLIC
ANTIDEPRESSANTS.
Proprietary preparation: Gamanil.

lofexidine hydrochloride A drug used to relieve the symptoms in
people who are undergoing withdrawal from physical *dependence on
opioids, such as heroin (*diamorphine). It acts on alpha-adrenoceptors in
the brain to reduce impulses in the *sympathetic nervous system.
Lofexidine is available as tablets on *prescription only.
Side effects: include drowsiness, dry mouth, throat, and nose, low blood
pressure, and slowing of the heart rate. Overdosage can cause sedation
and coma.
Precautions: lofexidine should not be taken by people who have certain
heart conditions or a slow heart rate. It should be used with caution in
people with a history of depression and by women who are pregnant or
breastfeeding. Treatment with lofexidine should be stopped gradually
(over several days) to prevent a sudden increase in blood pressure.
Interactions with other drugs:
  Anxiolytic and hypnotic drugs: lofexidine increases their sedative effects.
Proprietary preparation: BritLofex.

Logynon (Schering Health Care) A proprietary combination of
*ethinyloestradiol <ethinylestradiol> and *levonorgestrel used as an
*oral contraceptive of the triphasic type. These tablets are packaged in
three phases, which differ in the amounts of the active ingredients they
contain. **Logynon ED** contains both active and dummy tablets, so that a
tablet is taken each day of a 28-day cycle. Both preparations are available
on *prescription only.
Side effects, precautions, and interactions with other drugs: see ORAL
CONTRACEPTIVES.

Lomexin (Dominion Pharma) See FENTICONAZOLE.

Lomotil (Searle) See CO-PHENOTROPE.

lomustine An *alkylating drug used for the treatment of Hodgkin's
disease and certain solid tumours (see CANCER). It is available as capsules
on *prescription only.
Side effects: include nausea and vomiting, which may be moderately
severe. See also CYTOTOXIC DRUGS.
Precautions: see CYTOTOXIC DRUGS.
Proprietary preparation: CCNU.

Loniten (Pharmacia & Upjohn) See MINOXIDIL.

loop diuretics The most powerful class of *diuretics. Loop diuretics
act rapidly, causing large volumes of urine to be excreted, but have a
short duration of action. The name comes from the fact that they inhibit

salt reabsorption in the loop of Henle, part of the tubular structure of the kidney. They are used for the treatment of *heart failure, nephrotic syndrome (a condition in which there is a large loss of protein in the urine, causing low blood protein and *oedema), and pulmonary oedema (fluid in the spaces of the lungs). Loop diuretics cause a marked loss of potassium, which may be corrected by the use of *potassium supplements or the addition of a *potassium-sparing diuretic. They start to act rapidly within one hour, and diuresis is complete within six hours. *See* BUMETANIDE; FRUSEMIDE <FUROSEMIDE>; TORASEMIDE.

Side effects: these diuretics can sometimes have too powerful an action, causing depletion of potassium, sodium, and water; these effects in turn can cause weakness, lethargy, cramps, and dizziness. The dizziness often occurs as a result of low blood pressure on standing up from a lying or sitting posture (postural hypotension). Other side effects include a loss of calcium. Loop diuretics may worsen diabetic control because they reduce insulin secretion and therefore increase blood sugar concentration. There is a risk of gout with loop diuretics due to their effect of reducing uric acid excretion. Large doses of frusemide <furosemide> intravenously can disturb hearing transiently. Rashes, pancreatitis, and thrombocytopenia (decreased number of platelets in the blood, causing easy bruising) are rare side effects of loop diuretics.

Precautions: potassium supplements will often be required. Loop diuretics should not be taken by people with advanced cirrhosis of the liver. They are not usually given to pregnant women and should be used with caution in men with an enlarged prostate gland and in people with diabetes or gout. Loop diuretics can increase the likelihood of dehydration and hangovers after drinking.

Interactions with other drugs:

ACE inhibitors: the blood-pressure-lowering effect of ACE inhibitors is enhanced; since ACE inhibitors cause potassium retention, the loss of potassium is not so great when these drugs are taken together.

Aminoglycoside antibiotics: increase the risk of hearing problems.

Anti-arrhythmic drugs: if potassium loss occurs, amiodarone, disopyramide, flecainide, and quinidine are more likely to have adverse effects on the heart and the action of lignocaine <lidocaine> and mexiletine are antagonized.

Antihistamines: the risk of *arrhythmias with astemizole and terfenadine is increased if potassium concentrations are low.

Antihypertensive drugs: their effects in lowering blood pressure are increased.

Corticosteroids: may further increase the loss of potassium.

Digitalis drugs: the adverse effects of these drugs is increased if potassium loss occurs.

Lithium: concentrations of lithium in the blood may be increased, causing adverse effects.

NSAIDs: may reduce the diuretic effect of loop diuretics.

Pimozide: if potassium loss occurs, pimozide is more likely to cause arrhythmias.

LoperaGen (Norgine) *See* LOPERAMIDE HYDROCHLORIDE.

loperamide hydrochloride An *opioid that slows down movements of the gut and is used in the treatment of acute diarrhoea in adults and children over four years old and chronic diarrhoea in adults only (*see* ANTIDIARRHOEAL DRUGS). Loperamide is available as capsules or a syrup on *prescription, but capsules for treating acute diarrhoea can be obtained from pharmacies without a prescription.
Side effects: abdominal cramps, bloating, and rashes may occur.
Precautions: loperamide should not be taken by people with acute ulcerative colitis, antibiotic-associated colitis, paralysis of the small intestine, or abdominal distension.
Proprietary preparations: Arret; Boots Diareze; Diasorb; Diocalm Ultra; Diocaps; Imodium (capsules or syrup); Lodiar; LoperaGen; Normaloe; Norimode.

Lopid (Parke-Davis Medical) *See* GEMFIBROZIL.

Lopranol LA (Opus) *See* PROPRANOLOL HYDROCHLORIDE.

loprazolam A short-acting *benzodiazepine used for the short-term treatment of insomnia. It is available as tablets on *prescription only.
Side effects and precautions: see BENZODIAZEPINES; DIAZEPAM.
Interactions with other drugs: see BENZODIAZEPINES.

Lopressor, Lopressor SR (Novartis Pharmaceuticals) *See* METOPROLOL TARTRATE.

loratadine One of the newer (non-sedating) *antihistamines, used to relieve the symptoms of such allergic conditions as hay fever and urticaria. It is available as tablets or a syrup on *prescription, and packs containing no more than 10 days' supply can be bought from pharmacies without a prescription.
Side effects and interactions with other drugs: see ANTIHISTAMINES.
Precautions: loratadine should not be taken by women who are pregnant or breastfeeding. *See also* ANTIHISTAMINES.
Proprietary preparations: Boots Hayfever Relief; Clarityn; Clarityn Allergy.

lorazepam A short-acting *benzodiazepine used for the short-term treatment of anxiety and insomnia and to relax patients before operations. It is also given by injection in the treatment of status epilepticus (repeated epileptic seizures). Lorazepam is available as tablets and an injection on *prescription only.
Side effects and precautions: see DIAZEPAM; BENZODIAZEPINES.

Interactions with other drugs: see BENZODIAZEPINES.
Proprietary preparation: Ativan.

lormetazepam A short-acting *benzodiazepine used for the short-term treatment of insomnia. It is available as tablets on *prescription only.
Side effects and precautions: see BENZODIAZEPINES; DIAZEPAM.
Interactions with other drugs: see BENZODIAZEPINES.

Loron (Roche Products) *See* SODIUM CLODRONATE.

losartan potassium An *angiotensin II inhibitor used in the treatment of *hypertension. It is available as tablets on *prescription only.
Side effects and precautions: see ANGIOTENSIN II INHIBITORS.
Interactions with other drugs: see ACE INHIBITORS.
Proprietary preparations: Cozaar; COZAAR-COMP (combined with hydrochlorothiazide).

Losec (AstraZeneca) *See* OMEPRAZOLE.

lotion A medicinal solution for washing or bathing the external parts of the body. Lotions usually have a cooling, soothing, or antiseptic action.

Lotriderm (Schering-Plough) A proprietary combination of *betamethasone dipropionate (a potent steroid) and *clotrimazole (an antifungal agent), used for the treatment of short-term fungal infections of the skin. It is available as a cream on *prescription only.
Side effects: there may be local mild burning, irritation, and allergic reactions. *See also* TOPICAL STEROIDS.
Precautions: see TOPICAL STEROIDS.

low molecular weight heparins Forms of *heparin that consist of smaller molecules than standard heparin. They have a longer duration of action than standard heparin and are used for the prevention and treatment of deep-vein *thrombosis and in the treatment of pulmonary embolism and unstable *angina. They are also used in patients undergoing kidney dialysis, in order to prevent the formation of blood clots. The low molecular weight heparins include *certoparin, *dalteparin sodium, *enoxaparin, and *tinzaparin sodium; they are administered by injection (usually subcutaneous) and are available on *prescription only. *See also* DANAPAROID SODIUM.
Side effects, precautions, and interactions with other drugs: see HEPARIN.

Loxapac (Wyeth Laboratories) *See* LOXAPINE.

loxapine An *antipsychotic drug used for the treatment of acute and chronic psychotic states. It is available as capsules on *prescription only.

Side effects: as for *chlorpromazine, but loxapine is less sedating and can cause nausea and vomiting.
Precautions and interactions with other drugs: see CHLORPROMAZINE HYDROCHLORIDE.
Proprietary preparation: Loxapac.

lozenge A medicinal tablet containing sugar. Lozenges are usually solid and rigid (compared to a *pastille, which is soft) and should be sucked, so that the medication is applied to the mouth and throat.

Luborant (Antigen Pharmaceuticals) *See* CARMELLOSE.

Lubri-Tears (Alcon Laboratories) A proprietary combination of *white soft paraffin, *liquid paraffin, and wool fat (anhydrous *lanolin), used for the lubrication of dry eyes. It is available as an eye ointment and can be obtained without a prescription, but only from pharmacies.

Ludiomil (Novartis Pharmaceuticals) *See* MAPROTILINE HYDROCHLORIDE.

Lugol's solution *See* IODINE.

Lustral (Pfizer) *See* SERTRALINE.

Lyclear Creme Rinse, **Lyclear Dermal Cream** (Warner-Lambert Consumer Healthcare) *See* PERMETHRIN.

lymecycline A tetracycline antibiotic used for the treatment of chronic bronchitis, brucellosis, chlamydial infections, and infections caused by mycoplasmas and rickettsias (*see* TETRACYCLINES). It is also used to treat mouth ulcers and acne. It is available on *prescription only as tablets or capsules.
Side effects, precautions, and interactions with other drugs: see TETRACYCLINES.
Proprietary preparation: Tetralysal 300.

lymphoma *See* CANCER.

lysuride maleate <lisuride maleate> A *dopamine receptor agonist, similar to *bromocriptine, that is used for the treatment of Parkinson's disease. It is available as tablets on *prescription only.
Side effects: include nausea and vomiting, dizziness, headache, lethargy, malaise, drowsiness, psychiatric problems (including hallucinations), and, occasionally, severe low blood pressure.
Precautions: lysuride maleate should not be taken by people with severe disturbances of blood circulation, especially in the limbs, or poor coronary function.
Interactions with other drugs:
 Antipsychotic drugs: antagonize the effect of lysuride.
Proprietary preparation: Revanil.

Maalox (Rhône-Poulenc Rorer) *See* CO-MAGALDROX.

Maalox Plus (Rhône-Poulenc Rorer) A proprietary combination of
*aluminium hydroxide and *magnesium hydroxide (antacids) and
activated *dimethicone <dimeticone> (an antifoaming agent), used for
the relief of indigestion (*see* ACID-PEPTIC DISEASES). It is freely available
*over the counter in the form of a suspension or tablets; the tablets
cannot be prescribed on the NHS.
Side effects, precautions, and interactions with other drugs: see ANTACIDS.

Mabthera (Roche Products) *See* RITUXIMAB.

Mackenzies Smelling Salts (Cox Pharmaceuticals) A proprietary
combination of strong *ammonia solution and *eucalyptus oil, used as
an aromatic inhalation for the relief of nasal congestion associated with
catarrh and head colds. It is freely available *over the counter.
Precautions: Mackenzies Smelling Salts should not be used in babies
under three months old.

Macrobid (Procter & Gamble) *See* NITROFURANTOIN.

Macrodantin (Procter & Gamble) *See* NITROFURANTOIN.

macrogols *See* POLYETHYLENE GLYCOLS.

macrolide antibiotics A group of antibiotics that are bacteriostatic,
i.e. they prevent bacteria from multiplying, but do not kill them. They
have a similar spectrum of activity to the *penicillins and are therefore
useful for treating infections in patients who are allergic to penicillin.
The original, and probably best known, macrolide is *erythromycin. Its
major drawback is that it can have gastrointestinal side effects; this effect
is not so marked with the other macrolide antibiotics, *azithromycin and
*clarithromycin.

Madopar, **Madopar CR** (Roche Products) *See* CO-BENELDOPA.

Magnapen (SmithKline Beecham Pharmaceuticals) *See* CO-FLUAMPICIL.

magnesia, cream of *See* MAGNESIUM HYDROXIDE.

magnesium alginate *See* ALGINIC ACID.

magnesium carbonate A salt of magnesium that is used as an *antacid for the relief of indigestion (*see* ACID-PEPTIC DISEASES). It is available in the form of a mixture and is also included as an ingredient in a variety of compound antacid preparations. Most preparations containing magnesium carbonate are freely available *over the counter.

Side effects and precautions: see MAGNESIUM SALTS.

Interactions with other drugs: see ANTACIDS.

Proprietary preparations: ACTONORM POWDER (combined with other antacids and atropine sulphate); ALGICON (combined with aluminium hydroxide, magnesium alginate, and potassium bicarbonate); ANDREWS ANTACID (combined with calcium carbonate); BIRLEYS (combined with aluminium hydroxide and magnesium trisilicate); BISMAG TABLETS (combined with sodium bicarbonate); BISODOL ANTACID POWDER (combined with sodium bicarbonate); BISODOL ANTACID TABLETS (combined with sodium bicarbonate and calcium carbonate); BISODOL EXTRA TABLETS (combined with sodium bicarbonate, calcium carbonate, and dimethicone <dimeticone>); DE WITT'S ANTACID POWDER (combined with sodium bicarbonate, calcium carbonate, magnesium trisilicate, kaolin, and peppermint oil); DE WITT'S ANTACID TABLETS (combined with calcium carbonate, magnesium trisilicate, and peppermint oil); DIJEX TABLETS (combined with aluminium hydroxide); MOORLAND (combined with aluminium hydroxide, bismuth, magnesium trisilicate, calcium carbonate, and kaolin); RENNIE (combined with calcium carbonate); RENNIE DEFLATINE (combined with calcium carbonate and dimethicone <dimeticone>); TOPAL (combined with aluminium hydroxide and alginic acid); URIFLEX R (combined with citric acid, gluconolactone, and disodium edetate).

magnesium citrate An *osmotic laxative used for total evacuation of the bowel before X-ray examination or surgery of the bowel. It is available without a prescription in the form of an effervescent powder to be dissolved in water.

Side effects and precautions: see BOWEL-CLEANSING SOLUTIONS.

Proprietary preparations: Citramag; PICOLAX (combined with sodium picosulphate).

magnesium hydroxide A salt of magnesium that is included as an ingredient in a variety of *antacid preparations for the relief of indigestion (*see* ACID-PEPTIC DISEASES). Magnesium hydroxide, in the form of a mixture (**cream of magnesia**), is also used as an *osmotic laxative. Most preparations containing magnesium hydroxide are freely available *over the counter. *See also* CO-MAGALDROX.

Side effects and precautions: see MAGNESIUM SALTS.

Interactions with other drugs: see ANTACIDS.

Proprietary preparations: Phillips' Milk of Magnesia (laxative); ACTONORM GEL (combined with aluminium hydroxide, dimethicone <dimeticone>, and peppermint oil); CARBELLON (combined with charcoal and peppermint oil); DIJEX SUSPENSION (combined with aluminium hydroxide); DIOVOL (combined with aluminium hydroxide and dimethicone <dimeticone>); Maalox (*see* CO-MAGALDROX); MAALOX PLUS (combined with aluminium hydroxide and dimethicone <dimeticone>); MIL-PAR (combined with liquid paraffin); MUCAINE (combined with oxethazaine <oxetacaine> and aluminium hydroxide); Mucogel (*see* CO-MAGALDROX).

magnesium oxide A salt of magnesium that has laxative properties and is therefore included as an ingredient in aluminium-containing *antacids, such as aluminium hydroxide, to reduce their constipating effect. Antacid preparations containing magnesium oxide are freely available *over the counter.

Side effects and precautions: see MAGNESIUM SALTS.

Interactions with other drugs: see ANTACIDS.

Proprietary preparations: ASILONE SUSPENSION (combined with aluminium hydroxide and dimethicone <dimeticone>); KOLANTICON GEL (combined with aluminium hydroxide, dimethicone <dimeticone>, and dicyclomine hydrochloride).

magnesium salts A group of magnesium-containing compounds. Magnesium salts used as *antacids include *magnesium carbonate, magnesium trisilicate, and *magnesium hydroxide. The latter is also an *osmotic laxative, as are *magnesium sulphate and *magnesium citrate; they are used to treat constipation or as *bowel-cleansing solutions.

Side effects: magnesium salts in antacid preparations can cause diarrhoea; in laxatives they can cause colic. *See also* ANTACIDS.

Precautions: magnesium salts should not be taken by people with kidney disease as this can cause dangerously high plasma concentrations of magnesium.

Interactions with other drugs: see ANTACIDS.

magnesium sulphate A salt of magnesium used as an *osmotic laxative; it produces rapid evacuation of the bowel. Magnesium sulphate given by intravenous infusion or intramuscular injection is used to treat magnesium deficiency. Intravenous injections of magnesium sulphate are used for the emergency treatment of serious *arrhythmias. Intravenous magnesium sulphate is also used to prevent the recurrence of seizures in eclampsia, a serious condition that can affect pregnant women. Magnesium sulphate paste can be used to treat boils. Laxatives (which include **Epsom salts**) and pastes containing magnesium sulphate are available without a prescription; injections are *prescription only medicines.

Side effects: colic and diarrhoea can occur when magnesium sulphate is taken by mouth. Injections of magnesium sulphate may cause nausea, vomiting, thirst, flushing, low blood pressure, and drowsiness.

Precautions: see MAGNESIUM SALTS.

Interactions with other drugs: see ANTACIDS.

Proprietary preparation: ORIGINAL ANDREWS SALTS (combined with sodium bicarbonate and citric acid).

magnesium trisilicate A salt of magnesium that is used as an *antacid for the relief of indigestion (*see* ACID-PEPTIC DISEASES). It is available in the form of tablets, a mixture, or a powder and is also an ingredient of a variety of compound antacid preparations. Preparations containing magnesium silicate can be obtained without a prescription.

Side effects and precautions: see MAGNESIUM SALTS.

Interactions with other drugs: see ANTACIDS.

Proprietary preparations: ASILONE HEARTBURN (combined with alginic acid, aluminium hydroxide, and sodium bicarbonate); BIRLEYS (combined with aluminium hydroxide and magnesium carbonate); DE WITT'S ANTACID POWDER (combined with sodium bicarbonate, calcium carbonate, magnesium carbonate, kaolin, and peppermint oil); DE WITT'S ANTACID TABLETS (combined with calcium carbonate, magnesium carbonate, and peppermint oil); GASTROCOTE (combined with alginic acid, aluminium hydroxide, and sodium bicarbonate); GAVISCON TABLETS (combined with aluminium hydroxide, alginic acid, and sodium bicarbonate); MOORLAND (combined with aluminium hydroxide, bismuth, magnesium carbonate, calcium carbonate, and kaolin); PYROGASTRONE (combined with carbenoloxone sodium, aluminium hydroxide, sodium bicarbonate, and alginic acid).

malaria An infectious disease due to the presence of parasitic protozoa of the genus *Plasmodium* within the red blood cells. *P. falciparum* causes **falciparum** (or **malignant**) **malaria** (the most serious kind); *P. vivax* (or less commonly *P. malariae* or *P. ovale*) cause **benign malarias**. Malaria is transmitted by the *Anopheles* mosquito and is confined mainly to tropical and subtropical areas.

When the mosquito bites an individual, parasites are injected into the bloodstream and migrate to the liver and other organs, where they multiply. After an incubation period varying from 12 days (*P. falciparum*) to 10 months (some varieties of *P. vivax*), parasites return to the bloodstream and invade the red blood cells. Rapid multiplication of the parasites results in destruction of the red cells and the release of more parasites capable of infecting other red cells. This causes a short bout of shivering, fever, and sweating, and the loss of healthy red cells results in *anaemia. When the next batch of parasites is released symptoms reappear. The interval between fever attacks varies in different types of malaria: two or three days in benign malarias, and from a few hours to two days in falciparum malaria.

Drugs used to treat falciparum malaria include *quinine, *mefloquine, *Malarone (a combination of *proguanil hydrochloride and atovaquone), and (rarely) *halofantrine hydrochloride (*see also* FANSIDAR; MALOPRIM). For benign malarias, *chloroquine is the treatment of choice. Drugs used to prevent travellers from contracting malaria include chloroquine, mefloquine, and proguanil hydrochloride.

Malarone (GlaxoWellcome) A proprietary combination of *proguanil hydrochloride and *atovaquone, used for the treatment of falciparum

*malaria that is thought to be resistant to other antimalarial drugs. It is available as tablets on *prescription only.

Side effects: include nausea, vomiting, and diarrhoea (which can reduce its absorption), abdominal pain, loss of appetite, headache, and cough.

Precautions: Malarone should be used with caution in people with acute kidney failure and in pregnant women. It should not be taken by women who are breastfeeding.

Interactions with other drugs: see PROGUANIL HYDROCHLORIDE; ATOVAQUONE.

malathion A pesticide that is used clinically to treat infestations of *lice and *scabies. It is available as a lotion or shampoo; lotions are preferable since contact time is longer (12 hours or overnight is recommended). Some lotions contain alcohol; these are not recommended for treating scabies or crab lice (see also precautions below). Hair treated with malathion preparations should be allowed to dry naturally. Malathion can be obtained without a prescription, but only from pharmacies.

Side effects: malathion may irritate the skin.

Precautions: malathion should not be applied near the eyes or on broken skin; treatment of infants under six months old should be supervised by a doctor. Lotions containing alcohol should not be used to treat scabies or crab lice; they should also not be used for treating head lice in young children or people with asthma (since inhalation of the fumes can be dangerous). Continuous or prolonged use of alcoholic lotions should be avoided.

Proprietary preparations: Derbac-M; Prioderm; Quellada-M; Suleo-M.

malic acid An acid present in apples, pears, and many other fruits. It is used as an ingredient in skin preparations (combined with *benzoic acid and *salicylic acid) for the removal of dead skin from ulcers, burns, and wounds. As it can cause increased salivation when taken by mouth, malic acid is also an ingredient in artifical saliva preparations.

Proprietary preparations: ASERBINE (combined with benzoic acid and salicylic acid); SALIVIX (combined with acacia).

Malix (Lagap Pharmaceuticals) *See* GLIBENCLAMIDE.

Maloprim (GlaxoWellcome) A proprietary combination of *dapsone and *pyrimethamine, used for the prevention of falciparum *malaria. It is available as tablets on *prescription only and is taken weekly.

Side effects, precautions, and interactions with other drugs: see DAPSONE; PYRIMETHAMINE.

Manerix (Roche Products) *See* MOCLOBEMIDE.

Manevac (Galen) A proprietary combination of *senna (a stimulant laxative) and *ispaghula husk (a bulk-forming laxative), used for the treatment of constipation. It is available as granules and can be obtained without a prescription, but only from pharmacies.

Side effects: there may be flatulence, abdominal distention, and diarrhoea.

Precautions: see ISPAGHULA HUSK.

Manusept (Seton Scholl Healthcare) *See* TRICLOSAN.

MAOIs *See* MONOAMINE OXIDASE INHIBITORS.

maprotiline hydrochloride An *antidepressant drug used for the treatment of depressive illness, especially when sedation is desirable. It is related to the *tricyclic antidepressants and blocks the reuptake of noradrenaline <norepinephrine> but not serotonin. It is available as tablets on *prescription only.

Side effects: similar to those of *amitriptyline hydrochloride, but antimuscarinic effects (dry mouth, blurred vision, difficulty in urinating) occur less frequently; rashes are more common and there is a higher risk of convulsions at high doses.

Precautions: maprotiline should not be taken by patients who are manic or who have liver or kidney disease, a history of epilepsy, or a recent heart attack. It should be used with caution in women who are pregnant or breastfeeding and in patients with schizophrenia or suicidal tendencies.

Interactions with other drugs: see TRICYCLIC ANTIDEPRESSANTS.

Proprietary preparation: Ludiomil.

Marevan (Goldshield Pharmaceuticals) *See* WARFARIN SODIUM.

Marvelon (Organon Laboratories) A proprietary combination of *ethinyloestradiol <ethinylestradiol> and *desogestrel used as an *oral contraceptive. It is available as tablets on *prescription only.

Side effects and interactions with other drugs: see ORAL CONTRACEPTIVES.

Precautions: Marvelon should not be used by women who are at risk of developing thromboembolism, for example because they are very overweight or have varicose veins or a history of thrombosis. It should therefore only be taken by women who cannot tolerate other brands and who are prepared to accept the increased risk. *See also* ORAL CONTRACEPTIVES.

Masnoderm (Dominion Pharma) *See* CLOTRIMAZOLE.

Maxalt, **Maxalt Melt** (Merck Sharp & Dohme) *See* RIZATRIPTAN.

Maxepa (Seven Seas) *See* OMEGA-3 MARINE TRIGLYCERIDES.

Maxidex (Alcon Laboratories) *See* DEXAMETHASONE.

Maximum Strength Aspro Clear (Roche Products) *See* ASPIRIN.

Maxitrol (Alcon Laboratories) A proprietary combination of
*dexamethasone (a corticosteroid), *neomycin sulphate and *polymyxin
B sulphate (antibiotics), and *hypromellose (a lubricant), used for the
treatment of local inflammation of the eye. It is available as drops or an
ointment on *prescription only.
Side effects: include increased pressure in the eye, thinning of the
cornea, cataracts, and fungal infections.
Precautions: Maxitrol should not be used when viral or fungal infections
are present, during pregnancy, or by children, people with glaucoma or a
perforated eardrum, or by wearers of soft contact lenses.

Maxivent (APS-Berk) *See* SALBUTAMOL.

Maxolon (Monmouth Pharmaceuticals) *See* METOCLOPRAMIDE.

Maxtrex (Pharmacia & Upjohn) *See* METHOTREXATE.

MCR-50 (Pharmacia & Upjohn) *See* ISOSORBIDE MONONITRATE.

mebendazole An *anthelmintic that immobilizes and kills parasitic
worms in the intestine; it is active against roundworms, threadworms,
whipworms, and hookworms. Mebendazole is available on *prescription
as tablets or a suspension, but packs of tablets containing no more than
800 mg mebendazole can be obtained from pharmacies without a
prescription.
Side effects: there may be diarrhoea and abdominal pain; otherwise side
effects are rare as the drug is poorly absorbed from the intestine.
Precautions: mebendazole should not be used during pregnancy.
Interactions with other drugs:
  Cimetidine: increases the plasma concentration (and therefore side
    effects) of mebendazole.
Proprietary preparations: Boots Threadworm Treatment; Ovex; Pripsen
Mebendazole; Vermox.

mebeverine hydrochloride An *antispasmodic drug used in the
treatment of irritable bowel syndrome (IBS) and other conditions marked
by gut spasms. It is available as tablets or a liquid on *prescription only,
but limited quantities of tablets can be obtained from pharmacies
without a prescription.
Precautions: mebeverine should be used with caution by people with
intestinal obstruction due to loss of intestinal movement and by women
who are pregnant or breastfeeding.
Proprietary preparations: Boots IBS Relief; Colofac; Colofac 100; Colofac
IBS; Equilon; Fomac; FYBOGEL MEBEVERINE (combined with ispaghula).

meclozine hydrochloride An *antihistamine, similar to *cyclizine hydrochloride, that is used for the treatment of motion sickness. It is available as tablets that can be obtained without a prescription, but only from pharmacies.

Side effects, precautions, and interactions with other drugs: see ANTIHISTAMINES.

Proprietary preparation: Sea-Legs.

Medicoal (Concord Pharmaceuticals) *See* ACTIVATED CHARCOAL.

Medihaler-Ergotamine (3M Health Care) *See* ERGOTAMINE TARTRATE.

Medijel (DDD) A proprietary combination of *aminacrine <aminoacridine> hydrochloride (an antiseptic) and *lignocaine <lidocaine> hydrochloride (a local anaesthetic), used to relieve the pain of mouth ulcers, sore gums, and ill-fitting dentures. It is available as a gel or pastilles. The pastilles are available without a prescription, but only from pharmacies; the gel is freely available *over the counter.

Medinol (Seton Scholl Healthcare) *See* PARACETAMOL.

Medised (Seton Scholl Healthcare) A proprietary combination of *paracetamol (an analgesic and antipyretic) and *promethazine (a sedative antihistamine), formulated for young children. It is used to relieve mild to moderate pain (including headache and toothache) and the symptoms of influenza, colds, and chickenpox. It is available as a liquid (standard or sugar-free) and can be obtained without a prescription, but only from pharmacies.

Side effects: see ANTIHISTAMINES.

Precautions: Medised should not be given to children under one year old. *See also* PARACETAMOL; ANTIHISTAMINES.

Interactions with other drugs: see ANTIHISTAMINES.

Medrone (Pharmacia & Upjohn) *See* METHYLPREDNISOLONE.

medroxyprogesterone A synthetic *progestogen used to treat menstrual disorders (including irregular bleeding and absence of periods), *endometriosis, breast cancer in postmenopausal women, and cancers of the kidney, endometrium (lining of the uterus), or (rarely) prostate gland. Deep intramuscular injections of medroxyprogesterone are used as a *depot contraceptive, providing contraception for periods of up to three months. Medroxyprogesterone is also used with oestrogens in *hormone replacement therapy. It is available as tablets or injections on *prescription only.

Side effects: include weight gain, fluid retention, and breast tenderness. Depot injections may also cause irregular, prolonged, or heavy vaginal bleeding during the first 2–3 cycles, headache, abdominal pain, dizziness, and weakness, and there may be temporary infertility when the treatment stops.

Precautions: medroxyprogesterone should not be used during pregnancy or by women with hormone-dependent cancer (some kinds of breast or genital cancer), undiagnosed vaginal bleeding, or liver disease. It should be used with caution in women with asthma, diabetes, epilepsy, migraine, a history of depression, heart disease, or clotting problems.

Interactions with other drugs: see PROGESTOGENS.

Proprietary preparations: Depo-Provera (depot injection); Farlutal (tablets or injection); Provera (tablets); IMPROVERA (packaged with estropipate); PREMIQUE CYCLE (packaged with conjugated oestrogens); PREMIQUE (combined with conjugated oestrogens); TRIDESTRA (combined with oestradiol <estradiol>).

mefenamic acid An *NSAID used for the treatment of mild to moderate pain in rheumatoid arthritis (including arthritis in children), osteoarthritis, period pains, and heavy periods. It is available, on prescription only, as capsules, tablets, and a suspension for children.

Side effects: see NSAIDS. Additional side effects may include a rash or diarrhoea (in which case a doctor should be informed as treatment may need to be discontinued) and drowsiness.

Precautions: see NSAIDS. In addition, mefenamic acid should not be taken by people with inflammatory bowel disease.

Interactions with other drugs: see NSAIDS.

Proprietary preparations: Contraflam; Dysman 250; Dysman 500; Ponstan; Ponstan Forte; Ponstan Paediatric Suspension.

mefloquine A drug used for the prevention of *malaria, especially in areas where chloroquine-resistant malaria parasites are common. It can also be used to treat falciparum malaria in people who have not used it previously for prevention. Mefloquine is available as tablets on *prescription only.

Side effects: mefloquine has a range of side effects, which should be reported to a doctor if they occur. These include nausea, vomiting, diarrhoea, abdominal pain, dizziness, loss of balance, headache, and sleep disorders, tremor, shaking with unsteady gait, anxiety, depression, panic attacks, agitation, and hallucinations. Other possible side effects are tinnitus, visual disturbances, circulatory disorders, slowing or increasing of the heart rate, muscle weakness, muscle or joint pain, itching, hair loss, malaise, fever, fatigue, loss of appetite, and blood disorders. If any of these side effects occur, medical advice should be obtained before the next dose.

Precautions: this drug should not be used for prevention of malaria in people who have liver or kidney disease. It should not be taken during pregnancy, and contraception should be used for three months after treatment has been stopped. It should not be taken by women who are breastfeeding or by people with a history of depression or other psychiatric disorders. Mefloquine should be used with caution in people with epilepsy or certain heart disorders. Dizziness or a disturbed sense of balance may impair the performance of such skilled tasks as driving.

Interactions with other drugs:

Anti-arrhythmic drugs: there is an increased risk of *arrhythmias with amiodarone (which should not be taken with mefloquine) and quinidine.

Antiepileptic drugs: their anticonvulsant effects are antagonized by mefloquine.

Antipsychotic drugs: there is an increased risk of arrhythmias; pimozide should not be taken with mefloquine.

Chloroquine and quinine: there is an increased risk of convulsions.

Halofantrine: there is a danger of abnormal heart rhythms.

Proprietary preparation: Lariam.

Mefoxin (Merck Sharp & Dohme) *See* CEFOXITIN.

mefruside A thiazide-like diuretic (*see* THIAZIDE DIURETICS) used for the treatment of *hypertension and *oedema. It is available as tablets on *prescription only.

Side effects, precautions, and interactions with other drugs: *see* THIAZIDE DIURETICS.

Proprietary preparation: Baycaron.

See also ANTIHYPERTENSIVE DRUGS; DIURETICS.

Megace (Bristol-Myers Squibb) *See* MEGESTROL ACETATE.

megestrol acetate A synthetic *progestogen used to treat breast *cancer, cancer of the endometrium (lining of the womb), and a type of kidney cancer. It is available as tablets on *prescription only.

Side effects and precautions: *see* MEDROXYPROGESTERONE.

Interactions with other drugs: *see* PROGESTOGENS.

Proprietary preparation: Megace.

Melleril (Novartis Consumer Health) *See* THIORIDAZINE.

Melo (Anglian Pharma) *See* IPECACUANHA.

meloxicam An *NSAID used for the short-term treatment of acute osteoarthritis and for the long-term treatment of rheumatoid arthritis and ankylosing spondylitis. It is available as tablets or suppositories on *prescription only.

Side effects and interactions with other drugs: *see* NSAIDS.

Precautions: *see* NSAIDS. The suppositories should not be used in people with haemorrhoids.

Proprietary preparation: Mobic.

melphalan An *alkylating drug used for the treatment of myeloma (cancer of the plasma cells of the bone marrow) and occasionally of solid tumours (ovarian and breast cancer) and lymphomas (*see* CANCER). It is available, on *prescription only, as a solution for injection or as tablets.

Side effects: these are rare, but *bone marrow suppression can occur. *See also* CYTOTOXIC DRUGS.

Precautions: see CYTOTOXIC DRUGS.

Interactions with other drugs:

Cyclosporin: the risk of this drug having adverse effects on the kidneys is increased.

Proprietary preparation: Alkeran.

Meltus Cough Control (Seton Scholl Healthcare) *See* DEXTROMETHORPHAN.

Meltus Dry Cough (Seton Scholl Healthcare) A proprietary combination of *dextromethorphan (a cough suppressant) and *pseudoephedrine (a decongestant), used for the relief of dry coughs and congestion associated with colds. It is available as a liquid without a prescription, but only from pharmacies. It cannot be prescribed on the NHS.

Side effects, precautions, and interactions with other drugs: see DEXTROMETHORPHAN; OPIOIDS; EPHEDRINE HYDROCHLORIDE; DECONGESTANTS.

Meltus Expectorant, Meltus Honey and Lemon (Seton Scholl Healthcare) *See* GUAIPHENESIN <GUAIFENESIN>.

menadiol sodium phosphate A synthetic form of *vitamin K that is given to correct vitamin K deficiency. It is available as tablets that can be obtained without a prescription, but only from pharmacies.

Precautions: menadiol should not be taken by newborn babies and infants or by women in the late stages of pregnancy. This vitamin should be used with caution by people with glucose-6-phosphate dehydrogenase (G6PD) deficiency and vitamin E deficiency.

Interactions with other drugs:

Oral anticoagulants: their effects may be reduced by menadiol sodium phosphate.

Menogon (Ferring Pharmaceuticals) *See* HUMAN MENOPAUSAL GONADOTROPHIN.

Menophase (Searle) A proprietary preparation of *mestranol tablets and combined mestranol/*norethisterone tablets used as sequential combined *hormone replacement therapy for the relief of menopausal symptoms and the prevention of osteoporosis in women who have not had a hysterectomy. The tablets, which are available on *prescription only, must be taken in the prescribed order.

Side effects, precautions, and interactions with other drugs: see HORMONE REPLACEMENT THERAPY.

Menorest (Rhône-Poulenc Rorer) *See* OESTRADIOL <ESTRADIOL>; HORMONE REPLACEMENT THERAPY.

menotrophin *See* HUMAN MENOPAUSAL GONADOTROPHIN.

menthol (levomenthol) An aromatic substance with a minty taste, extracted from peppermint oil. It is commonly used, with or without *eucalyptus oil, *camphor, and *turpentine oil, in vapour inhalations, vapour rubs, and cough remedies to relieve nasal or catarrhal congestion associated with colds, influenza, rhinitis, or sinusitis and it is also included, together with more active ingredients, in many other proprietary cough medicines. Menthol is used as a counterirritant (*see* RUBEFACIENTS) in preparations that are rubbed into the skin to relieve muscle or joint pain, and is included in oral preparations to treat gallstones or kidney stones.
Proprietary preparations: Deep Freeze Cold Gel; Hill's Balsam Nasal Congestion Pastilles; Vicks Vaposyrup for Tickly Coughs; VICKS INHALER (combined with camphor); VICKS VAPORUB (combined with turpentine oil, camphor, and eucalyptus oil); plus many other proprietary medicines (see individual entries).

Mepranix (Ashbourne Pharmaceuticals) *See* METOPROLOL TARTRATE.

meprobamate An *anxiolytic drug used for the short-term treatment of anxiety. It is not recommended, since it is less effective than the *benzodiazepines, has a higher incidence of side effects, and is more dangerous in overdosage. Combined with analgesics, it is used for the treatment of muscle pain. Meprobamate is available as tablets; it is a *controlled drug.
Side effects: include drowsiness (the most common effect), light-headedness, confusion, shaky movements, unsteadiness, amnesia, paradoxical overexcitedness, headache, blurred vision, nausea, vomiting, diarrhoea, low blood pressure, 'pins and needles', and weakness. *Dependence can develop.
Precautions: meprobamate should not be taken by people with respiratory depression or severe breathing problems, or by women who are breastfeeding; it is not recommended for children. Meprobamate should be used with caution in pregnant women, elderly or debilitated people, and in people with lung disease, muscle weakness, epilepsy, liver or kidney disease, a history of drug or alcohol abuse, or a marked personality disorder. Drowsiness can affect driving and the performance of other skilled tasks and is increased by alcohol. Treatment should be stopped gradually; sudden withdrawal can lead to convulsions.
Interactions with other drugs: the sedative effect of meprobamate is increased by a number of drugs, including anaesthetics, opioid analgesics, antidepressants, antihistamines, and antipsychotic drugs.
Proprietary preparation: EQUAGESIC (combined with ethoheptazine and aspirin).

meptazinol An *opioid analgesic used for the treatment of moderate to severe pain, including postoperative pain. It is available as tablets or an injection on *prescription only.

Side effects and precautions: see MORPHINE.
Interactions with other drugs: see OPIOIDS.
Proprietary preparation: Meptid.

Meptid (Monmouth Pharmaceuticals) *See* MEPTAZINOL.

mepyramine An *antihistamine that is used topically to relieve the irritation and itching caused by insect bites or stings and allergic skin conditions, such as urticaria (nettle rash). It is available in the form of creams and sprays that can be obtained from pharmacies without a prescription.

Side effects: mepyramine may occasionally cause allergic reactions.
Precautions: preparations containing mepyramine should not be used for longer than three days and should not be applied to broken skin.
Proprietary preparations: Anthisan (cream); Boots Bite and Sting Antihistamine Cream; ANTHISAN PLUS (combined with benzocaine); WASP-EZE SPRAY (combined with benzocaine).

mequitazine One of the original (sedating) *antihistamines, used to relieve the symptoms of such allergic conditions as hay fever and urticaria. It is available as tablets on *prescription only or as an elixir that can be bought from pharmacies without a prescription.

Side effects: see ANTIHISTAMINES; mequitazine may also cause extrapyramidal reactions.
Precautions and interactions with other drugs: see ANTIHISTAMINES.
Proprietary preparation: Primalan.

Merbentyl, Merbentyl 20 (Hoechst Marion Roussel) *See* DICYCLOMINE <DICYCLOVERINE> HYDROCHLORIDE.

mercaptopurine An *antimetabolite used to prevent the recurrence of acute leukaemia, particularly in children (*see* CANCER). It is available as tablets on *prescription only.

Side effects: include *bone marrow suppression, loss of appetite, nausea and vomiting, and liver damage. *See also* CYTOTOXIC DRUGS.
Precautions: mercaptopurine should not be taken by pregnant women and should be used with caution in people with kidney or liver disease. *See also* CYTOTOXIC DRUGS.
Interactions with other drugs:

Allopurinol: the dosage of mercaptopurine should be reduced if it is taken with allopurinol since this drug increases the adverse effects of mercaptopurine.
Proprietary preparation: Puri-Nethol.

Mercilon (Organon Laboratories) A proprietary combination of *ethinyloestradiol <ethinylestradiol> and *desogestrel used as an *oral contraceptive. It is available as tablets on *prescription only.

Side effects and interactions with other drugs: see ORAL CONTRACEPTIVES.

Precautions: Mercilon should not be used by women who are at risk of developing thromboembolism, for example because they are very overweight or have varicose veins or a personal or family history of thrombosis. It should therefore only be taken by women who cannot tolerate other brands and who are prepared to accept the increased risk. *See also* ORAL CONTRACEPTIVES.

Merocaine (Hoechst Marion Roussel) A proprietary combination of *benzocaine (a local anaesthetic) and *cetylpyridinium chloride (an antiseptic), used for the treatment of mouth and throat infections and as an *adjunct for tonsillitis, pharyngitis, and dental procedures. It is available as lozenges and can be obtained without a prescription, but only from pharmacies.

Precautions: Merocaine is not recommended for children under 12 years old.

Merocet, **Merocets** (Hoechst Marion Roussel) *See* CETYLPYRIDINIUM CHLORIDE.

Meronem (AstraZeneca) *See* MEROPENEM.

meropenem A beta-lactam antibiotic, similar to *penicillins, that is used for the treatment of pneumonia, urinary-tract, intra-abdominal, and gynaecological infections, skin and soft-tissue infections, septicaemia, and fevers associated with a low white blood cell count. It is also used to treat chronic lower respiratory-tract infections in those with cystic fibrosis. It is given by intravenous infusion and is available on *prescription only.

Side effects: include nausea, vomiting, diarrhoea, abdominal pain, blood disorders, headache, 'pins and needles', rash, itching, urticaria (nettle rash), and pain at the injection site.

Precautions: meropenem should not be given to people who are allergic to it and should be used with caution in anyone allergic to other beta-lactam antibiotics. It should also be used with caution in patients who have liver or kidney disease and in women who are pregnant or breastfeeding.

Proprietary preparation: Meronem.

mesalazine An *aminosalicylate used for the treatment of mild to moderate attacks of ulcerative colitis and to maintain remission in ulcerative colitis and colitis due to Crohn's disease. It is available, on *prescription only, as tablets, *modified-release tablets, suppositories, or an enema.

Side effects: include nausea, diarrhoea, headache, abdominal pain, blood disorders (see precautions below), and kidney damage.

Precautions: mesalazine should not be taken by people with severe liver disease or a blood-clotting disorder; any unexplained bleeding, bruising, sore throat, or malaise should be reported immediately to a doctor, as this may indicate a blood disorder. *See* AMINOSALICYLATES.

Proprietary preparations: Asacol; Pentasa; Salofalk.

mesna A drug that is given in conjunction with *cyclophosphamide or *ifosfamide to prevent the adverse effects of these cytotoxic drugs on the bladder. It is available, on *prescription only, as a solution for injection or as tablets.

Proprietary preparation: Uromitexan.

mesterolone A drug used for the treatment of *androgen deficiency and male infertility. It is available as tablets on *prescription only.

Side effects: include excessive frequency and duration of penile erection, fluid retention and weight gain, and liver disorders.

Precautions and interactions with other drugs: see TESTOSTERONE.

Proprietary preparation: Pro-Viron.

Mestinon (Roche Products) *See* PYRIDOSTIGMINE.

mestranol A synthetic *oestrogen that is used in combination with *norethisterone (a progestogen) in *oral contraceptives and in *hormone replacement therapy. It is available as tablets on *prescription only.

Side effects, precautions, and interactions with other drugs: see OESTROGENS; ORAL CONTRACEPTIVES; HORMONE REPLACEMENT THERAPY.

Proprietary preparations: MENOPHASE; NORINYL-1.

Metanium (Roche Products) A proprietary combination of *titanium dioxide, titanium peroxide, and titanium salicylate in a cream base that includes *dimethicone <dimeticone>, light *liquid paraffin, and *white soft paraffin. It is used as a *barrier preparation for the prevention and treatment of napkin rash and is freely available *over the counter in the form of an ointment.

metaraminol A *sympathomimetic drug that causes blood vessels to constrict and therefore raises blood pressure. It is used to restore or maintain blood pressure in patients undergoing surgery, especially those who have low blood pressure due to spinal anaesthesia. It is available as a solution for intravenous injection or infusion on *prescription only.

Side effects, precautions, and interactions with other drugs: see NORADRENALINE <NOREPINEPHRINE>.

Proprietary preparation: Aramine.

metastases *See* CANCER.

Metatone (Warner-Lambert Consumer Healthcare) A proprietary combination of calcium glycerophosphate, manganese glycerophosphate, potassium glycerophosphate, sodium glycerophosphate, and *thiamine hydrochloride (vitamin B$_1$) in the form of a *tonic, used to stimulate the appetite. The glycerophosphates are believed to be readily absorbed into the brain where they exert their tonic effects, but there is no evidence for this action. Metatone is freely available *over the counter and cannot be prescribed on the NHS.

Meted (DermaPharm) A proprietary combination of *sulphur and *salicylic acid (both keratolytics), used for the treatment of scaly disorders of the scalp, such as seborrhoeic *eczema, *psoriasis, and dandruff. It is available as a shampoo and can be obtained without a prescription, but only from pharmacies.
Side effects: Meted may cause local irritation.

Metenix (Hoechst Marion Roussel) *See* METOLAZONE.

metered-dose inhaler *See* INHALER.

metformin hydrochloride An *oral hypoglycaemic drug that lowers blood-glucose concentrations by increasing the uptake of glucose into the body's tissues and reducing its release from the liver. It belongs to a group of drugs called **biguanides** and is the only drug of this group that is currently available. Metformin is used for the treatment of noninsulin-dependent (type II) *diabetes mellitus and is of particular value in obese people. It is available as tablets on *prescription only.
Side effects: include loss of appetite, nausea, vomiting, and diarrhoea (usually transient). Uptake of vitamin B$_{12}$ is reduced, and prolonged treatment may cause anaemia. Occasionally metformin causes lactic acidosis (resulting in coma); this risk is increased in people with kidney or liver disease and in certain other vulnerable groups, in whom metformin should be avoided (see below).
Precautions: metformin should not be taken by people with liver or kidney disease, heart failure, or severe infections, after surgery or injury, by those who are dehydrated, or by women who are pregnant or breastfeeding. Alcohol should be avoided, as it increases the risk of *hypoglycaemia and may cause lactic acidosis.
Interactions with other drugs:
  Cimetidine: increases the plasma concentration of metformin and therefore the risk of hypoglycaemia.
Proprietary preparations: Glucamet; Glucophage.

methadone hydrochloride An *opioid analgesic used in the treatment of people who are physically dependent on diamorphine (heroin) or other opioids, in whom it prevents the occurrence of withdrawal symptoms (*see* DEPENDENCE). It is also sometimes used to treat severe pain in people who cannot tolerate morphine and occasionally to control coughing in terminally ill patients. Methadone is a *controlled drug; it is available as tablets, a liquid, or an injection.

Side effects and precautions: *see* MORPHINE.

Interactions with other drugs:

 Carbamazepine: reduces the effects of methadone.

 Phenytoin: reduces the effects of methadone and may cause withdrawal symptoms.

 Zidovudine: its plasma concentration may be increased by methadone.

 See also OPIOIDS.

Proprietary preparations: Methadose; Metharose; Methex; Physeptone.

Methadose (Rosemont Pharmaceuticals) *See* METHADONE HYDROCHLORIDE.

Metharose (Rosemont Pharmaceuticals) *See* METHADONE HYDROCHLORIDE.

methenamine hippurate *See* HEXAMINE HIPPURATE.

Methex (Generics) *See* METHADONE HYDROCHLORIDE.

methocarbamol A *muscle relaxant that is used for the short-term relief of muscle spasms. It is available as tablets or an injection on *prescription only.

Side effects: include lassitude, light-headedness, drowsiness, dizziness, restlessness, anxiety, confusion, nausea, and an allergic rash.

Precautions: methocarbamol should not be given to anyone who is in a coma or who has brain damage, epilepsy, or myasthenia gravis. It should be used with caution in people with impaired liver or kidney function. Drowsiness may affect driving or the ability to operate machinery, and methocarbamol can enhance the sedative effects of alcohol.

Proprietary preparation: Robaxin.

methotrexate An *antimetabolite that is used for the treatment of acute lymphoblastic leukaemia in children and adults and of choriocarcinoma (a form of cancer occurring in the uterus during or after pregnancy), non-Hodgkin's lymphoma, and a number of solid tumours in adults (*see* CANCER). Methotrexate is also used as an *immunosuppressant to treat severe *psoriasis and rheumatoid arthritis that have not responded to other treatments. It may be taken orally or injected into a vein, a muscle, or around the spinal cord, and *folinic acid is often given afterwards to prevent side effects. It is available as tablets or solutions for injection on *prescription only.

Side effects: include *bone marrow suppression, inflammation and ulceration of the mucous membranes, especially the mouth, and rarely inflammation of the lungs. It can also cause liver damage. *See* CYTOTOXIC DRUGS.

Precautions: methotrexate should not be given to people with severe kidney or liver disease or to pregnant women. *See* CYTOTOXIC DRUGS.

Interactions with other drugs:

Acitretin: increases the plasma concentrations of methotrexate and the risk of adverse effects on the liver.

Aspirin: increases the risk of adverse effects of methotrexate.

Cyclosporin: the adverse effects of both methotrexate and cyclosporin are increased.

NSAIDs: increase the risk of adverse effects of methotrexate; azaproprazone should not be taken with methotrexate.

Probenecid: increases the risk of adverse effects of methotrexate.

Proprietary preparation: Maxtrex.

methotrimeprazine <levomepromazine> A phenothiazine *antipsychotic drug used for the treatment of schizophrenia and manic-depressive psychosis, especially when sedation is desirable. It is also given to terminally ill patients to relieve restlessness, distress, or vomiting. Methotrimeprazine is available as tablets or an injection on *prescription only.

Side effects: as for *chlorpromazine, but methotrimeprazine is more sedating.

Precautions and interactions with other drugs: see CHLORPROMAZINE HYDROCHLORIDE.

Proprietary preparation: Nozinan.

methoxamine hydrochloride A *sympathomimetic drug that causes blood vessels to constrict and therefore raises blood pressure. It is used to restore blood pressure in patients undergoing surgery, especially those who have dangerously low blood pressure resulting from spinal or epidural anaesthesia. Methoxamine is available as an injection on *prescription only.

Side effects and precautions: as for *noradrenaline <norepinephrine>. However, methoxamine is longer acting than noradrenaline <norepinephrine> and may cause a prolonged rise in blood pressure.

Proprietary preparation: Vasoxine.

methylcellulose A synthetic *bulk-forming laxative used for treating constipation and for managing chronic diarrhoea in bowel disease. It is also used in the treatment of *obesity to reduce food intake, since its bulk-forming properties are supposed to induce feelings of fullness. Methylcellulose is freely available *over the counter in the form of tablets.

Side effects and precautions: see ISPAGHULA HUSK.

Proprietary preparation: Celevac.

methylcysteine hydrochloride A *mucolytic drug that reduces the viscosity of bronchial secretions by liquefying mucus. It is used to relieve congestion of the airways, for example in bronchitis. Methylcysteine is available as tablets without a prescription, but only from pharmacies. It cannot be prescribed on the NHS.

Side effects: stomach and bowel upsets may occur.

Proprietary preparation: Visclair.

methyldopa An alpha stimulant (*see* SYMPATHOMIMETIC DRUGS) that acts centrally (on receptors in the brain). It is used in the treatment of all grades of *hypertension, sometimes in combination with *diuretics. It is available on *prescription only, as tablets, a suspension, or a solution for injection.

Side effects: include sedation, headache, depression, nasal congestion, dry mouth, and gastrointestinal upsets; rarely it can cause anaemia.

Proprietary preparation: Aldomet.

See also ANTIHYPERTENSIVE DRUGS.

methyl nicotinate A drug that is used as a *rubefacient for the relief of aches and pains in muscles, tendons, and joints. It is an ingredient of creams, ointments, and sprays most of which are freely available *over the counter.

Side effects and precautions: see RUBEFACIENTS.

Proprietary preparations: ALGIPAN RUB (combined with capsicum oleoresin and glycol salicylate); CREMALGIN (combined with capsicum oleoresin and glycol salicylate); DEEP HEAT SPRAY (combined with ethyl salicylate, methyl salicylate, and glycol salicylate); DUBAM SPRAY (combined with ethyl salicylate, methyl salicylate, and glycol salicylate); FIERY JACK CREAM (combined with capsicum oleoresin, diethylamine salicylate, and glycol salicylate); NELLA RED OIL (combined with clove oil and mustard oil); RALGEX CREAM (combined with capsicum oleoresin and glycol monosalicylate); RALGEX HEAT SPRAY (combined with glycol salicylate) TRANSVASIN HEAT SPRAY (combined with diethylamine salicylate and 2-hydroxyethyl salicylate)

methylphenidate hydrochloride A *stimulant of the central nervous system, similar to *dexamphetamine <dexamfetamine>, that is used for the treatment of attention deficit disorder in children. A *controlled drug, it is available as tablets.

Side effects: see DEXAMPHETAMINE <DEXAMFETAMINE> SULPHATE. In addition, rashes, urticaria, fever, muscle aches, hair loss, and dermatitis can occur.

Precautions and interactions with other drugs: see DEXAMPHETAMINE <DEXAMFETAMINE> SULPHATE.

Proprietary preparation: Ritalin.

methylphenobarbitone <methylphenobarbital> An *anticonvulsant drug very similar to *phenobarbitone <phenobarbital>. A *controlled drug, it is available as tablets.

Side effects and precautions: see PHENOBARBITONE <PHENOBARBITAL>.

Interactions with other drugs: see BARBITURATES.
Proprietary preparation: Prominal.

methylprednisolone A *corticosteroid used for treatment of inflammatory disorders (including rheumatic disease), cerebral oedema (swelling of the brain), and eczematous skin conditions. It is available, on *prescription only, as tablets, as a solution for injection, or as a cream for topical application.

Side effects, precautions, and interactions with other drugs: see CORTICOSTEROIDS; TOPICAL STEROIDS.

Proprietary preparations: Depo-Medrone (*depot injection into a muscle or a joint); Medrone (tablets); Solu-Medrone (injection); DEPO-MEDRONE WITH LIDOCAINE (combined with lignocaine <lidocaine> hydrochloride).

methylrosanilinium chloride See CRYSTAL VIOLET.

methyl salicylate (oil of wintergreen) A *salicylate that is an ingredient of many *rubefacient creams and sprays for the relief of aches, pains, and stiffness in muscles, tendons, and joints. It is also used in preparations for treating fungal skin infections, relieving congestion due to colds and catarrh, and soothing *haemorrhoids. Preparations containing methyl salicylate are available without a prescription, but some can only be obtained from pharmacies.

Side effects and precautions: see SALICYLATES.

Proprietary preparations: BALMOSA (combined with camphor, capsicum oleoresin, and menthol); BOOTS PAIN RELIEF WARMING SPRAY (combined with camphor and ethyl nicotinate); BOOTS SUPPOSITORIES FOR HAEMORRHOIDS (combined with benzyl alcohol, glycol monosalicylate, and zinc oxide); CHYMOL EMOLLIENT BALM (combined with eucalyptus oil, phenol, and terpineol); DEEP HEAT MASSAGE LINIMENT (combined with menthol); DEEP HEAT RUB (combined with eucalyptus oil, menthol, and turpentine oil); DEEP HEAT SPRAY (combined with ethyl salicylate, glycol salicylate, and methyl nicotinate); DUBAM CREAM (combined with menthol and cineole); DUBAM SPRAY (combined with ethyl salicylate, glycol salicylate, and methyl nicotinate); GERMOLENE OINTMENT (combined with zinc oxide, octaphonium <octafonium> chloride, phenol, and emollients); MONPHYTOL (combined with chlorbutol <chlorobutanol>, methyl undecenoate, salicylic acid, propyl salicylate, and propyl undecenoate); OLBAS OIL (combined with eucalyptus oil, menthol, cajuput oil, clove oil, and juniper berry oil); OLBAS PASTILLES (combined with eucalyptus oil, menthol, peppermint oil, clove oil, and juniper berry oil); PHYTEX (combined with borotannic acid complex, salicylic acid, and acetic acid); PR HEAT SPRAY (combined with ethyl nicotinate and camphor); RADIAN-B MUSCLE RUB (combined with camphor, capsicin, and menthol); RALGEX STICK (combined with capsicum oleoresin, ethyl salicylate, glycol salicylate, and menthol); SALONAIR (combined with benzyl nicotinate, camphor, menthol, glycol salicylate, and squalane);

SALONPAS PLASTERS (combined with glycol salicylate, camphor, and menthol).

methyl violet *See* CRYSTAL VIOLET.

methysergide A drug that antagonizes the action of the neurotransmitter *serotonin (5-hydroxytryptamine). It is used for preventing attacks in severe recurrent *migraine and other headaches with vascular causes that do not respond to standard treatments. In much higher doses it is used to treat diarrhoea associated with carcinoid syndrome (caused by a tumour that secretes serotonin). Methysergide is available as tablets on *prescription only; patients taking it should be closely monitored in hospitals because of the severity of its side effects.
Side effects: nausea, vomiting, abdominal discomfort, drowsiness, and dizziness often occur at the start of treatment; other side effects include mental and behavioural disturbances, insomnia, fluid retention and weight gain, and – after prolonged treatment – abnormal development of fibrous tissue within the abdomen and elsewhere.
Precautions: methysergide should not be given to people with high blood pressure or heart, lung, liver, or kidney disease, or to women who are pregnant or breastfeeding. It should be used with caution in patients with a history of peptic ulceration.
Proprietary preparation: Deseril.

metipranolol A *beta blocker used in the form of eye drops for treating chronic (open-angle) *glaucoma in people who are allergic to the preservatives (such as benzalkonium chloride) that are included in similar preparations and people who wear soft contact lenses (who should not use eye drops containing benzalkonium chloride). Metipranolol is available on *prescription only.
Side effects, precautions, and interactions with other drugs: see BETA BLOCKERS.
Proprietary preparation: Minims Metipranolol.

metirosine A drug that inhibits the enzyme tyrosine hydroxylase, which is required for the synthesis of adrenaline <epinephrine>, noradrenaline <norepinephrine>, and dopamine. It is used to treat phaeochromocytoma, a tumour of the adrenal gland that unpredictably secretes excessive amounts of adrenaline <epinephrine> and noradrenaline <norepinephrine>, causing sudden attacks of raised blood pressure. Metirosine is available as capsules on *prescription only.
Side effects: include sedation, *extrapyramidal reactions, possibly severe diarrhoea, and allergic reactions.
Precautions: a high fluid intake is necessary when taking metirosine to maintain blood volume. The ability to drive or operate machinery may be impaired in those taking metirosine.
Interactions with other drugs:

Antipsychotic drugs: the risk of extrapyramidal reactions is increased if these drugs are taken with metirosine.

Proprietary preparation: Demser.

metoclopramide A drug that antagonizes the action of *dopamine. It is an *antiemetic used to prevent or treat nausea and vomiting, including that produced by radiotherapy or cytotoxic chemotherapy for cancer, when it is usually given together with other drugs. It is also included in some preparations for the treatment of *migraine, to alleviate the nausea and vomiting that can accompany migraine headaches and to hasten the absorption of analgesic drugs. It is not effective for motion sickness. Metoclopramide also stimulates gastric motility (*see* PROKINETIC DRUGS) and is used for the treatment of various gastrointestinal disorders, including indigestion (apart from that caused by peptic ulceration) and gastro-oesophageal reflux (*see* ACID-PEPTIC DISEASES). It is available, on *prescription only, as tablets, *modified-release capsules or tablets, a syrup, or a solution for intravenous injection.

Side effects: metoclopramide can cause abnormal facial and body movements, such as twisting of the neck (*see* EXTRAPYRAMIDAL REACTIONS); these effects are more common in children and young adults (under 20 years old). Other side effects include raised serum prolactin, which causes breast enlargement and milk production.

Precautions: in people under 20 years old, metoclopramide should only be used for treating vomiting caused by radiotherapy or chemotherapy, severe vomiting of known cause that is resistant to other drugs, or to facilitate the insertion of a nasogastric tube (through the nose to the stomach). It should not be used for 3–4 days after gastrointestinal surgery and should be used with caution in people with impaired liver or kidney function, women who are pregnant or breastfeeding, and the elderly.

Interactions with other drugs:

Analgesics: the effects of aspirin and paracetamol are enhanced by metoclopramide.

Antipsychotics: the risk of extrapyramidal reactions is increased.

Proprietary preparations: Gastrobid Continus (modified-release tablets); Gastroflux; Gastromax (modified-release capsules); Maxolon; Maxolon High Dose; Maxolon SR (modified-release capsules); Parmid; Primperan; MIGRAVESS (combined with aspirin); PARAMAX (combined with paracetamol).

metolazone A thiazide-like diuretic (*see* THIAZIDE DIURETICS) used for the treatment of *hypertension and *oedema. It is available as tablets on *prescription only.

Side effects, precautions, and interactions with other drugs: *see* THIAZIDE DIURETICS.

Proprietary preparation: Metenix.

See also ANTIHYPERTENSIVE DRUGS; DIURETICS.

Metopirone (Alliance Pharmaceuticals) *See* METYRAPONE.

metoprolol tartrate A cardioselective *beta blocker used for the treatment and prevention of heart *arrhythmias and the treatment of *hypertension. It is also used to treat *angina and is taken after a heart attack to prevent worsening of the condition. It is available as tablets, *modified-release tablets, or an injection on *prescription only.

Side effects and precautions: see BETA BLOCKERS.

Interactions with other drugs:

Lercanidipine: may increase the effect of metoprolol in lowering blood pressure.

Propafenone: increases the plasma concentration of metoprolol.

For other interactions, *see* BETA BLOCKERS.

Proprietary preparations: Arbralene; Betaloc; Betaloc SA (modified-release tablets); Lopressor; Lopressor SR (modified-release tablets); Mepranix; CO-BETALOC (combined with hydrochlorothiazide).

See also ANTI-ARRHYTHMIC DRUGS; ANTIHYPERTENSIVE DRUGS.

Metosyn, Metosyn Scalp Lotion (AstraZeneca) *See* FLUOCINONIDE.

Metrodin High Purity (Serono Laboratories) *See* UROFOLLITROPHIN <UROFOLLITROPIN>.

Metrogel (Novartis Consumer Health) *See* METRONIDAZOLE.

Metrolyl (Lagap Pharmaceuticals) *See* METRONIDAZOLE.

metronidazole An *antibiotic with activity against certain types of bacteria and protozoa. It is used to treat trichomonal vaginitis (a sexually transmitted protozoal infection of the vagina) and bacterial vaginitis. It is also active against *Entamoeba histolytica*, the cause of amoebic dysentry and ulcers of the gut wall, and *Giardia*, which causes diarrhoea. The drug is also used to treat or prevent surgical and gynaecological infections and to treat dental and gum infections (including gingivitis). Metronidazole is effective in the treatment of pseudomembranous colitis, an infection of the large bowel caused by overgrowth of the microbes normally occurring in the gut, which is often caused by the use of broad-spectrum antibiotics. Topical metronidazole is used to prevent the odour associated with infected tumours and to treat rosacea (a chronic inflammatory condition of the face). A *prescription only medicine, it is available as tablets or a suspension for oral use, a solution for *intravenous infusion, and as a gel, solution, cream, or suppositories for topical use.

Side effects: include nausea, vomiting, an unpleasant taste in the mouth, furred tongue, gastrointestinal disturbances, rashes, and swelling of the face. Rare side effects are drowsiness, headache, dizziness, and darkening of urine; on prolonged therapy transient epileptic seizures may occur. Topical preparations may cause local irritation.

Precautions: alcohol should be avoided during treatment as the combination may lead to vomiting. The drug should be used with caution in women who are pregnant or breastfeeding.

Interactions with other drugs (unlikely with topical preparations):

Anticoagulants: the effects of warfarin and nicoumalone <acenocoumarol> are enhanced.

Cimetidine: increases plasma concentrations of metronidazole.

Lithium: concentrations of lithium may be increased and cause toxic effects.

Phenobarbitone <phenobarbital>: reduces plasma concentrations of metronidazole.

Phenytoin: the effects of phenytoin are increased.

Proprietary preparations: Anabact (topical solution); Elyzol (gel); Flagyl; Metrogel (gel); Metrolyl; Metrotop (gel); Noritate (cream); Rozex (gel); Vaginyl (tablets); Zidoval (gel); FLAGYL COMPAK (packaged with nystatin).

Metrotop (Seton Scholl Healthcare) *See* METRONIDAZOLE.

metyrapone A drug that inhibits the hormone aldosterone, which acts on the kidneys to regulate salt and water balance. Its action results in increased volumes of urine being excreted. It thus acts as a *diuretic, but by a mechanism different from that of most of the common diuretics. It is used to treat Cushing's syndrome or given in combination with glucocorticoids (*see* CORTICOSTEROIDS) to treat resistant *oedema. Metyrapone is available as capsules on *prescription only.

Side effects: include nausea, vomiting, hypotension (low blood pressure), and allergic reactions.

Precautions: metyrapone should not be taken by people suffering from pituitary disorders or adrenal insufficiency.

Proprietary preparation: Metopirone.

mexiletine A class I *anti-arrhythmic drug used for the treatment of ventricular *arrhythmias. It is available as capsules on *prescription only.

Side effects: include nausea, vomiting, constipation, a slow heart rate, low blood pressure, drowsiness, and confusion.

Precautions and interactions with other drugs: *see* ANTI-ARRHYTHMIC DRUGS.

Proprietary preparation: Mexitil.

Mexitil (Boehringer Ingelheim) *See* MEXILETINE.

Miacalcic (Novartis Consumer Health) *See* SALCATONIN <CALCITONIN (SALMON)>.

mianserin hydrochloride An *antidepressant drug, similar to the *tricyclic antidepressants, used for the treatment of depressive illness, particularly when sedation is required. It is available as tablets on *prescription only.

Side effects: similar to *amitriptyline hydrochloride, but mianserin has fewer antimuscarinic effects (e.g. dry mouth, difficulty in urinating, blurred vision); it can cause blood disorders.

Precautions: a full blood count should be taken every four weeks during the first three months of treatment. Treatment should be stopped if signs of infection (e.g. fever, sore throat) develop. *See also* TRICYCLIC ANTIDEPRESSANTS.

Interactions with other drugs: *see* TRICYCLIC ANTIDEPRESSANTS.

Micanol (Medeva) *See* DITHRANOL.

Micolette Micro-enema (Dominion Pharma) A proprietary combination of *sodium citrate (an osmotic laxative), *sodium lauryl sulphoacetate (a wetting agent), and glycerol (*see* GLYCERIN), used for the treatment of constipation. It can be obtained without a prescription, but only from pharmacies.

Precautions: *see* SODIUM CITRATE.

miconazole An imidazole *antifungal drug similar to *ketoconazole. It is used to treat and prevent a wide range of fungal infections, including candidiasis (thrush), especially of the vulva and vagina, tinea (ringworm), acne, and gastrointestinal infections. It may also be used as a solution to wash out the bladder in cases of *Candida* infection. It is available as tablets, vaginal capsules, pessaries, a mouth gel, a cream, a powder, a spray powder, and a denture lacquer. Tablets, pessaries, and vaginal capsules are available on *prescription only; topical preparations may be bought without a prescription, but only from pharmacies.

Side effects: the tablets and gel may cause nausea, vomiting, and rashes. Topical preparations may produce skin irritation.

Precautions: miconazole should not be used by people with porphyria and should be used with caution by women who are pregnant or breastfeeding.

Interactions with other drugs:

Anticoagulants: the effects of warfarin and nicoumalone <acenocoumarol> are enhanced.

Antidiabetic drugs: plasma concentrations of the sulphonylureas are increased.

Astemizole: should not be taken with miconazole because of the risk of irregular heart rhythms.

Cisapride: should not be taken with miconazole because of the risk of irregular heart rhythms.

Phenytoin: its effect is enhanced.

Terfenadine: should not be taken with miconazole because of the risk of irregular heart rhythms.

Proprietary preparations: Daktarin; Daktarin Oral Gel; Dumicoat (denture lacquer); Femeron (cream and pessaries); Gyno-Daktarin (vaginal cream); ACNIDAZIL (combined with benzoyl peroxide); DAKTACORT (combined with hydrocortisone).

Micralax Micro-enema (Medeva) A proprietary combination of
*sodium citrate (an osmotic laxative) and sodium alkylsulphoacetate (a
wetting agent) used for the treatment of constipation. It can be obtained
without a prescription, but only from pharmacies.
Precautions: see SODIUM CITRATE.

Microgynon 30 (Schering Health Care) A proprietary combination of
*ethinyloestradiol <ethinylestradiol> (30 micrograms) and
*levonorgestrel used as an *oral contraceptive. **Microgynon 30 ED**
contains both active and dummy tablets, so that a tablet is taken each
day of a 28-day cycle. Both preparations are available as tablets on
*prescription only.
Side effects, precautions, and interactions with other drugs: see ORAL
CONTRACEPTIVES.

Micronor (Janssen-Cilag) *See* NORETHISTERONE; ORAL CONTRACEPTIVES.

Micronor-HRT (Janssen-Cilag) *See* NORETHISTERONE; HORMONE
REPLACEMENT THERAPY.

Microval (Wyeth Laboratories) *See* LEVONORGESTREL; ORAL
CONTRACEPTIVES.

Mictral (Sanofi Winthrop) A proprietary combination of *nalidixic acid
(a quinolone antibiotic), *sodium citrate, *citric acid, and *sodium
bicarbonate (all alkalizing agents), used for the treatment of cystitis and
other infections of the lower urinary tract. It is available, on
*prescription only, as effervescent granules.
Side effects: include nausea, vomiting, abdominal pain, diarrhoea, visual
disturbances, seizures, and allergic reactions.
Precautions: Mictral should not be taken by people with a history of
epilepsy or seizures, poor kidney function, or by women who are
pregnant or breastfeeding. People who are taking Mictral should avoid
exposure to sunlight.
Interactions with other drugs: see QUINOLONES.

midazolam A *benzodiazepine that is used to produce sedation in
patients about to undergo surgery. It also causes amnesia, so that patients
do not remember the preoperative period, and recovery from its effects
after surgery is more rapid than with *diazepam. Midazolam is available
as an injection on *prescription only.
Side effects and precautions: high dosages given by intravenous injection
may cause profound sedation and depression of breathing. *See also*
BENZODIAZEPINES.
Interactions with other drugs:
  Antifungal drugs: itraconazole, ketoconazole, and fluconazole inhibit the
    breakdown of midazolam, causing profound sedation.
  Antiviral drugs: ritonavir, indinavir and nelfinavir increase the risk of

profound sedation and depression of breathing and should not be used with midazolam.

Erythromycin: inhibits the breakdown of midazolam, causing profound sedation.

See also BENZODIAZEPINES.

Proprietary preparation: Hypnovel.

Midrid (Shire Pharmaceuticals) A proprietary combination of *paracetamol (an analgesic) and *isometheptene mucate (a vasoconstrictor) in the form of capsules, used for the treatment of *migraine attacks. Packs containing 100 capsules are available on *prescription only, but 15-capsule packs can be obtained from pharmacies without a prescription.

Side effects and precautions: *see* PARACETAMOL; ISOMETHEPTENE MUCATE.

Interactions with other drugs: *see* ISOMETHEPTENE MUCATE.

Mifegyne (Exelgyn Laboratories) *See* MIFEPRISTONE.

mifepristone A drug that blocks the action of *progesterone, a hormone that is essential for maintaining a pregnancy. Mifepristone is used to induce abortion up to the 20th week of pregnancy. It is taken by mouth under medical supervision; if the pregnancy is more advanced than 9 weeks *gemeprost pessaries may need to be given in addition. Mifepristone is also used for softening and dilating the cervix (neck of the uterus) before mechanical termination of pregnancy. It is available as tablets on *prescription only.

Side effects: include malaise, faintness, headache, nausea, vomiting, rashes, vaginal bleeding (sometimes severe), and (especially after gemeprost) pain in the uterus.

Precautions: mifepristone should not be used if an ectopic pregnancy is suspected or in women with chronic adrenal failure or taking long-term corticosteroids or anticoagulants. It should not be used in combination with gemeprost by women over 35 who smoke. Alcohol and smoking must be avoided for two days before gemeprost treatment and on the day of this treatment. Mifepristone should be used with caution by women with asthma, heart, liver or kidney disease, and during breastfeeding.

Interactions with other drugs:

Aspirin and NSAIDs: should not be taken for at least 8–12 days after mifepristone treatment.

Proprietary preparation: Mifegyne.

Migrafen (Chatfield) *See* IBUPROFEN.

migraine A recurrent headache that is usually throbbing and typically affects one side of the head. Some attacks are preceded by a warning (**aura**) consisting of visual disturbances and numbness and/or weakness of the limbs. The headache is often accompanied by nausea and vomiting. Migraine may be precipitated or exacerbated by certain foods (such as cheese or chocolate), red wine, or stress. It is thought to be caused by changes in the blood vessels around the brain and eyes and in the scalp, which constrict and then become overdilated.

A variety of drugs is available for the treatment of migraine attacks. Analgesics, for pain relief, usually contain *aspirin, *paracetamol, and/or *codeine; if these are ineffective, *tolfenamic acid (an NSAID) may be tried. For people who fail to respond to these analgesics, *5HT$_1$ agonists, such as *sumatriptan or *zolmitriptan, are the recommended treatment for an acute attack. They act by reversing the overdilatation of the blood vessels in the brain. *Ergotamine tartrate also constricts blood vessels, but it is less selective in this action than the 5HT$_1$ agonists and has more severe side effects. Antiemetics, such as *metoclopramide, *cyclizine, or *buclizine hydrochloride, may be required to relieve the nausea and vomiting associated with a migraine headache. These may be used alone or combined with an analgesic. *See also* ISOMETHEPTENE MUCATE.

For people who experience frequent migraine attacks (more than one a month), a preventive approach is needed. The drugs used for this purpose include *beta blockers (such as *propranolol, *metoprolol, *nadolol, and *timolol), the antihistamines *pizotifen and *cyproheptadine (which antagonize the effects of *serotonin), and *tricyclic antidepressants (such as *amitriptyline). Since long-term treatment with these drugs is not advisable, the patient's condition should be assessed at six-monthly intervals to see if treatment needs to be continued. Some individuals benefit from the herbal remedy feverfew. *See also* METHYSERGIDE.

Migraleve (Pfizer Consumer Healthcare) A proprietary preparation consisting of a combination of the analgesics *paracetamol and *codeine phosphate and the antiemetic antihistamine *buclizine hydrochloride in the form of **pink tablets**, packaged with a combination of paracetamol and codeine phosphate (**yellow tablets**), used for the treatment of *migraine. Two pink tablets taken at the start of a migraine attack are followed by two yellow tablets at four-hourly intervals. Migraleve can be obtained without a prescription, but only from pharmacies.

Side effects: Migraleve causes drowsiness.

Precautions: Migraleve should not be taken by children under 10 years old, except under medical supervision. *See also* PARACETAMOL; ANTIHISTAMINES.

Interactions with other drugs: see ANTIHISTAMINES; OPIOIDS.

Migravess (Bayer) A proprietary combination of *aspirin (an analgesic) and *metoclopramide (an antiemetic), used for the relief of migraine. **Migravess Forte** contains a higher dose of aspirin. Both preparations are available as effervescent tablets on *prescription only.

Side effects, precautions, and interactions with other drugs: see ASPIRIN; METOCLOPRAMIDE.

Migril (GlaxoWellcome) A proprietary combination of *ergotamine tartrate, *cyclizine hydrochloride (an antiemetic antihistamine), and *caffeine hydrate, used for the treatment of *migraine. It is available as tablets on prescription only.

Side effects and precautions: *see* ERGOTAMINE TARTRATE; CYCLIZINE; ANTIHISTAMINES; CAFFEINE.

Interactions with other drugs: *see* ERGOTAMINE TARTRATE; ANTIHISTAMINES.

Mildison Lipocream (Yamanouchi Pharma) *See* HYDROCORTISONE.

Mil-Par (Merck Consumer Health) A proprietary combination of *liquid paraffin (a faecal softener) and *magnesium hydroxide (an osmotic laxative), used for the treatment of constipation. It is available as a liquid and can be obtained without a prescription, but only from phamacies.

Side effects and precautions: *see* LIQUID PARAFFIN; MAGNESIUM SALTS.

Interactions with other drugs: *see* ANTACIDS.

milrinone A drug, similar to *enoximone, that acts on the heart muscles to strengthen the heartbeat. It is used for the short-term treatment of severe congestive *heart failure, especially in people who have not responded to standard therapy, and acute heart failure occurring after heart surgery. Milrinone is available as an injection on *prescription only.

Side effects, precautions, and interactions with other drugs: *see* ENOXIMONE.

Proprietary preparation: Primacor.

Minadex (Seven Seas) A proprietary combination of *vitamin A, *vitamin C, and *vitamin D, used as a vitamin supplement for children. It is freely available *over the counter in the form of oral drops.

Side effects, precautions, and interactions with other drugs: *see* VITAMIN A.

mineralocorticoids *See* CORTICOSTEROIDS.

Minihep, Minihep Calcium (Leo Pharmaceuticals) *See* HEPARIN.

Min-I-Jet Adrenaline (International Medication Systems) *See* ADRENALINE <EPINEPHRINE>.

Min-I-Jet Atropine (International Medication Systems) *See* ATROPINE SULPHATE.

Min-I-Jet Calcium Chloride (International Medication Systems; Aurum Pharmaceuticals) *See* CALCIUM CHLORIDE.

Min-I-Jet Morphine Sulphate (International Medication Systems) *See* MORPHINE).

Min-I-Jet Naloxone (International Medication Systems) *See* NALOXONE HYDROCHLORIDE.

Min-I-Jet Sodium Bicarbonate (International Medication Systems) *See* SODIUM BICARBONATE.

Minims Amethocaine Hydrochloride (Chauvin Pharmaceuticals) *See* AMETHOCAINE <TETRACAINE>.

Minims Artificial Tears (Chauvin Pharmaceuticals) A proprietary combination of *sodium chloride and *hydroxyethylcellulose, used as a lubricant for dry eyes. It is available as single-dose eye drops and can be obtained without a prescription, but only from pharmacies.

Minims Atropine Sulphate (Chauvin Pharmaceuticals) *See* ATROPINE SULPHATE.

Minims Chloramphenicol (Chauvin Pharmaceuticals) *See* CHLORAMPHENICOL.

Minims Cyclopentolate (Chauvin Pharmaceuticals) *See* CYCLOPENTOLATE HYDROCHLORIDE.

Minims Dexamethasone (Chauvin Pharmaceuticals) *See* DEXAMETHASONE.

Minims Fluorescein Sodium (Chauvin Pharmaceuticals) *See* FLUORESCEIN SODIUM.

Minims Gentamicin (Chauvin Pharmaceuticals) *See* GENTAMICIN.

Minims Homatropine Hydrobromide (Chauvin Pharmaceuticals) *See* HOMATROPINE HYDROBROMIDE.

Minims Lignocaine and Fluorescein (Chauvin Pharmaceuticals) A proprietary combination of *lignocaine <lidocaine> hydrochloride (a local anaesthetic) and *fluorescein sodium (a dye), used for locating damaged areas of the cornea and foreign bodies in the eye. It is available as single-dose eye drops on *prescription only.

Minims Metipranolol (Chauvin Pharmaceuticals) *See* METIPRANOLOL.

Minims Neomycin (Chauvin Pharmaceuticals) *See* NEOMYCIN SULPHATE.

Minims Phenylephrine (Chauvin Pharmaceuticals) *See* PHENYLEPHRINE.

Minims Pilocarpine (Chauvin Pharmaceuticals) *See* PILOCARPINE.

Minims Prednisolone (Chauvin Pharmaceuticals) *See* PREDNISOLONE.

Minims Rose Bengal (Chauvin Pharmaceuticals) *See* ROSE BENGAL.

Minims Sodium Chloride (Chauvin Pharmaceuticals) *See* SODIUM CHLORIDE.

Minims Tropicamide (Chauvin Pharmaceuticals) *See* TROPICAMIDE.

Minitran (3M Health Care) *See* GLYCERYL TRINITRATE.

Minocin, **Minocin MR** (Wyeth Laboratories) *See* MINOCYCLINE.

minocycline A tetracycline antibiotic used for the treatment of chronic bronchitis, brucellosis, chlamydial infections, and infections caused by mycoplasmas and rickettsias (*see* TETRACYCLINES). It is also used to treat mouth ulcers and acne. Unlike most tetracyclines, minocycline does not exacerbate kidney disease and may be used by people with kidney impairment. It is available, on *prescription only, as tablets, capsules, or a gel for oral (topical) application.

Side effects: see TETRACYCLINES. In addition, this drug may cause dizziness and vertigo, severe rashes, and pigmentation (sometimes irreversible). Local irritation can occur with topical application.

Precautions: see TETRACYCLINES. In addition, liver function should be monitored if this drug is used for more than six months.

Interactions with other drugs: see TETRACYCLINES.

Proprietary preparations: Aknemin (capsules); Blemix (tablets); Cyclomin (tablets); Dentomycin (gel); Minocin (tablets); Minocin MR (modified-release capsules).

Minodiab (Pharmacia & Upjohn) *See* GLIPIZIDE.

minoxidil A *vasodilator drug used for the treatment of severe *hypertension and also to promote hair growth in male-pattern baldness (for both men and women). For treating hypertension minoxidil is supplied as tablets on *prescription only. For the treatment of baldness minoxidil is available as a solution for topical application and can be obtained from pharmacies without a prescription; it cannot be prescribed on the NHS.

Side effects: the tablets can cause fluid retention, weight gain, *oedema, excessive hair growth, and an increase in heart rate. These side effects are less likely to occur with the solution as only a small percentage of the drug is absorbed; local side effects include dermatitis.

Precautions: monoxidil tablets should not be taken by people with phaeochromocytoma (a tumour of the adrenal glands that can unpredictably release large amounts of adrenaline <epinephrine> or noradrenaline <norepinephrine>, raising blood pressure). They must be used with caution in pregnant women and people with certain heart

conditions. The solution should not be allowed to come into contact with the eyes, mouth, and mucous membranes, or with broken, infected, or inflamed skin. It should be used with caution by people with hypertension.
Proprietary preparations: Loniten (tablets); Regaine (solution).

Mintec (Monmouth Pharmaceuticals) *See* PEPPERMINT OIL.

Mintezol (Merck Sharp & Dohme) *See* THIABENDAZOLE <TIABENDAZOLE>.

Minulet (Wyeth Laboratories) A proprietary combination of *ethinyloestradiol <ethinylestradiol> and *gestodene used as an *oral contraceptive. It is available as tablets on *prescription only.
Side effects and interactions with other drugs: see ORAL CONTRACEPTIVES.
Precautions: Minulet should not be used by women who are at risk of developing thromboembolism, for example because they are very overweight or have varicose veins or a history of thrombosis. It should therefore only be taken by women who cannot tolerate other brands and who are prepared to accept the increased risk. *See also* ORAL CONTRACEPTIVES.

Miochol (CIBA Vision Ophthalmics) *See* ACETYLCHOLINE CHLORIDE.

miotics Drugs that cause the pupil of the eye to contract by constricting the muscle of the iris. This pulls the iris away from the cornea and thus increases the angle between the iris and cornea, through which fluid (aqueous humour) drains from the front chamber of the eye. Miotics are used to improve the outflow of fluid from the eye (and therefore reduce the pressure) in the treatment of *glaucoma. *See* CARBACHOL; PILOCARPINE.

Miradol (B & S Durbin) *See* PARACETAMOL.

Mirena (Schering Health Care) *See* LEVONORGESTREL.

mirtazapine An *antidepressant drug that enhances the effects of *serotonin and *noradrenaline <norepinephrine> in the brain. It has fewer antimuscarinic side effects than the *tricyclic antidepressants and does not cause the nausea and other gastrointestinal upsets associated with *SSRIs; however, sedation can occur at the start of treatment. Mirtazapine is available as tablets on *prescription only.
Side effects: include an increase in appetite, weight gain, and drowsiness; if jaundice develops, treatment should be stopped. Signs of infection (such as fever and sore throat) should be reported to a doctor as this may indicate a blood disorder.
Precautions: mirtazapine is not recommended for women who are pregnant or breastfeeding. It should be used with caution in people with epilepsy, impaired liver or kidney function, heart disease, low blood

pressure, diabetes, glaucoma, an enlarged prostate, psychotic illness, or a history of manic depressive illness. Alcohol increases the sedative effect of mirtazapine.

Interactions with other drugs:

Anxiolytics and hypnotics: enhance the sedative effect of mirtazapine.

Apraclonidine and brimonidine: should not be taken with mirtazapine.

MAOIs: mirtazapine should not be started until two weeks after stopping MAOIs; MAOIs should not be started until one week after mirtazapine has been stopped.

Proprietary preparation: Zispin.

misoprostol An *analogue of *prostaglandins that has *cytoprotectant action and is used in the treatment of duodenal, gastric, and *NSAID-induced ulcers (*see* ACID-PEPTIC DISEASES). It is given in combination with NSAIDs to avoid the gastrointestinal problems that these drugs can cause. Misoprostol is available as tablets on *prescription only.

Side effects: include diarrhoea, abdominal pain, indigestion, flatulence, nausea and vomiting, and abnormal vaginal bleeding.

Precautions: misoprostol should not be taken by women who are pregnant, planning to become pregnant, or breastfeeding. It should only be used in premenopausal women if they require NSAID therapy and are at high risk of ulceration induced by NSAIDs; these women must take effective contraception measures.

Proprietary preparations: Cytotec; ARTHROTEC (combined with diclofenac sodium); CONDROTEC (combined with naproxen); NAPRATEC (packaged with naproxen).

mitomycin A *cytotoxic antibiotic used for the treatment of cancer of the mouth, oesophagus, and stomach, breast cancer, and recurrent superficial bladder tumours. It is injected intravenously for gastrointestinal or breast cancer and instilled directly into the bladder to treat bladder cancer; it is usually given at six-weekly intervals because it causes delayed *bone marrow suppression. Mitomycin is available as a form for injection on *prescription only.

Side effects: include bone marrow suppression (long-term use may permanently damage the bone marrow) and damage to the lung and kidneys. *See also* CYTOTOXIC DRUGS.

Precautions: *see* CYTOTOXIC DRUGS. Mitomycin is irritant to the skin and must be handled with caution.

Proprietary preparation: Mitomycin C Kyowa.

Mitomycin C Kyowa (Kyowa Hakko) *See* MITOMYCIN.

Mitoxana (ASTA Medica) *See* IFOSFAMIDE.

mitoxantrone *See* MITOZANTRONE.

mitozantrone <mitoxantrone> A *cytotoxic antibiotic used for the treatment of breast *cancer. It is also used for the treatment of leukaemias and lymphomas and is instilled directly into the bladder to treat bladder cancer. Mitozantrone is available, on *prescription only, as a solution for intravenous infusion or bladder instillation.

Side effects: *bone marrow suppression is the most likely side effect; high doses can have adverse effects on the heart. *See also* DOXORUBICIN; CYTOTOXIC DRUGS.

Precautions: *see* DOXORUBICIN; CYTOTOXIC DRUGS.

Proprietary preparation: Novantrone.

mizolastine One of the newer (non-sedating) *antihistamines, used to relieve the symptoms of such allergic conditions as hay fever and urticaria (nettle rash). It is available as tablets on *prescription only.

Side effects: *see* ANTIHISTAMINES. Mizolastine may also cause weight gain.

Precautions: mizolastine should not be taken by people with heart disease or by women who are pregnant or breastfeeding. *See also* ANTIHISTAMINES.

Interactions with other drugs:

Anti-arrhythmic drugs: these drugs should not be taken with mizolastine, as this increases the risk of ventricular *arrhythmias.

Erythromycin: should not be taken with mizolastine, as this combination increases the risk of ventricular arrhythmias.

Sotalol: the risk of ventricular arrhythmias is increased if sotalol is taken with mizolastine.

Proprietary preparation: Mizollen.

Mizollen (Lorex Synthélabo) *See* MIZOLASTINE.

Mobic (Boehringer Ingelheim) *See* MELOXICAM.

Mobiflex (Roche Products) *See* TENOXICAM.

moclobemide A reversible *monoamine oxidase inhibitor (MAOI) used for the treatment of severe depression. It does not have such a severe reaction as most MAOIs when interacting with food and beverages that contain tyramine (including cheese and wine), but people taking moclobemide should still moderate their intake of these foods and drinks and be aware of the potential danger. Moclobemide is available as tablets on *prescription only.

Side effects, precautions, and interactions with other drugs: *see* MONOAMINE OXIDASE INHIBITORS.

Proprietary preparation: Manerix.

modafinil A drug that acts on the brain as a *stimulant and is used to treat narcolepsy (an extreme tendency to fall asleep). It is available as tablets on *prescription only.

Side effects: include loss of appetite, abdominal pain, headache, insomnia, excitation, euphoria, nervousness, dry mouth, palpitations, a fast heart rate, hypertension (high blood pressure), tremor, nausea, stomach discomfort, rashes, and itching.

Precautions: modafinil should not be taken by women who are pregnant or breastfeeding or by people with moderate to severe hypertension or certain heart conditions. It should be used with caution in people with liver or kidney disease. Long-term treatment with modafinil may cause *dependence.

Interactions with other drugs:

Oral contraceptives: modafinil reduces their contraceptive effect; alternative methods of contraception should be considered.

Proprietary preparation: Provigil.

Modalim (Sanofi Winthrop) *See* CIPROFIBRATE.

Modaplate (APS-Berk) *See* DIPYRIDAMOLE.

Modecate (Sanofi Winthrop) *See* FLUPHENAZINE HYDROCHLORIDE.

modified-release preparation (sustained-release preparation; continuous-release preparation) A formulation of a drug taken orally that releases the active component slowly over a long period. Drugs taken by mouth are usually absorbed in minutes or hours from the gut into the blood, where they are removed by excretory mechanisms – often via the liver. As a result, plasma concentrations of the drug rise and fall, then rise again when the next dose is taken. For some drugs this fluctuating plasma concentration is not desirable. In such cases, modified-release tablets or capsules enable the drug to be released over several hours, so that a relatively constant plasma concentration of the drug can be maintained. The terms 'modified release', 'sustained release', or 'continuous release' are often incorporated into the proprietary names of these preparations in the forms 'MR', 'SR', 'CR', or 'Continus'.

Modisal XL (Lagap Pharmaceuticals) *See* ISOSORBIDE MONONITRATE.

Moditen (Sanofi Winthrop) *See* FLUPHENAZINE HYDROCHLORIDE.

Modrasone (Schering-Plough) *See* ALCLOMETASONE DIPROPIONATE.

Modrenal (Wanskerne) *See* TRILOSTANE.

Moducren (Merck Sharp & Dohme) A proprietary combination of *hydrochlorothiazide (a thiazide diuretic), *amiloride hydrochloride (a potassium-sparing diuretic), and *timolol maleate (a beta blocker), used for the treatment of mild to moderate *hypertension. It is available as tablets on *prescription only.

Side effects, precautions, and interactions with other drugs: see THIAZIDE
DIURETICS; POTASSIUM-SPARING DIURETICS; BETA BLOCKERS.
See also ANTIHYPERTENSIVE DRUGS; DIURETICS.

Moduret 25 (Du Pont Pharmaceuticals) *See* CO-AMILOZIDE.

Moduretic (Du Pont Pharmaceuticals) *See* CO-AMILOZIDE.

moexipril hydrochloride An *ACE inhibitor used alone, or as an
adjunct to *diuretics or *calcium antagonists, for the treatment of
*hypertension. It is available as tablets on *prescription only.
Side effects, precautions, and interactions with other drugs: see ACE
INHIBITORS.
Proprietary preparation: Perdix.
See also ANTIHYPERTENSIVE DRUGS.

Mogadon (Roche Products) *See* NITRAZEPAM.

Moisture-Eyes (Co-Pharma) *See* HYPROMELLOSE.

Molcer (Wallace Manufacturing) *See* DOCUSATE SODIUM.

molgramostim Recombinant human granulocyte macrophage-colony
stimulating factor, a form of GM-CSF (*see* GRANULOCYTE-COLONY
STIMULATING FACTOR) produced by genetic engineering. It is used for the
treatment of neutropenia (a decrease in the number of neutrophils, a
type of white blood cell) that is induced by *cytotoxic drug treatment for
*cancer (except cancer affecting the bone marrow), or results from
treatment to destroy the bone marrow prior to bone marrow
transplantation, or occurs as a side effect to *ganciclovir therapy.
Molgramostim is available as a form for injection on *prescription only;
its use is restricted to specialist units.
Side effects: include nausea, diarrhoea, vomiting, loss of appetite,
breathlessness, fatigue, rash, fever, chills, flushing, and pain in muscles
or bones; serious side effects that have been reported include
*anaphylaxis and heart failure.
Precautions: serum albumin (a blood protein) and full blood counts
should be monitored during treatment. Molgramostim should be used
with caution in women who are pregnant or breastfeeding and in people
with lung disease.
Proprietary preparation: Leucomax.

Molipaxin, **Molipaxin CR** (Hoechst Marion Roussel) *See* TRAZODONE.

mometasone furoate A potent *topical steroid used for the
treatment of *psoriasis and allergic dermatitis and for the prevention and
treatment of allergic rhinitis, including hay fever. It is available, on

*prescription only, as a cream, ointment, scalp lotion, or metered-dose nasal spray.

Side effects and precautions: *see* TOPICAL STEROIDS. The nasal spray may cause headache, sore throat, and nasal irritation.

Proprietary preparations: Elocon (cream, ointment, or lotion); Nasonex (nasal spray).

Monit, Monit SR (Lorex Synthélabo) *See* ISOSORBIDE MONONITRATE.

monoamine oxidase inhibitors (MAOIs) A class of *antidepressant drugs that act by inhibiting monoamine oxidases, enzymes that break down noradrenaline <norepinephrine> and serotonin, and thus increase the activity of these neurotransmitters in the brain. Because they also inhibit enzymes that break down certain other chemicals (especially tyramine), they interact, sometimes quite dangerously, with other drugs and certain foods and beverages (see precautions and interactions with other drugs below). For this reason MAOIs are used less often than other types of antidepressants, although they are useful for treating people who do not respond to *tricyclic antidepressants or *SSRIs. They are most commonly given to patients who have depression with hypochondriacal or hysterical features. The MAOIs are *isocarboxazid, *phenelzine, and *tranylcypromine (which is the most hazardous). *Moclobemide is a newer type of MAOI that reversibly inhibits monoamine oxidase type A; it is less likely than traditional MAOIs to cause adverse effects due to tyramine.

Side effects: include a sudden fall in blood pressure on standing (causing faintness), dizziness, drowsiness, insomnia, weakness and fatigue, dryness of the mouth, and constipation and other gastrointestinal disturbances; less common side effects are headache, oedema, skin rashes, blood disorders, sexual disturbances, jaundice, weight gain, and mania.

Precautions: foods and beverages rich in tyramine (e.g. cheese, hung meat or game, meat or yeast extracts, pickled herrings, flavoured textured vegetable proteins, and wine) should be avoided as they can cause dramatic and dangerous rises in blood pressure. This effect can persist for some two weeks after stopping the MAOI. MAOIs should be stopped gradually at the end of treatment.

Interactions with other drugs:

  Analgesics: opioid analgesics (especially pethidine) can cause severe reactions and should not be taken with MAOIs. The non-opioid analgesic nefopam should also be avoided.

  Antidepressants: it is dangerous to take MAOIs with other antidepressants, and this should only be done under specialist supervision. Clomipramine should never be taken with tranylcypromine. Other antidepressants should not be started for two weeks after treatment with MAOIs has stopped, and MAOIs should not be started for at least one week after treatment with other antidepressants has stopped.

Antihypertensive drugs: their effect in lowering blood pressure is enhanced; indoramin should not be taken with MAOIs.

Antipsychotics: stimulation of the central nervous system and increased blood pressure can occur with oxypertine and clozapine.

Carbamazepine: there is an increased risk of convulsions.

Levodopa: causes a dangerous rise in blood pressure; it should not be taken until two weeks after stopping MAOIs.

Sympathomimetics: the following drugs cause a dangerous rise in blood pressure if taken with MAOIs: dexamphetamine <dexamfetamine>, dopamine, isometheptene, methylphenidate, pemoline, phentermine, and ephedrine, phenylephrine, phenylpropanolamine, and pseudoephedrine (which are present in many cough mixtures and decongestants).

Mono-Cedocard (Pharmacia & Upjohn) *See* ISOSORBIDE MONONITRATE.

Monoclate-P (Armour) *See* FACTOR VIII.

monoclonal antibody An antibody produced by genetic engineering techniques from a cell clone (i.e. numerous identical cells originally derived from a single parent cell) and therefore consisting of a single type of *immunoglobulin. Monoclonal antibodies have recently been developed for targeting specific tissues for use in treating certain cancers (*see* RITUXIMAB). *See also* ABCIXIMAB.

Monocor (Wyeth Laboratories) *See* BISOPROLOL FUMARATE.

monofluorophosphate *See* FLUORIDE.

Monomax SR (Trinity Pharmaceuticals) *See* ISOSORBIDE MONONITRATE.

Mononine (Armour) *See* FACTOR IX.

Monoparin, **Monoparin Calcium** (CP Pharmaceuticals) *See* HEPARIN.

Monosorb XL 60 (Dexcel Pharma) *See* ISOSORBIDE MONONITRATE.

Monotrim (Solvay Healthcare) *See* TRIMETHOPRIM.

Monovent (Lagap Pharmaceuticals) *See* TERBUTALINE SULPHATE.

Monozide 10 (Wyeth Laboratories) A proprietary combination of *bisoprolol fumarate (a cardioselective beta blocker), and *hydrochlorothiazide (a thiazide diuretic), used for the treatment of *hypertension. It is available as tablets on *prescription only.
Side effects, precautions, and interactions with other drugs: *see* BETA BLOCKERS; THIAZIDE DIURETICS.
See also ANTIHYPERTENSIVE DRUGS; DIURETICS.

Monphytol (Laboratories for Applied Biology) A proprietary combination of the antiseptic *chlorbutol <chlorobutanol>, the antifungal drugs methyl undecenoate and propyl undecenoate (*see* UNDECENOIC ACID), and the keratolytics *salicylic acid, *methyl salicylate, and propyl salicylate, used for the treatment of athlete's foot. It is available as a paint and can be obtained without a prescription, but only from pharmacies.

Precautions: Monphytol should not be used during pregnancy. It is not recommended for children except on medical advice.

montelukast A *leukotriene receptor antagonist used as an *adjunct for the treatment of mild to moderate *asthma that is not adequately controlled by the usual combination of an inhaled *corticosteroid and a beta stimulant (such as *salbutamol). It can also be used to prevent an attack of asthma being brought on by exercise, but it should not be used to treat acute attacks. Montelukast is available as tablets or chewable tablets on *prescription only.

Side effects: include abdominal pain, headache, diarrhoea, and dizziness.

Precautions: the chewable tablets contain aspartame and should be used with caution by people who have phenylketonuria. Montelukast should be used with caution by women who are pregnant or breastfeeding.

Interactions with other drugs:

Phenobarbitone <phenobarbital>: can reduce the effectiveness of montelukast.

Proprietary preparation: Singulair.

Moorland (Torbet Laboratories) A proprietary combination of *bismuth aluminate, *magnesium trisilicate, *aluminium hydroxide, *magnesium carbonate, and *calcium carbonate (all antacids), and light *kaolin (an adsorbent), used for the relief of indigestion and flatulence. It is freely available *over the counter in the form of tablets.

Side effects and interactions with other drugs: see ANTACIDS.

Precautions: this medicine is not recommended for children under six years old.

moracizine (moricizine) A class I *anti-arrhythmic drug used to treat *arrhythmias. It is available as tablets on *prescription only.

Side effects: include dizziness, nervousness, 'pins and needles', gastrointestinal upset, dry mouth, sweating, chest pain, muscle pain, sleep disorders, blurred vision.

Precautions: moracizine should not be taken by people with liver or kidney disease, if congestive *heart failure is present, or by pregnant women. *See also* ANTI-ARRHYTHMIC DRUGS.

Morcap SR (Sanofi Winthrop) *See* MORPHINE.

Morhulin (Seton Scholl Healthcare) A proprietary combination of cod liver oil (an *emollient) and *zinc oxide (an astringent protective agent) in the form of an ointment, used for the prevention and treatment of napkin rash, pressure sores, and leg ulcers and for the relief of *eczema and minor wounds and abrasions. It is freely available *over the counter.

morphine An opiate that is the most commonly used of the *opioid analgesics for treating severe pain, including that caused by surgery. It is particularly valuable for controlling pain in terminal illnesses; as well as pain relief, it also induces feelings of well-being and mental detachment. Morphine is also used to control coughing in terminally ill patients. Because it is constipating, low doses of morphine are used in some *antidiarrhoeal preparations. Morphine is a *controlled drug; it is available as tablets, *modified-release tablets or capsules, oral solutions, suppositories, and solutions for injection.

Side effects: nausea and vomiting, drowsiness, and constipation frequently occur (morphine may need to be given with a laxative or an antiemetic); higher doses cause depression of breathing and low blood pressure. Other side effects can include difficulty in passing urine, dry mouth, sweating, constriction of the pupils, a feeling of faintness on standing, palpitations, confusion, and hallucinations.

Precautions: morphine should be used with caution in people with asthma or other respiratory disorders (it can exacerbate asthma and should not be used during an attack), low blood pressure, an underactive thyroid gland, an enlarged prostate gland, liver or kidney disease, or epilepsy, and in women who are pregnant or breastfeeding. It should not be used in people with severely depressed breathing or acute alcoholism, or in those who have a head injury. Treatment with morphine must be stopped gradually in those who have been taking it on a long-term basis in order to avoid withdrawal reactions. *See also* OPIOIDS.

Interactions with other drugs: see OPIOIDS.

Proprietary preparations: Min-I-Jet Morphine Sulphate (injection); Morcap SR (modified-release capsules); Morphine Sulphate Rapiject (injection); MST Continus (modified-release tablets); MXL (modified-release capsules); Oramorph (oral solution); Oramorph SR (modified-release tablets); Sevredol (tablets); Zomorph (modified-release capsules); CYCLIMORPH (combined with cyclizine tartrate); ENTEROSAN (combined with belladonna and kaolin); J COLLIS BROWNE'S MIXTURE (combined with peppermint oil); J COLLIS BROWNE'S TABLETS (combined with calcium carbonate and kaolin); OPAZIMES (combined with kaolin, aluminium hydroxide, and belladonna).

Morphine Sulphate Rapiject (Medeva) *See* MORPHINE.

Motens (Boehringer Ingelheim) *See* LACIDIPINE.

Mothers' and Children's Vitamin Drops (Cupal) A proprietary combination of *vitamin A, *vitamin D, and *vitamin C, used as a vitamin supplement for pregnant women and children under five years old. It is available without a prescription.

Side effects, precautions, and interactions with other drugs: see VITAMIN A.

Motifene 75 mg (Sankyo Pharma) See DICLOFENAC SODIUM.

Motilium (Sanofi Winthrop) See DOMPERIDONE.

Motipress (Sanofi Winthrop) A proprietary combination of *fluphenazine hydrochloride (an antipsychotic drug) and *nortriptyline (a tricyclic antidepressant), used for the treatment of mild to moderate anxiety. It is available as tablets on *prescription only.

Side effects: see FLUPHENAZINE HYDROCHLORIDE; AMITRIPTYLINE HYDROCHLORIDE.

Precautions see FLUPHENAZINE HYDROCHLORIDE; CHLORPROMAZINE HYDROCHLORIDE; TRICYCLIC ANTIDEPRESSANTS.

Interactions with other drugs: see CHLORPROMAZINE HYDROCHLORIDE; TRICYCLIC ANTIDEPRESSANTS.

Motival (Sanofi Winthrop) A proprietary combination of *fluphenazine hydrochloride (an antipsychotic drug) and *nortriptyline (a tricyclic antidepressant), used for the treatment of mild to moderate anxiety. It is available as tablets on *prescription only.

Side effects: see FLUPHENAZINE HYDROCHLORIDE; AMITRIPTYLINE HYDROCHLORIDE.

Precautions see FLUPHENAZINE HYDROCHLORIDE; CHLORPROMAZINE HYDROCHLORIDE; TRICYCLIC ANTIDEPRESSANTS.

Interactions with other drugs: see CHLORPROMAZINE HYDROCHLORIDE; TRICYCLIC ANTIDEPRESSANTS.

Motrin (Pharmacia & Upjohn) See IBUPROFEN.

Movelat (Sankyo Pharma) A proprietary combination of *salicylic acid and mucopolysaccharide polysulphate (a *heparinoid), used for the relief of rheumatic, muscular, and mild arthritic pain, sprains, and strains (*see* RUBEFACIENTS). It is available as a cream (which also contains *thymol) and a gel, both of which can be obtained from pharmacies without a prescription.

Side effects and precautions: see SALICYLATES.

Movicol (Norgine) A proprietary combination of macrogol '3350' (*see* POLYETHYLENE GLYCOLS), *sodium bicarbonate, *sodium chloride, and *potassium chloride, used as an *osmotic laxative for the treatment of chronic constipation and impacted faeces. It is available as an oral powder to be dissolved in water and can be obtained without a prescription, but only from pharmacies.

Side effects and precautions: see POLYETHYLENE GLYCOLS.

moxisylyte *See* THYMOXAMINE.

moxonidine A drug that acts in the brain to reduce activity in the
*sympathetic nervous system, causing a fall in the resistance of the blood
vessels and a decrease in blood pressure. Thus, it has similar actions to
*alpha blockers, but does not cause the side effects of dry mouth and
sedation seen with these drugs. It is used for the treatment of mild to
moderate *hypertension. It is available as tablets on *prescription only.
Side effects: include headache, weakness, dizziness, sleep disturbances,
and nausea.
Precautions: moxonidine should be used with caution in patients with
certain types of heart disease or with liver or kidney disease.
Proprietary preparation: Physiotens.
See also ANTIHYPERTENSIVE DRUGS.

MST Continus (Napp Pharmaceuticals) *See* MORPHINE.

Mucaine (Wyeth Laboratories) A proprietary combination of
*aluminium hydroxide and *magnesium hydroxide (antacids) and
oxethazaine <oxetacaine> (a *local anaesthetic), used in the treatment of
oesophagitis and acid reflux associated with a hiatus hernia (*see* ACID-
PEPTIC DISEASES). It is available as a sugar-free suspension on
*prescription only.
Side effects, precautions, and interactions with other drugs: see ANTACIDS.

Mucodyne (Rhône-Poulenc Rorer) *See* CARBOCISTEINE.

Mucogel (Pharmax) *See* CO-MAGALDROX.

mucolytic drugs Agents that dissolve or break down mucus and thus
facilitate expectoration. Mucolytics are used to treat chest conditions
involving excessive or thickened mucus secretions. *See* ACETYLCYSTEINE;
CARBOCISTEINE; DORNASE ALFA; METHYLCYSTEINE HYDROCHLORIDE. *Compare*
EXPECTORANTS.

Mu-Cron Tablets (Novartis Consumer Health) A proprietary
combination of *phenylpropanolamine (a decongestant) and
*paracetamol (an analgesic and antipyretic), used for the treatment of
nasal congestion, sinus pain, and other symptoms of colds and influenza.
It can be obtained without a prescription, but only from pharmacies.
Side effects: see EPHEDRINE HYDROCHLORIDE.
Precautions: these tablets should not be taken by children. *See also*
EPHEDRINE HYDROCHLORIDE; PARACETAMOL.
Interactions with other drugs: see PHENYLPROPANOLAMINE; EPHEDRINE
HYDROCHLORIDE.

Multiparin (CP Pharmaceuticals) *See* HEPARIN.

mupirocin A broad-spectrum *antibiotic that is not related to any of the other antibiotics. It is used for treating bacterial skin infections and is especially useful for nasal infections, since it is active against methicillin-resistant *Staphylococcus aureus* (MRSA), a bacterium that is resistant to many antibiotics and may be carried in the nostrils. Mupirocin is available, on *prescription only, as an ointment to be applied to the skin or nostrils.

Side effects: the ointment may cause stinging on application; contact with the eyes should be avoided.

Precautions: mupirocin should be used with caution by people with kidney disease.

Proprietary preparations: Bactroban; Bactroban Nasal.

muscle relaxants Drugs that reduce the tension in skeletal muscles. They are used to treat muscle spasms (involuntary and often painful contractions of muscles caused by injury or disease) and spasticity, in which the muscles are continually in a state of increased tension or rigidity due to such disorders as multiple sclerosis and cerebral palsy.

Muscle relaxants either act centrally (i.e. on the brain or spinal cord), to inhibit the nerve signals that cause the muscles to contract (*see* BACLOFEN; CARISOPRODOL; DIAZEPAM; METHOCARBAMOL; TIZANIDINE), or directly on the muscles themselves, to prevent the activity in the cells that cause the muscles to contract (*see* DANTROLENE SODIUM). The dosage of these drugs may need some adjustment to obtain the optimum that controls symptoms but does not cause muscle weakness. Skeletal muscle relaxants should not be stopped abruptly or stiffness may be worse than before treatment.

The muscle relaxants used in surgery during general anaesthesia work in a different way. They act at neuromuscular junctions (where the nerve fibre meets the muscle it supplies) to block the transmission of nerve impulses, either by binding to receptor sites normally occupied by the chemical transmitter *acetylcholine (nondepolarizing muscle relaxants, such as **pancuronium** and **mivacurium**) or by mimicking the action of acetylcholine, making the muscle no longer receptive to stimulation by this transmitter (depolarizing muscle relaxants, such as **suxamethonium**).

Drugs that relax smooth muscle include *antispasmodics, *bronchodilators, and *vasodilators.

MUSE (AstraZeneca) *See* ALPROSTADIL.

mustard oil An oil distilled from mustard seeds. It is a powerful irritant and is used as a *rubefacient.

Side effects and precautions: see RUBEFACIENTS.

Proprietary preparation: NELLA RED OIL (combined with clove oil and methyl nicotinate).

mustine hydrochloride <chlormethine hydrochloride> An

*alkylating drug used for the treatment of Hodgkin's disease (*see* CANCER). Since it is very toxic, mustine is now rarely used. It is available, on *prescription only, as a form for fast intravenous infusion.

Side effects: see CYTOTOXIC DRUGS; mustine can cause severe vomiting, and it can seriously damage surrounding tissues if it leaks out during infusion.

Precautions: see CYTOTOXIC DRUGS; mustine is extremely irritant to tissues and must be handled with care.

MXL (Napp Pharmaceuticals) *See* MORPHINE.

Mycardol (Sanofi Winthrop) *See* PENTAERYTHRITOL <PENTAERITHRITYL> TETRANITRATE.

Mycifradin (Pharmacia & Upjohn) *See* NEOMYCIN SULPHATE.

Mycil Foot Spray (Crookes Healthcare) *See* TOLNAFTATE.

Mycil Gold (Crookes Healthcare) *See* CLOTRIMAZOLE.

Mycil Ointment (Crookes Healthcare) A proprietary combination of *tolnaftate (an antifungal drug) and *benzalkonium chloride (an antiseptic), used for the treatment of tinea (ringworm), including athlete's foot, and prickly heat. It is freely available *over the counter.

Mycil Powder (Crookes Healthcare) A proprietary combination of *tolnaftate (an antifungal drug) and *chlorhexidine (an antiseptic), used for the treatment of tinea (ringworm), including athlete's foot, and prickly heat. It is freely available *over the counter.

Mycobutin (Pharmacia & Upjohn) *See* RIFABUTIN.

mycophenolate mofetil An *immunosuppressant drug used in conjunction with *cyclosporin and *corticosteroids for the prevention of rejection in kidney transplant patients. It is available, on *prescription only, as capsules, tablets, or a form for intravenous infusion.

Side effects: include diarrhoea, vomiting, constipation, nausea, abdominal pain, high blood pressure, chest pain, breathlessness, cough, dizziness, insomnia, headache, and tremor.

Precautions: full blood counts must be performed during therapy. Mycophenolate should not be given to patients with active gastrointestinal disease or to women who are pregnant or breastfeeding.

Interactions with other drugs:

  Aciclovir: plasma concentrations of both drugs are increased.

  Antacids: reduce the absorption of mycophenolate.

  Cholestyramine <colestyramine>: reduces the absorption of mycophenolate.

Proprietary preparation: CellCept.

Mycota (Seton Scholl Healthcare) *See* UNDECENOIC ACID.

Mydriacyl (Alcon Laboratories) *See* TROPICAMIDE.

Mydrilate (Boehringer Ingelheim) *See* CYCLOPENTOLATE HYDROCHLORIDE.

Myleran (GlaxoWellcome) *See* BUSULPHAN <BUSULFAN>.

Myocrisin (Rhône-Poulenc Rorer) *See* SODIUM AUROTHIOMALATE.

Myotonine (Glenwood Laboratories) *See* BETHANECHOL CHLORIDE.

Mysoline (AstraZeneca) *See* PRIMIDONE.

myxoedema *See* THYROID HORMONES.

N

nabilone A synthetic derivative of cannabis that is used to prevent or treat the nausea and vomiting caused by *cytotoxic drug treatment for cancer. It is used in patients who have not responded to other *antiemetics, but treatment needs to be carefully supervised, since some people can experience disorientation and mood changes as side effects (see below). Nabilone is available as capsules on *prescription only.

Side effects: include drowsiness, vertigo, euphoria, shaky movements, dry mouth, visual disturbances, difficulty in concentrating, sleep disturbances, confusion, disorientation, hallucinations, psychosis, depression, lack of coordination, tremor, a fast heart rate, and loss of appetite. Mood changes and other mental side effects may persist for up to three days after stopping the treatment.

Precautions: nabilone should not be taken by people with severe liver disease or by women who are pregnant or breastfeeding. It should be used with caution in people with a history of psychiatric disorders and in the elderly. Nabilone may affect driving ability, and its sedative effects are increased by alcohol.

Interactions with other drugs:

Anxiolytics and hypnotics: enhance the sedative effects of nabilone.

nabumetone An *NSAID used for the treatment of pain and inflammation in osteoarthritis and rheumatoid arthritis. It is available as tablets or a suspension on *prescription only.

Side effects, precautions, and interactions with other drugs: see NSAIDS.

Proprietary preparation: Relifex.

nadolol A *beta blocker used for the treatment and prevention of heart *arrhythmias and *angina. It is also used for the prevention of *migraine and, combined with a diuretic, for the treatment of *hypertension. It is available as tablets on *prescription only.

Side effects, precautions, and interactions with other drugs: see BETA BLOCKERS.

Proprietary preparations: Corgard; CORGARETIC 40, CORGARETIC 80 (combined with bendrofluazide <bendroflumethiazide>).

nafarelin An analogue of *gonadorelin used to treat *endometriosis and to suppress the release of gonadotrophins by the pituitary gland before inducing ovulation in women undergoing fertility treatment. Nafarelin is available, on *prescription only, as a nasal spray or a solution for injection.

Side effects: include hot flushes, loss of libido, vaginal dryness, emotional upset, headache, changes in breast size, breast tenderness, ovarian cysts, depression, muscle aches, tingling in the fingers or toes, acne, migraine, bouts of palpitation, and blurred vision. The spray may cause transient nasal irriation.

Precautions: see BUSERELIN.

Proprietary preparation: Synarel (nasal spray).

naftidrofuryl oxalate A drug used for the treatment of disorders of the peripheral arteries, such as intermittent claudication (poor circulation in the legs giving rise to cramping pain on exercise), and cerebrovascular disease, although its value is not proven. It is available as capsules on *prescription only.

Side effects: include nausea, pains in the stomach region, and rashes.

Proprietary preparation: Praxilene.

nalbuphine hydrochloride An *opioid analgesic used for the treatment of moderate to severe pain, including pain relief before and during surgery. It causes less nausea and vomiting than other opioids. Nalbuphine is available as an injection on *prescription only.

Side effects and precautions: see MORPHINE.

Interactions with other drugs: see OPIOIDS.

Proprietary preparation: Nubain.

Nalcrom (Pantheon Healthcare) *See* SODIUM CROMOGLYCATE <CROMOGLICATE>.

nalidixic acid A *quinolone antibiotic, similar to *ciprofloxacin, that is used for the treatment of urinary-tract infections. It is available, on *prescription only, as tablets, capsules, granules, or a suspension.

Side effects, precautions, and interactions with other drugs: see QUINOLONES.

Proprietary preparations: Negram; Uriben; MICTRAL (combined with sodium citrate, citric acid, and sodium bicarbonate).

Nalorex (Du Pont Pharmaceuticals) *See* NALTREXONE HYDROCHLORIDE.

naloxone hydrochloride A drug that opposes the action of *opioids. It is used to treat overdosage with opioids and also to reverse the depression of breathing caused by the use of opioid analgesics during surgery. Naloxone is available as an injection on *prescription only.

Side effects: nausea and vomiting, an increase in heart rate, and abnormal heartbeats may occur.

Precautions: naloxone should be used with caution in patients who are physically dependent on opioids, who have cardiovascular disease, or who are receiving other drugs that can have adverse effects on the heart. When given after surgery, the dosage should be calculated to reverse the respiratory effects of the opioids without interfering with their pain-relieving effects.

Proprietary preparations: Min-I-Jet Naloxone; Narcan; Narcan Neonatal.

naltrexone hydrochloride A drug that opposes the action of *opioids (such as heroin) and is used to help maintain a drug-free habit in people who were formerly dependent on opioids. Naltrexone is usually started after the individual has abstained from taking opioid drugs for at least 7–10 days. It is available as tablets on *prescription only.

Side effects: include nausea, vomiting, abdominal pain, anxiety, nervousness, difficulties in sleeping, headache, reduced energy, and joint and muscle pain. Less frequently there may be mood changes and decreased potency.

Precautions: naltrexone should not be taken by people who are still dependent on opioids or by those with severe liver disease.

Proprietary preparation: Nalorex.

nandrolone decanoate An *anabolic steroid that is sometimes used as an *adjunct in the treatment of aplastic *anaemias (types of anaemia resulting from a failure of the bone marrow to produce blood cells). It is available as a solution for injection on *prescription only.

Side effects: include acne, oedema (accumulation of fluid in the tissues) due to sodium retention, masculinization in women, and high plasma calcium concentrations.

Precautions: nandrolone should not be used during pregnancy or in men with suspected prostate cancer or breast cancer. It should be used with caution in people with liver or kidney disease, high blood pressure, epilepsy, migraine, or diabetes.

Interactions with other drugs: see ANABOLIC STEROIDS.

Proprietary preparation: Deca-Durabolin 100.

Napratec (Searle) A proprietary preparation consisting of tablets of *naproxen (an NSAID) packaged with tablets of *misoprostol (a prostaglandin analogue). It is used for the treatment of rheumatoid arthritis, osteoarthritis, and ankylosing spondylitis; the misoprostol is included to prevent the bleeding and ulceration of the stomach or duodenum that may result from the use of naproxen alone. Napratec is available on *prescription only.

Side effects and precautions: see NSAIDS; MISOPROSTOL.

Interactions with other drugs: see NSAIDS.

Naprosyn, **Naprosyn SR** (Roche Products) *See* NAPROXEN.

naproxen An *NSAID used for the treatment of pain and inflammation in rheumatoid arthritis (including arthritis in children), acute gout, and other disorders of the joints or muscles. It is also used to relieve period pains. Naproxen is available, on *prescription only, as tablets, *enteric-coated tablets, *modified-release tablets, a suspension, and suppositories.

Side effects: see NSAIDS. Suppositories may cause local irritation and occasionally bleeding.

Precautions and interactions with other drugs: see NSAIDS.

Proprietary preparations: Arthrosin; Arthroxen; Naprosyn (tablets, suspension, and suppositories); Naprosyn EC (enteric-coated tablets); Naprosyn SR (modified-release tablets); Nycopren (enteric-coated tablets); Synflex; Timpron; Timpron EC (enteric-coated tablets); CONDROTEC (packaged with misoprostol); NAPRATEC (packaged with misoprostol).

Naramig (GlaxoWellcome) *See* NARATRIPTAN.

naratriptan A *5HT$_1$ agonist used to treat acute attacks of *migraine. A single dose can relieve a migraine headache at any stage of the attack. Naratriptan is available as tablets on *prescription only.

Side effects: include sensations of tingling, heat, heaviness, pressure, or tightness; if tightness in the chest or throat is severe, treatment should be discontinued. Other side effects may include a slow or fast heart rate, disturbed vision, flushing, dizziness, and weakness.

Precautions: naratriptan should not be taken by people with certain heart conditions, uncontrolled high blood pressure, or disease of the peripheral blood vessels or by those who have previously had a heart attack. It should be used with caution by women who are pregnant or breastfeeding and by people with impaired liver or kidney function.

Proprietary preparation: Naramig.

Narcan, Narcan Neonatal (Du Pont Pharmaceuticals) *See* NALOXONE HYDROCHLORIDE.

Nardil (Parke-Davis Medical) *See* PHENELZINE.

Narphen (Napp Pharmaceuticals) *See* PHENAZOCINE HYDROBROMIDE.

Nasacort (Rhône-Poulenc Rorer) *See* TRIAMCINOLONE ACETONIDE.

Nasciodine Massage Cream (Health Aid Pharmadass) A proprietary combination of *iodine, *menthol, *methyl salicylate, *turpentine oil, and *camphor, used as a *rubefacient for the relief of mild muscular aches and pains, chilblains, sprains, and bruises. It is freely available *over the counter.

Side effects and precautions: see RUBEFACIENTS.

Naseptin (AstraZeneca) A proprietary combination of *chlorhexidine (an antiseptic) and *neomycin sulphate (an antibiotic), used for the treatment of nasal infections caused by bacteria and to eradicate *Staphylococcus* bacteria that may be carried in the nostrils. It is available as a cream on *prescription only.

Side effects: allergic rashes may develop.

Precautions: prolonged use should be avoided.

Nasobec (Norton Healthcare) *See* BECLOMETHASONE <BECLOMETASONE> DIPROPIONATE.

Nasonex (Schering-Plough) *See* MOMETASONE FUROATE.

Natramid (Trinity Pharmaceuticals) *See* INDAPAMIDE HEMIHYDRATE.

Natrilix, Natrilix SR (Servier Laboratories) *See* INDAPAMIDE HEMIHYDRATE.

Navelbine (Pierre Fabre) *See* VINORELBINE

Navidrex (Alliance Pharmaceuticals) *See* CYCLOPENTHIAZIDE.

Navispare (Alliance Pharmaceuticals) A proprietary combination of *cyclopenthiazide (a thiazide diuretic) and *amiloride hydrochloride (a potassium-sparing diuretic), used for the treatment of *hypertension. It is available as tablets on *prescription only.
Side effects, precautions, and interactions with other drugs: see THIAZIDE DIURETICS; POTASSIUM-SPARING DIURETICS.
See also ANTIHYPERTENSIVE DRUGS; DIURETICS.

Navoban (Novartis Consumer Health) *See* TROPISETRON.

Nazo-Mist (Co-Pharma) *See* XYLOMETAZOLINE.

Nebcin (Eli Lilly & Co) *See* TOBRAMYCIN.

nebulizer A device that forces compressed air through a solution of a drug so that a fine spray is delivered to a face mask and can be inhaled. Nebulizers are often used to administer drugs to children who lack the coordination to use a metered-dose or breath-activated *inhaler.

nedocromil sodium A *chromone drug used to prevent attacks in the treatment of *asthma and other allergic conditions. It is available as a suspension or liquid in metered-dose aerosols for inhalation, as a pump spray for the nose, and as eye drops. Nedocromil is a *prescription only medicine.
Side effects: with a nasal spray and eye drops there may be mild local irritation and taste disturbances. When inhaled it may cause coughing, occasionally headache and stomach upsets, and rarely transient wheezing.
Proprietary preparations: Rapitil (eye drops); Tilade (aerosol inhaler), Tilade Syncroner (with spacer device); Tilarin (nasal spray).

nefazodone hydrochloride An *antidepressant drug related to the *SSRI group; it inhibits the reuptake of *serotonin and selectively blocks serotonin receptors. It is used for the treatment of depressive illness and depressive syndromes accompanied by anxiety or sleep disturbance. Nefazodone is available as tablets on *prescription only.

Side effects: include weakness, dry mouth, nausea, drowsiness, and dizziness.

Precautions: nefazodone should not be taken by women who are breastfeeding and it should be used with caution during pregnancy and in those with epilepsy, a history of mania, impaired liver or kidney function, and in elderly women. Driving ability may be impaired.

Interactions with other drugs:

  Antihistamines: there is an increased risk of *arrhythmias with astemizole and terfenadine and these drugs should not be taken with nefazodone.

  Cisapride: there is an increased risk of ventricular *arrhythmias and cisapride should not be taken with nefazodone.

  MAOIs: nefazodone increases the risk of adverse effects of MAOIs; if nefazodone is started shortly after stopping MAOIs, the dosage should be low initially and increased gradually.

Proprietary preparation: Dutonin.

nefopam An *analgesic used for the relief of persistent pain that has not responded to other non-opioid analgesics; the way in which it works is not completely understood. Nefopam is used to treat moderate pain, including that occurring after operations or dental procedures or associated with cancer; it does not reduce fever or inflammation. Nefopam is available as tablets or an injection on *prescription only.

Side effects: include nausea, nervousness, dry mouth, urinary retention, and dizziness.

Precautions: nefopam should not be used to relieve the pain of a heart attack and should not be taken by people with epilepsy or other convulsive disorders. It should be used with caution in people with liver or kidney disease or urinary retention, in elderly people, and in women who are pregnant or breastfeeding.

Interactions with other drugs:

  MAOIs: should not be taken with nefopam.

  Tricyclic antidepressants: may increase the side effects of nefopam.

Proprietary preparation: Acupan.

Negram (Sanofi Winthrop) *See* NALIDIXIC ACID.

nelfinavir A protease inhibitor (*see* ANTIVIRAL DRUGS) that is used in combination with the nucleoside analogues for the treatment of *HIV infection. It is available, on *prescription only, as tablets or a powder to be mixed with water or milk.

Side effects: include diarrhoea, flatulence, nausea, rashes, reduced white-blood-cell count, and hepatitis.

Precautions: nelfinavir should not be taken by women who are pregnant or breastfeeding. It should be used with caution in people with kidney or liver disease, haemophilia, or diabetes.

Interactions with other drugs: nelfinavir is a potent inhibitor of several enzyme systems in the liver that are involved in metabolizing drugs; it therefore has the potential to interact with many drugs. A doctor should be consulted before taking nelfinavir with any other drug.

Proprietary preparation: Viracept.

Nella Red Oil (Nella) A proprietary combination of *clove oil, *mustard oil, and *methyl nicotinate, used as a *rubefacient for the relief of muscular aches and pains. It is freely available *over the counter.

Side effects and precautions: see RUBEFACIENTS.

Neo-Bendromax (Ashbourne Pharmaceuticals) *See* BENDROFLUAZIDE <BENDROFLUMETHIAZIDE>.

Neo-Cortef (Dominion Pharma) A proprietary combination of *neomycin sulphate (an antibiotic) and *hydrocortisone (a corticosteroid), used for the treatment of infections of the ears and eyes. It is available as drops or an ointment on *prescription only.

Side effects: see TOPICAL STEROIDS.

Precautions: this preparation should not be used on perforated eardrums. *See also* TOPICAL STEROIDS.

Neo-Cytamen (Medeva) *See* HYDROXOCOBALAMIN.

Neogest (Schering Health Care) *See* NORGESTREL; ORAL CONTRACEPTIVES.

Neo Gripe Mixture (Wallace Manufacturing) A proprietary combination of *sodium bicarbonate, *dill seed oil, and *ginger tincture, used for the relief of wind pain. It is suitable for infants but may also be taken by adults, such as pregnant women and nursing mothers. The mixture is freely available *over the counter.

Neo-Mercazole (Roche Products) *See* CARBIMAZOLE.

neomycin sulphate An *aminoglycoside antibiotic that is used to sterilize the bowel before surgery. Given by mouth a few hours before surgery, it acts locally on the gut but is not absorbed. It is also used to treat infections of the skin, ears, and eyes but is too toxic to be injected. Available on *prescription only, it is administered orally as tablets or topically as a solution, nose, ear, or eye drops, an ear or eye ointment, or by nasal spray.

Side effects, precautions, and interactions with other drugs: similar to those of *gentamicin, but as very little of the drug is absorbed into the body problems rarely occur.

Proprietary preparations: Minims Neomycin (single-dose eye drops); Mycifradin (tablets); Nivemycin (tablets); NEOSPORIN (combined with polymyxin B sulphate); ADCORTYL WITH GRANEODIN (combined with triamcinolone acetonide and gramicidin); AUDICORT (combined with triamcinolone); BETNESOL-N and BETNOVATE-N (combined with betamethasone); CICATRIN (combined with bacitracin); DERMOVATE-NN (combined with clobetasol and nystatin); FML-NEO (combined with fluorometholone); GRANEODIN (combined with gramicidin); GREGODERM (combined with nystatin, polymyxin B sulphate, and hydrocortisone); MAXITROL (combined with dexamethasone); NASEPTIN (combined with chlorhexidine); NEO-CORTEF (combined with hydrocortisone); NEOSPORIN (combined with polymyxin B and gramicidin); OTOMIZE (combined with dexamethasone); OTOSPORIN (combined with polymyxin B sulphate and hydrocortisone); PREDSOL-N (combined with prednisolone); SYNALAR N (combined with fluocinolone acetonide); TRI-ADCORTYL OTIC (combined with triamcinolone, gramicidin, and nystatin); VISTA-METHASONE N (combined with betamethasone).

Neo-Naclex (Goldshield Pharmaceuticals) *See* BENDROFLUAZIDE <BENDROFLUMETHIAZIDE>.

Neo-Naclex-K (Goldshield Pharmaceuticals) A proprietary combination of *bendrofluazide <bendroflumethiazide> (a thiazide diuretic) and *potassium chloride, used for the treatment of *hypertension and *oedema associated with heart failure, liver disease, or kidney disease. It is available as *modified-release tablets on *prescription only.
Side effects, precautions, and interactions with other drugs: see THIAZIDE DIURETICS.
See also ANTIHYPERTENSIVE DRUGS; DIURETICS.

Neoral (Novartis Pharmaceuticals) *See* CYCLOSPORIN.

Neorecormon (Roche Products) *See* ERYTHROPOIETIN.

Neosporin (Dominion Pharma) A proprietary combination of *gramicidin, *neomycin, and *polymyxin B sulphate, used for the treatment of bacterial infections of the eye and for the prevention of infection after eye surgery. It is available as eye drops on *prescription only.
Side effects, precautions, and interactions with other drugs: see NEOMYCIN SULPHATE.

neostigmine An *anticholinesterase drug used for the treatment of myasthenia gravis. It is also injected by anaesthetists after surgery to reverse the action of drugs that have been used to paralyse or relax muscles during surgical procedures; for this purpose it is used in conjunction with *glycopyrronium bromide or (less commonly) *atropine sulphate. Neostigmine is available as tablets or an injection on *prescription only.
Side effects: nausea and vomiting, increased salivation, diarrhoea, and abdominal cramps are the most common side effects. Overdosage

worsens these effects and can cause slowing of the heart rate and low blood pressure.

Precautions: neostigmine should not be given to people with intestinal or urinary obstruction or to those with asthma. It should be used with caution in those with low blood pressure, peptic ulcers, epilepsy, Parkinson's disease, or kidney disease.

Interactions with other drugs:

Anti-arrhythmic drugs: procainamide and quinidine antagonize the action of neostigmine.

Antibiotics: aminoglycosides, clindamycin, and colistin antagonize the action of neostigmine.

Beta blockers: the risk of arrhythmia is increased; propranolol antagonizes the action of neostigmine.

Chloroquine: increases the symptoms of myasthenia gravis and thus diminishes the effect of neostigmine.

Hydroxychloroquine: increases the symptoms of myasthenia gravis and thus diminishes the effect of neostigmine.

Lithium: antagonizes the effect of neostigmine.

Proprietary preparation: ROBINUL-NEOSTIGMINE (combined with glycopyrronium).

Neotigason (Roche Products) *See* ACITRETIN.

Nephril (Pfizer) *See* POLYTHIAZIDE.

Nericur (Schering Health Care) *See* BENZOYL PEROXIDE.

Nerisone, **Nerisone Forte** (Schering Health Care) *See* DIFLUCORTOLONE VALERATE.

Netillin (Schering-Plough) *See* NETILMICIN.

netilmicin An *aminoglycoside antibiotic used for the treatment of serious infections that are resistant to *gentamicin. It is given as an *intramuscular or *intravenous injection and is available on *prescription only.

Side effects, precautions, and interactions with other drugs: *see* GENTAMICIN.

Proprietary preparation: Netillin.

Neulactil (JHC Healthcare) *See* PERICYAZINE.

Neupogen (Amgen) *See* FILGRASTIM.

neuroleptic drugs *See* ANTIPSYCHOTIC DRUGS.

Neurontin (Parke-Davis Medical) *See* GABAPENTIN.

Neutrexin (Ipsen) *See* TRIMETREXATE.

Neutrogena Long Lasting Dandruff Control Shampoo (Johnson & Johnson) *See* KETOCONAZOLE.

nevirapine A non-nucleoside *antiviral drug that inhibits reverse transcriptase by binding directly to the enzyme, thus blocking the synthesis of retroviral DNA and preventing viral replication. It is used in combination therapy for the treatment of infections in patients with advanced or progressive *HIV disease. Nevirapine is available as tablets on *prescription only.
Side effects: include rash (which should be reported to a doctor), nausea, fatigue, fever, headache, somnolence, and hepatitis.
Precautions: nevirapine should be used with caution in people with kidney or liver disease and in women who are pregnant or breastfeeding.
Interactions with other drugs:
  Ketoconazole: nevirapine reduces the plasma concentration of ketoconazole and the two drugs should not be taken together.
  Oral contraceptives: their contraceptive effect is reduced.
Proprietary preparation: Viramune.

nicardipine A class II *calcium antagonist used for the treatment of chronic stable *angina and *hypertension. It is available as capsules on *prescription only.
Side effects: *see* CALCIUM ANTAGONISTS.
Precautions: nicardipine should not be used to treat unstable or acute angina or to treat patients who have had a heart attack during the previous month. It should not be taken by women who are pregnant or breastfeeding. *See also* CALCIUM ANTAGONISTS.
Interactions with other drugs:
  Cyclosporin: its plasma concentration is increased by nicardipine.
  Digoxin: its plasma concentration is increased by nicardipine.
  See also CALCIUM ANTAGONISTS.
Proprietary preparations: Cardene; Cardene SR (modified-release capsules).
See also ANTIHYPERTENSIVE DRUGS.

niclosamide An *anthelmintic used for the treatment of tapeworm infestations. It is available as tablets on *prescription only.
Side effects: include nausea, retching, abdominal pain, light-headedness, and itching.
Proprietary preparation: Yomesan.

nicorandil A *potassium channel activator that is used for the prevention and long-term treatment of *angina. It is available as tablets on *prescription only.
Side effects: include headache (especially at the start of treatment),

flushing, nausea, vomiting, dizziness, and weakness. High dosages of nicorandil may cause a fall in blood pressure and/or an increase in heart rate.

Precautions and interactions with other drugs: nicorandil should not be taken by people with low blood pressure. It should be used with caution in people with certain types of heart or lung disease and in women who are pregnant or breastfeeding. Nicorandil's effects in lowering blood pressure may be increased if it is taken with alcohol, tricyclic antidepressants, or vasodilators.

Sildenafil: significantly enhances the effects of nicorandil in lowering blood pressure; the two drugs should not be taken together.

Proprietary preparation: Ikorel.

Nicorette, **Nicorette Microtab**, **Nicorette Plus** (Pharmacia & Upjohn) *See* NICOTINE.

nicotinamide A vitamin of the B group (*see* VITAMIN B COMPLEX). It is a derivative of *nicotinic acid, another B vitamin, and both forms of the vitamin are equally active in the body, being required for many metabolic reactions. Deficiency can lead to pellagra, symptoms of which include dermatitis. Supplements of nicotinamide in the form of tablets or multivitamin preparations are used to treat or prevent deficiency; most of them are available without a prescription. Nicotinamide is also used for the *topical treatment of mild to moderate inflamed acne; it is available as a gel and can be obtained without a prescription, but only from pharmacies.

Side effects: the gel may cause dryness, itching, redness, or irritation of the skin.

Precautions: the gel should not be applied near the eyes, nostrils or mouth.

Proprietary preparations: Papulex (gel); PABRINEX (combined with other B vitamins and vitamin C).

nicotine An *alkaloid that occurs in tobacco and is absorbed into the body when tobacco is chewed or smoked, causing an increase in blood pressure and heart rate and stimulating the brain and central nervous system. The effects of nicotine are responsible for the psychological *dependence of regular smokers on cigarettes; heavy smokers can experience withdrawal symptoms if they stop smoking abruptly.

Various nicotine products are available to help smokers give up the habit. Such products contain nicotine in precise amounts and are used to replace the nicotine usually obtained from cigarettes when a person is trying to give up smoking. The dosage of nicotine can then be reduced in a controlled manner to avoid the problem of withdrawal. Nicotine products in the form of chewing gum, inhalators ('mock cigarettes'), *transdermal (skin) patches, and *sublingual tablets can be obtained from pharmacies without a prescription; they cannot be prescribed on the NHS. A nasal spray is available on *prescription only.

Side effects: include nausea, dizziness, headache, influenza-like symptoms, palpitations, indigestion, insomnia and vivid dreams, and muscle aches. Skin patches may cause local reactions. Sprays can cause throat and nasal irritation, nose bleeds, watery eyes, and sensations in the ear. Gums can irritate the throat and cause mouth ulcers and sometimes swelling of the tongue. Inhalators can cause a sore mouth or throat, mouth ulcers, a swollen tongue, cough, running nose, and sinusitis.

Precautions: nicotine products should not be used by people with severe heart disease or after a heart attack or a recent stroke, or by women who are pregnant or breastfeeding. Patches are not suitable for occasional smokers and should never be placed on broken skin. People should not smoke while they are using nicotine products.

Interactions with other drugs:

  Theophylline: nicotine products may reduce the effectiveness of theophylline.

Proprietary preparations: Nicorette (chewing gum, skin patches, nasal spray, inhalator); Nicorette Microtab (sublingual tablets); Nicorette Plus (higher strength chewing gum); Nicotinell (chewing gum, skin patches); NiQuitin CQ (skin patches).

Nicotinell (Novartis Consumer Health) *See* NICOTINE.

nicotinic acid A member of the *vitamin B complex. Nicotinic acid is used as a *lipid-lowering drug: it reduces concentrations of *cholesterol and *triglycerides in the blood and increases HDL-cholesterol (*see* LIPOPROTEINS). However, it causes *vasodilatation and other side effects that may limit its use. Nicotinic acid is available as tablets; it is a *prescription only medicine if used as a lipid-lowering drug.

  Nicotinic acid derivatives are used as *vasodilators to treat peripheral vascular disease and other disorders of circulation, including Raynaud's syndrome (*see* INOSITOL NICOTINATE; NICOTINYL ALCOHOL). They can reduce concentrations of fibrinogen (an agent involved in the clotting of blood) and lower blood viscosity (the fluidity of the blood). The nicotinic acid derivative *acipimox is used as a lipid-lowering drug.

Side effects: include flushing, dizziness, headache, nausea and vomiting, palpitations, and itching.

Precautions and interactions with other drugs: nicotinic acid should not be taken by women who are pregnant or breastfeeding, and it should be used with caution in people with diabetes, gout, liver disease, or a peptic ulcer. It should also be used with caution if taken with *statins, since the combination of these two types of lipid-lowering drugs can affect the muscles.

nicotinyl alcohol A *nicotinic acid derivative used for the treatment of circulatory disorders and peripheral vascular disease. It is available as tablets or *modified-release tablets and can be obtained from pharmacies without a prescription.

Side effects: as for *nicotinic acid, but side effects are less severe and occur less frequently.

Precautions: nicotinyl alcohol should not be taken in the long term by people with diabetes.

Proprietary preparations: Ronicol; Ronicol Timespan (modified-release tablets).

nicoumalone <acenocoumarol> An oral *anticoagulant used for the prevention and treatment of deep-vein *thrombosis and pulmonary embolism and for the prevention of embolism in people with atrial fibrillation (*see* ARRHYTHMIA) and in those who have received an artificial heart valve. It is available as tablets on *prescription only.

Side effects, precautions, and interactions with other drugs: see WARFARIN SODIUM.

Proprietary preparation: Sinthrome.

nifedipine A class II *calcium antagonist used for the prevention of *angina and the treatment of *hypertension. It is also used to treat Raynaud's phenomenon (pallor and numbness of the fingers). A *prescription only medicine, it is available as capsules or tablets, some of which are *modified-release formulations.

Side effects: see CALCIUM ANTAGONISTS.

Precautions: nifedipine should not be used to treat unstable angina and should not be given to patients who have had a heart attack in the previous month. *See also* CALCIUM ANTAGONISTS.

Interactions with other drugs:

Digoxin: its plasma concentration may be increased by nifedipine.

Phenytoin: its plasma concentration is increased by nifedipine.

Quinidine: its plasma concentration is reduced by nifedipine.

Rifampicin: reduces the effects of nifedipine.

See also CALCIUM ANTAGONISTS.

Proprietary preparations: Adalat (capsules); Adalat LA (modified-release tablets); Adalat Retard (modified-release tablets); Adipine MR (modified-release tablets); Angiopine MR (modified-release tablets); Calanif (capsules); Cardilate MR (modified-release tablets); Coracten (modified-release tablets); Coroday MR (modified-release tablets); Fortipine LA 40 (modified-release tablets); Hypolar Retard 20 (modified-release tablets); Nifedipress MR (modified-release tablets); Nifedotard 20 MR (modified-release tablets); Nifelease (modified-release tablets); Nimodrel MR (modified-release tablets); Nivaten Retard (modified-release tablets); Slofedipine XL (modified-release tablets); Tensipine MR (modified-release tablets); Unipine XL (modified-release tablets); BETA-ADALAT (combined with atenolol); TENIF (combined with atenolol).

See also ANTIHYPERTENSIVE DRUGS.

Nifedipress MR (Lagap Pharmaceuticals) *See* NIFEDIPINE.

Nifedotard 20 MR (Ashbourne Pharmaceuticals) *See* NIFEDIPINE.

Nifelease (Trinity Pharmaceuticals) *See* NIFEDIPINE.

Niferex, Niferex Drops (Tillomed Laboratories) *See* POLYSACCHARIDE–IRON COMPLEX.

Night Nurse (SmithKline Beecham Consumer Healthcare) A proprietary combination of *paracetamol (an analgesic and antipyretic), *promethazine hydrochloride (an antihistamine that induces drowsiness), and *dextromethorphan (a cough suppressant), taken at night to relieve the symptoms of colds, chills, and influenza. It is available as a liquid or capsules and can be obtained without a prescription, but only from pharmacies.
Side effects: see DEXTROMETHORPHAN; ANTIHISTAMINES.
Precautions: Night Nurse should not be given to children under six years old except on medical advice. *See also* PARACETAMOL; ANTIHISTAMINES; OPIOIDS.
Interactions with other drugs: see ANTIHISTAMINES; OPIOIDS.

nimodipine A class II *calcium antagonist that relaxes the cerebral arteries, which supply blood to the brain. It is used to prevent spasm of these arteries following a subarachnoid haemorrhage (bleeding into the spaces around the brain caused by a rupture of one of the cerebral arteries), and thus prevents further interruption of the blood supply to the brain. Nimodipine is available, as tablets or a solution for infusion, on *prescription only.
Side effects: include low blood pressure, flushing, headache, and gastrointestinal upset (including nausea).
Precautions: nimodipine should be used with caution in patients with swelling of the brain, raised pressure within the brain, or poor kidney function. *See also* CALCIUM ANTAGONISTS.
Interactions with other drugs: see CALCIUM ANTAGONISTS.
Proprietary preparation: Nimotop.

Nimodrel MR (Opus) *See* NIFEDIPINE.

Nimotop (Bayer) *See* NIMODIPINE.

Nindaxa 2.5 (Ashbourne Pharmaceuticals) *See* INDAPAMIDE HEMIHYDRATE.

Nipent (Wyeth Laboratories) *See* PENTOSTATIN.

NiQuitin CQ (SmithKline Beecham Consumer Healthcare) *See* NICOTINE.

Nirolex Chesty Cough Linctus (Boots) *See* GUAIPHENESIN <GUAIFENESIN>.

Nirolex for Chesty Coughs with Decongestant (Boots) A proprietary combination of *pseudoephedrine (a decongestant) and *guaiphenesin <guaifenesin> (an expectorant), used to relieve the symptoms of productive coughs and congestion. It is available as a liquid without a prescription, but only from Boots.

Side effects, precautions, and interactions with other drugs: see EPHEDRINE HYDROCHLORIDE; DECONGESTANTS; GUAIPHENESIN.

Nirolex for Dry Coughs with Decongestant (Boots) A proprietary combination of *dextromethorphan (a cough suppressant) and *pseudoephedrine (a decongestant), used to relieve the symptoms of dry irritating coughs and congestion. It is available as a liquid without a prescription, but only from Boots.

Side effects, precautions, and interactions with other drugs: see DEXTROMETHORPHAN; OPIOIDS; EPHEDRINE HYDROCHLORIDE; DECONGESTANTS.

Nirolex Lozenges (Boots) *See* DEXTROMETHORPHAN.

nisoldipine A class II *calcium antagonist used for the treatment of mild to moderate *hypertension and for preventive treatment in chronic stable *angina. It is available as *modified-release tablets on *prescription only.

Side effects and interactions with other drugs: see CALCIUM ANTAGONISTS.

Precautions: nisoldipine should not be taken by people with liver disease or by women who are pregnant or breastfeeding. *See also* CALCIUM ANTAGONISTS.

Proprietary preparation: Syscor MR.

See also ANTIHYPERTENSIVE DRUGS.

nitrates *Vasodilator drugs used in the treatment of *angina, and also as adjuncts to *cardiac glycosides and *diuretics in the treatment of congestive *heart failure. Nitrates dilate large veins, which reduces the amount of blood returning to the heart and therefore decreases the workload on the heart. The drugs in this group are *isosorbide mononitrate, *isosorbide dinitrate, *glyceryl trinitrate, and *pentaerythritol <pentaerithrityl> tetranitrate. Nitrates are available in a variety of formulations: sublingual tablets (which dissolve in the mouth when placed under the tongue), buccal tablets (which dissolve when inserted between teeth and cheek), oral tablets (which are swallowed), *modified-release tablets and capsules, chewable tablets, a sublingual spray (which is absorbed across the lining of the mouth), ointment or skin patches (both of which are applied to the chest wall and absorbed through the skin), and intravenous solutions. The choice of product depends on the onset and duration of action required.

Side effects: headache, flushing, and dizziness are the most common side effects; less commonly fainting may occur. Side effects decrease with long-term use.

Precautions: some patients on long-acting nitrates or transdermal patches rapidly develop *tolerance. Therefore longer acting tablets and modified-release preparations are usually administered so that there is a 'nitrate-free' period at night, and transdermal patches should be removed for several consecutive hours during each 24 hours. This helps to avoid tolerance and increases the efficacy of the nitrate in preventing angina attacks.

Interactions with other drugs:

Antihypertensive drugs: can cause a further lowering of blood pressure.

Heparin: its anticoagulant effect is reduced by nitrates.

Sildenafil: causes significant lowering of blood pressure and should not be used with nitrates.

nitrazepam A long-acting *benzodiazepine used for the short-term treatment of insomnia. It is available as tablets or an oral suspension on *prescription only; certain proprietary preparations cannot be prescribed on the NHS.

Side effects and precautions: see BENZODIAZEPINES; DIAZEPAM.

Interactions with other drugs: see BENZODIAZEPINES.

Proprietary preparations: Mogadon; Remnos; Somnite.

Nitrocine (Schwartz Pharma) *See* GLYCERYL TRINITRATE.

Nitro-Dur (Schering-Plough) *See* GLYCERYL TRINITRATE.

nitrofurantoin An *antibiotic used for the treatment of urinary-tract infections and to prevent infection during surgery of the genitourinary tract. It is especially useful for treating kidney infections that are resistant to other antibiotics. It is available, on *prescription only, as tablets, capsules, *modified-release capsules, or a suspension.

Side effects: include gastrointestinal upset, breathing difficulties, rash, and itching. Rare side effects are jaundice, inflammation of the liver, and blood disorders. The drug should be withdrawn if signs of breathing problems, jaundice, or liver problems occur.

Precautions: nitrofurantoin should not be taken by people with impaired kidney function or by women at the end of pregnancy or who are breastfeeding.

Interactions with other drugs:

Magnesium trisilicate: reduces absorption of nitrofurantoin.

Probenecid: increases the potential toxicity of nitrofurantoin.

Proprietary preparations: Furadantin; Macrobid; Macrodantin.

Nitrolingual Pumpspray (Merck Pharmaceuticals) *See* GLYCERYL TRINITRATE.

Nitromin (Dominion Pharma) *See* GLYCERYL TRINITRATE.

Nitronal (Merck Pharmaceuticals) *See* GLYCERYL TRINITRATE.

Nivaquine (Rhône-Poulenc Rorer) *See* CHLOROQUINE.

Nivaten Retard (Cox Pharmaceuticals) *See* NIFEDIPINE.

Nivemycin (Knoll) *See* NEOMYCIN SULPHATE.

nizatidine An *H$_2$-receptor antagonist used in the treatment of
duodenal or gastric ulcers, ulcers caused by use of *NSAIDs, and gastro-
oesophageal reflux disease, and for the prevention of ulcer recurrence
(*see* ACID-PEPTIC DISEASES). It is available as capsules or an injection on
*prescription only. Packs containing no more than two weeks' supply of
capsules, for the treatment and prevention of indigestion and heartburn
in those over 16 years old, can be obtained from pharmacies without a
prescription.
Side effects: include anaemia, sweating, itching, hepatitis, and jaundice.
See also H$_2$-RECEPTOR ANTAGONISTS.
Precautions: nizatidine should be used with caution by people with liver
or kidney disease and by women who are pregnant or breastfeeding.
Proprietary preparations: Axid; Zinga.

Nizoral (Janssen-Cilag) *See* KETOCONAZOLE.

Nolvadex-D, **Nolvadex Forte** (AstraZeneca) *See* TAMOXIFEN.

nonoxinol-9 (nonoxynol-9) A drug that kills sperm and is the active
ingredient of *spermicidal contraceptives. It is freely available *over the
counter in the form of a cream, a gel, a foam, or pessaries.
Side effects: see SPERMICIDAL CONTRACEPTIVES.
Proprietary preparations: Delfen (foam aerosol); Double Check (pessary);
Duragel (gel); Gynol-II (jelly); Ortho-Creme; Orthoforms (pessaries).

non-steroidal anti-inflammatory drugs *See* NSAIDS.

nonylic acid vanillylamide A drug that is used as a *rubefacient for
the relief of muscular aches and pains. It is an ingredient of a cream that
is freely available *over the counter.
Side effects and precautions: see RUBEFACIENTS.
Proprietary preparation: BOOTS PAIN RELIEF BALM (combined with ethyl
nicotinate and glycol salicylate).

Nootropil (UCB Pharma) *See* PIRACETAM.

noradrenaline <norepinephrine> A substance that transmits messages
in the *sympathetic nervous system. It acts on *adrenoceptors to have
effects on the heart, blood vessels, intestines, lungs, salivary glands, and
bladder. It is also available as a drug (**noradrenaline acid tartrate**

<norepinephrine bitartrate>), which is used in an emergency to restore
dangerously low blood pressure or to treat cardiac arrest. Noradrenaline
is given by intravenous infusion (for low blood pressure) or by rapid
injection into a vein or the heart (for cardiac arrest). Available on
*prescription only, it is only used in a hospital setting.

Side effects: include hypertension (high blood pressure), headache, and
arrhythmias (irregular heartbeat).

Precautions: noradrenaline should be used with caution in patients with
thrombosis, diabetes, thyroid disease, or following a heart attack.

Interactions with other drugs:

  Beta blockers: may cause severe hypertension.

  Dopexamine: may increase the effect of noradrenaline.

  Entacapone: may increase the effects of noradrenaline.

  Tricyclic antidepressants: hypertension and arrhythmias may occur if
    noradrenaline is given to patients who are taking these drugs.

Proprietary preparations: Levophed; Levophed Special.

Norditropin (Novo Nordisk Pharmaceutical) *See* SOMATROPIN.

norepinephrine *See* NORADRENALINE.

norethisterone A synthetic *progestogen. Combined with
*oestrogens it is used in *oral contraceptives, and as an *adjunct to
oestrogens it is used as part of *hormone replacement therapy (HRT). It
can be used alone as a progestogen-only contraceptive pill and – but only
for a limited period – to delay menstruation, to treat heavy or painful
periods, or to relieve premenstrual tension. Norethisterone is also used as
a *depot contraceptive, which is given by intramuscular injection and
lasts for up to eight weeks. It is also used to treat certain cancers.
Norethisterone is available, on *prescription only, as tablets, skin
patches, or as a solution for injection.

Side effects, precautions, and interactions with other drugs: see ORAL
CONTRACEPTIVES; PROGESTOGENS.

Proprietary preparations: Micronor (contraceptive pill); Micronor-HRT (in
hormone replacement therapy); Noriday (contraceptive pill); Noristerat
(depot contraceptive); Primolut N (tablets); Utovlan (tablets); BINOVUM
(combined with ethinyloestradiol <ethinylestradiol>); BREVINOR
(combined with ethinyloestradiol <ethinylestradiol>); CLIMAGEST
(packaged with oestradiol <estradiol> valerate); CLIMESSE (combined with
oestradiol <estradiol> valerate); ELLESTE DUET (packaged with oestradiol
<estradiol>); ELLESTE DUET CONTI (combined with oestradiol <estradiol>);
ESTRACOMBI (combined with oestradiol <estradiol>); EVOREL CONTI
(combined with oestradiol <estradiol>); EVOREL-PAK (packaged with
oestradiol <estradiol>); EVOREL SEQUI (combined with oestradiol
<estradiol>); KLIOFEM (combined with oestradiol <estradiol>); KLIOVANCE
(combined with oestradiol <estradiol>); LOESTRIN 20 and LOESTRIN 30
(combined with ethinyloestradiol <ethinylestradiol>); MENOPHASE
(combined with mestranol); NORIMIN (combined with ethinyloestradiol

<ethinylestradiol>); NORINYL-1 (combined with mestranol); OVYSMEN (combined with levonorgestrel); SYNPHASE (combined with ethinyloestradiol <ethinylestradiol>); TRINOVUM (combined with ethinyloestradiol <ethinylestradiol>); TRISEQUENS (combined with oestradiol <estradiol>).

norfloxacin A *quinolone antibiotic, similar to *ciprofloxacin, that is used for the treatment and prevention of urinary-tract infections. It is available as capsules on *prescription only.
Side effects, precautions, and interactions with other drugs: see QUINOLONES.
Proprietary preparation: Utinor.

Norgalax Micro-enema (Norgine) *See* DOCUSATE SODIUM.

norgestimate A synthetic *progestogen used as an ingredient in combined *oral contraceptives. It is available on *prescription only.
Side effects, precautions, and interactions with other drugs: see ORAL CONTRACEPTIVES.
Proprietary preparation: CILEST (combined with ethinyloestradiol <ethinylestradiol>).

Norgeston (Schering Health Care) *See* LEVONORGESTREL; ORAL CONTRACEPTIVES.

norgestrel A synthetic *progestogen that is used as a progestogen-only *oral contraceptive. In combination with an *oestrogen, it is used to provide postcoital ('morning-after') contraception or for treating symptoms of the menopause and preventing osteoporosis in postmenopausal women (*see* HORMONE REPLACEMENT THERAPY).
Side effects, precautions, and interactions with other drugs: see PROGESTOGENS; ORAL CONTRACEPTIVES.
Proprietary preparations: Neogest (contraceptive pill); SCHERING PC4 (combined with ethinyloestradiol <ethinylestradiol>).

Noriday (Searle) *See* NORETHISTERONE; ORAL CONTRACEPTIVES.

Norimin (Searle) A proprietary combination of *ethinyloestradiol <ethinylestradiol> and *norethisterone used as an *oral contraceptive. It is available as tablets on *prescription only.
Side effects, precautions, and interactions with other drugs: see ORAL CONTRACEPTIVES.

Norimode (Tillomed Laboratories) *See* LOPERAMIDE HYDROCHLORIDE.

Norinyl-1 (Searle) A proprietary combination of *mestranol and *norethisterone used as an *oral contraceptive. It is available as tablets on *prescription only.

Side effects, precautions, and interactions with other drugs: see ORAL CONTRACEPTIVES.

Noristerat (Schering Health Care) *See* NORETHISTERONE.

Noritate (Kestrel Healthcare) *See* METRONIDAZOLE.

Normacol (Norgine) *See* STERCULIA.

Normacol Plus (Norgine) A proprietary combination of *sterculia and frangula (both *bulk-forming laxatives), used for treating constipation and for encouraging bowel movement after haemorrhoidectomy. It is freely available *over the counter in the form of granules.
Side effects and precautions: see ISPAGHULA HUSK.

normal immunoglobulin *See* IMMUNOGLOBULINS.

Normaloe (Tillomed Laboratories) *See* LOPERAMIDE HYDROCHLORIDE.

Normasol (Seton Scholl Healthcare) *See* SODIUM CHLORIDE.

Normax (Medeva) *See* CO-DANTHRUSATE.

Normegon (Organon Laboratories) *See* HUMAN MENOPAUSAL GONADOTROPHIN.

Norphyllin SR (Norton Healthcare) *See* AMINOPHYLLINE.

Norplant (Hoechst Marion Roussel) *See* LEVONORGESTREL.

Norprolac (Novartis Pharmaceuticals) *See* QUINAGOLIDE.

nortriptyline A *tricyclic antidepressant drug used for the treatment of depressive illness and also bedwetting in children; it is less sedative than *amitriptyline. It is available as tablets on *prescription only.
Side effects, precautions, and interactions with other drugs: see AMITRIPTYLINE HYDROCHLORIDE; TRICYCLIC ANTIDEPRESSANTS.
Proprietary preparations: Allegron; MOTIPRESS (combined with fluphenazine hydrochloride); MOTIVAL (combined with fluphenazine hydrochloride).

Norvir (Abbott Laboratories) *See* RITONAVIR.

Novantrone (Wyeth Laboratories) *See* MITOZANTRONE <MITOXANTRONE>.

NovoNorm (Novo Nordisk Pharmaceutical) *See* REPAGLINIDE.

NovoSeven (Novo Nordisk Pharmaceutical) *See* FACTOR VIIA.

Nozinan (Link Pharmaceuticals) *See* METHOTRIMEPRAZINE
<LEVOMEPROMAZINE>.

NSAIDs (non-steroidal anti-inflammatory drugs) A large group of drugs
that reduce inflammation. NSAIDs act by inhibiting the enzymes (cyclo-
oxygenases) required for the production of *prostaglandins, which are
involved in inflammation. They also have *analgesic (pain-relieving)
activity. NSAIDs are used for the long-term treatment of inflammatory
rheumatic diseases and back pain; they are particularly appropriate for
the relief of chronic pain and stiffness in inflammatory diseases of the
joints, such as rheumatoid arthritis. NSAIDs are also used to relieve acute
pain, such as that occurring after operations or associated with acute
gout or heavy periods (in which they reduce the production of
prostaglandins that are thought to be responsible for the increased blood
flow and painful contractions of the uterus). In cancer patients, NSAIDs
may reduce the need for *opioid analgesics; they are particularly suitable
for the pain associated with secondary tumours (metastases) in bones.

Many of the side effects of NSAIDs are related to their suppression of
prostaglandins, which – in addition to their role in the inflammatory
response – also protect the lining of the stomach against attack by gastric
acid (*see* ACID-PEPTIC DISEASES). Therefore many NSAIDs have adverse
effects on the stomach and intestines (see Side effects below). However,
these effects vary in severity with different NSAIDs; there is also
considerable variation in how individuals respond to the different drugs
in this group. It may therefore take a period of 'trial and error' before the
NSAID that suits a particular individual is found.

NSAIDs are available in a variety of forms, including tablets, capsules,
*modified-release formulations, injections, and suppositories. Some are
also available as gels or creams to be applied to the skin to relieve
sprains, strains, aches, and pains. Most preparations are *prescription
only medicines, but some can be obtained without a prescription.

See ACECLOFENAC; ACEMETACIN; AZAPROPAZONE; BENZYDAMINE
HYDROCHLORIDE; DICLOFENAC SODIUM; DIFLUNISAL; ETODOLAC; FELBINAC;
FENBUFEN; FENOPROFEN; FLURBIPROFEN; IBUPROFEN; INDOMETHACIN
<INDOMETACIN>; KETOPROFEN; KETOROLAC TROMETAMOL; MEFENAMIC ACID;
MELOXICAM; NABUMETONE; NAPROXEN; PHENYLBUTAZONE; PIROXICAM;
SULINDAC; TENOXICAM; TIAPROFENIC ACID; TOLFENAMIC ACID.

Side effects: gastrointestinal effects can include indigestion, nausea,
diarrhoea, and occasionally bleeding and ulceration. Indigestion can be
prevented by taking NSAIDs with milk or food; to reduce the likelihood
of bleeding and ulceration, NSAIDs can be taken with an *antacid, *H$_2$-
receptor antagonist, or *proton pump inhibitor, or with *misoprostol.
NSAIDs can cause allergic reactions, such as rashes, an asthma attack, or
(rarely) swelling of the face and constriction of the airways (*see*
ANAPHYLAXIS). Other side effects may include headache, dizziness,
vertigo, tinnitus (the sensation of noises in the ear), and sensitivity to
sunlight (especially with topical preparations).

Precautions: NSAIDs should not be taken by people who have had
allergic reactions to aspirin or other NSAIDs (including an asthma attack,

itching, or a running nose) or by people who have peptic ulcers, except on medical advice. They should not be taken by women who are pregnant or breastfeeding. NSAIDs should only be prescribed for people with a history of peptic ulcers and for elderly people after other treatments have been carefully considered. NSAIDs should be used with caution in people who have liver, kidney, or heart disease. Topical NSAIDs are usually not recommended for children. They should not come into contact with the eyes, lips, or other mucous membranes or with broken skin. Prolonged exposure of treated skin to sunlight should be avoided.

Interactions with other drugs:

ACE inhibitors: NSAIDs may reduce the effect of ACE inhibitors in lowering blood pressure.

Analgesics: aspirin should not be taken with other NSAIDs and two or more NSAIDs should not be taken together, since this is likely to increase their gastrointestinal side effects.

Antibiotics: NSAIDs may increase the risk of convulsions with quinolones.

Anticoagulants: the risk of bleeding may be increased if anticoagulants are taken with NSAIDs.

Antidiabetic drugs: NSAIDs may enhance the effects of the sulphonylureas.

Cyclosporin: there is an increased risk of kidney damage if cyclosporin is taken with NSAIDs.

Lithium: its excretion is reduced by NSAIDs, so that it builds up in the bloodstream and is more likely to cause adverse effects.

Methotrexate: its excretion is reduced by NSAIDs, so that it builds up in the bloodstream and is more likely to cause adverse effects.

Probenecid: may increase the effects of NSAIDs.

Nubain (Du Pont Pharmaceuticals) *See* NALBUPHINE HYDROCHLORIDE.

nucleoside analogues *See* ANTIVIRAL DRUGS.

Nuelin, **Nuelin SA** (3M Health Care) *See* THEOPHYLLINE.

Numark Cold Relief Capsules with Decongestant (Numark) A proprietary combination of *paracetamol (an analgesic and antipyretic) and *phenylephrine (a decongestant), used to relieve the fever, congestion, and other symptoms of colds and influenza. It is freely available *over the counter.
Side effects, precautions, and interactions with other drugs: *see* PARACETAMOL; PHENYLEPHRINE; DECONGESTANTS.

Numark Cold Relief Powders (Numark) *See* PARACETAMOL.

Nurofen, **Nurofen for Children** (Crookes Healthcare) *See* IBUPROFEN.

Nurofen Colds & Flu (Crookes Healthcare) A proprietary combination of *ibuprofen (an NSAID) and *pseudoephedrine (a decongestant), used to relieve the symptoms of colds and influenza, including nasal congestion, aches and pains, headache, fever, and sore throat. It is available as tablets and can be obtained without a prescription, but only from pharmacies.
Side effects, precautions, and interactions with other drugs: see NSAIDS; DECONGESTANTS; EPHEDRINE HYDROCHLORIDE.

Nurofen Plus (Crookes Healthcare) A proprietary combination of *ibuprofen (an NSAID) and *codeine phosphate (an opioid analgesic), used for the relief of migraine, tension headaches, toothache, period pains, sciatica, lumbago, and rheumatism. It is available as tablets and can be obtained without a prescription, but only from pharmacies.
Side effects, precautions, and interactions with other drugs: see IBUPROFEN; NSAIDS; CODEINE; OPIOIDS.

Nurse Harvey's Gripe Mixture (Harvey-Scruton) *See* SODIUM BICARBONATE.

Nurse Sykes Bronchial Balsam (Anglian Pharma) *See* GUAIPHENESIN <GUAIFENESIN>.

Nurse Sykes Powders (Anglian Pharma) A proprietary combination of *aspirin and *paracetamol (analgesics and antipyretics) and *caffeine (a stimulant), used to relieve mild to moderate pain and fever and the symptoms of colds and influenza. It is available without a prescription, but larger packs can only be obtained from pharmacies.
Side effects and interactions with other drugs: see ASPIRIN.
Precautions: this medicine should not be given to children, except on medical advice. *See also* ASPIRIN; CAFFEINE; PARACETAMOL.

Nu-Seals Aspirin (Eli Lilly & Co) *See* ASPIRIN.

Nutraplus (Galderma) *See* UREA.

Nutrizyme GR, **Nutrizyme 10**, **Nutrizyme 22** (Merck Pharmaceuticals) *See* PANCREATIN.

Nuvelle (Schering Health Care) A proprietary preparation of *oestradiol <estradiol> tablets and combined oestradiol/*levonorgestrel tablets used as sequential combined *hormone replacement therapy for the relief of menopausal symptoms and the prevention of osteoporosis in women who have not had a hysterectomy. The tablets must be taken in the prescribed order. **Nuvelle TS** is available in the form of skin patches. Both preparations are available on *prescription only.
Side effects, precautions, and interactions with other drugs: see HORMONE REPLACEMENT THERAPY.

Nycopren (Ardern Healthcare) *See* NAPROXEN.

Nylax with Senna (Crookes Healthcare) *See* SENNA.

Nystadermal (Bristol-Myers Squibb) A proprietary combination of *triamcinolone acetonide (a potent steroid) and *nystatin (an antifungal drug), used for treating *Candida* infections of the skin and eczema when these are associated with inflammation. It is available as a cream on *prescription only.
Side effects and precautions: see TOPICAL STEROIDS; NYSTATIN.

Nystaform (Bayer) A proprietary combination of *nystatin (an antifungal drug) and *chlorhexidine (an antiseptic), used for the treatment of skin infections. It is available as a cream on *prescription only.
Side effects and precautions: see NYSTATIN.

Nystaform-HC (Bayer) A proprietary combination of *nystatin (an antifungal agent), *chlorhexidine (an antiseptic), and *hydrocortisone (a corticosteroid), used for the treatment of a variety of skin conditions in which infection is present or suspected. It is available as a cream or ointment on *prescription only.
Side effects and precautions: see TOPICAL STEROIDS.

Nystamont (Rosemont Pharmaceuticals) *See* NYSTATIN.

Nystan (Bristol-Myers Squibb) *See* NYSTATIN.

nystatin An *antifungal drug that is particularly effective in treating candidiasis (thrush). Since it is not absorbed from the gastrointestinal tract, it is particularly useful for treating candidiasis of the mouth, throat, and gut, as well as the genital area. As it is too toxic to be administered intravenously, it is not suitable for treating systemic (generalized) infections. Nystatin is available, on *prescription only, in a variety of formulations, including tablets, a suspension, pastilles, and a mouthwash for oral administration, pessaries, creams, a gel, and an ointment.
Side effects: high doses may cause nausea, vomiting, and diarrhoea. Oral preparations may cause local irritation and (rarely) allergic reactions, and a rash may rarely occur after topical application.
Precautions: nystatin should be used with caution by women who are pregnant or breastfeeding.
Proprietary preparations: Infestat; Nystamont; Nystan; DERMOVATE-NN (combined with clobetasol and neomycin); FLAGYL COMPAK (packaged with metronidazole); GREGODERM (combined with neomycin, polymyxin B, and hydrocortisone); NYSTADERMAL (combined with triamcinolone acetonide); NYSTAFORM (combined with chlorhexidine); NYSTAFORM-HC (combined with chlorhexidine and hydrocortisone); TERRA-CORTRIL NYSTATIN (combined with oxytetracycline and hydrocortisone); TIMODINE

(combined with hydrocortisone, benzalkonium chloride and dimethicone <dimeticone>); TINADERM-M (combined with tolnaftate); TRI-ADCORTYL (combined with triamcinolone, neomycin, and gramicidin); TRI-ADCORTYL OTIC (combined with triamcinolone acetonide, neomycin, and gramicidin); TRIMOVATE (combined with clobetasone butyrate and oxytetracycline).

Nytol (Stafford-Miller) *See* DIPHENHYDRAMINE.

O

obesity The condition in which excess fat has accumulated in the body (mostly in the tissues beneath the skin), which is usually caused by the consumption of more food than is required for producing enough energy for daily activities. Obesity is usually considered to be present when a person is 20% above the recommended weight for his or her height and build. It is measured by means of the body mass index (BMI), which is calculated by dividing a person's weight by the square of their height. A BMI of 18.5–25 kg/m^2 is regarded as within the normal range; someone with a BMI of over 25 would be considered to be overweight, and a BMI of 30 or more indicates clinical obesity.

Obesity is the most common nutritional disorder of Western societies and predisposes to many health problems, including heart disease and diabetes. The main treatment is dietary restriction; drug treatment (if considered necessary) should only be used in conjunction with a carefully controlled diet. Anti-obesity drugs that act on the digestive tract include *orlistat and *methylcellulose; *phentermine acts on the brain to suppress appetite and should only be used on selected patients for short periods.

Occlusal (DermaPharm) *See* SALICYLIC ACID.

Octagam (Octapharma) *See* IMMUNOGLOBULINS.

octaphonium chloride <octafonium chloride> An antiseptic, similar to *cetrimide, that is an ingredient of an ointment for the treatment of minor wounds, cuts, grazes, burns, scalds, and blisters.
Proprietary preparation: GERMOLENE OINTMENT (combined with zinc oxide, methyl salicylate, phenol, and emollients).

octocog alfa *See* FACTOR VIII.

octreotide A long-acting *analogue of somatostatin, a hormone that is produced in the brain, gastrointestinal tract, and pancreas and inhibits the release of *growth hormone. It is used for the treatment of acromegaly (a conditon due to excessive secretion of growth hormone by a tumour in the pituitary gland), either in the short term for patients awaiting pituitary surgery and for the long-term treatment of those individuals with acromegaly who do not respond to surgery, *dopamine antagonists, or radiotherapy. It may also be used until radiotherapy is effective. Octreotide is also used to inhibit the secretions (and thus relieve the symptoms) of hormone-secreting tumours of the gastrointestinal tract. It is available as a solution for injection on *prescription only.
Side effects: include pain, stinging, and swelling at the injection site and

gastrointestinal upsets, such as loss of appetite, nausea, vomiting, and abdominal pain; gallstones may develop with long-term treatment.

Precautions: octreotide should not be given to women who are pregnant or breastfeeding. Diabetic patients may need to reduce their dosage of insulin or oral antidiabetic drugs. Gall bladder function should be monitored throughout treatment. The drug should be stopped gradually at the end of treatment.

Interactions with other drugs:

Antidiabetic drugs: doses of these may need to be reduced (see precautions).

Cimetidine: octreotide delays the absorption of cimetidine.

Cyclosporin: octreotide reduces the absorption of cyclosporin.

Proprietary preparation: Sandostatin.

Ocufen (Allergan) *See* FLURBIPROFEN.

Ocusert Pilo (Dominion Pharma) *See* PILOCARPINE.

Odrik (Hoechst Marion Roussel) *See* TRANDOLAPRIL.

oedema Excessive accumulation of fluid in the body tissues. The resultant swelling may be local, as occurs after injury or with inflammation, or it may be more general, as in *heart failure. In generalized oedema there may be accumulation of fluid within the chest cavity (pleural effusion) or abdomen (ascites). Oedema can also occur within the spaces of the lungs (**pulmonary oedema**). Other causes of oedema include varicose veins, cirrhosis of the liver, acute inflammation of the kidney or other kidney disease, starvation, and (rarely) diabetes. Allergic reactions may be accompanied by local oedema. It can also be produced in response to some drugs. In all these cases the kidneys can be stimulated to excrete more urine by using a *diuretic. Temporary oedema can occur before menstruation or on long-haul flights, when it typically affects the legs, ankles, and feet.

oestradiol <estradiol> One of the female sex hormones produced by the ovaries (*see* OESTROGENS). It is used mainly for *hormone replacement therapy (HRT), either alone or in combination with a *progestogen. Oestradiol is available, on *prescription only, as tablets, a gel or patches to be applied to the skin, or as a vaginal ring or tablets.

Side effects, precautions, and interactions with other drugs: *see* HORMONE REPLACEMENT THERAPY.

Proprietary preparations: Climavall; Dermestril; Elleste Solo; Elleste Solo MX; Estraderm TTS, Estraderm MX; Estring; Evorel; Fematrix; FemSeven; Menorest; Oestrogel; Progynova; Progynova TS; Sandrena; Vagifem; Zumenon; CLIMAGEST (packaged with norethisterone); CLIMESSE (combined with norethisterone); CYCLO-PROGYNOVA (combined with levonorgestrel); ELLESTE DUET (packaged with norethisterone); ELLESTE DUET CONTI (combined with norethisterone); ESTRACOMBI (combined with norethisterone); ESTRAPAK (packaged with norethisterone); EVOREL CONTI (combined with norethisterone); EVOREL-PAK (packaged with norethisterone); EVOREL SEQUI (combined with norethisterone); FEMAPAK (packaged with dydrogesterone); FEMOSTON (packaged with dydrogesterone); HORMONIN (combined with oestriol <estriol> and oestrone <estrone>); KLIOFEM (combined with norethisterone); KLIOVANCE (combined with norethisterone); NUVELLE (packaged with levonorgestrel); TRIDESTRA (packaged with medroxyprogesterone); TRISEQUENS (packaged with norethisterone). See table at HORMONE REPLACEMENT THERAPY.

Oestrifen (Ashbourne Pharmaceuticals) *See* TAMOXIFEN.

oestriol <estriol> One of the female sex hormones produced by the ovaries (*see* OESTROGENS). It is used in *hormone replacement therapy, mainly for the local relief of wasting or inflammation of the vagina, shrinkage or itching of the vulva (external genitals), or pain on intercourse, in menopausal and postmenopausal women. Oestriol is available as tablets or a cream on *prescription only.

Side effects, precautions, and interactions with other drugs: see OESTROGENS; HORMONE REPLACEMENT THERAPY.

Proprietary preparations: Ortho-Gynest (pessaries or cream); Ovestin (tablets or cream); HORMONIN (combined with oestradiol <estradiol> and oestrone <estrone>); TRISEQUENS (combined with oestradiol <estradiol>).

Oestrogel (Hoechst Marion Roussel) *See* OESTRADIOL <ESTRADIOL>; HORMONE REPLACEMENT THERAPY.

oestrogen antagonists (anti-oestrogens) Drugs that oppose the action of oestrogens, the female sex hormones. The main anti-oestrogens are *clomiphene citrate <clomifene citrate>, *tamoxifen, and *toremifene. In the brain, oestrogen normally prevents the release of *gonadotrophins from the pituitary gland. Oestrogen antagonists block this action, so that the pituitary is stimulated to produce greater amounts of gonadotrophins, which (in women) stimulate the ovaries to produce egg cells. Anti-oestrogens are therefore used in the treatment of infertility in women. Tamoxifen and toremifene can also block the action of oestrogen in other cells of the body, including cancer cells, and are therefore also used to treat tumours that require oestrogen for their continued growth. *See also* AROMATASE INHIBITORS.

oestrogens A group of steroid hormones, including *oestradiol <estradiol>, *oestriol <estriol>, and *oestrone <estrone>, that control female sexual development, promoting growth and function of the female sex organs and female secondary sex characteristics (such as breast development and growth of pubic hair). Oestrogens are synthesized mainly by the ovaries; small amounts are produced by the adrenal glands, testes, and placenta. Naturally occurring oestrogens and **conjugated oestrogens** (mixtures of natural oestrogens obtained from the urine of pregnant mares) are used mainly to treat a deficiency of these hormones (resulting in lack of sexual development and absence of periods) and symptoms of the menopause (*see* HORMONE REPLACEMENT THERAPY). Synthetic oestrogens (*see* ETHINYLOESTRADIOL <ETHINYLESTRADIOL>; MESTRANOL) are used mainly in *oral contraceptives, in which they are combined with *progestogens, but some preparations are used in HRT (*see also* DIENOESTROL <DIENESTROL>; ESTROPIPATE; STILBOESTROL <DIETHYLSTILBESTROL>). Oestrogens are also used to treat some menstrual disorders and certain types of prostate and breast cancer.

Side effects: include nausea and vomiting, swelling and tenderness of the breasts, weight gain due to fluid and salt retention, abdominal cramps, headache and dizziness, and irregular vaginal bleeding. There may be changes in libido and depression, and contact lenses may irritate.

Precautions: prolonged treatment with oestrogens alone may increase the risk of cancer of the endometrium (lining of the uterus). For this reason women with an intact uterus who are undergoing hormone replacement therapy are usually given oestrogens in combination with a progestogen. Oestrogens should not be used during pregnancy or breastfeeding or by women with cancer of the breast, uterus, or genital tract (or a history of these oestrogen-dependent cancers), thrombosis, liver disorders, or undiagnosed vaginal bleeding. Oestrogens should be used with caution by women with a history of migraine (or migraine-like headaches) or breast lumps. Oestrogens can increase the size of existing fibroids and exacerbate the symptoms of *endometriosis.

Interactions with other drugs:

ACE inhibitors: their effect in lowering blood pressure is reduced.

Antibiotics: ampicillin, tetracyclines, rifabutin, and rifampicin reduce the effects of oestrogens.

Anticoagulants: the effects of warfarin, nicoumalone <acenocoumarol>, and phenindione are antagonized.

Antiepileptic drugs: carbamazepine, phenobarbitone <phenobarbital>, phenytoin, primidone, and topiramate reduce the effects of oestrogens.

Antifungal drugs: griseofulvin, fluconazole, itraconazole, and ketoconazole can reduce the effects of oestrogens.

Beta blockers: their effect in lowering blood pressure is reduced.

Bile acids: oestrogens increase the elimination of cholesterol in bile.

Cyclosporin: oestrogens increase the plasma concentration (and therefore side effects) of cyclosporin.

Modafinil: reduces the effects of oestrogens.

Retinovir: reduces the effects of oestrogens.

oestrone <estrone> One of the female sex hormones produced by the ovaries (*see* OESTROGENS). Combined with other oestrogens, it is used in *hormone replacement therapy for the relief of menopausal symptoms and prevention of osteoporosis. It is available on *prescription only. *See also* ESTROPIPATE.

Side effects, precautions, and interactions with other drugs: see HORMONE REPLACEMENT THERAPY.

Proprietary preparation: HORMONIN (combined with oestriol <estriol> and oestradiol <estradiol>).

ofloxacin A *quinolone antibiotic, similar to *ciprofloxacin, that is used for the treatment of infections of the urinary tract, respiratory tract, and skin. It is also used to treat infections of the genital tract (including gonorrhoea and nongonococcal urethritis) and bacterial infections of the eye. It is available, on *prescription only, as tablets, a solution for *intravenous infusion, or eye drops.

Side effects, precautions, and interactions with other drugs: see QUINOLONES.

Proprietary preparations: Exocin (eye drops); Tarvid.

Oilatum Bath Formula, Oilatum Junior Bath Formula (Stiefel Laboratories) *See* LIQUID PARAFFIN.

Oilatum Cream (Stiefel Laboratories) *See* ARACHIS OIL.

Oilatum Emollient (Stiefel Laboratories) *See* LIQUID PARAFFIN.

Oilatum Hand Aquagel (Stiefel Laboratories) *See* LIQUID PARAFFIN.

Oilatum Junior Flare Up (Stiefel Laboratories) A proprietary combination of *triclosan and *benzalkonium chloride (both antiseptics) and *liquid paraffin (an emollient) in the form of a bath additive, used for treating *eczema in children. It is freely available *over the counter.

Oilatum Plus (Stiefel Laboratories) A proprietary combination of *benzalkonium chloride and *triclosan (both antiseptics) and *liquid paraffin (an emollient), to be added to the bath for the treatment of *eczema, particularly if there is a risk of this becoming infected. It is also available as a shower gel. Oilatum Plus is freely available *over the counter.

oil of wintergreen *See* METHYL SALICYLATE.

ointment A greasy preparation that is applied to the skin or mucous membranes; it may or may not contain pharmacologically active ingredients. Ointments are usually insoluble in water and not easily removed from the surface to which they are applied (*compare* CREAM). Skin ointments commonly contain soft paraffin and/or liquid paraffin. *See* EMOLLIENTS.

olanzapine An atypical *antipsychotic drug used for the treatment of schizophrenia. It is available as tablets on *prescription only.
Side effects: include weight gain, dizziness, low blood pressure on standing (which can cause fainting in some people), drowsiness,

increased appetite, and mild antimuscarinic effects (*see* CHLORPROMAZINE HYDROCHLORIDE). Occasionally olanzapine causes blood disorders.

Precautions: olanzapine should not be taken by people with acute glaucoma or by women who are breastfeeding. It should be used with caution by pregnant women, men with an enlarged prostate gland, and by anyone with liver or kidney disease, a low white blood cell count, or bone marrow suppression.

Interactions with other drugs:

Anaesthetics: their effect in lowering blood pressure is enhanced.

Antidepressants: there is an increased risk of antimuscarinic effects and arrhythmias if olanzapine is taken with tricyclic antidepressants.

Antiepileptic drugs: their anticonvulsant effects are antagonized by olanzapine; carbamazepine reduces the effects of olanzapine.

Antihistamines: there is an increased risk of arrhythmias if olanzapine is taken with astemizole or terfenadine.

Halofantrine: there is an increased risk of arrhythmias if this drug is taken with olanzapine.

Ritonavir: may increase the effects of olanzapine.

Sedatives: the sedative effects of olanzapine are increased if it is taken with anxiolytic or hypnotic drugs, or any other drug that causes sedation.

Proprietary preparation: Zyprexa.

Olbas Inhaler (Lane Health Products) A proprietary combination of *eucalyptus oil, *menthol, *cajuput oil, and *peppermint oil, used for the relief of blocked sinuses, colds and influenza, catarrh, and hay fever. It is freely available *over the counter in the form of a stick to be placed in the nostril before inhaling.

Olbas Oil (Lane Health Products) A proprietary combination of *eucalyptus oil, *menthol, *cajuput oil, *clove oil, *juniper berry oil, and oil of wintergreen (*methyl salicylate). It can be inhaled (from a handkerchief or dissolved in hot water) to relieve bronchial and nasal congestion due to colds, influenza, catarrh, and hay fever or applied topically to relieve muscular aches and pains or stiffness due to backache, sciatica, lumbago, or fibrositis. Olbas Oil is freely available *over the counter.

Precautions: Olbas Oil is not recommended for children under two years old.

Olbas Pastilles (Lane Health Products) A proprietary combination of *eucalyptus oil, *menthol, *peppermint oil, *clove oil, *juniper berry oil, and oil of wintergreen (*methyl salicylate), used for the relief of colds, coughs, catarrh, sore throats, influenza, nasal congestion, and catarrhal headaches. These pastilles are freely available *over the counter.

Precautions: Olbas Pastilles are not recommended for children under seven years old.

Olbetam (Pharmacia & Upjohn) *See* ACIPIMOX.

olsalazine sodium An *aminosalicylate used for the treatment of mild ulcerative colitis and to maintain patients in remission from it. It is available as capsules or tablets on *prescription only.
Side effects: include diarrhoea and joint pains; *see also* AMINOSALICYLATES.
Precautions: see AMINOSALICYLATES.
Proprietary preparation: Dipentum.

omega-3 marine triglycerides A preparation of fish oils that is rich in omega-3, a type of *triglyceride. It reduces plasma concentrations of triglycerides and is used in treating people with very high plasma triglyceride concentrations. It is available as capsules and can be obtained from pharmacies without a prescription.
Side effects: fish oils can cause occasional nausea and belching.
Precautions: fish oils should not be taken by people who have bleeding disorders.
Proprietary preparation: Maxepa.

omeprazole A *proton pump inhibitor used for the treatment of reflux oesophagitis, gastric and duodenal ulcers (including those associated with *Helicobacter pylori* infection and the use of *NSAIDs), Zollinger-Ellison syndrome, and other kinds of *acid-peptic disease. It is available as capsules on *prescription only.
Side effects: include nausea, headache, diarrhoea, constipation, dizziness, itching, rashes, allergic reactions, sensitivity of the skin to sunlight, and 'pins and needles'.
Precautions: see PROTON PUMP INHIBITORS.
Interactions with other drugs:
  Antifungal drugs: the absorption of ketoconazole and itraconazole may be reduced by omeprazole.
  Diazepam: its effects may be increased by omeprazole.
  Digoxin: its absorption is increased by omeprazole.
  Phenytoin: its effect is enhanced by omeprazole.
  Warfarin: its effect is enhanced by omeprazole.
Proprietary preparation: Losec.

Omnopon *See* PAPAVERETUM.

Oncovin (Eli Lilly & Co) *See* VINCRISTINE SULPHATE.

ondansetron An *antiemetic used for the prevention or treatment of nausea and vomiting associated with *cytotoxic chemotherapy or radiotherapy or occurring after surgery. It acts by opposing the action of the neurotransmitter 5-hydroxytryptamine (*serotonin) at receptors in the central nervous system and in the gut. It is available, on *prescription only, as tablets, suppositories, syrup, or an intravenous injection.

Side effects: include headache, constipation, a sense of flushing or warmth, and hiccups.

Precautions: ondansetron should be used with caution by people with liver disease and by women who are pregnant or breastfeeding.

Proprietary preparation: Zofran.

One Alpha (Leo Pharmaceuticals) *See* ALFACALCIDOL.

Opas (Co-Pharma) A proprietary combination of *sodium bicarbonate, *calcium carbonate, and *magnesium trisilicate, used as an antacid for the relief of indigestion (*see* ACID-PEPTIC DISEASES). It is freely available *over the counter in the form of tablets.

Side effects, precautions, and interactions with other drugs: see ANTACIDS; MAGNESIUM SALTS.

Opazimes (Co-Pharma) A proprietary combination of *kaolin (an adsorbent), *aluminium hydroxide (an antacid), *belladonna extract (an antispasmodic drug), and *morphine (which reduces gut motility), used for the treatment of diarrhoea and stomach upsets (*see* ANTIDIARRHOEAL DRUGS. It is available as chewable tablets and can be obtained without a prescription, but only from pharmacies.

Side effects, precautions, and interactions with other drugs: see MORPHINE; KAOLIN.

opiates *See* OPIOIDS.

Opilon (Parke-Davis Medical) *See* THYMOXAMINE <MOXISYLYTE>.

opioids A group of *analgesics that includes the **opiates** – naturally occurring compounds, such as morphine, found in the opium poppy (*Papaver somniferum*) and their derivatives – together with synthetic drugs that have similar effects. Opioids are extremely effective pain-killers, but people are often reluctant to use them because of fears of addiction and associations with illicit 'street drugs'. When taken repeatedly, opioids can cause *dependence, and *tolerance to their action may develop, so that increased doses are required to produce the same analgesic effect (see side effects and precautions below). However, when used in a clinical setting for the control of acute pain, there is little risk of opioids causing dependence.

Opioids are classified as **weak opioids** or **strong opioids**. Weak opioids, such as *codeine, *dextropropoxyphene, and *dihydrocodeine, are used for the treatment of mild to moderate pain. Strong opioids, which include morphine, *diamorphine, *dextromoramide, *fentanyl, and *phenazocine, are particularly useful in controlling severe pain, such as that associated with major surgery or advanced cancer. For chronic pain, treatment will often start with weak opioids (usually in combination with other analgesics) and then progress to strong opioids, either alone or in combination with other analgesics. The advantage of including other analgesics is to reduce the dosages and therefore the side effects of the opioids.

Some opioids are used to suppress coughing and to treat diarrhoea. Opioid *cough suppressants include codeine, *dextromethorphan, and *pholcodine (the last two have no analgesic activity). Opioids used as *antidiarrhoeal drugs include codeine, morphine, *loperamide hydrochloride, and **diphenoxylate hydrochloride** (combined with atropine in *co-phenotrope).

Because of their potential for abuse, many opioids are *controlled drugs, i.e. their prescription and use is strictly regulated.

Side effects and precautions: the most common side effects of opioids are nausea and vomiting, constipation, and drowsiness (which may affect driving ability and the performance of other skilled tasks. The effects of alcohol may be enhanced by opioids. People taking opioids should be warned that there may be withdrawal symptoms (including sweating, hallucinations, and strange dreams) when the drug is stopped, particularly if high dosages have been used. *See also* MORPHINE.

Interactions with other drugs: because the effects of opioids can be additive, opioids should not be used in combination with each other. Opioids enhance the sedative effects of anxiolytic drugs, hypnotics, and antipsychotics.

MAOIs: taking these antidepressants with opioids may have severe effects on blood pressure; opioids should therefore not be taken with MAOIs or for two weeks after stopping MAOIs.

Ritonavir: may increase the plasma concentration of opioids (and therefore may enhance their effects).

Details of specific interactions are listed at entries for individual opioids.

Oprisine (Trinity Pharmaceuticals) *See* AZATHIOPRINE.

Opticrom (Pantheon Healthcare) *See* SODIUM CROMOGLYCATE <CROMOGLICATE>.

Optilast (ASTA Medica) *See* AZELASTINE HYDROCHLORIDE.

Optimax (Merck Pharmaceuticals) *See* TRYPTOPHAN.

Optimine (Schering-Plough) *See* AZATADINE MALEATE.

Optrex (Crookes Healthcare) *See* HAMAMELIS.

Optrex Hayfever Allergy Eye Drops (Crookes Healthcare) *See* SODIUM CROMOGLYCATE <CROMOGLICATE>.

Opumide (Opus) *See* INDAPAMIDE HEMIHYDRATE.

Orabase (ConvaTec) A proprietary combination of *carmellose sodium (a protective agent) and pectin and gelatine (which thicken the preparation and encourage its adherence to the lining of the mouth). It is used to protect mouth sores and ulcers against abrasions and the action of saliva. Orabase is available as an ointment and can be obtained without a prescription, but only from pharmacies.

Oragard (Colgate-Palmolive) A proprietary combination of *cetylpyridinium chloride (an antiseptic) and *lignocaine <lidocaine> hydrochloride (a local anaesthetic), used to relieve the pain caused by mouth ulcers, ill-fitting dentures, and teething problems. It is freely available *over the counter in the form of a gel.

oral Taken by mouth. *Compare* PARENTERAL.

oral antidiabetic drugs *See* ORAL HYPOGLYCAEMIC DRUGS.

Oralbalance (Ethical Research Marketing) A proprietary combination of *xylitol (a sugar) and oxidase enzymes (to replace normal salivary enzymes), used as an artificial saliva for the relief of dry mouth, which occurs, for example, after radiotherapy. It is freely available *over the counter in the form of a gel.

oral contraceptives Tablets consisting of one or more synthetic female sex hormones taken by women to prevent pregnancy. Most oral contraceptives are **combined pills** (known colloquially as 'the pill'), consisting of an *oestrogen and a *progestogen, which suppress ovulation by, respectively, blocking the release of follicle-stimulating hormone and blocking the release of luteinizing hormone from the pituitary gland (*see* GONADOTROPHINS). Progestogens also alter the lining of the uterus and the viscosity of mucus in the cervix, so that conception is less likely. The oestrogens used in combined pills are *ethinyloestradiol <ethinylestradiol> and *mestranol (which is converted to ethinyloestradiol in the body); a variety of progestogens are used, including *desogestrel, *gestodene, *levonorgestrel, *norgestimate, and *norethisterone. **Biphasic** and **triphasic pills** are taken in two or three phases during the menstrual cycle. The tablets in each phase contain different amounts of oestrogen and progestogen to be taken on different days of the cycle; therefore the pills must be taken in the right order: packaging usually makes this a simple procedure. Phasic pills are designed to reduce the total amount of hormones taken, but still retain the same efficacy. Combined pills are usually taken for 21 days, with a gap of 7 days before starting the next cycle during which the 'period' occurs. Some combined pills, known as **everyday** (**ED**) **pills**, are packaged with placebo (dummy) pills for these 7 days so that a tablet is taken every day and thus the need to remember when to start the next pack is eliminated. It is best to take combined pills at the same time every day to maintain their efficacy. A pill that is taken more than 12 hours late is regarded as 'missed', and the normal cycle of pill taking should be resumed as soon as possible by taking the missed pill and continuing with the rest of the pack; in addition, extra contraception should be used for 7 days. If the 7 days of extra precautions run past the end of a pack, a new pack should be started immediately; i.e. without the usual 7-day gap in pill taking or without taking the 7 dummy pills in ED preparations. Most of the side effects of the pill (see below) are related to the oestrogen content. There is a small risk that blood clots may form in the veins, especially the deep veins of the legs (deep-vein *thrombosis), which may be carried in the bloodstream and block a blood vessel in another part of the body (thromboembolism), most often in the lungs. This risk is greater with some oral contraceptives than with others, depending on which progestogen is used in the preparation. However, the risk of a thromboembolism is actually higher during pregnancy.

Progestogen-only pills contain only a synthetic progestogen and no oestrogen. In some women these pills suppress ovulation completely; in others the normal menstrual cycle occurs. Because they cause fewer side effects than the combined pill, progestogen-only pills are more acceptable to some women, especially those who are breastfeeding, who have diabetes, who are at risk of developing thromboembolism (see precautions below), or who cannot take oestrogens. These pills should be taken every day of the cycle, at the same time each day – preferably several hours before intercourse. A pill should be regarded as missed if only 3 hours late, in which case the pills should be resumed as soon as possible and extra contraception should be used for the following week.

A combined pill containing high doses of an oestrogen and a progestogen is available for postcoital contraception – the so-called 'morning-after pill' (see SCHERING PC4). Oral contraceptives may also be given to regulate the menstrual cycle, to relieve very heavy or painful periods, and to treat premenstrual tension. They are available on *prescription only.

Side effects: with combined pills, these include breast enlargement, fluid retention with a bloated feeling, weight gain, cramps and pains in the legs, headache, nausea, vomiting, depression, loss of libido, vaginal discharge, skin changes (including brown patches on the face), and breakthrough bleeding. There may be changes in libido, depression, an increase in blood pressure, and irritation from contact lenses. The occurrence of a migraine-like headache for the first time, frequent severe headaches, or visual disturbance should be reported immediately to a doctor. For side effects of progestogen-only pills, *see* PROGESTOGENS.

Precautions: combined pills should not be used during breastfeeding or by women with a history of thrombosis, heart disease, or angina, sickle-cell anaemia, a history of jaundice during pregnancy or any liver disease, breast or genital cancer, or undiagnosed vaginal bleeding; they should not be taken during pregnancy and must be stopped if pregnancy occurs. Combined pills should be used with caution by women with high blood pressure, Raynaud's syndrome, diabetes, varicose veins, asthma, severe depression, or multiple sclerosis and by those on dialysis. The risk of thombosis is increased with age, smoking, and obesity. Breast examination should be carried out before and during treatment. For precautions with progestogen-only pills, *see* PROGESTOGENS.

Oral contraceptives

Proprietary preparation	Ingredients	Formulation (per 28-day pack)
Combined pills		
Brevinor	†ethinyloestradiol norethisterone	21 active tablets
Cilest	ethinyloestradiol norgestimate	21 active tablets
Eugynon 30	ethinyloestradiol levonorgestrel	21 active tablets
Femodene	ethinyloestradiol gestodene	21 active tablets
Femodene ED	ethinyloestradiol gestodene	21 active tablets + 7 dummy tablets
Loestrin 20	ethinyloestradiol (20 mcg) norethisterone	21 active tablets
Loestrin 30	ethinyloestradiol norethisterone	21 active tablets
Marvelon	ethinyloestradiol desogestrel	21 active tablets
Mercilon	ethinyloestradiol (20 mcg) desogestrel	21 active tablets
Microgynon 30	ethinyloestradiol levonorgestrel	21 active tablets
Microgynon 30 ED	ethinyloestradiol levonorgestrel	21 active tablets + 7 dummy tablets
Minulet	ethinyloestradiol gestodene	21 active tablets
Norimin	ethinyloestradiol norethisterone	21 active tablets
Norinyl-1	mestranol (50 mcg) norethisterone	21 active tablets
Ovran	ethinyloestradiol (50 mcg) levonorgestrel	21 active tablets
Ovran 30	ethinyloestradiol levonorgestrel	21 active tablets
Ovranette	ethinyloestradiol levonorgestrel	21 active tablets
Ovysmen	ethinyloestradiol norethisterone	21 active tablets
Phasic combined pills		
BiNovum	ethinyloestradiol norethisterone	2 phases (7 + 14) of active tablets
Logynon	ethinyloestradiol levonorgestrel	3 phases (6 + 5 + 10) of active tablets

Phasic combined pills (cont)

Logynon ED	ethinyloestradiol levonorgestrel	3 phases (6 + 5 + 10) of active tablets + 7 dummy tablets
Synphase	ethinyloestradiol norethisterone	3 phases (7 + 9 + 5) of active tablets
Triadene	ethinyloestradiol gestodene	3 phases (6 + 5 + 10) of active tablets
Tri-Minulet	ethinyloestradiol gestodene	3 phases (6 + 5 + 10) of active tablets
Trinordiol	ethinyloestradiol levonorgestrel	3 phases (6 + 5 + 10) of active tablets
TriNovum	ethinyloestradiol norethisterone	3 phases (7 + 7 + 7) of active tablets

Progestogen-only pills

Femulen	ethynodiol diacetate	28 active tablets
Micronor	norethisterone	28 active tablets
Microval	levonorgestrel	28 active tablets
Neogest	norgestrel	28 active tablets
Norgeston	levonorgestrel	28 active tablets
Noriday	norethisterone	28 active tablets

† doses of ethinyloestradiol/mestranol are 30–35 mcg (standard strength) except where otherwise stated

Interactions with other drugs (of combined pills):

ACE inhibitors: their effect in lowering blood pressure is reduced.

Antibiotics: ampicillin, tetracycline, rifabutin, and rifampicin reduce the contraceptive effect of combined pills. Additional contraception should be used while taking a short course of broad-spectrum antibiotics and for 7 days after stopping treatment; for women taking rifampicin, additional contraception should be continued for 4–8 weeks after stopping this drug. Women taking a longer course of these antibiotics are advised to use an oral contraceptive containing a higher dose (50 micrograms) of ethinyloestradiol <ethinylestradiol>; for women taking a longer course of rifampicin, an alternative method of contraception may be advised.

Anticoagulants: the effects of warfarin, nicoumalone <acenocoumarol>, and phenindione are antagonized.

Antiepileptic drugs: carbamazepine, phenobarbitone <phenobarbital>, phenytoin, primidone, and topiramate reduce the contraceptive effect of combined pills. Additional contraception should be used while taking a short course of these drugs and for 7 days after stopping treatment. Women taking a longer course of these drugs are advised to use an oral contraceptive containing a higher dose (50 micrograms) of ethinyloestradiol <ethinylestradiol>.

Antifungal drugs: griseofulvin, fluconazole, itraconazole, and ketoconazole can reduce the contraceptive effect of combined pills. Additional contraception should be used while taking a short course of these drugs and for 7 days after stopping treatment. Women taking a longer course of these drugs are advised to use an oral contraceptive containing a higher dose (50 micrograms) of ethinyloestradiol <ethinylestradiol>.

Antiviral drugs: reduce the contraceptive effect of combined pills.

Beta blockers: their effect in lowering blood pressure is reduced.

Cyclosporin: combined pills increase the plasma concentration (and therefore side effects) of cyclosporin.

Modafinil: reduces the contraceptive effect of combined pills.

Tretinoin: when taken orally, tretinoin may reduce the contraceptive effect of combined pills.

Proprietary preparations: see table (pp 451–452).

See also DEPOT CONTRACEPTIVES.

Oraldene (Warner-Lambert Consumer Healthcare) *See* HEXETIDINE.

oral hypoglycaemic drugs (oral antidiabetic drugs) Drugs that are taken by mouth to reduce the concentration of glucose (sugar) in the blood; they act in various ways. Oral hypoglycaemic drugs are usually prescribed for people with noninsulin-dependent (type II) *diabetes mellitus, in whom there is still some natural insulin production by the pancreas. The main oral hypoglycaemic drugs used are the *sulphonylureas and *metformin hydrochloride (a biguanide); *acarbose, *guar gum, and *repaglinide are also taken orally.

oral rehydration therapy (ORT) Solutions designed to replace fluids and *electrolytes lost in cases of dehydration, especially caused by diarrhoea. ORT solutions contain salts, such as *sodium chloride, *potassium chloride, *sodium citrate, and *sodium bicarbonate, together with glucose or other forms of carbohydrate, which enhance their absorption. ORT preparations are available as powders or effervescent tablets to be dissolved in water and taken by mouth; they can be obtained without a prescription, but only from pharmacies.

Proprietary preparations: DIOCALM REPLENISH (glucose, sodium chloride, sodium citrate, and potassium chloride); DIORALYTE NATURAL (glucose, sodium chloride, potassium chloride, and disodium hydrogen citrate); DIORALYTE RELIEF (sodium chloride, potassium chloride, sodium citrate, and precooked rice powder); DIORALYTE TABLETS (sodium bicarbonate, citric acid, glucose, sodium chloride, and potassium chloride); ELECTROLADE (sodium chloride, potassium chloride, sodium bicarbonate, and glucose); REHIDRAT (potassium chloride, sodium bicarbonate, citric acid, and sugars).

Oramorph, Oramorph SR (Boehringer Ingelheim) *See* MORPHINE.

Orap (Janssen-Cilag) *See* PIMOZIDE.

orciprenaline sulphate A *sympathomimetic drug that stimulates beta *adrenoceptors in the airways and – to a lesser extent – in the heart. It is used mainly as a *bronchodilator in the treatment of *asthma, bronchitis, and emphysema. Orciprenaline is available as tablets or a syrup on *prescription only.
Side effects: similar to those of *salbutamol, but orciprenaline is more likely to have adverse effects on the heart.
Precautions and interactions with other drugs: see SALBUTAMOL.
Proprietary preparation: Alupent.

Orelox (Hoechst Marion Roussel) *See* CEFPODOXIME.

Orgafol (Organon Laboratories) *See* UROFOLLITROPHIN <UROFOLLITROPIN>.

Orgaran (B & S Durbin) *See* DANAPAROID SODIUM.

Original Andrews Salts (SmithKline Beecham Consumer Healthcare) A proprietary combination of *sodium bicarbonate, *magnesium sulphate, and *citric acid, used as an *antacid for the relief of stomach upset and indigestion, and as a laxative. It is freely available *over the counter in the form of an effervescent powder.
Side effects and interactions with other drugs: see ANTACIDS.
Precautions: Andrews Salts are not recommended for children under three years old.

Orimeten (Novartis Pharmaceuticals) *See* AMINOGLUTETHIMIDE.

Orlept (CP Pharmaceuticals) *See* SODIUM VALPROATE.

orlistat A drug that inhibits pancreatic lipases, digestive enzymes that are secreted by the pancreas and break down dietary fat so that it can be absorbed. Orlistat acts in the stomach and small intestine to prevent the absorption of up to one-third of the dietary intake of fat. It is used in conjunction with a low-calorie diet in the treatment of *obesity, but it should only be taken by people who are clinically obese or by those who are severely overweight in whom obesity is causing medical problems, such as diabetes. People taking orlistat must demonstrate that they have previously been able to adhere to a low-calorie diet for a period of four weeks, which has resulted in a weight loss of 2.5 kg. Orlistat is available as capsules on *prescription only.
Side effects: include the frequent passage of copious liquid oily stools, flatulence, and stomach upset (all of which are less marked if fat intake is reduced), headache, menstrual irregularity, anxiety, and fatigue.
Precautions: orlistat should not be taken by women who are pregnant or breastfeeding, by people with obstructed bile ducts or other conditions in

which secretion of bile into the intestine is reduced, or by those in whom absorption from the intestine is reduced. Orlistat should be used with caution by people with diabetes.

Interactions with other drugs:

Antidiabetic drugs: acarbose and metformin should not be used with orlistat.

Clofibrate and related drugs: should not be taken with orlistat.

Pravastatin: its plasma concentration is increased by orlistat and therefore its dosage should be reduced.

Vitamin supplements: orlistat may impair the absorption of fat-soluble vitamins (A, D, E, and K), therefore multivitamin preparations should not be taken for at least two hours after taking orlistat.

Proprietary preparation: Xenical.

Orovite Complement B6 (Seton Scholl Healthcare) *See* PYRIDOXINE.

orphenadrine An *antimuscarinic drug that has pronounced skeletal *muscle relaxant properties. It is used for the treatment of Parkinson's disease and the reversal of drug-induced *extrapyramidal reactions (*see* ANTIPARKINSONIAN DRUGS) and also for the short-term relief of muscle spasm. A *prescription only medicine, it is available as tablets, a solution, or an elixir for oral use and as a solution for injection.

Side effects: include dry mouth, gastrointestinal disturbances, dizziness, and blurred vision; less common side effects are difficulty in urinating, slow heart rate, nervousness, euphoria, and insomnia. In high doses and in susceptible individuals, mental confusion, excitement, and psychiatric disturbances can occur.

Precautions and interactions with other drugs: *see* BENZHEXOL ⟨TRIHEXYPHENIDYL⟩ HYDROCHLORIDE.

Proprietary preparations: Biorphen; Disipal.

ORT *See* ORAL REHYDRATION THERAPY.

Ortho-Creme (Janssen-Cilag) *See* NONOXINOL-9.

Ortho Dienoestrol (Janssen-Cilag) *See* DIENOESTROL ⟨DIENESTROL⟩.

Orthoforms (Janssen-Cilag) *See* NONOXINOL-9.

Ortho-Gynest (Janssen-Cilag) *See* OESTRIOL ⟨ESTRIOL⟩.

Orudis (Rhône-Poulenc Rorer) *See* KETOPROFEN.

Oruvail (Rhône-Poulenc Rorer) *See* KETOPROFEN.

Osmolax (Ashbourne Pharmaceuticals) *See* LACTULOSE.

osmotic laxatives *Laxatives that act by retaining water in the colon (large bowel). Osmotic laxatives include magnesium salts (such as *magnesium hydroxide and *magnesium sulphate) and *lactulose, which are taken orally for the treatment of constipation; *phosphate laxatives, which are given as suppositories or enemas for constipation or for clearing the bowel before surgery or examination; and *sodium citrate, which is given rectally to treat constipation. *See also* BOWEL-CLEANSING SOLUTIONS.

Ossopan (Sanofi Winthrop) *See* HYDROXYAPATITE.

Ostram (Merck Pharmaceuticals) *See* CALCIUM PHOSPHATE.

OTC *See* OVER THE COUNTER.

Otex (DDD) *See* UREA HYDROGEN PEROXIDE.

Otomize (Stafford-Miller) A proprietary combination of *dexamethasone (a corticosteroid), *acetic acid, and *neomycin sulphate (an antibiotic), used for the treatment of inflammation and infections of the outer ear. It is available as a pump-action spray on *prescription only.
Side effects: there may be transient stinging or burning on application.
Precautions: Otomize should not be used on perforated eardrums or by pregnant women.

Otosporin (GlaxoWellcome) A proprietary combination of *polymyxin B sulphate and *neomycin sulphate (both antibiotics) and *hydrocortisone (a corticosteroid), used for the treatment of bacterial infections and inflammation of the outer ear. It is available as ear drops on *prescription only.
Side effects: a secondary infection may occur (*see* CORTICOSTEROIDS).
Precautions: long-term use of these drops in infants should be avoided. Otosporin should not be used by people with perforated eardrums or untreated viral, fungal, or tuberculous infections.

Otrivine (Novartis Consumer Health) *See* XYLOMETAZOLINE.

Otrivine-Antistin (CIBA Vision Ophthalmics) A proprietary combination of *xylometazoline (a sympathomimetic drug) and *antazoline sulphate (an antihistamine), used for the treatment of allergic conjunctivitis. It is available as eye drops without a prescription.
Side effects: include transient stinging, headache, drowsiness, blurred vision, and rebound congestion (*see* DECONGESTANTS).
Precautions: the drops should not to be used by people with acute glaucoma or by wearers of contact lenses.

over the counter Denoting or relating to drugs that can be obtained without a *prescription. There are two legal categories of such drugs: those that can only be bought from a pharmacy when a registered pharmacist is present – these pharmacy medicines are designated P; and those that can be bought from the self-service displays of pharmacies or from any other retail outlet, designated GSL (general sales list). For some OTC drugs there may be a restriction on the quantity that can be purchased from a GSL outlet or at one time. The term 'over the counter' can be applied to either P drugs or GSL drugs, although it is more properly restricted to GSL items (in this dictionary described as "freely available over the counter"). Some drugs may be classified as GSL or P at low doses, but as POM (*prescription only medicine) at higher doses. A medical practitioner can prescribe OTC medicines, although some are restricted and cannot be prescribed at NHS expense.

Ovestin (Organon Laboratories) *See* OESTRIOL <ESTRIOL>.

Ovex (Johnson & Johnson) *See* MEBENDAZOLE.

Ovran (Wyeth Laboratories) A proprietary combination of *ethinyloestradiol <ethinylestradiol> and *levonorgestrel used as an *oral contraceptive. **Ovran 30** contains a lower dose (30 micrograms) of ethinyloestradiol <ethinylestradiol>. Both preparations are available as tablets on *prescription only.
Side effects, precautions, and interactions with other drugs: see ORAL CONTRACEPTIVES.

Ovranette (Wyeth Laboratories) A proprietary combination of *ethinyloestradiol <ethinylestradiol> and *levonorgestrel used as an *oral contraceptive. It is available as tablets on *prescription only.
Side effects, precautions, and interactions with other drugs: see ORAL CONTRACEPTIVES.

Ovysmen (Janssen-Cilag) A proprietary combination of *ethinyloestradiol <ethinylestradiol> and *norethisterone used as an *oral contraceptive. It is available as tablets on *prescription only.
Side effects, precautions, and interactions with other drugs: see ORAL CONTRACEPTIVES.

oxazepam A short-acting *benzodiazepine used for short-term treatment of anxiety. It is available as tablets on *prescription only.
Side effects and precautions: see DIAZEPAM; BENZODIAZEPINES.
Interactions with other drugs: see BENZODIAZEPINES.

OxBipp, **OxBipp-G** (Aurum Pharmaceuticals; Oxford Pharmaceuticals) *See* BISMUTH SUBNITRATE AND IODOFORM.

oxerutins Naturally occurring compounds used for the relief of heavy aching legs, night cramp, and other symptoms associated with poor circulation, although their value is not proven. They are available as capsules and can be obtained without a prescription, but only from pharmacies.

Side effects: include gastrointestinal upset, flushes, and headache.

Proprietary preparation: Paroven.

oxethazaine <oxetacaine> *See* MUCAINE.

Oxis Turbohaler (AstraZeneca) *See* EFORMOTEROL <FORMOTEROL> FUMARATE.

oxitropium bromide An *antimuscarinic drug used as a *bronchodilator for the treatment of *asthma and conditions associated with chronic obstruction of the airways. It is available as a metered-dose or breath-activated aerosol *inhaler on *prescription only.

Side effects: see ANTIMUSCARINIC DRUGS. There may also be local irritation and nausea.

Precautions: oxitropium should not be used by people who are sensitive to atropine or ipratropium bromide or by women who are pregnant or breastfeeding. It is not recommended for children, and should be used with caution by individuals with glaucoma or an enlarged prostate gland. The drug should be discontinued if wheeze or cough occurs.

Proprietary preparations: Oxivent; Oxivent Autohaler.

Oxivent (Boehringer Ingelheim) *See* OXITROPIUM BROMIDE.

oxpentifylline <pentoxifylline> A *xanthine used in the treatment of peripheral vascular disease, such as Raynaud's syndrome. It is available as *modified-release tablets on *prescription only.

Side effects: include gastrointestinal disturbances, dizziness, and headache. *See also* XANTHINES.

Precautions: oxpentifylline should not be taken by people with the acute porphyrias. *See also* XANTHINES.

Interactions with other drugs:

Ketorolac: may increase the risk of gastrointestinal bleeding.

See also XANTHINES.

Proprietary preparation: Trental.

oxprenolol hydrochloride A *beta blocker used to treat *angina, *arrhythmias, and anxiety. It is also used as a *modified-release formulation for the treatment of *hypertension. It is available as tablets, capsules, or modified-release tablets on *prescription only.

Side effects, precautions, and interactions with other drugs: see BETA BLOCKERS.

Proprietary preparations: Trasicor; Slow-Trasicor (modified-release tablets); TRASIDREX (combined with cyclopenthiazide).

See also ANTIHYPERTENSIVE DRUGS; ANTI-ARRHYTHMIC DRUGS.

Oxy (SmithKline Beecham Consumer Healthcare) *See* BENZOYL PEROXIDE.

oxybuprocaine *See* LOCAL ANAESTHETICS.

oxybutynin hydrochloride An *antimuscarinic drug used to treat abnormal frequency and urgency in passing urine, urinary incontinence, and bedwetting. It acts by reducing instability in the muscle of the bladder wall. However, oxybutynin has a high level of side effects, which limits its usefulness, and the dosage must be carefully assessed in older people. It is available as tablets or an *elixir on *prescription only.
Side effects: include dry mouth, constipation, blurred vision, nausea, abdominal discomfort, flushing (more marked in children), difficulty in passing urine, headache, dizziness, drowsiness, dry skin, rash, increased sensitivity to sunlight, diarrhoea, restlessness, disorientation, hallucination, and convulsions. Children are more susceptible to the disorientating or hallucinatory effects of oxybutynin.
Precautions: oxybutynin should not be taken by people with obstruction of the gut, severe ulcerative colitis, or glaucoma, or by people in whom the outlet of the bladder is obstructed (for example, by an enlarged prostate gland). It should be used with caution in frail elderly people, in people with liver or kidney disease, some types of heart disease, or an overactive thyroid gland, and in women who are pregnant or breastfeeding.
Interactions with other drugs: see ANTIMUSCARINIC DRUGS.
Proprietary preparations: Contimin; Cystrin; Ditropan (tablets or elixir).

oxycodone An *opioid analgesic that is used for the relief of pain in patients who are terminally ill. A *controlled drug, it is available as suppositories.
Side effects and precautions: see MORPHINE; OPIOIDS.
Interactions with other drugs: see OPIOIDS.

oxymetazoline A *sympathomimetic drug that constricts blood vessels and is used as a nasal *decongestant. It is available as a nasal spray without a prescription.
Side effects, precautions, and interactions with other drugs: see XYLOMETAZOLINE; DECONGESTANTS.
Proprietary preparations: Afrazine; Dristan Nasal Spray; Sudafed Nasal Spray; VICKS SINEX (combined with menthol and eucalyptol).

oxymetholone *See* ANABOLIC STEROIDS.

Oxymycin (DDSA Pharmaceuticals) *See* OXYTETRACYCLINE.

oxypertine An *antipsychotic drug used for the treatment of schizophrenia and other psychotic illnesses and mania. It is available as tablets or capsules on *prescription only.
Side effects: similar to those of *chlorpromazine, but extrapyramidal

reactions (such as abnormal face and body movements) occur less frequently; agitation may develop with low doses, and sedation with high doses.

Precautions: *see* CHLORPROMAZINE HYDROCHLORIDE.

Interactions with other drugs:

Anaesthetics: their effect in lowering blood pressure is increased.

Antidepressants: there is an increased risk of antimuscarinic effects and arrhythmias if oxypertine is taken with tricyclic antidepressants; stimulation of the central nervous system and high blood pressure occur if oxypertine is taken with MAOIs.

Antiepileptic drugs: oxypertine antagonizes the effects of these drugs in controlling seizures.

Antihistamines: there is an increased risk of arrhythmias if oxypertine is taken with astemizole or terfenadine.

Halofantrine: there is an increased risk of arrhythmias if this drug is taken with oxypertine.

Ritonavir: may increase the effects of oxypertine.

Sedatives: the sedative effects of oxypertine are increased if it is taken with anxiolytic or hypnotic drugs, or any other drug that causes sedation.

oxyphenisatin <oxyphenisatine> A *stimulant laxative used to evacuate the bowel before diagnostic procedures or surgery. It is available as a powder to be dissolved for use as an enema and can be obtained without a prescription, but only from pharmacies.

Side effects and precautions: *see* STIMULANT LAXATIVES.

Proprietary preparation: Veripaque.

oxytetracycline A tetracycline antibiotic used for the treatment of chronic bronchitis, brucellosis, chlamydial infections, and infections caused by mycoplasmas and rickettsias (*see* TETRACYCLINES). It is also used to treat mouth ulcers and *acne. It is available, on *prescription only, as tablets or capsules.

Side effects and interactions with other drugs: *see* TETRACYCLINES.

Precautions: *see* TETRACYCLINES. In addition, oxytetracycline should not to be taken by people with porphyria.

Proprietary preparations: Berkmycin (tablets); Oxymycin (tablets); Oxytetramix (tablets); Terramycin (capsules); TERRA-CORTRIL (combined with hydrocortisone).

Oxytetramix (Ashbourne Pharmaceuticals) *See* OXYTETRACYCLINE.

oxytocin A hormone produced by the pituitary gland that causes contractions of the uterus during labour and also stimulates milk production in nursing mothers. It is used therapeutically to induce labour and to prevent or treat bleeding from the uterus after childbirth. Since high doses may overstimulate the uterus, posing a threat to the fetus, oxytocin should only be used to induce labour under medical supervision. It may also be used in certain cases to assist abortion. Oxytocin is available, on *prescription only, as a solution for slow intravenous infusion; it is usually used only in hospitals.

Side effects: include spasm of the uterus, nausea, vomiting, irregular heart rhythms, and rashes or other allergic reactions.

Precautions: oxytocin should not be used when there is any mechanical obstruction to delivery or when a vaginal delivery is not appropriate. It should be used with caution in women who are over 35 years old or who have had a previous Caesarean section.

Interactions with other drugs:

Anaesthetics: may possibly reduce the effect of oxytocin.

Prostaglandins: enhance the effect of oxytocin.

Vasoconstrictor sympathomimetic drugs: their effects in constricting blood vessels and increasing blood pressure are enhanced.

Proprietary preparations: Syntocinon; SYNTOMETRINE (combined with ergometrine maleate).

P

P (pharmacy medicine) *See* OVER THE COUNTER.

Pabrinex (Link Pharmaceuticals) A proprietary combination of *thiamine hydrochloride, *nicotinamide, *pyridoxine hydrochloride, and *riboflavine (all of which are B vitamins) and ascorbic acid (*see* VITAMIN C), used for the treatment of severe vitamin B deficiency states, such as those caused by alcoholism or occurring after acute infections, surgery, or in some psychiatric conditions. It may also be needed by people undergoing kidney dialysis. Pabrinex is available as an intramuscular or intravenous injection on *prescription only.
Side effects and precautions: since severe allergic reactions can occur during or after injection, Pabrinex should be reserved for those patients unable to take the vitamins by mouth. When given intravenously, the injection should be slow (over 10 minutes).

Pacifene, Pacifene Maximum Strength (Sussex Pharmaceutical) *See* IBUPROFEN.

paclitaxel A *taxane that is used in conjunction with *cisplatin for the treatment of primary ovarian *cancer; it is used alone for treating ovarian cancer that has spread to other parts of the body and has not responded to platinum-containing drugs. It is also used for treating advanced breast cancer when standard therapy has failed. Paclitaxel may cause severe allergic reactions: drugs to prevent this, including *corticosteroids and *antihistamines, are therefore usually given before treatment starts. Paclitaxel is available as a solution for intravenous infusion on *prescription only.
Side effects: include severe allergic reactions (see above), a fall in blood pressure, slowing of heart rate, *bone marrow suppression, hair loss, muscle pain, nerve damage, nausea, and vomiting. *See also* CYTOTOXIC DRUGS.
Precautions: paclitaxel should not be given to pregnant women or people with severe liver disease. *See also* CYTOTOXIC DRUGS.
Interactions with other drugs:
  Ketoconazole: may enhance the effect of paclitaxel.
Proprietary preparation: Taxol.

paint A liquid preparation that is applied to the skin or mucous membranes. Paints usually contain antiseptics, astringents, caustics, or analgesics.

Paldesic (Rosemont Pharmaceuticals) *See* PARACETAMOL.

Palfium (Roche Products) *See* DEXTROMORAMIDE.

Palladone, **Palladone SR** (Napp Pharmaceuticals) *See* HYDROMORPHONE HYDROCHLORIDE.

Paludrine (AstraZeneca) *See* PROGUANIL HYDROCHLORIDE.

Paludrine/Avloclor (AstraZeneca) A proprietary preparation consisting of 14 tablets of *chloroquine phosphate packaged with 98 tablets of *proguanil hydrochloride (the recommended dosages), used for the prevention of malaria. It is available without a prescription, but only from pharmacies.
Side effects, precautions, and interactions with other drugs: see CHLOROQUINE; PROGUANIL HYDROCHLORIDE.

Pamergan P100 (Martindale Pharmaceuticals) *See* PETHIDINE HYDROCHLORIDE.

pamidronate disodium *See* DISODIUM PAMIDRONATE.

Panadeine (SmithKline Beecham Consumer Healthcare) *See* CO-CODAMOL.

Panadol (SmithKline Beecham Consumer Healthcare) *See* PARACETAMOL.

Panadol Extra (SmithKline Beecham Consumer Healthcare) A proprietary combination of *paracetamol (an analgesic and antipyretic) and *caffeine (a stimulant), used for the relief of headache (including migraine), toothache, neuralgia, rheumatic pain, backache, period pains, and the symptoms of influenza and colds. It is available as tablets or soluble tablets and can be obtained without a prescription, but larger packs are only available from pharmacies.
Precautions: Panadol Extra should not be given to children, except on medical advice. *See also* PARACETAMOL; CAFFEINE.

Panadol Night (SmithKline Beecham Consumer Healthcare) A proprietary combination of *paracetamol (an analgesic) and *diphenhydramine (a sedative antihistamine), used for the short-term treatment of pains that are disturbing sleep, such as rheumatic and muscle pain, backache, neuralgia, toothache, migraine, and period pains. It is available as tablets and can be obtained without a prescription, but only from pharmacies.
Side effects: see ANTIHISTAMINES.
Precautions: Panadol Night should not be taken for more than seven consecutive nights without medical advice; it is not recommended for children except on medical advice. *See also* PARACETAMOL; ANTIHISTAMINES.
Interactions with other drugs: see ANTIHISTAMINES.

Panadol Ultra (SmithKline Beecham Consumer Healthcare) A proprietary combination of *paracetamol (a non-opioid analgesic) and *codeine (an opioid analgesic), used for the relief of rheumatic pains, sciatica, lumbago, strains and sprains, neuralgia, and migraine. It is available as tablets and can be obtained without a prescription, but only from pharmacies.

Side effects: see CODEINE.

Precautions: Panadol Ultra should not be given to children under 12 years old. *See also* PARACETAMOL.

Interactions with other drugs: see OPIOIDS.

Pancrease, Pancrease HL (Janssen-Cilag) *See* PANCREATIN.

pancreatin An extract of the pancreas (usually obtained from pigs) that contains the pancreatic enzymes amylase, lipase, and protease, which aid the digestion and absorption of starch, fat, and protein. Pancreatin is used as replacement therapy when the body's natural pancreatic enzymes are lacking. A lack of enzymes may be due to inherited conditions, such as cystic fibrosis, or disease, such as chronic pancreatitis, or it may occur following surgical removal of the pancreas. Pancreatin should be taken before or with meals and the dosage adjusted according to absorption of food – judged by the size, number, and consistency of stools and lack of diarrhoea. Preparations should be swallowed without chewing; if they are mixed with food, the food should not be too hot, since the enzymes may be inactivated. Pancreatin is available as granules, capsules, tablets, or powder; some preparations are *enteric-coated, which enables a higher concentration of enzymes to reach the duodenum. Pancreatin preparations of standard strength can be obtained from pharmacies without a prescription; higher-strength preparations are *prescription only medicines.

Side effects: include nausea, vomiting, and abdominal discomfort. Irritation of the mouth or anal region can occur if the enzymes are taken without food or are used in excessive dosage.

Precautions: a high intake of fluids must be maintained, particularly in those taking higher-strength preparations. Individuals taking high dosages should report unusual abdominal symptoms to a doctor.

Proprietary preparations: Creon; Creon 10 000; Creon 25 000 (high-strength); Nutrizyme GR; Nutrizyme 10; Nutrizyme 22 (high-strength); Pancrease; Pancrease HL (high-strength); Pancrex; Pancrex V.

Pancrex, Pancrex V (Paines & Byrne) *See* PANCREATIN.

PanOxyl (Stiefel Laboratories) *See* BENZOYL PEROXIDE.

panthenol *See* VITAMIN B COMPLEX.

pantoprazole A *proton pump inhibitor used for the treatment of duodenal or gastric ulcers and moderate to severe reflux oesophagitis (*see*

ACID-PEPTIC DISEASES). It is available, on *prescription only, as *enteric-coated tablets or an injection.

Side effects: include headache, diarrhoea, rashes, itching, dizziness, nausea and vomiting, and constipation.

Precautions: see PROTON PUMP INHIBITORS.

Proprietary preparation: Protium.

pantothenic acid *See* VITAMIN B COMPLEX.

papaveretum An *opioid analgesic consisting of a mixture of *morphine hydrochloride, *papaverine hydrochloride, and *codeine hydrochloride in fixed amounts. It is used for the treatment of pain following surgery and also as part of premedication for the control of existing pain before surgery. Papaveretum was formerly known by the proprietary name **Omnopon**. A combination of papaveretum and *hyoscine hydrobromide is also used in premedication. Both preparations are available as injections; they are *controlled drugs.

Side effects and precautions: see MORPHINE; OPIOIDS.

Interactions with other drugs: see OPIOIDS.

Proprietary preparation: ASPAV (combined with aspirin).

papaverine An alkaloid, derived from opium, that relaxes smooth muscle. It is an ingredient of *papaveretum. Alone, papaverine is used in the treatment of impotence, being injected directly into the penis to achieve an erection, although it does not have a *licence for this purpose. Papaverine is available as a solution for injection on *prescription only.

Side effects and precautions: there may be a burning pain and bruising at the injection site. An erection that lasts for longer than four hours is a medical emergency and requires prompt treatment (by withdrawing blood from the penis followed, if necessary, by injections of phenylephrine or adrenaline <epinephrine>).

Papulex (Bioglan Laboratories) *See* NICOTINAMIDE.

paracetamol A drug that relieves pain (*see* ANALGESICS) and also reduces fever (but has no anti-inflammatory activity). Paracetamol provides effective relief of mild to moderate pain, including headache, toothache, period pains, backache, and rheumatic pains, and is useful for reducing high temperatures in colds, influenza, and other feverish conditions. Unlike *aspirin, it does not irritate the stomach lining and is preferred to aspirin for elderly people and young children (under 12 years old). Paracetamol is available as tablets, soluble tablets, capsules, solutions, and suppositories; there are also suspensions and solutions specially formulated for babies and young children, often as flavoured sugar-free syrups. Paracetamol can be obtained without a prescription, but because it can have serious effects in overdosage (see below) there are restrictions on the quantities of tablets or capsules that can be supplied. Packs containing 16 tablets or capsules are freely available *over the counter; packs containing up to 32 (or exceptionally up to 100) tablets or capsules can only be obtained from pharmacies. Larger quantities are available on *prescription only. Paracetamol is combined with aspirin, codeine, or other ingredients in a variety of compound analgesic preparations and cold remedies. *See also* BENORYLATE; CO-CODAMOL; CO-DYDRAMOL; CO-PROXAMOL.

Side effects and precautions: side effects of recommended doses (up to 8 tablets/capsules a day in adults) are rare, but rashes or other allergic reactions may rarely occur; pancreatitis has been reported after prolonged use. In higher than recommended doses paracetamol causes liver damage, which may not be apparent for two days or more and can be fatal unless treated immediately with the antidote (methionine or acetylcysteine). For this reason it is important not to mix preparations containing paracetamol, in case the recommended dose is accidentally exceeded, and paracetamol should be taken with caution by people with liver disease. One proprietary preparation (*Paradote) contains paracetamol in combination with methionine in an attempt to avoid the problems of overdosage.

Proprietary preparations: Alvedon; Anadin Paracetamol; Boots Children's Pain Relief Syrup; Boots Cold Relief Hot Blackcurrant, Hot Lemon; Boots Infant Pain Relief; Calpol; Disprol; Fanalgic; Fennings Children's Cooling Powders; Hedex Caplets; Infadrops; Medinol; Miradol; Numark Cold Relief Powders; Paldesic; Panadol; Panadol Soluble; Paracets; Paraclear; Paramin; Placidex; Resolve; Salzone; Tramil 500. For details of these and other preparations of which paracetamol is an ingredient, see Appendix.

Paracets (Sussex Pharmaceutical) *See* PARACETAMOL.

Paraclear (Roche Products) *See* PARACETAMOL.

Paraclear Extra Strength (Roche Products) A proprietary combination of *paracetamol (an analgesic) and *caffeine (a stimulant), used for the relief of minor aches and pains. It is freely available *over the counter in the form of soluble tablets.
Precautions: these tablets are not recommended for children under 12 years old. *See also* PARACETAMOL; CAFFEINE.

Paracodol (Roche Products) *See* CO-CODAMOL.

Paradote (Penn Pharmaceuticals) A proprietary combination of *paracetamol (an analgesic and antipyretic) and methionine (its antidote); this mixture is called **co-methiamol**. Paradote is used to relieve pain and reduce fever; the methionine is included in an attempt to prevent liver damage caused by overdosage of paracetamol. It is available as tablets without a prescription, but only from pharmacies.
Side effects and precautions: see PARACETAMOL.

Parake (Galen) *See* CO-CODAMOL.

paraldehyde An *anticonvulsant drug used to treat status epilepticus, a medical emergency in which epileptic seizures occur repeatedly without the person recovering consciousness between them. Paraldehyde is available on *prescription only; it is given by intramuscular injection or as an enema.

Side effects: paraldehyde may cause rashes. There may be pain and abscess formation after injection; the enema may irritate the rectum.

Precautions: paraldehyde should be used with caution in people with disease of the airways or lungs.

Paramax (Lorex Synthélabo) A proprietary combination of *paracetamol (an analgesic) and *metoclopramide (an antiemetic), used for the relief of migraine. It is available as tablets or effervescent powder on *prescription only.

Side effects, precautions, and interactions with other drugs: see PARACETAMOL; METOCLOPRAMIDE.

Paramin (The Wallis Laboratory) *See* PARACETAMOL.

Paramol (Seton Scholl Healthcare) A proprietary combination of *paracetamol (an analgesic and antipyretic) and *dihydrocodeine (an opioid analgesic), used for the relief of headache, migraine, fevers, period pains, toothache, backache, and other muscular aches and pains. It is available as tablets and can be obtained without a prescription, but only from pharmacies.

Side effects: see MORPHINE.

Precautions: Paramol is not recommended for children. *See also* PARACETAMOL; MORPHINE.

Interactions with other drugs: see OPIOIDS.

Paraplatin (Bristol-Myers Squibb) *See* CARBOPLATIN.

parasympathetic nervous system A part of the nervous system that works in conjunction with another series of nerves (the *sympathetic nervous system) to control certain functions of the heart, lungs, intestines and pancreas, salivary glands, bladder, and genitalia. In general, the actions of the parasympathetic nervous system oppose those of the sympathetic nervous system. Both the parasympathetic and sympathetic nervous systems function automatically – we are not aware of their actions and have no voluntary control over them.

The substance that relays information in the parasympathetic nervous system is *acetylcholine, which acts on very small specialized areas of the cells of the target tissues called receptors. Many drugs act on the parasympathetic nervous system, either by mimicking the actions of acetylcholine (*see* CHOLINERGIC DRUGS) or by opposing them (*see* ANTIMUSCARINIC DRUGS).

parasympathomimetic drugs *See* CHOLINERGIC DRUGS.

parathyroid hormone (parathormone) A hormone that is synthesized and released by the parathyroid glands, situated at the base of the neck behind the thyroid gland, in response to low concentrations of *calcium in the blood. It acts in opposition to *calcitonin to control the distribution of calcium and phosphate in the body. Parathyroid hormone promotes the transfer of calcium from the bones to the blood; it also converts *vitamin D to its active form, which increases absorption of calcium from the intestine. A deficiency of parathyroid hormone results in reduced concentrations of calcium in the blood, causing tetany (spasm and twitching of the muscles). This condition may be treated with forms of vitamin D.

Pardelprin (Cox Pharmaceuticals) *See* INDOMETHACIN <INDOMETACIN>.

parenteral Introduced into the body by any way other than through the mouth. The term is applied, for example, to administration of drugs by injection.

Pariet (Janssen-Cilag) *See* RABEPRAZOLE SODIUM.

Parkinson's disease *See* ANTIPARKINSONIAN DRUGS.

Parlodel (Novartis Pharmaceuticals) *See* BROMOCRIPTINE.

Parmid (Lagap Pharmaceuticals) *See* METOCLOPRAMIDE.

Parnate (SmithKline Beecham Pharmaceuticals) *See* TRANYLCYPROMINE.

Paroven (Novartis Consumer Health) *See* OXERUTINS.

paroxetine An *antidepressant drug of the *SSRI group. It is used for the treatment of depressive illness, obsessive-compulsive disorder, panic disorder, and agoraphobia. Paroxetine is available as tablets or liquid on *prescription only.
Side effects: see SSRIS.
Precautions: see SSRIS. In addition, dosage of this drug should be reduced gradually at the end of treatment.
Interactions with other drugs:
  Phenytoin: reduces the plasma concentration of paroxetine.
  Sertindole: its plasma concentration is increased by paroxetine.
  Terfenadine: there is an increased risk of *arrhythmias and paroxetine should not be taken with terfenadine.
  See also SSRIS.
Proprietary preparation: Seroxat.

Parstelin (SmithKline Beecham Pharmaceuticals) A proprietary combination of *tranylcypromine (a monoamine oxidase inhibitor) and

*trifluoperazine (an antipsychotic drug), used for the treatment of depression with anxiety. It is available as tablets on *prescription only.
Side effects: see MONOAMINE OXIDASE INHIBITORS; TRIFLUOPERAZINE.
Precautions and interactions with other drugs: see MONOAMINE OXIDASE INHIBITORS; CHLORPROMAZINE HYDROCHLORIDE.

Partobulin (Baxter Healthcare) *See* ANTI-D (RH$_0$) IMMUNOGLOBULIN.

Parvolex (Medeva) *See* ACETYLCYSTEINE.

paste A medicinal preparation of a thick and stiff consistency, which is applied to the skin. It contains a high proportion of insoluble powder (e.g. zinc oxide or starch) in an *ointment base.

pastille A medicinal tablet that contains gelatine and glycerin (and is therefore soft); it is usually coated with sugar. Pastilles should be sucked, so that the medication is applied to the mouth and throat.

Pavacol D (Boehringer Ingelheim) *See* PHOLCODINE.

peanut oil *See* ARACHIS OIL.

pediculicides *See* LICE.

Penbritin (SmithKline Beecham Pharmaceuticals) *See* AMPICILLIN.

penciclovir A nucleoside analogue (*see* ANTIVIRAL DRUGS) used for the treatment of cold sores. It is available as a cream on *prescription only.
Side effects: there may be transient burning or stinging.
Precautions: penciclovir should be used with caution by those whose immune systems are functioning poorly (due to disease or drug therapy) and by women who are pregnant or breastfeeding. The cream should not come into contact with the eyes or mucous membranes.
Proprietary preparation: Vectavir.

Pendramine (ASTA Medica) *See* PENICILLAMINE.

penicillamine A drug used for the treatment of active progressive rheumatoid arthritis and having similar actions to gold (*see* SODIUM AUROTHIOMALATE). Side effects are frequent, which may restrict its use. It must be started at a low dosage, which is gradually increased over months; improvement may not be seen for 6–12 weeks after treatment starts. Penicillamine is also used for the treatment of Wilson's disease (in which copper accumulates in the body), copper or lead poisoning, chronic active hepatitis, and cystinuria (a kidney disease). It is available as tablets on *prescription only.
Side effects: include nausea at the start of treatment, which resolves with

further use; loss of appetite and taste; and fever, rash, and bloody or cloudy urine (which should all be reported to a doctor).

Precautions and interactions with other drugs: blood counts must be performed in the early stages of treatment. Concurrent treatment with gold, chloroquine, hydroxychloroquine, or immunosuppressants should be avoided. Penicillamine should be used with caution in people with kidney disease and in women who are pregnant or breastfeeding.

Proprietary preparations: Distamine; Pendramine.

penicillins A group of bactericidal beta-lactam *antibiotics that act by interfering with bacterial cell wall synthesis. They penetrate well into most body tissues and fluids, but do not enter the cerebrospinal fluid (surrounding the brain and spinal cord) unless there is inflammation of cerebrospinal tissues. The drug *probenecid is very occasionally given with some penicillins to prevent their excretion by the kidneys and thus raise the concentration of penicillins retained in the body. Some penicillins are broken down by enzymes called beta-lactamases (or penicillinases), which are produced by some types of bacteria, so they are sometimes given with *clavulanic acid or *tazobactam, which inhibit these enzymes; alternatively, penicillinase-resistant penicillins must be used. The ability of a drug to resist attack by these enzymes is an important factor in determining which drug is effective against specific types of bacteria.

The most important side effect of penicillins is hypersensitivity (allergy), which can cause rashes and occasionally an extreme and potentially fatal allergic reaction (*see* ANAPHYLAXIS). If an individual is allergic to one type of penicillin he or she will be allergic to all penicillins. It is important, therefore, that anyone with known sensitivity always tells a doctor who is prescribing antibiotics. Otherwise penicillins are relatively free from severe side effects, but they may cause diarrhoea. Penicillins are classified according to their spectrum of antibacterial activity; for example **broad-spectrum penicillins** are active against a wide range of bacteria.

See AMOXYCILLIN <AMOXICILLIN>; AMPICILLIN; AZLOCILLIN; BENZYLPENICILLIN (PENCILLIN G); CO-AMOXICLAV; CO-FLUAMPICIL; FLUCLOXACILLIN; PHENOXYMETHYLPENICILLIN (PENICILLIN V); PIPERACILLIN; PROCAINE PENICILLIN <PROCAINE BENZYLPENICILLIN>; TICARCILLIN.

Pentacarinat (JHC Healthcare) *See* PENTAMIDINE ISETHIONATE <ISETIONATE>.

pentaerythritol tetranitrate <pentaerithrityl tetranitrate> A *nitrate drug used to prevent angina. It is available as tablets and can be obtained without a prescription, but only from pharmacies.

Side effects, precautions, and interactions with other drugs: *see* NITRATES.

Proprietary preparation: Mycardol.

pentamidine isethionate <pentamidine isetionate> A drug used for the treatment of pneumonia caused by *Pneumocystis carinii*, especially in people who cannot tolerate, or have not responded to, *co-trimoxazole. Pentamidine has also been used for treating certain other serious infections, such as leishmaniasis. It has the potential for causing severe side effects, including a dangerous fall in blood pressure (see below), and should therefore only be used by specialists. Pentamidine is available, on *prescription only, as a form for injection or as a solution to be used in a *nebulizer.

Side effects: when given by injection pentamidine can have serious side effects, including severe hypotension (low blood pressure), low blood glucose (*see* HYPOGLYCAEMIA), *arrhythmias, and reduced numbers of white blood cells and platelets. Other side effects include nausea, vomiting, dizziness, fainting, flushing, rash, taste disturbances, and pain or other reactions at the injection site. If given by inhalation side effects are reduced because less of the drug is absorbed, but there may be constriction of the airways, cough, wheezing, and shortness of breath.

Precautions: pentamidine should be used with caution in women who are pregnant or breastfeeding and in people with high or low blood pressure, high or low blood sugar, or blood disorders.

Interactions with other drugs: pentamidine should not be given to patients who are taking amiodarone, cisapride, or terfenadine, since these drugs increase the risk of arrhythmias occurring.

Proprietary preparation: Pentacarinat.

Pentasa (Ferring Pharmaceuticals) *See* MESALAZINE.

pentazocine An *opioid analgesic used for the treatment of moderate to severe pain. When injected, it is more potent than dihydrocodeine or codeine but has additional side effects and is not suitable for some patients (see below). Pentazocine is a *controlled drug; it is available as tablets, capsules, an injection, or suppositories.

Side effects: see MORPHINE. In addition, it may cause hallucinations.

Precautions: pentazocine should not be given to patients who are regularly taking other opioids, since it antagonizes their action and can cause withdrawal symptoms; it should not be used in people who have had a heart attack or who have heart failure. *See also* MORPHINE.

Interactions with other drugs: see OPIOIDS.

Proprietary preparations: Fortral; FORTAGESIC (combined with paracetamol).

pentostatin A *cytotoxic drug that is highly effective in the treatment of hairy cell leukaemia (*see* CANCER). It is available as an injection on *prescription only and is most usually used in specialist centres.

Side effects: include *bone marrow suppression and decreased activity of the immune system, which reduces the body's resistance to infection.

Precautions: see CYTOTOXIC DRUGS.

Interactions with other drugs:

Fludarabine: the adverse effects of fludarabine on the lungs are increased if it is taken with pentostatin.

Proprietary preparation: Nipent.

pentoxifylline *See* OXPENTIFYLLINE.

Pentrax (DermaPharm) *See* COAL TAR.

Pepcid (Merck Sharp & Dohme) *See* FAMOTIDINE.

peppermint oil An oil extracted from the peppermint plant, used for its *antispasmodic effect on the gut to relieve the symptoms of irritable bowel syndrome, especially abdominal colic. It is also included as an ingredient in many *antacid preparations and in preparations to relieve nasal congestion. Peppermint oil is available as *enteric-coated capsules or *modified-release capsules, which can be obtained without a prescription, but only from pharmacies.

Side effects: peppermint oil may cause heartburn and (rarely) allergic reactions.

Proprietary preparations: Colpermin (modified-release capsules); Mintec (enteric-coated capsules); plus many other proprietary preparations of which it is an ingredient.

Peptac (Norton Healthcare) A proprietary combination of sodium alginate (*see* ALGINIC ACID), *sodium bicarbonate, and *calcium carbonate, used as an antacid in the treatment of heartburn and reflux (*see* ACID-PEPTIC DISEASES). It is available as a sugar-free suspension and can be obtained without a prescription, but only from pharmacies.

Side effects, precautions, and interactions with other drugs: *see* ANTACIDS.

peptic ulcers *See* ACID-PEPTIC DISEASES.

Peptimax (Ashbourne Pharmaceuticals) *See* CIMETIDINE.

Pepto-Bismol (Procter & Gamble) *See* BISMUTH SUBSALICYLATE.

Percutol (Dominion Pharma) *See* GLYCERYL TRINITRATE.

Perdix (Schwartz Pharma) *See* MOEXIPRIL HYDROCHLORIDE.

Perfan (Hoechst Marion Roussel) *See* ENOXIMONE.

pergolide A *dopamine receptor agonist, similar to *bromocriptine, used as an *adjunct to *levodopa in the treatment of Parkinson's disease. It is available as tablets on *prescription only.

Side effects: include hallucinations, confusion, involuntary abnormal movements, somnolence, abdominal pain, nausea, dyspepsia, double vision, breathlessness, lung problems, and insomnia.

Precautions: pergolide should not be taken by people with heart disease, abnormal heart rhythms (*see* ARRHYTHMIA), or a history of hallucinations or by women who are pregnant or breastfeeding (it stops production of breast milk). Dosage should be reduced gradually at the end of treatment.

Interactions with other drugs:

Antipsychotics: antagonize the effect of pergolide.

Metoclopramide: antagonizes the effect of pergolide.

Proprietary preparation: Celance.

Pergonal (Serono Laboratories) *See* HUMAN MENOPAUSAL GONADOTROPHIN.

Periactin (Merck Sharp & Dohme) *See* CYPROHEPTADINE HYDROCHLORIDE.

pericyazine A phenothiazine *antipsychotic drug used for the treatment of schizophrenia and as an *adjunct for the short-term treatment of severe anxiety or agitation and violent or dangerously impulsive behaviour. It is available as tablets or a syrup on *prescription only.

Side effects: as for *chlorpromazine, but pericyazine is more sedating, has more pronounced antimuscarinic effects (e.g. dry mouth, constipation, difficulty in passing urine, blurred vision), but fewer *extrapyramidal reactions. Low blood pressure may occur at the start of treatment.

Precautions and interactions with other drugs: see CHLORPROMAZINE HYDROCHLORIDE.

Proprietary preparation: Neulactil.

Perinal (Dermal Laboratories) A proprietary combination of *hydrocortisone (a corticosteroid) and *lignocaine <lidocaine> hydrochloride (a local anaesthetic), used for the relief of pain or itching in or around the anus. It is available in a metered-dose spray and can be obtained without a prescription, but only from pharmacies.

Side effects: see CORTICOSTEROIDS.

Precautions: Perinal should not be used when viral or fungal infection is present; prolonged use should be avoided. Perinal is not recommended for children under 14 years old.

perindopril An *ACE inhibitor used as an adjunct to *diuretics for the treatment of *heart failure; it is also licensed for use in the treatment of *hypertension. It is available as tablets on *prescription only.

Side effects, precautions, and interactions with other drugs: see ACE INHIBITORS.

Proprietary preparation: Coversyl.

permethrin A pesticide that is used clinically to treat infestations of head *lice and *scabies. It is available as a lotion (for eradicating lice) or a cream (for eradicating scabies mites) and can be obtained without a prescription, but only from pharmacies.

Side effects: permethrin may cause itching, redness, and stinging of the skin.

Precautions: permethrin should not be applied near the eyes or on broken skin; treatment of children under two years old should be supervised by a doctor. Permethrin should be used with caution by women who are pregnant or breastfeeding.

Proprietary preparations: Lyclear Creme Rinse; Lyclear Dermal Cream.

Permitabs (Bioglan Laboratories) *See* POTASSIUM PERMANGANATE.

Peroxyl (Colgate-Palmolive) *See* HYDROGEN PEROXIDE.

perphenazine A phenothiazine *antipsychotic drug used for the treatment of schizophrenia and mania and for the short-term management of severe anxiety or agitation and violent or dangerously impulsive behaviour. It is also used as an *antiemetic to treat severe nausea and vomiting. Perphenazine is available as tablets on *prescription only.

Side effects: as for *chlorpromazine, but perphenazine is less sedating and has fewer antimuscarinic effects, and *extrapyramidal reactions are more frequent.

Precautions: perphenazine should not be used to treat agitated elderly patients. *See also* CHLORPROMAZINE HYDROCHLORIDE.

Interactions with other drugs: see CHLORPROMAZINE HYDROCHLORIDE.

Proprietary preparation: Fentazin.

Persantin, **Persantin Retard** (Boehringer Ingelheim) *See* DIPYRIDAMOLE.

Peru balsam (balsam of Peru) A balsam exuded from the trunk of the tree *Myroxylon balsamum*. It has mild antiseptic properties by virtue of its content of cinnamic acid and *benzoic acid. Peru balsam can be used diluted with castor oil to soothe bedsores and chronic venous ulcers, and it is included as an ingredient in some topical preparations for the treatment of *eczema and in preparations to relieve the pain and itching of *haemorrhoids.

Proprietary preparations: ANUGESIC-HC (combined with zinc oxide, bismuth oxide, hydrocortisone acetate, and benzyl benzoate); ANUGESIC-HC SUPPOSITORIES (combined with zinc oxide, bismuth oxide, bismuth subgallate, pramoxine <pramocaine> hydrochloride, and hydrocortisone acetate); ANUSOL (combined with zinc oxide, bismuth subgallate, and bismuth oxide); ANUSOL-HC (combined with zinc oxide, bismuth subgallate, bismuth oxide, hydrocortisone acetate, and benzyl benzoate).

pessary (vaginal suppository) A bullet-shaped plug containing a drug that is administered by insertion into the vagina. Pessaries are used when the drug needs to be delivered to the vaginal wall or the cervix; examples of drugs administered as pessaries are antibiotics used in the treatment of vaginal infections or prostaglandins used to induce labour or abortion.

pethidine hydrochloride An *opioid analgesic used for the treatment of moderate to severe pain and for pain relief during labour and before, during, or after surgery. Pethidine is a *controlled drug; it is available as tablets or an injection.

Side effects: see MORPHINE. In addition, overdosage may cause convulsions.

Precautions: see MORPHINE. In addition, pethidine should not be given to people with severe kidney disease.

Interactions with other drugs:

  MAOIs: should not be taken with pethidine.

  Ritonavir: increases the plasma concentration of pethidine; these two drugs should not be taken together.

  Selegiline: should not be taken with pethidine as the combination of these two drugs can cause a high fever and have severe effects on the central nervous system.

  See also OPIOIDS.

Proprietary preparation: Pamergan P100.

petroleum jelly *See* WHITE SOFT PARAFFIN; YELLOW SOFT PARAFFIN.

Pevaryl (Janssen-Cilag) *See* ECONAZOLE NITRATE.

Pevaryl TC (Janssen-Cilag) A proprietary combination of *econazole nitrate (an antifungal drug) and *triamcinolone acetonide (a potent steroid), used for the treatment of inflammatory fungal or bacterial infections of the skin. It is available as a cream on *prescription only.

Side effects, precautions, and interactions with other drugs: see ECONAZOLE NITRATE; TOPICAL STEROIDS.

pharmacy medicine *See* OVER THE COUNTER.

Pharmorubicin (Pharmacia & Upjohn) *See* EPIRUBICIN.

phenazocine hydrobromide An *opioid analgesic used for the treatment of severe pain. Phenazocine is a *controlled drug; it is available as tablets to be swallowed or dissolved under the tongue.

Side effects and precautions: see MORPHINE.

Interactions with other drugs: see OPIOIDS.

Proprietary preparation: Narphen.

phenelzine A *monoamine oxidase inhibitor used for the treatment of depressive illness. It is available as tablets on *prescription only.

Side effects and interactions with other drugs: see MONOAMINE OXIDASE INHIBITORS.

Precautions: see MONOAMINE OXIDASE INHIBITORS. In addition, phenelzine should not be taken by people with liver disease or by those who have had a stroke.

Proprietary preparation: Nardil.

Phenergan (Rhône-Poulenc Rorer) *See* PROMETHAZINE HYDROCHLORIDE.

phenindamine tartrate One of the original (sedating) *antihistamines, used to relieve the symptoms of such allergic conditions as hay fever and urticaria (nettle rash). It is available as tablets and can be obtained from pharmacies without a *prescription.

Side effects, precautions, and interactions with other drugs: see ANTIHISTAMINES.

Proprietary preparation: Thephorin.

phenindione An oral *anticoagulant used for the prevention and treatment of deep-vein *thrombosis and pulmonary embolism and for the prevention of embolism in people with atrial fibrillation (*see* ARRHYTHMIA) and in those who have received an artificial heart valve. It is available as tablets on *prescription only.

Side effects: see WARFARIN SODIUM. Phenindione is more likely than warfarin to cause allergic reactions, such as rashes, fever, blood disorders, diarrhoea, and damage to the liver or kidneys.

Precautions and interactions with other drugs: see WARFARIN SODIUM.

Proprietary preparation: Dindevan.

pheniramine maleate One of the original (sedating) *antihistamines, which is included as an ingredient in cough and decongestant preparations. Preparations containing pheniramine maleate can be bought from pharmacies without a prescription.

Side effects, precautions, and interactions with other drugs: see ANTIHISTAMINES.

Proprietary preparation: TRIOMINIC (combined with phenylpropanolamine).

phenobarbital *See* PHENOBARBITONE.

phenobarbitone <phenobarbital> A *barbiturate that is used mainly as an *anticonvulsant drug for the treatment of all forms of epilepsy except absence seizures, although newer antiepileptics are now usually preferred. It has a sedating effect in adults and may cause behavioural problems in children. A *controlled drug, it is available as tablets or an elixir for oral use and as a form for injection.

Side effects: include drowsiness, lethargy, mental depression, and allergic skin reactions. Paradoxical excitement, restlessness, and confusion can occur in the elderly and hyperactivity in children.

Precautions: phenobarbitone should be used with caution in people who have liver or kidney disease and in women who are pregnant or breastfeeding; women who are planning to become pregnant should seek specialist advice.

Interactions with other drugs: see BARBITURATES.

phenol A *disinfectant that is used in diluted solutions as an ingredient in some *antiseptic preparations. Oily phenol is used in *sclerotherapy for treating *haemorrhoids; it is available as a solution for injection on *prescription only.

Side effects: injection of phenol may cause local irritation and if it leaks from the injection site it may damage surrounding tissue.

Proprietary preparations: GERMOLENE CREAM (combined with chlorhexidine); TCP LIQUID ANTISEPTIC (halogenated phenols).

phenothiazines A group of chemically related compounds that are used mainly as *antipsychotic drugs, although some of them have other uses as well (for example, as *antiemetics). *See* CHLORPROMAZINE HYDROCHLORIDE; FLUPHENAZINE HYDROCHLORIDE; PERICYAZINE; PERPHENAZINE; PIPOTHIAZINE <PIPOTIAZINE> PALMITATE; PROCHLORPERAZINE; PROMAZINE HYDROCHLORIDE; THIORIDAZINE; TRIFLUOPERAZINE.

phenothrin An insecticide that is used clinically to treat infestations of head *lice. It is available as a lotion or a shampoo and can be obtained without a prescription, but only from pharmacies.

Side effects: phenothrin may irritate the skin.

Precautions: phenothrin should not be applied near the eyes or on broken skin; treatment of infants under six months old should be supervised by a doctor. Lotions containing alcohol should not be used for treating young children or people with asthma or severe eczema. Continuous or prolonged use of alcoholic lotions should be avoided.

Proprietary preparation: Full Marks.

phenoxybenzamine hydrochloride A powerful *alpha blocker that is used in conjunction with a *beta blocker to treat episodes of *hypertension associated with phaeochromocytoma, a tumour of the adrenal gland that unpredictably secretes large amounts of adrenaline <epinephrine> and noradrenaline <norepinephrine>, causing sudden attacks of raised blood pressure. Phenoxybenzamine is available, on *prescription only, as capsules or a form for intravenous infusion.

Side effects: include low blood pressure on standing (with dizziness and a fast heart rate), tiredness, nasal congestion, constriction of the pupils, and failure of ejaculation; decreased sweating and a dry mouth can occur after infusion.

Precautions: phenoxybenzamine should not be given to people who have had a stroke or are recovering from a heart attack. It should be used with caution in the elderly, in people with heart failure or other heart disease or kidney disease, and in pregnant women.

Proprietary preparation: Dibenyline (capsules).

phenoxymethylpenicillin (penicillin V) A *penicillin that has a similar spectrum of action to *benzylpenicillin but is less active and is therefore not used for serious infections. It has the advantage that it can be taken by mouth. It is available as tablets or a syrup on *prescription only.

Side effects: include diarrhoea, nausea, and allergic reactions (*see* BENZYLPENICILLIN).

Precautions: *see* BENZYLPENICILLIN; PENICILLINS.

Interactions with other drugs: *see* BENZYLPENICILLIN.

Proprietary preparations: Apsin; Tenkicin.

Phensic (SmithKline Beecham Consumer Healthcare) A proprietary combination of *aspirin (an analgesic) and *caffeine (a stimulant), used for the relief of mild to moderate pain. It is available as tablets without a prescription, but larger packs can only be obtained from pharmacies.

Side effects and interactions with other drugs: *see* ASPIRIN.

Precautions: these tablets should not be given to children, except on medical advice. *See also* ASPIRIN; CAFFEINE.

phentermine A drug that acts on the brain to suppress appetite; it has effects similar to those produced by *adrenaline <epinephrine> and *noradrenaline <norepinephrine>. Phentermine is used in conjunction with a low-calorie diet for the short-term treatment of *obesity in selected patients. It should not be used for more than 12 weeks since *tolerance to its effects develops (i.e. its ability to suppress the appetite soon wears off) and *dependence can occur. It is not suitable for the management of severe obesity. Phentermine is available as capsules; it is a *controlled drug.

Side effects: include dry mouth, headache, rashes, euphoria, insomnia, restlessness, nervousness, agitation, nausea, vomiting, dizziness, depression, hallucinations, palpitations and fast heart rate, hypertension (high blood pressure), constipation, and an increase in the frequency of passing urine. If breathlessness occurs, this should be reported to a doctor and treatment will be stopped, as it may indicate pulmonary hypertension, which has serious effects on the heart.

Precautions: phentermine should not be taken by people with high blood pressure or other cardiovascular disease, glaucoma, an overactive thyroid gland, epilepsy, a history of psychiatric illness or drug or alcohol abuse, or by women who are pregnant or breastfeeding. It is not recommended for children.

Interactions with other drugs:

MAOIs: there is a risk of a dangerous rise in blood pressure.

Proprietary preparations: Duromine; Ionamin.

phentolamine An *alpha blocker used for the treatment of episodes of hypertension in phaeochromocytoma, a tumour of the adrenal gland that can release large amounts of noradrenaline <norepinephrine> and adrenaline <epinephrine> unpredictably and thereby cause raised blood pressure. It is also used to treat the hypertension caused by *monoamine oxidase inhibitors and related substances. It is available as a solution for injection on *prescription only.

Side effects, precautions, and interactions with other drugs: see ALPHA BLOCKERS.

Proprietary preparation: Rogitine.

See also ANTIHYPERTENSIVE DRUGS.

phenylbutazone An *NSAID used for the treatment of ankylosing spondylitis (a type of arthritis affecting the spine) when this has not responded to other drugs. It is used only under supervision in hospital because it occasionally causes severe side effects. Phenylbutazone is available as tablets on *prescription only.

Side effects: see NSAIDS. Additional side effects of phenylbutazone may include inflammation of the lining of the mouth and salivary glands, enlargement of the thyroid gland (goitre), hepatitis, and blood disorders. Anyone taking phenylbutazone who develops a sore throat, mouth ulcers, bruising, fever, malaise, or a rash should inform a doctor immediately.

Precautions: see NSAIDS.

Interactions with other drugs: see NSAIDS. In addition:

Phenytoin: its effects are enhanced by phenylbutazone.

Warfarin: should not be taken with phenylbutazone, as phenylbutazone greatly increases its anticoagulant effects.

Proprietary preparation: Butacote.

phenylephrine A *sympathomimetic drug that constricts blood vessels. It is widely used as a nasal *decongestant and is an ingredient in many cough and cold preparations. Phenylephrine can be administered by injection or infusion to increase blood pressure and is sometimes used for this purpose in emergencies until blood or plasma transfusions can be given. It is also used in eye drops to dilate the pupils in order to facilitate ophthalmic examinations and is combined with local anaesthetics in topical preparations to restrict the action of the anaesthetic to the area of application. Phenylephrine for injection or infusion is a *prescription only medicine; other preparations are available without a prescription.

Side effects: include headache and high blood pressure, changes in heart rate, vomiting, and tingling and coolness of the skin.

Precautions: phenylephrine should not be taken by people with an overactive thyroid gland or severe hypertension. *See also* NORADRENALINE <NOREPINEPHRINE>.

Interactions with other drugs:

Antihypertensive drugs: phenylephrine antagonizes the effect of alpha blockers and possibly other antihypertensives drugs in lowering blood pressure.

MAOIs: may cause a dangerous rise in blood pressure.

Proprietary preparations: Fenox (nasal drops and spray); Minims Phenylephrine (eye drops); BEECHAMS ALL-IN-ONE (combined with guaiphenesin <guaifenesin> and paracetamol); BEECHAMS FLU-PLUS CAPLETS (combined with paracetamol and caffeine); BEECHAMS FLU-PLUS HOT LEMON, HOT BERRY FRUITS (combined with paracetamol); BEECHAMS POWDERS CAPSULES (combined with paracetamol and caffeine); BETNOVATE RECTAL (combined with betamethasone and lignocaine <lidocaine>); BOOTS COLD AND 'FLU RELIEF TABLETS (combined with caffeine, paracetamol, and ascorbic acid); CATARRH-EX (combined with paracetamol and caffeine); COLDREX BLACKCURRANT POWDERS, COLDREX HOT LEMON POWDERS (combined with paracetamol); COLDREX TABLETS (combined with caffeine and paracetamol); DIMOTAPP (combined with brompheniramine and phenylpropanolamine); DRISTAN DECONGESTANT TABLETS (combined with aspirin, caffeine, and chlorpheniramine <chlorphenamine>); ISOPTO FRIN (combined with hypromellose); LEMSIP COLD + FLU COMBINED RELIEF CAPSULES (combined with caffeine and paracetamol); LEMSIP COLD + FLU ORIGINAL LEMON (combined with paracetamol and vitamin C); NUMARK COLD RELIEF CAPSULES WITH DECONGESTANT (combined with paracetamol); SP COLD RELIEF CAPSULES (combined with caffeine and paracetamol); UNIFLU WITH GREGOVITE C (combined with codeine, diphenhydramine, and paracetamol).

phenylpropanolamine A *sympathomimetic drug that constricts blood vessels. It is incorporated into a number of oral preparations for treating colds and coughs, hay fever, and asthma, in which it acts as a *decongestant on the nose and upper airways. It is usually freely available without a prescription but some preparations may be bought only from a pharmacy, depending on the other ingredients.

Side effects and precautions: *see* EPHEDRINE HYDROCHLORIDE.

Interactions with other drugs:

Bromocriptine: there is an increased risk of adverse effects if this drug is given with phenylpropanolamine.

For other interactions, *see* EPHEDRINE HYDROCHLORIDE.

Proprietary preparations: ALLER-EZE PLUS (combined with clemastine); BENYLIN DAY & NIGHT TABLETS (day tablets; combined with paracetamol); CONTAC 400 (combined with chlorpheniramine <chlorphenamine>); DAY NURSE (combined with dextromethorphan and paracetamol); DIMOTAPP (combined with brompheniramine and phenylephrine); ESKORNADE (combined with diphenylpyraline); MU-CRON TABLETS (combined with paracetamol); SINUTAB (combined with paracetamol); SINUTAB NIGHT-TIME (combined with paracetamol and phenyltoloxamine); TRIOGESIC (combined with paracetamol); TRIOMINIC (combined with pheniramine); VICKS COLDCARE (combined with paracetamol and dextromethorphan).

phenytoin An *anticonvulsant used to treat epilepsy (major and partial seizures) and status epilepticus (repeated seizures with no recovery of consciousness between them) and to control or prevent seizures following neurosurgery or head injury. It is also used to treat trigeminal neuralgia. Phenytoin is available on *prescription only, either as an injection for use under medical supervision or as tablets, chewable tablets, capsules, or a suspension for oral use.

Side effects: include nausea, vomiting, headache, tremor, nervousness, and insomnia; less common effects are unsteadiness, shakiness, slurred speech, acne, increased growth of body hair, overgrowth of the gums, and rashes (if rashes develop the treatment should be discontinued). Rapid involuntary eye movements and blurred vision are signs of overdosage.

Precautions: phenytoin should be used with caution in women who are pregnant or breastfeeding and in people with impaired liver function. Women who are planning to become pregnant should seek specialist advice. When given intravenously, continuous monitoring of the electrocardiogram is essential and resuscitative equipment should be available.

Interactions with other drugs:

Analgesics: the plasma concentration of phenytoin is increased by aspirin, azapropazone (which should not be taken with phenytoin), and phenylbutazone; the effects of methadone are reduced by phenytoin.

Anti-arrhythmic drugs: amiodarone increases the plasma concentration of phenytoin; the plasma concentrations of disopyramide, mexiletine, and quinidine are reduced by phenytoin.

Antibiotics: the plasma concentration of phenytoin is increased by chloramphenicol, cycloserine, isoniazid, metronidazole, co-trimoxazole, and trimethoprim and reduced by rifampicin. The plasma concentration of doxycycline is reduced by phenytoin.

Anticoagulants: the metabolism of warfarin and nicoumalone <acenocoumarol> is increased by phenytoin, which may reduce their anticoagulant effect (but in some cases has enhanced it).

Anticonvulsants: taking two or more anticonvulsants together may enhance their adverse effects: phenytoin often reduces plasma concentrations of clonazepam, carbamazepine, lamotrigine, topiramate, and sodium valproate and increases the plasma concentration of phenobarbitone <phenobarbital>.

Antidepressants: antagonize the anticonvulsant effect of phenytoin. Fluoxetine, fluvoxamine, and viloxazine increase the plasma concentration of phenytoin; the plasma concentrations of mianserin, paroxetine, and tricyclic antidepressants are reduced by phenytoin.

Antifungal drugs: fluconazole and miconazole increase the plasma concentration of phenytoin; the plasma concentrations of itraconazole and ketoconazole are reduced by phenytoin.

Antimalarial drugs: antagonize the anticonvulsant effect of phenytoin; the antifolate effect of pyrimethamine is enhanced by phenytoin.

Antipsychotics: antagonize the anticonvulsant effect of phenytoin; the plasma concentrations of clozapine, quetiapine, and sertindole are reduced by phenytoin.

Antiviral drugs: the plasma concentrations of indinavir, nelfinavir, and saquinavir may be reduced by phenytoin; zidovudine either increases or reduces plasma concentrations of phenytoin.

Calcium antagonists: diltiazem and nifedipine increase the plasma concentration of phenytoin; phenytoin reduces the effects of felodipine, isradipine, and probably also of nicardipine, nifedipine, diltiazam, and verapamil.

Corticosteroids: their effects are reduced by phenytoin.

Cyclosporin: its plasma concentration is reduced by phenytoin.

Disulfiram: increases the plasma concentration of phenytoin.

Oral contraceptives: their contraceptive effect is reduced by phenytoin.

Sulphinpyrazone <sulfinpyrazone>: increases the plasma concentration of phenytoin.

Ulcer-healing drugs: cimetidine increases the plasma concentration of phenytoin; sucralfate reduces the absorption of phenytoin; omeprazole increases the effects of phenytoin.

Proprietary preparations: Epanutin; Epanutin Ready-Mixed Parenteral.

Phillips' Milk of Magnesia (SmithKline Beecham Consumer Healthcare) *See* MAGNESIUM HYDROXIDE.

Phimetin (BHR Pharmaceuticals) *See* CIMETIDINE.

pHiso-Med (Sanofi Winthrop) *See* CHLORHEXIDINE.

pholcodine A weak *opioid that acts as a *cough suppressant but has no appreciable analgesic activity. It is therefore used for the treatment of dry or painful coughs and is available as a linctus and as an ingredient of many cough medicines. Pholcodine is usually freely available *over the counter, although some preparations can be bought only from a pharmacy, depending on the other ingredients.

Side effects: as for *codeine, but side effects are rare. Pholcodine is not addictive.

Precautions: *see* CODEINE.

Interactions with other drugs: *see* OPIOIDS.

Proprietary preparations: Benylin Children's Dry Coughs; Boots Daytime Cough Relief; Famel Linctus; Galenphol, Galenphol Paediatric, and Galenphol Strong; Hill's Balsam Dry Cough Liquid; Pavacol D; Tixylix Daytime; BOOTS CHILDREN'S 1 YEAR PLUS NIGHT TIME COUGH SYRUP (combined with diphenhydramine); BOOTS DAY COLD COMFORT (combined with paracetamol and pseudoephedrine); BOOTS NIGHT COLD COMFORT (combined with paracetamol, diphenhydramine, and pseudoephedrine); BOOTS NIGHT-TIME COUGH RELIEF (combined with diphenhydramine); EXPULIN (combined with chlorpheniramine <chlorphenamine>, menthol,

and pseudoephedrine); EXPULIN DRY (combined with menthol); EXPULIN
PAEDIATRIC (combined with chlorpheniramine <chlorphenamine> and
menthol); TIXYLIX COUGH & COLD (combined with chlorpheniramine
<chlorphenamine> and pseudoephedrine); TIXYLIX NIGHT-TIME (combined
with promethazine).

PhorPain (Goldshield Pharmaceuticals) *See* IBUPROFEN.

Phosex (Vitaline Pharmaceuticals) *See* CALCIUM ACETATE.

phosphate-binding agents Aluminium- and calcium-containing
salts that are used to bind to phosphates in the diet and stop them from
being absorbed. This is important in people who have kidney disease,
especially those who are on kidney dialysis, since high concentrations of
phosphate in the blood can cause bone disease. Phosphate-binding
agents, which are taken before food, include *aluminium hydroxide,
*calcium carbonate, and *calcium acetate.

phosphate laxatives A group of phosphate salts used as *osmotic
laxatives to evacuate the bowel before abdominal X-ray examinations or
before investigative procedures or surgery of the bowel. They are also
used to relieve postoperative constipation and in obstetrics. The common
phosphate laxatives are *sodium acid phosphate and **sodium phosphate**
which are available as enemas or suppositories and can be obtained
without a prescription, but only from pharmacies. **Sodium dihydrogen
phosphate dihydrate** and **disodium phosphate dodecahydrate** are
ingredients in *bowel-cleansing solutions.
Side effects: there may be local irritation.
Precautions: phosphates should be used with caution in elderly people
and should not be used in patients with acute gastrointestinal disorders.

Phosphate-Sandoz (HK Pharma) A proprietary combination of
*sodium acid phosphate, *sodium bicarbonate, and *potassium
bicarbonate, used as a *phosphate supplement. It is also occasionally
used to reduce high plasma calcium concentrations that result from
overproduction of *parathyroid hormone by the parathyroid gland or
occur with certain cancers. Phosphate-Sandoz is available as effervescent
tablets and can be obtained without a prescription, but only from
pharmacies.
Side effects and precautions: see PHOSPHATE SUPPLEMENTS. When used to
reduce plasma calcium, this medicine may bind to calcium to form
calcium phosphate in the tissues, leading to kidney impairment and the
formation of kidney stones (*see also* SODIUM CELLULOSE PHOSPHATE).

phosphate supplements Preparations containing phosphate salts
(usually *sodium acid phosphate) used to treat conditions of phosphate
deficiency. Supplementary phosphate may be required in addition to
*vitamin D for treating patients with a type of rickets or osteomalacia in
which plasma phosphate concentrations are very low. A lack of

phosphate is occasionally also seen in people with diabetic ketoacidosis (a condition that can occur in poorly controlled *diabetes mellitus) and in alcoholics. Phosphate supplements are usually taken by mouth, but infusions may be required for treating severe cases of phosphate depletion.

Side effects: diarrhoea is the most common side effect.

Precautions: plasma concentrations of electrolytes should be monitored during phosphate therapy.

phosphodiesterase inhibitors Compounds that inhibit the enzyme phosphodiesterase and thereby allow the accumulation of the substance cAMP (cyclic adenosine monophosphate). cAMP is produced when the *sympathetic nervous system is stimulated (among other circumstances). Thus an accumulation of cAMP has a similar effect to stimulating the sympathetic nervous system (*see* SYMPATHOMIMETIC DRUGS). There are two types of phosphodiesterase (PDE) inhibitor: the *xanthines, which are *bronchodilators used for treating asthma; and the PDE type III inhibitors (such as *enoximone and *milrinone), which have been used in the treatment of congestive *heart failure.

Phyllocontin Continus (Napp Pharmaceuticals) *See* AMINOPHYLLINE.

Phyllosan (Seton Scholl Healthcare) A proprietary combination of *ferrous fumarate, B vitamins (*see* VITAMIN B COMPLEX), and *vitamin C, used for the prevention of deficiencies of iron, B vitamins, and vitamin C. It is not recommended for children, except on medical advice. Phyllosan tablets are freely available *over the counter.

Side effects, precautions, and interactions with other drugs: see IRON.

Physeptone (Martindale Pharmaceuticals) *See* METHADONE HYDROCHLORIDE.

Physiotens (Solvay Healthcare) *See* MOXONIDINE.

Phytex (Pharmax) A proprietary combination of the antifungal agent borotannic acid complex (consisting of tannic acid and boric acid), *salicylic acid, *methyl salicylate, and *acetic acid, used for the treatment of fungal infections of the skin and nails. It is available as a solution for painting on the nails and can be obtained without a prescription, but only from pharmacies.

Precautions: Phytex should not be used during pregnancy.

phytomenadione (vitamin K₁) A form of *vitamin K that is used in the prevention and treatment of haemorrhage (severe bleeding) in low-birth-weight babies. It is also used to reverse the effects of *warfarin sodium if too large a dosage has been used. Phytomenadione is available as a solution for intramuscular or intravenous injection on *prescription only, or as tablets that can be obtained from pharmacies without a prescription.

Proprietary preparations: Konakion; Konakion MM; Konakion MM Paediatric.

Picolax (Ferring Pharmaceuticals) A proprietary combination of *sodium picosulphate <picosulfate> (a stimulant laxative) and *magnesium citrate (an osmotic laxative), used to evacuate the bowel before radiological procedures, investigation, or surgery. It is available as an oral powder to be dissolved in water and can be obtained without a prescription, but only from pharmacies.
Side effects and precautions: see BOWEL-CLEANSING SOLUTIONS.

piles *See* HAEMORRHOIDS.

pilocarpine A *cholinergic drug that is used (in the form of drops or gel) to improve the drainage of fluid from the front chamber of the eye (*see* MIOTICS) in the treatment of *glaucoma. Because it stimulates the salivary glands, pilocarpine is also used (as tablets) to prevent the dry mouth caused by radiation treatment. It is available, on *prescription only, as eye drops, *modified-release inserts placed beneath the eyelid, eye gel, or tablets.
Side effects: eye formulations commonly cause temporary blurring of vision, and there may be brow ache and headache. The tablets (and rarely the eye formulations) may cause watering eyes, sweating, chills, diarrhoea, nausea, abdominal pain, and increased frequency of urination.
Precautions: eye formulations should not be used by people with inflammation of the iris or by those who wear soft contact lenses. Pilocarpine tablets should be used with caution by people with impaired liver or kidney function, heart or circulatory disease, asthma, or gall-bladder or bile-duct disease and by women who are pregnant or breastfeeding.
Interactions with other drugs:
  Beta blockers: the risk of abnormal heart rhythms is increased.
Proprietary preparations: Minims Pilocarpine (preservative-free single-dose eye drops); Ocusert Pilo (ocular inserts); Pilogel (eye gel); Salagen (tablets); ISOPTO CARPINE (combined with hypromellose).

Pilogel (Alcon Laboratories) *See* PILOCARPINE.

pimozide An *antipsychotic drug used for the treatment of schizophrenia and some other psychoses. It is available as tablets on *prescription only.
Side effects: as for *chlorpromazine but pimozide is less sedating, has more pronounced *extrapyramidal reactions, and can cause serious abnormalities in heart rhythm (*arrhythmias).
Precautions: pimozide should not be taken by women who are breastfeeding or by people who have, or have had, heart arrhythmias. People who are being treated with pimozide will need periodic heart monitoring.

Interactions with other drugs: pimozide should not be used with other antipsychotic drugs or with certain other drugs (see below), as this increases the risk of serious effects on the heart.

Anaesthetics: their effect in lowering blood pressure is enhanced.

Anti-arrhythmic drugs: amiodarone, disopyramide, procainamide, and quinidine should not be taken with pimozide.

Antibiotics: pimozide should not be taken with clarithromycin or erythromycin.

Antidepressants: tricyclic antidepressants should not be taken with pimozide.

Antiepileptic drugs: their anticonvulsant effects are antagonized by pimozide.

Antihistamines: pimozide should not be taken with astemizole or terfenadine.

Antimalarial drugs: pimozide should not be taken with mefloquine or quinine.

Cisapride: should not be taken with pimozide.

Diuretics: should not be taken with pimozide.

Ritonavir: should not be taken with pimozide.

Sedatives: the sedative effects of pimozide are increased if it is taken with anxiolytic or hypnotic drugs, or any other drug that causes sedation.

Proprietary preparation: Orap.

pindolol A non-cardioselective *beta blocker used for the treatment of *angina or *hypertension. It is available as tablets on *prescription only.

Side effects, precautions, and interactions with other drugs: see BETA BLOCKERS.

Proprietary preparations: Visken; VISKALDIX (combined with clopamide). *See also* ANTIHYPERTENSIVE DRUGS.

piperacillin A broad-spectrum *penicillin that is active against *Pseudomonas* and *Proteus* bacteria. It is used for the treatment of systemic and local infections (such as infected wounds or burns) and respiratory or urinary-tract infections. Given by injection or infusion, it is available on *prescription only. It is sometimes used in conjunction with an *aminoglycoside antibiotic.

Side effects, precautions, and interactions with other drugs: see BENZYLPENICILLIN.

Proprietary preparations: Pipril; TAZOCIN (combined with tazobactam).

piperazine An *anthelmintic that acts by paralysing intestinal worms so that they can be eliminated from the body. It is used for the treatment of roundworm and threadworm infestations. Piperazine is available as an elixir and as a powder combined with sennosides (to aid elimination of the worms) and can be obtained without a prescription, but only from pharmacies.

Side effects: include nausea, vomiting, colic, diarrhoea, allergic reactions (including itching), and rarely visual disturbances, vertigo, and dizziness.

Precautions: piperazine should not be taken by people with liver disease, severe kidney disease, or epilepsy or by pregnant women; it should be used with caution by women who are breastfeeding.

Proprietary preparations: De Witt's Worm Syrup; Pripsen Worm Elixir; PRIPSEN (combined with sennosides).

Piportil Depot (Rhône-Poulenc Rorer) *See* PIPOTHIAZINE <PIPOTIAZINE> PALMITATE.

pipothiazine palmitate <pipotiazine palmitate> A phenothiazine *antipsychotic drug used for the maintenance treatment of schizophrenia and other psychoses. It is available as a *depot injection on *prescription only.

Side effects, precautions, and interactions with other drugs: see CHLORPROMAZINE HYDROCHLORIDE.

Proprietary preparation: Piportil Depot.

Pipril (Wyeth Laboratories) *See* PIPERACILLIN.

piracetam An *anticonvulsant drug used to treat myoclonus – a sudden spasm of the muscles that occurs in people with certain other neurological illnesses. It is available, on *prescription only, as tablets or an oral solution.

Side effects: include diarrhoea, weight gain, somnolence, insomnia, nervousness, and depression.

Precautions: piracetam should not be taken by people who have liver or kidney disease or by women who are pregnant or breastfeeding. The drug should be withdrawn gradually at the end of treatment.

Proprietary preparation: Nootropil.

Piriton (Stafford-Miller) *See* CHLORPHENIRAMINE <CHLORPHENAMINE> MALEATE.

piroxicam An *NSAID used for the treatment of pain and inflammation in rheumatoid arthritis (including arthritis in children) and other disorders of the joints and muscles and to relieve the pain of acute gout. It is available, on *prescription only, as tablets, dispersible tablets, capsules, an injection, suppositories, and a gel for topical application (a gel formulation can be obtained from pharmacies without a prescription).

Side effects: see NSAIDS. Suppositories may cause local irritation and occasionally bleeding; there may be pain at the site of the injection.

Precautions: see NSAIDS.

Interactions with other drugs: see NSAIDS. In addition:

Ritonavir: should not be used with piroxicam since it increases plasma concentrations of piroxicam to an extent that might cause toxic effects.

Proprietary preparations: Feldene; Feldene Melt (tablets that readily dissolve in the mouth); Feldene P Gel; Flamatrol; Kentene; Larapam; Pirozip.

Pirozip (Ashbourne Pharmaceuticals) *See* PIROXICAM.

Pitressin (Parke-Davis Medical) *See* VASOPRESSIN.

Piz Buin (Novartis Consumer Health) A proprietary *sunscreen preparation consisting of a lotion containing ethylhexyl *p*-methoxycinnamate, avobenzone, and *titanium dioxide. It protects against both UVA and UVB (SPF 20) and can be prescribed on the NHS or obtained without a prescription.

pizotifen An *antihistamine that also opposes the action of *serotonin; it is used for the prevention of *migraine or recurrent vascular headaches. Pizotifen is available as tablets or an elixir on *prescription only.
Side effects: include drowsiness, increased appetite, and weight gain.
Precautions: drowsiness may affect driving performance or other skilled tasks. Pizotifen should be used with caution by people with glaucoma, urinary retention, or kidney disease and by women who are pregnant or breastfeeding.
Proprietary preparation: Sanomigran.

placebo A medicine that is ineffective but may help to relieve a condition because the patient has faith in its powers. New drugs are tested against placebos in clinical trials: the drug's effect is compared with the **placebo response**, which occurs even in the absence of any pharmacologically active substance in the placebo.

Placidex (E. C. De Witt & Co) *See* PARACETAMOL.

Plaquenil (Sanofi Winthrop) *See* HYDROXYCHLOROQUINE SULPHATE.

Plavix (Bristol-Myers Squibb; Sanofi Winthrop) *See* CLOPIDOGREL.

Plendil (AstraZeneca) *See* FELODIPINE.

Plesmet (Link Pharmaceuticals) *See* FERROUS GLYCINE SULPHATE.

podophyllotoxin A caustic agent (*see* KERATOLYTICS) that is the main active constituent of *podophyllum. It is used to treat and dissolve warts affecting the penis or female genitalia. It is available, on *prescription only, as a solution for topical application.
Side effects: local irritation may occur.

Precautions: podophyllotoxin should not be used on open wounds or by women who are pregnant or breastfeeding. It is very irritant to the eyes.
Proprietary preparations: Condyline; Warticon.

podophyllum A caustic resin (*see* KERATOLYTICS) that is used in the form of **compound podophyllin paint** for treating warts on the penis or external female genitalia. It is available on *prescription only.
Side effects and precautions: podophyllum can irritate the treated area and should be washed off after six hours. If many warts are to be treated, only a few should be treated at any one time, since podophyllum is extremely toxic if absorbed. It should not be applied to healthy skin (skin surrounding the wart should be protected during application) or to open wounds, and should not come into contact with the face (it is very irritant to the eyes). It should not be used by women who are pregnant or breastfeeding.
Proprietary preparation: POSALFILIN (combined with salicylic acid).

polyacrylic acid *See* CARBOMER.

polyethylene glycols (macrogols) Polymers that are hydrophilic and are used as bases for ointments. Macrogol '3350' (polyethylene glycol '3350') is an *osmotic laxative that is used, in combination with other ingredients, for treating chronic constipation or clearing the bowel (*see* BOWEL-CLEANSING SOLUTIONS).
Side effects: macrogols can cause abdominal distension and pain and nausea.
Precautions: preparations containing macrogols should not be used in people with perforated or obstructed intestines and severe inflammatory bowel disease (such as Crohn's disease or ulcerative colitis). They should be used with caution during pregnancy and breastfeeding.
Proprietary preparations: KLEAN-PREP (combined with sodium sulphate, sodium bicarbonate, sodium chloride, and potassium chloride); MOVICOL (combined with sodium chloride, sodium bicarbonate, and potassium chloride).

Polyfax (Dominion Pharma) A proprietary combination of the antibiotics *polymyxin B sulphate and *bacitracin zinc, used to treat styes, conjunctivitis, and inflammation of the eyelids and to prevent infection after eye surgery or removal of foreign bodies. It is also used for treating skin infections, impetigo, and burns. Polyfax is available as separate ointments for the eyes and skin on *prescription only.
Side effects: there may be local irritation due to allergic reactions.
Precautions: if large areas of skin are treated the ointment may be absorbed, giving rise to hearing impairment. This is more likely to occur in children, the elderly, and people with kidney disease.

Polymer Gel Corn Removers (Seton Scholl Healthcare) *See* SALICYLIC ACID.

polymyxin B sulphate An antibacterial drug that is used in combination with a variety of other *antibiotics to treat a wide range of bacterial infections.

Side effects, precautions, and interactions with other drugs: see entries for individual combined preparations.

Proprietary preparations: GREGODERM (combined with nystatin and hydrocortisone); MAXITROL (combined with dexamethasone, hypromellose, and neomycin sulphate); NEOSPORIN (combined with neomycin sulphate); OTOSPORIN (combined with neomycin sulphate and hydrocortisone); POLYFAX (combined with bacitracin); POLYTRIM (combined with trimethoprim).

polysaccharide–iron complex A combination of *iron and a polysaccharide (a complex sugar) used for the treatment of iron-deficiency anaemia. It is available as an *elixir and can be obtained without a prescription, but only from pharmacies. A formulation for use in children can be prescribed on the NHS, but only for treating premature babies.

Side effects, precautions, and interactions with other drugs: see IRON.

Proprietary preparations: Niferex; Niferex Drops (for children).

Polytar (Stiefel Laboratories) A proprietary combination of *tar, *coal tar extract, *arachis oil, *cade oil, coal tar solution, and oleyl alcohol, used for the treatment of scaly and itching scalp disorders, including *psoriasis, *eczema, and dandruff. It is freely available *over the counter in the form of a liquid.

Side effects and precautions: see COAL TAR.

Polytar AF (Stiefel Laboratories) A proprietary combination of *tar, *coal tar extract, *arachis oil, *cade oil, coal tar solution, pine tar, and pyrithione zinc, used for the treatment of scaly scalp disorders, including *psoriasis, *eczema, and dandruff. It is freely available *over the counter in the form of a shampoo.

Side effects and precautions: see COAL TAR.

Polytar Plus (Stiefel Laboratories) A proprietary combination of *tar, *coal tar extract, *arachis oil, cade oil, coal tar solution, oleyl alcohol, and hydrolysed animal protein, used for the treatment of scaly and itching scalp disorders, including *psoriasis, *eczema, and dandruff. It is freely available *over the counter in the form of a liquid.

Side effects and precautions: see COAL TAR.

polythiazide A *thiazide diuretic used for the treatment of *hypertension and *oedema associated with heart failure, liver disease, or kidney disease. It is available as tablets on *prescription only.

Side effects, precautions, and interactions with other drugs: see THIAZIDE DIURETICS.

Proprietary preparation: Nephril.
See also ANTIHYPERTENSIVE DRUGS; DIURETICS.

Polytrim (Dominion Pharma) A proprietary combination of the antibiotics *trimethoprim and *polymyxin B sulphate, used for the treatment of bacterial eye infections. It is available as drops or an ointment on *prescription only.
Side effects: there may be local irritation due to allergic effects.

polyvinyl alcohol An agent that is used in the treatment of dry eyes to thicken the natural film of tears that covers the eyes. It is available as eye drops and can be obtained without a prescription, but only from pharmacies.
Side effects: there may be transient stinging and blurred vision on application.
Precautions: polyvinyl alcohol should not be used with soft contact lenses.
Proprietary preparations: Hypotears; Liquifilm Tears; Refresh Ophthalmic Solution; Sno Tears.

POM *See* PRESCRIPTION ONLY MEDICINE.

Ponstan (Elan Pharma) *See* MEFENAMIC ACID.

poractant alfa A synthetic pulmonary *surfactant that is used to treat breathing difficulties in premature babies who are receiving mechanical ventilation (*see* VENTILATOR). It is also used to prevent breathing difficulties in premature babies. Poractant alfa is available, on *prescription only, as a suspension that is administered through a tube placed in the trachea (windpipe).
Precautions: constant monitoring of heart rate and blood gases is necessary during treatment as poractant alfa can cause a rapid improvement in the baby's condition and high concentrations of oxygen in the tissues have toxic effects.
Proprietary preparation: Curosurf.

Pork Insulatard (Novo Nordisk Pharmaceutical) *See* INSULIN.

Pork Mixtard 30 (Novo Nordisk Pharmaceutical) *See* INSULIN.

Pork Velosulin (Novo Nordisk Pharmaceutical) *See* INSULIN.

Posalfilin (Norgine) A proprietary combination of *salicylic acid (a keratolytic) and *podophyllum resin (a caustic agent), used for the treatment of verrucas. It is available as an ointment and can be obtained without a prescription, but only from pharmacies.
Side effects and precautions: see SALICYLIC ACID; PODOPHYLLUM.

Posiject (Eli Lilly & Co) *See* DOBUTAMINE HYDROCHLORIDE.

postcode prescribing The practice in the National Health Service of blacklisting certain expensive drugs in some regions, although doctors in other regions may be allowed to prescribe them. Thus whether or not a patient can benefit from these drugs may depend on their postcode.

PostMI 75EC (Ashbourne Pharmaceuticals) *See* ASPIRIN.

Potaba (Glenwood Laboratories) *See* POTASSIUM AMINOBENZOATE.

potassium A mineral element necessary for the functioning of all cells of the body (*see* ELECTROLYTE). Together with *sodium, it is essential for the conduction of impulses in nerves and the functioning of muscles. Low concentrations of potassium can cause weakness, confusion, and in severe cases abnormal heart rhythms (*see* ARRHYTHMIA). **Potassium supplements** are salts of potassium given to prevent or treat potassium deficiency. This is particularly necessary during treatment with *anti-arrhythmic drugs or *digoxin, when low concentrations of potassium in the blood may induce irregularities in heart rhythm; in patients with certain kidney diseases, cirrhosis of the liver, or heart failure; and in cases of severe or chronic diarrhoea. Potassium supplements may also be required by the elderly and by people taking *corticosteroids or certain *diuretics, but in the latter case a *potassium-sparing diuretic may be given instead of a potassium supplement. Potassium supplements are given in the form of oral *potassium chloride, but if potassium depletion is severe potassium chloride can be given intravenously.
Side effects: include nausea and vomiting.
Precautions: potassium salts may cause ulceration of the bowel or oesophagus (gullet) and should be discontinued if there is discomfort or bleeding. They should generally not be used by people with severe kidney disease or those taking ACE inhibitors (see below), except in rare cases under specialist supervision, and should be used with caution by those with mild or moderate kidney disease. *Modified-release preparations must always be swallowed whole and never chewed or broken up.
Interactions with other drugs:
  ACE inhibitors: can cause high concentrations of potassium in the blood.
  Cyclosporin: can cause high concentrations of potassium in the blood.
  Potassium-sparing diuretics: can cause high concentrations of potassium in the blood.

potassium aminobenzoate The potassium salt of *aminobenzoic acid, one of the B group vitamins. It is used for the treatment of various disorders associated with excessive thickening or scarring of connective tissue, such as scleroderma, but its therapeutic value is doubtful. Potassium aminobenzoate is available as capsules, tablets, or sachets of powder to be dissolved in water; it can be obtained from pharmacies without a prescription.

Proprietary preparation: Potaba.

potassium benzoate A *potassium salt used in combination with other salts as an oral potassium supplement.

Side effects, precautions, and interactions with other drugs: see POTASSIUM.

Proprietary preparation: KLOREF.

potassium bicarbonate A *potassium salt that is an ingredient of oral potassium supplements and other preparations (in which it provides effervescence) and of some *antacid preparations.

Side effects, precautions, and interactions with other drugs: see POTASSIUM.

Proprietary preparations: GAVISCON ADVANCE (combined with sodium alginate); KLOREF (combined with betaine hydrochloride, potassium benzoate, and potassium chloride); SANDO-K (combined with potassium chloride); PHOSPHATE-SANDOZ (combined with sodium bicarbonate and sodium acid phosphate).

potassium canrenoate A diuretic that has the same action as *spironolactone but has a longer duration of action (both drugs are converted to canrenone, which is responsible for their diuretic activity). It is given by intravenous injection for the treatment of *oedema associated with cirrhosis of the liver, kidney disorders, and primary hyperaldosteronism. Potassium canrenoate is available on *prescription only.

Side effects, precautions, and interactions with other drugs: see POTASSIUM-SPARING DIURETICS.

Proprietary preparation: Spiroctan-M.

See also DIURETICS.

potassium channel activators A new class of drugs that dilate both veins and arteries. They are used for the prevention and long-term treatment of *angina. The main drug in this class is *nicorandil.

potassium chloride A salt of *potassium used as a potassium supplement. It may be combined with *diuretics to maintain potassium balance. Potassium chloride is available as tablets or a syrup without a prescription, but some preparations can only be obtained from pharmacies. *Modified-release tablets of potassium chloride should be swallowed whole with plenty of water while sitting or standing. Preparations for intravenous infusions are available on *prescription only.

Side effects, precautions, and interactions with other drugs: see POTASSIUM.

Proprietary preparations: Kay-Cee-L (syrup); Slow-K (modified-release tablets); BURINEX K (combined with bumetanide); DIARREST (combined with codeine phosphate, dicyclomine <dicycloverine> hydrochloride, sodium chloride, and sodium citrate); DIOCALM REPLENISH (combined with glucose, sodium citrate, and sodium chloride); DIORALYTE NATURAL (combined with glucose, sodium chloride, and disodium hydrogen citrate); DIORALYTE RELIEF (combined with sodium chloride, sodium citrate, and precooked rice powder); DIORALYTE TABLETS (combined with sodium bicarbonate, citric acid, glucose, sodium chloride, and potassium chloride); DIUMIDE-K CONTINUS (combined with frusemide <furosemide>); ELECTROLADE (combined with sodium chloride, sodium bicarbonate, and glucose); KLEAN-PREP (combined with macrogol '3350', sodium sulphate, sodium bicarbonate, and sodium chloride); KLOREF (combined with betaine hydrochloride, potassium benzoate, and potassium bicarbonate); LASIKAL (combined with frusemide <furosemide>); MOVICOL (combined with polyethylene glycol, sodium bicarbonate, and sodium chloride); NEO-NACLEX-K (combined with bendrofluazide <bendroflumethiazide>); SANDO-K (combined with potassium bicarbonate).

potassium citrate A drug used for the treatment of cystitis: it acts by making the urine alkaline. It is available, without a prescription, as an oral solution, effervescent tablets, or granules.

Side effects: there may be stomach irritation and increased urine production.

Precautions: potassium citrate should be used with caution by people with kidney disease.

Interactions with other drugs:

Potassium-sparing diuretics: there is a risk of increased plasma concentrations of *potassium.

Proprietary preparations: Cystopurin (granules); Effercitrate (tablets).

potassium hydroxyquinoline sulphate A drug with *antifungal, antibacterial, and deodorant properties. It is used, often in conjunction with *benzoyl peroxide, in the *topical treatment of fungal infections, minor bacterial infections, and acne.

Proprietary preparations: QUINOCORT (combined with hydrocortisone); QUINODERM (combined with benzoyl peroxide); QUINOPED (combined with benzoyl peroxide).

potassium permanganate A salt of potassium that forms a purple solution with *antiseptic and *astringent properties. It is used to cleanse and deodorize the skin in people with weeping *eczema and to cleanse wounds. Potassium permanganate is available as a solution or as tablets to be dissolved in water; it can be obtained without a prescription, but only from pharmacies.

Side effects: potassium permanganate can irritate mucous membranes; it also stains skin and clothing.

Proprietary preparation: Permitabs (tablets).

potassium-sparing diuretics (K⁺-sparing diuretics) A class of mild
*diuretics that act on the kidneys to promote loss of water. They are
different from other diuretics in that they do not cause the loss of
*potassium ions (thus there is no need for potassium supplements) and
they do not worsen diabetes or gout. They are often combined with other
types of diuretics to offset or prevent potassium loss in the treatment of
*hypertension. They are also used (rarely) in the treatment of nephrotic
syndrome (a kidney disease characterized by protein loss in the urine and
*oedema) and oedema that has not responded to other diuretics. The
effect of these diuretics lasts for several hours and therefore they should
not be taken during the late afternoon or early evening or there may be a
need to pass urine during the night. *See* AMILORIDE HYDROCHLORIDE;
POTASSIUM CANRENOATE; SPIRONOLACTONE; TRIAMTERENE.

Side effects: potassium may be retained in the body, causing muscle
weakness and abnormal heartbeat. Nausea and gastrointestinal upsets are
quite common. For more specific side effects, see entries individual
drugs.

Precautions: potassium-sparing diuretics should be used with great
caution in people taking *ACE inhibitors, preferably under close medical
supervision. They should not be given to people taking potassium
supplements. Patients taking potassium-sparing diuretics should be
warned not to use potassium-containing salt substitutes as this could lead
to high blood concentrations of potassium.

Interactions with other drugs:

 ACE inhibitors: increase the risk of raised blood concentrations of
    potassium (see above).

 Cyclosporin: increases the risk of raised concentrations of potassium.

 Lithium: its plasma concentration is increased.

Potter's Cleansing Herb (Potter's Herbal Supplies) A proprietary
combination of the stimulant laxatives aloes (*see* ALOIN), *cascara, and
*senna, used as a traditional herbal remedy for constipation. It is freely
available *over the counter in the form of tablets.

Side effects: see STIMULANT LAXATIVES.

Precautions: this laxative is not recommended for children. *See also*
STIMULANT LAXATIVES.

povidone–iodine An *antiseptic used for the treatment of a range of
bacterial infections. It works by slowly releasing *iodine. It is available as
a vaginal cleansing kit containing pessaries, a gel, and a solution for the
treatment of inflammation of the vagina and/or cervix. A dilute solution
is used as a mouthwash and gargle. For skin infections, or to disinfect the
skin before surgery, the drug is available in varying strengths as a paint, a
lotion, a scalp and skin cleanser, and a shampoo. It is also available as a
powder or an ointment that can be applied to the skin to treat infections
or ulcers or to dress cuts and abrasions. Povidone–iodine can be obtained
without a *prescription.

Side effects: rarely, the drug may cause allergic reactions.

Precautions: providone–iodine should be used with caution in people with certain kidney diseases, in women who are pregnant or breastfeeding, and on broken skin.

Proprietary preparations: Betadine; Betadine Gargle and Mouthwash; Betadine Scalp Cleanser; Savlon Dry Powder.

Powergel (Searle) *See* KETOPROFEN.

Powerin (Whitehall Laboratories) A proprietary combination of *aspirin and *paracetamol (analgesics) and *caffeine (a stimulant), used for the relief of headaches and minor aches and pains. It is freely available *over the counter in the form of tablets.

Side effects, precautions, and interactions with other drugs: see ASPIRIN; PARACETAMOL.

Pragmatar (Bioglan Laboratories) A proprietary combination of *coal tar distillate, *sulphur, and *salicylic acid (all keratolytics), used for the treatment of greasy scalp conditions and scaly skin disorders. It is available as a cream and can be obtained without a prescription, but only from pharmacies.

Side effects: Pragmatar may irritate the skin.

Precautions: the cream should not be applied to the groin or inflamed skin and contact with the eyes and mouth should be avoided.

pramocaine hydrochloride *See* PRAMOXINE HYDROCHLORIDE.

pramoxine hydrochloride <pramocaine hydrochloride> A *local anaesthetic that is included as an ingredient in preparations for relieving the pain and itching associated with minor skin conditions and *haemorrhoids.

Side effects: pramoxine may cause initial burning or stinging.

Precautions: preparations containing pramoxine should not be applied to the eyes or nose.

Proprietary preparations: ANUGESIC-HC (combined with zinc oxide, hydrocortisone acetate, Peru balsam, and benzyl benzoate); ANUGESIC-HC SUPPOSITORIES (combined with zinc oxide, hydrocortisone acetate, Peru balsam, bismuth subgallate, bismuth oxide, and benzyl benzoate); PROCTOFOAM HC and PROTOCREAM HC (combined with hydrocortisone acetate).

pravastatin A *statin used for the treatment of primary hypercholesterolaemia (*see* HYPERLIPIDAEMIA) that has not responded to dietary measures. It is also used to prevent the progression of *atherosclerosis in patients with coronary artery disease and to reduce the incidence of coronary thrombosis in those at risk. It is available as tablets on *prescription only.

Side effects and precautions: see STATINS.

Interactions with other drugs:

Orlistat: increases the plasma concentration of pravastatin, whose dosage should therefore be reduced.

See also STATINS.

Proprietary preparation: Lipostat.

Praxilene (Merck Pharmaceuticals) *See* NAFTIDROFURYL OXALATE.

prazosin An *alpha blocker that produces peripheral *vasodilatation. It is used to treat *hypertension, congestive *heart failure, and Raynaud's syndrome (poor circulation in the hands and feet). It is also used as an *adjunct in the treatment of the symptoms of urinary obstruction due to an enlarged prostate gland. Because it can cause a dramatic drop in blood pressure, the initial doses are low and should be given while the patient is lying down. Doses are then increased as necessary. Prazosin is available as tablets on *prescription only.

Side effects and interactions with other drugs: *see* ALPHA BLOCKERS.

Precautions: alcohol may increase the side effects of this drug. Driving and hazardous work should be undertaken with caution until people are aware of whether or not the drug causes them to feel dizzy or faint.

Proprietary preparation: Hypovase.

See also ANTIHYPERTENSIVE DRUGS; VASODILATORS.

Preconceive (Lane Health Products) *See* FOLIC ACID.

Precortisyl Forte (Hoechst Marion Roussel) *See* PREDNISOLONE.

Predenema (Pharmax) *See* PREDNISOLONE.

Predfoam (Pharmax) *See* PREDNISOLONE.

Pred Forte (Allergan) *See* PREDNISOLONE.

Prednesol (GlaxoWellcome) *See* PREDNISOLONE.

prednisolone A *corticosteroid with anti-inflammatory and anti-allergic activity. It is used to treat *asthma, inflammatory bowel disease, rheumatic disease, and inflammatory conditions of the eyes and ears. Prednisolone is widely used in *cancer treatment, as it has a marked effect against some types of leukaemia, Hodgkin's disease, and non-Hodgkin's lymphomas. It is also active in hormone-sensitive breast cancer and has a role in the palliative care of patients in the terminal stages of cancer, in whom it may produce a sense of wellbeing. Prednisolone is available, on *prescription only, as tablets, *enteric-coated tablets, an enema or suppositories, eye or ear drops, or as a solution for local injection into joints or around tendons.

Side effects: *see* CORTICOSTEROIDS; TOPICAL STEROIDS.

Precautions and interactions with other drugs: *see* CORTICOSTEROIDS.

Proprietary preparations: Deltacortril Enteric; Deltastab (injection);

Minims Prednisolone (eye drops); Precortisyl Forte; Predenema (enema); Predfoam (rectal foam); Pred Forte (eye drops); Prednesol; Predsol (eye or ear drops, enema, suppositories); PREDSOL-N (combined with neomycin sulphate); SCHERIPROCT (combined with cinchocaine hydrochloride).

prednisone A glucocorticoid (*see* CORTICOSTEROIDS), similar to *prednisolone, used for the treatment of inflammatory and allergic disorders, including rheumatoid conditions. It is available as tablets on *prescription only.
Side effects and interactions with other drugs: see CORTICOSTEROIDS.
Precautions: see CORTICOSTEROIDS. In addition, this drug should not be used by those with liver disease.

Predsol (Medeva) *See* PREDNISOLONE.

Predsol-N (Medeva) A proprietary combination of *prednisolone (a corticosteroid) and *neomycin sulphate (an antibiotic), used for the treatment of inflammation of the outer ear with infection and eczema and inflammation of the eye. It is available as drops on *prescription only.
Side effects: there may be local irritation due to allergic reactions.
Precautions: prolonged use of the drops should be avoided.

Pregaday (Medeva) A proprietary combination of *ferrous fumarate and *folic acid, used to prevent deficiencies of iron and folic acid during pregnancy. It is available as tablets and can be obtained without a prescription, but only from pharmacies.
Side effects, precautions, and interactions with other drugs: see IRON.

Pregnacare (Robinson Healthcare) A proprietary combination of *folic acid and a wide range of vitamins and minerals, including vitamins C, E, B_{12}, B_2, B_6, B_1, iodine, iron, vitamin K, β-carotene, and zinc. It is used as a dietary supplement for women who are trying to conceive or who are pregnant or breastfeeding and is freely available as capsules *over the counter.

Pregnyl (Organon Laboratories) *See* HUMAN CHORIONIC GONADOTROPHIN.

Premarin (Wyeth Laboratories) *See* HORMONE REPLACEMENT THERAPY.

Premique (Wyeth Laboratories) A proprietary combination of conjugated *oestrogens and *medroxyprogesterone used as continuous combined *hormone replacement therapy for the relief of menopausal symptoms and prevention of osteoporosis in women who have not had a hysterectomy and who have not had a period for a year. It is available as tablets on *prescription only.
Side effects, precautions, and interactions with other drugs: see HORMONE REPLACEMENT THERAPY.

Premique Cycle (Wyeth Laboratories) A proprietary preparation of conjugated *oestrogen tablets and *medroxyprogesterone tablets used as sequential combined *hormone replacement therapy for the relief of menopausal symptoms and the prevention of osteoporosis in women who have not had a hysterectomy. It is available on *prescription only.
Side effects, precautions, and interactions with other drugs: see HORMONE REPLACEMENT THERAPY.

Prempak-C (Wyeth Laboratories) A proprietary preparation of conjugated *oestrogen tablets and *norgestrel tablets used as sequential combined *hormone replacement therapy for the relief of menopausal symptoms and prevention of osteoporosis in women who have not had a hysterectomy. The tablets, which are available on *prescription only, must be taken in the prescribed order.
Side effects, precautions, and interactions with other drugs: see HORMONE REPLACEMENT THERAPY.

Prepadine (APS-Berk) *See* DOTHIEPIN <DOSULEPIN> HYDROCHLORIDE.

Preparation H (Whitehall Laboratories) A proprietary combination of shark liver oil and yeast cell extract, used to relieve the discomfort of *haemorrhoids and anal itching and also as a lubricant for easing painful bowel movements. It is freely available *over the counter in the form of an ointment or suppositories.

Prepidil (Pharmacia & Upjohn) *See* DINOPROSTONE.

Prepulsid, **Prepulsid Quicklet** (Janssen-Cilag) *See* CISAPRIDE.

Prescal (Novartis Pharmaceuticals) *See* ISRADIPINE.

prescription A document giving the details of a medication, including the dosage and quantity, to be dispensed by a pharmacist for an identified patient. A prescription must be signed in ink by a registered medical practitioner, although a few items may now be prescribed by certain nurses. A drug that can only be issued on prescription has the legal category of **prescription only medicine** (**POM**), which must be stated on the packaging. Medical practitioners may also prescribe items that do not legally require a prescription (*see* OVER THE COUNTER). Some 'blacklisted' drugs cannot be prescribed on the National Health Service; if they fall in the POM category they must be issued on a private prescription. *See also* POSTCODE PRESCRIBING.

prescription only medicine (POM) A legal category denoting a drug that can only be dispensed with a *prescription.

Preservex (UCB Pharma) *See* ACECLOFENAC.

Prestim (Leo Pharmaceuticals) A proprietary combination of *timolol maleate (a beta blocker) and *bendrofluazide <bendroflumethiazide> (a thiazide diuretic), used in the treatment of mild to moderate *hypertension. It is available as tablets on *prescription only. **Prestim Forte** is a similar preparation twice the strength of Prestim.

Side effects, precautions, and interactions with other drugs: see BETA BLOCKERS; THIAZIDE DIURETICS.

See also ANTIHYPERTENSIVE DRUGS; DIURETICS.

PR Heat Spray (Crookes Healthcare) A proprietary combination of *methyl salicylate, *ethyl nicotinate, and *camphor, used as a *rubefacient for the relief of muscular and rheumatic pains and stiffness, including backache, sciatica, lumbago, and fibrositis, bruises, sprains, and chilblains. It is freely available *over the counter.

Side effects and precautions: see RUBEFACIENTS.

Priadel (Delandale Laboratories) *See* LITHIUM CARBONATE; LITHIUM CITRATE.

prilocaine A *local anaesthetic that is similar to *lignocaine <lidocaine> and has similar uses. It is combined with lignocaine in a topical preparation. Prilocaine is available on *prescription only.

Side effects and precautions: see LIGNOCAINE <LIDOCAINE>. In addition, high doses can cause methaemoglobinaemia (the presence in the blood of an abnormal form of haemoglobin that cannot carry oxygen around the body), and prilocaine should not be given to patients with anaemia. It should be used with caution in patients with kidney disease.

Proprietary preparations: Citanest (injection); EMLA (combined with lignocaine <lidocaine>).

Primacor (Sanofi Winthrop) *See* MILRINONE.

Primalan (Rhône-Poulenc Rorer) *See* MEQUITAZINE.

primaquine A drug that is used in the treatment of benign *malaria; it is given after *chloroquine has been used to eliminate the malaria parasites that may still be present in the liver. Primaquine is available as tablets on special order since it does not currently have a *licence.

Side effects: include nausea, vomiting, and abdominal pain.

Precautions: primaquine should be used with caution by women who are pregnant or breastfeeding and by people with rheumatoid arthritis.

Interactions with other drugs:

Mepacrine: increases the risk of side effects from primaquine.

Primaxin (Merck Sharp & Dohme) *See* IMIPENEM.

primidone An *anticonvulsant drug that may be used for the treatment of all forms of epilepsy except absence seizures. It is converted to *phenobarbitone <phenobarbital> in the body. A *prescription only medicine, it is available for oral use as tablets or a liquid.

Side effects: see BARBITURATES.

Precautions: women who are pregnant, or who are planning to become pregnant, should seek specialist advice. *See also* BARBITURATES.

Interactions with other drugs: taking two or more anticonvulsants together may increase their adverse effects. Other interactions are those of barbiturates used for treating epilepsy (*see* BARBITURATES).

Proprietary preparation: Mysoline.

Primolut N (Schering Health Care) *See* NORETHISTERONE.

Primoteston Depot (Schering Health Care) *See* TESTOSTERONE.

Primperan (APS-Berk) *See* METOCLOPRAMIDE.

Prioderm (Seton Scholl Healthcare) *See* MALATHION.

Pripsen (Seton Scholl Healthcare) A proprietary combination of *piperazine (an anthelmintic) and sennosides (a laxative; *see* SENNA), used to treat infestations of roundworms or threadworms; sennosides are included to aid elimination of the worms. It is available as an oral powder to be mixed with water or milk and can be obtained without a prescription, but only from pharmacies.

Side effects and precautions: see PIPERAZINE.

Pripsen Mebendazole (Seton Scholl Healthcare) *See* MEBENDAZOLE.

Pripsen Worm Elixir (Seton Scholl Healthcare) *See* PIPERAZINE.

Pro-Banthine (Norton Healthcare) *See* PROPANTHELINE BROMIDE.

probenecid A drug used for the prevention and long-term treatment of gout; it acts by increasing the amount of uric acid excreted in the urine. It is not used to control acute attacks, and may in fact exacerbate symptoms if started during an attack. It may be used in conjunction with *allopurinol. Probenecid also reduces the excretion of *penicillins by the kidneys, and may occasionally be given in conjunction with certain penicillins to increase the concentration of penicillin in the body. It is available as tablets on *prescription only.

Side effects: these are infrequent but may include nausea and vomiting, frequent urination, headache, flushing, dizziness, and sore gums. Occasionally allergic rashes may occur.

Precautions: people taking probenecid must maintain an adequate fluid intake (at least 2 litres a day) to prevent crystals of uric acid being passed in the urine (which can cause pain and bleeding). Probenecid should not be taken by people with kidney stones and it should be used with caution in those with peptic ulcers or kidney disease and in pregnant women.

Interactions with other drugs:

Antibacterials: probenecid increases plasma concentrations of penicillins, cephalosporins, and quinolones.

Antiviral drugs: probenecid increases plasma concentrations of aciclovir, ganciclovir, and zidovudine and may cause toxic effects.

Aspirin: antagonizes the effect of probenecid.

Methotrexate: probenecid increases plasma concentrations of methotrexate and may cause toxic effects.

NSAIDs: probenecid increases plasma concentrations of NSAIDs.

Proprietary preparation: Benemid.

Probeta LA (Trinity Pharmaceuticals) *See* PROPRANOLOL HYDROCHLORIDE.

procainamide hydrochloride A class I *anti-arrhythmic drug for the treatment of *arrhythmias. It is available as tablets on *prescription only.

Side effects: include nausea, diarrhoea, rashes, and fever. *See also* ANTI-ARRHYTHMIC DRUGS.

Precautions: see ANTI-ARRHYTHMIC DRUGS.

Interactions with other drugs: procainamide interacts with a number of drugs to increase the risk of ventricular arrhythmias. These drugs should therefore not be taken with procainamide (see below).

Amiodarone: should not be taken with procainamide.

Antibiotics: trimethoprim increases the plasma concentration of procainamide.

Antihistamines: procainamide should not be taken with astemizole, terfenadine, or mizolastine.

Antipsychotic drugs: procainamide should not be taken with thioridazine, pimozide, or sertindole.

Cimetidine: increases the plasma concentration of procainamide.

Cisapride: should not be taken with procainamide.

Halofantrine: the risk of arrhythmias is increased if this drug is taken with procainamide.

Muscle relaxants: their effects are increased by procainamide.

Sotalol: should not be taken with procainamide.

Tricyclic antidepressants: the risk of arrhythmias is increased if these drugs are taken with procainamide.

Proprietary preparation: Pronestyl.

procaine penicillin <procaine benzylpenicillin> A long-acting form of *benzylpenicillin that may be used in the treatment of syphilis. A *prescription only medicine, it is given by intramuscular injection.

Side effects, precautions, and interactions with other drugs: see BENZYLPENICILLIN; PENICILLINS.

Proprietary preparation: BICILLIN (combined with benzylpenicillin).

procarbazine A *cytotoxic drug used for the treatment of Hodgkin's disease (*see* CANCER), usually in combination with other drugs. It is available as capsules on *prescription only.

Side effects: include nausea and *bone marrow suppression (*see* CYTOTOXIC DRUGS); if an allergic rash develops, treatment may need to be discontinued.

Precautions: see CYTOTOXIC DRUGS. In addition, procarbazine should be used with caution in people with impaired kidney function. Alcohol should not be taken with procarbazine as this combination may result in a severe reaction (including a throbbing headache, palpitation, nausea, and vomiting).

prochlorperazine A phenothiazine *antipsychotic drug used for the treatment of schizophrenia and other psychoses and mania and for the short-term management of severe anxiety. It is also used as an *antiemetic to treat severe nausea and vomiting, especially that produced by chemotherapy or radiotherapy or associated with migraine, and to treat and prevent the vertigo and nausea caused by Ménière's disease or other disorders of the middle ear. Prochlorperazine is available, on *prescription only, as tablets, *buccal tablets, effervescent granules, a syrup, an injection, or suppositories.

Side effects: as for *chlorpromazine, but prochlorperazine is less sedating, produces fewer antimuscarinic effects, and has more pronounced *extrapyramidal reactions.

Precautions, and interactions with other drugs: see CHLORPROMAZINE HYDROCHLORIDE.

Proprietary preparations: Buccastem (buccal tablets); Prozière; Stemetil.

Proctocream HC (Stafford-Miller) *See* PROCTOFOAM HC.

Proctofoam HC (Stafford-Miller) A proprietary combination of *hydrocortisone acetate (a corticosteroid) and *pramoxine <pramocaine> hydrochloride (a local anaesthetic), used in the treatment of *haemorrhoids, inflammation of the bowel, and anal fissures. It is available as a foam in an aerosol on *prescription only; **Proctocream HC** is a cream that can be obtained from pharmacies without a prescription.

Side effects: see CORTICOSTEROIDS.

Precautions: Proctofoam and Proctocream should not be used when viral or fungal infection is present and should not be used for longer than seven days. Proctofoam is not recommended for children.

Proctosedyl (Hoechst Marion Roussel) A proprietary combination of *hydrocortisone (a corticosteroid) and *cinchocaine hydrochloride (a local anaesthetic), used for the treatment of *haemorrhoids and anal inflammation and itching. It is available as an ointment or suppositories on *prescription only.

Side effects: see CORTICOSTEROIDS.

Precautions: Proctosedyl should not be used when viral or fungal infection is present and should not be used for longer than seven days.

procyclidine An *antimuscarinic drug used for the treatment of Parkinson's disease and for the reversal of drug-induced *extrapyramidal reactions (*see* ANTIPARKINSONIAN DRUGS). It is available as tablets or a syrup on *prescription only.
Side effects, precautions, and interactions with other drugs: see BENZHEXOL <TRIHEXYPHENIDYL> HYDROCHLORIDE.
Proprietary preparations: Arpicolin; Kemadrin.

Profasi (Serono Laboratories) *See* HUMAN CHORIONIC GONADOTROPHIN.

Proflex (Novartis Consumer Health) *See* IBUPROFEN.

progesterone A steroid hormone secreted by the ovaries and placenta and also in small amounts by the adrenal glands and the testes. It is responsible for preparing the lining of the uterus (endometrium) for pregnancy. If fertilization occurs progesterone maintains the pregnancy and inhibits the further release of eggs from the ovaries. It is used therapeutically to treat abnormal vaginal bleeding, premenstrual syndrome, and postnatal depression. It is also used to maintain early pregnancies and to treat infertility in *in vitro* fertilization procedures. Progesterone is used as an *adjunct to oestrogens in *hormone replacement therapy (HRT). Progesterone is available, on *prescription only, as a solution for intramuscular injection, a vaginal cream or gel, or *pessaries: because it is rapidly absorbed from the intestine and broken down in the liver it cannot be taken orally. Synthetic versions of progesterone have a variety of therapeutic uses and are major ingredients of hormonal contraceptives (*see* PROGESTOGENS).
Side effects: include acne, urticaria (nettle rash), fluid retention, weight changes, stomach upsets, changes in libido, breast discomfort, premenstrual symptoms, menstrual disturbances, pigmentation of the face, depression, fever, insomnia, sleepiness, loss of hair on the head, and increase in body hair. Local reactions can occur on injection; diarrhoea and flatulence can occur with rectal administration.
Precautions: progesterone should not be given to women with undiagnosed vaginal bleeding and should be used with caution in women with liver disease, diabetes, or epilepsy and in those who suffer from migraine.
Interactions with other drugs: see PROGESTOGENS.
Proprietary preparations: Crinone (vaginal gel for HRT); Cyclogest (pessaries); Gestone (injection).

progestogens A group of steroids that includes the naturally occurring hormone *progesterone, which maintains the normal course of pregnancy, and synthetic equivalents of progesterone: the term is usually restricted to synthetic forms. Synthetic progestogens are used to treat menstrual disorders, including heavy, painful, or irregular periods. Because they prevent the release of egg cells from the ovary, they are major constituents of *oral contraceptives, either alone (in progestogen-only pills) or combined with an *oestrogen. They are also used in other forms of hormonal contraception (*see* DEPOT CONTRACEPTIVES) and in *hormone replacement therapy, and some are used in the treatment of breast and endometrial cancer and *endometriosis. Synthetic progestogens may be taken by mouth, by injection, by implants, or as skin patches. The commonly used progestogens are *desogestrel, *dydrogesterone, *ethynodiol <etynodiol>, *gestodene, *levonorgestrel, *medroxyprogesterone, *norethisterone, and *norgestimate.

Side effects: include irregular menstrual bleeding, breast discomfort, acne, cysts in the ovary, headache, nausea, and weight gain; there may be changes in libido.

Precautions: progestogens should not be taken by women with a history of heart disease, arterial disease, thrombosis, undiagnosed vaginal bleeding, or previous ectopic pregnancy. They should not be taken during pregnancy. They should be used with caution by women with high blood pressure, breast or genital cancer, liver disease, ovarian cysts, or migraine.

Interactions with other drugs:

Antibiotics: rifampicin and rifabutin reduce the contraceptive effects of progestogens. *See* ORAL CONTRACEPTIVES.

Antiepileptic drugs: carbamazepine, phenobarbitone <phenobarbital>, phenytoin, primidone, and topiramate reduce the contraceptive effects of progestogens. *See* ORAL CONTRACEPTIVES.

Cyclosporin: progestogens increase the plasma concentration (and therefore side effects) of cyclosporin.

Griseofulvin: reduces the effects of progestogens. *See* ORAL CONTRACEPTIVES.

Nevirapine: reduces the effects of progestogens.

Tretinoin: when taken orally, tretinoin reduces the contraceptive effects of progestogens.

Prograf (Fujisawa) *See* TACROLIMUS.

proguanil hydrochloride A drug used, usually in combination with *chloroquine, for the prevention of *malaria. It is also used in combination with *atovaquone for the treatment of falciparum malaria. Proguanil is available as tablets and can be obtained from pharmacies without a prescription.

Side effects: these are rare, but may include mild stomach upsets and diarrhoea and, occasionally, mouth ulcers and soreness, rashes, and hair loss.

Precautions: proguanil should be used with caution in people with impaired kidney function. Pregnant women should take folic acid supplements.

Interactions with other drugs:
  Warfarin: the anticoagulant effect of this drug may be enhanced.
Proprietary preparations: Paludrine; MALARONE (combined with atovaquone); PALUDRINE/AVLOCLOR (packaged with chloroquine).

Progynova, Progynova TS (Schering Health Care) *See* OESTRADIOL <ESTRADIOL>; HORMONE REPLACEMENT THERAPY.

prokinetic drugs A group of drugs that act on the gut to stimulate the emptying of the stomach. They therefore prevent reflux of acid and stomach contents (which can cause heartburn) and they also increase the motility of the oesophagus. The common drugs in this group are *metoclopramide and *domperidone, which are *dopamine receptor antagonists. *Cisapride is also prokinetic, but has a different pharmacological action.

Proleukin (Chiron) *See* ALDESLEUKIN.

Proluton Depot (Schering Health Care) *See* HYDROXYPROGESTERONE HEXANOATE <HYDROXYPROGESTERONE CAPROATE>.

promazine hydrochloride A phenothiazine *antipsychotic drug used as an *adjunct for the short-term treatment of moderate or severe agitation, including agitation and restlessness in elderly patients. It is available, on *prescription only, as tablets, a suspension, or an injection.
Side effects, precautions, and interactions with other drugs: see CHLORPROMAZINE HYDROCHLORIDE.

promethazine hydrochloride One of the original (sedating) *antihistamines, used to relieve the symptoms of such allergic conditions as hay fever and urticaria. It is also used as an *antiemetic and as a *hypnotic drug for the short-term treatment of insomnia. Promethazine is available as tablets or an elixir that can be bought from pharmacies without a *prescription, and as a solution for injection on *prescription only.
Side effects: see ANTIHISTAMINES; promethazine may also cause *extrapyramidal reactions.
Precautions and interactions with other drugs: see ANTIHISTAMINES.
Proprietary preparations: Phenergan; Phenergan Nightime (tablets for insomnia); Q-Mazine; Sominex (tablets for insomnia); MEDISED (combined with paracetamol); NIGHT NURSE (combined with paracetamol and dextromethorphan).

promethazine theoclate <promethazine teoclate> An *antihistamine used for the treatment of nausea, vomiting, vertigo, and motion sickness. It is available as tablets without a *prescription.
Side effects: drowsiness is the most common side effect; *see* ANTIHISTAMINES.

Precautions and interactions with other drugs: see ANTIHISTAMINES.
Proprietary preparation: Avomine.

Prominal (Sanofi Winthrop) *See* METHYLPHENOBARBITONE
<METHYLPHENOBARBITAL>.

Pronestyl (Bristol-Myers Squibb) *See* PROCAINAMIDE HYDROCHLORIDE.

Propaderm (GlaxoWellcome) *See* BECLOMETHASONE <BECLOMETASONE>
DIPROPIONATE.

propafenone hydrochloride A class I *anti-arrhythmic drug, that is
also a *beta blocker; it is used in the prevention and treatment of
*arrhythmias. It is available as tablets on *prescription only.
Side effects: include dizziness, nausea, vomiting, bitter taste,
constipation, blurred vision, dry mouth, diarrhoea, headache, fatigue,
and allergic skin reactions.
Precautions: therapy should be initiated under hospital supervision.
Propafenone should be used with caution in patients with liver or kidney
disease or asthma. *See also* ANTI-ARRHYTHMIC DRUGS.
Interactions with other drugs:
  Anticoagulants: the effects of warfarin and nicoumalone
    <acenocoumarol> are enhanced by propafenone.
  Antidepressants: there is an increased risk of arrhythmias if tricyclic
    antidepressants are taken with propafenone.
  Antihistamines: there is an increased risk of arrhythmias if astemizole or
    terfenadine are taken with propafenone.
  Cimetidine: increases the plasma concentration of propafenone.
  Digoxin: propafenone increases the plasma concentration of digoxin,
    whose dosage will therefore need to be reduced.
  Rifampicin: reduces the plasma concentration (and therefore effect) of
    propafenone.
  Ritonavir: should not be taken with propafenone as it increases the
    plasma concentration of propafenone, which increases the risk of
    arrhythmias.
Proprietary preparation: Arythmol.

Propain (Sankyo Pharma) A proprietary combination of *paracetamol
and *codeine (analgesics), *diphenhydramine (an antihistamine), and
*caffeine (a stimulant), used for the relief of headache, migraine,
muscular pains, period pains, and toothache. It is available as tablets and
can be obtained without a prescription, but only from pharmacies.
Side effects: see CODEINE; DIPHENHYDRAMINE; ANTIHISTAMINES.
Precautions: Propain should not be taken by children. *See also*
PARACETAMOL; ANTIHISTAMINES; CAFFEINE.
Interactions with other drugs: see ANTIHISTAMINES.

propamidine isethionate <propamidine isetionate> An *antibiotic used for the treatment of conjunctivitis and infections of the eyelids caused by bacteria. It is available as eye drops or ointment and can be obtained without a prescription, but only from pharmacies.
Proprietary preparations: Brolene (eye drops or ointment); Golden Eye (drops); Golden Eye Ointment.

Propanix, **Propanix SR** (Ashbourne Pharmaceuticals) *See* PROPRANOLOL HYDROCHLORIDE.

propantheline bromide An *antimuscarinic drug used for the relief of gut spasms (*see* ANTISPASMODICS). It is available as tablets on *prescription only.
Side effects and precautions: see ANTIMUSCARINIC DRUGS.
Proprietary preparation: Pro-Banthine.

Propess-RS (Ferring Pharmaceuticals) *See* DINOPROSTONE.

Propine (Allergan) *See* DIPIVEFRIN.

propiverine hydrochloride An *antimuscarinic drug used to treat urinary incontinence and abnormal frequency or urgency in passing urine. It is available as tablets on *prescription only.
Side effects: include dry mouth, blurred vision, and (less frequently) nausea, abdominal discomfort, low blood pressure, drowsiness, difficulty in passing urine, and fatigue. A fast heart rate, restlessness, irritability, hot flushes, and rash are rare side effects.
Precautions: propiverine should not be taken by people with obstruction of the gut, severe ulcerative colitis, glaucoma, impaired liver function, severely impaired kidney function, or by people in whom the outlet of the bladder is obstructed (for example by an enlarged prostate gland), or by women who are pregnant or breastfeeding. It should be used with caution in frail elderly people and in people with heart disease, an overactive thyroid gland, or reflux oesophagitis caused by a hiatus hernia.
Interactions with other drugs: see ANTIMUSCARINIC DRUGS.
Proprietary preparation: Detrunorm.

propranolol hydrochloride A non-cardioselective *beta blocker used for the treatment and prevention of heart *arrhythmias and *angina and for the treatment of *hypertension. It is used after a heart attack to prevent worsening of the condition. It is also used for the prevention of *migraine, the treatment of anxiety, and to relieve the acute symptoms of hyperthyroidism before surgery. It is available, on *prescription only, as tablets, *modified-release capsules, an oral solution, or a solution for injection.
Side effects and precautions: see BETA BLOCKERS; ANTIHYPERTENSIVE DRUGS.
Interactions with other drugs:

Anti-arrhythmic drugs: the adverse effects of lignocaine <lidocaine> are increased if it is taken with propranolol; propafenone increases the plasma concentration of propranolol. *See also* BETA BLOCKERS.

Chlorpromazine: the plasma concentrations of both drugs may be increased if they are taken together.

Fluvoxamine: increases the plasma concentration of propranolol.

Lercanipidine: may increase the effect of propranolol in lowering blood pressure.

Rifampicin: reduces the plasma concentration of propranolol.

For other interactions, *see* BETA BLOCKERS.

Proprietary preparations: Angilol; Apsolol; Bedranol SR (modified-release capsules); Berkolol; Beta-Prograne (modified-release capsules); Cardinol; Half-Beta Prograne (half the strength of Beta-Prograne); Inderal; Inderal LA (modified-release capsules); Half-Inderal LA (half the strength of Inderal LA); Lopranol LA (modified-release capsules); Probeta LA (modified-release capsules); Propanix; Propanix SR (modified-release capsules); INDERETIC and INDEREX (combined with bendrofluazide <bendroflumethiazide>).

proprietary name The trade name of a drug: the name assigned to it by the company who manufactures it. For example, Zantac is a proprietary name for ranitidine. When drugs are first introduced by a pharmaceutical company they are under patent and may only be dispensed or sold under the trade name. On expiry of the patent (usually after ten years) any other company may manufacture the drug, although they will still need a *licence, granted by the Medicines Control Agency, in order to sell the drug under its generic name. Most generic drugs are cheaper than the corresponding proprietary preparations. This is particularly apparent with *over the counter medicines, such as aspirin and paracetamol.

propylthiouracil An antithyroid drug similar to *carbimazole. It is used to treat thyrotoxicosis (overproduction of *thyroid hormones) and also to reduce hormone concentrations before surgery to remove part of an overactive thyroid gland. Propylthiouracil is available as tablets on *prescription only.

Side effects and precautions: *see* CARBIMAZOLE.

Proscar (Merck Sharp & Dohme) *See* FINASTERIDE.

prostaglandins A large group of hormone-like substances that exert their effects close to where they are produced. They are produced by many organs and tissues and have a wide range of actions. For example, they cause contraction of smooth muscle, such as the uterus or intestines, and dilatation of blood vessels, and they are mediators of the inflammatory response (*aspirin and other *NSAIDs act by blocking their production). They are also involved in the production of mucus in the stomach, which provides protection against gastric acid. Synthetic forms

(*analogues) of prostaglandins are used for the treatment of peptic ulcers (*see* MISOPROSTOL), to induce labour and abortion and to treat bleeding after childbirth (*see* CARBOPROST; DINOPROST; DINOPROSTONE; GEMEPROST), and to treat men with erectile dysfunction and babies with congenital heart disease (*see* ALPROSTADIL) and people with glaucoma (*see* LATANOPROST).

Prostap SR, **Prostap 3** (Wyeth Laboratories) *See* LEUPRORELIN.

Prostin E2 (Pharmacia & Upjohn) *See* DINOPROSTONE.

Prostin F2 alpha (Pharmacia & Upjohn) *See* DINOPROST.

Prostin VR (Pharmacia & Upjohn) *See* ALPROSTADIL.

Prosulf (CP Pharmaceuticals) *See* PROTAMINE SULPHATE.

protamine sulphate A drug used to counteract overdosage with *heparin. It is available as a solution for injection on *prescription only.
Side effects: include nausea, vomiting, flushing, low blood pressure, slow heart rate, and breathlessness.
Precautions: there can be allergic reactions in people who have had previous treatment with protamine *insulin or who are allergic to fish.
Proprietary preparation: Prosulf.

protease inhibitors *See* ANTIVIRAL DRUGS.

Prothiaden (Knoll) *See* DOTHIEPIN <DOSULEPIN> HYDROCHLORIDE.

protirelin Thyrotrophin-releasing hormone, which is secreted by the hypothalamus (in the brain) and controls the secretion of thyrotrophin, a hormone that is secreted by the pituitary gland and acts on the thyroid gland to stimulate production of *thyroid hormones. Protirelin is given intravenously to assess the function of the thyroid gland, although its use has largely been superseded by other techniques. Failure of protirelin to produce a rise in plasma thyrotrophin concentrations indicates hyperthyroidism (excessive production of thyroid hormones). Protirelin is available as an injection on *prescription only.
Side effects: an increased desire to pass urine, flushing, dizziness, nausea, and a strange taste in the mouth can occur after rapid injection.
Precautions: protirelin should be used with caution in pregnant women, and in people with an underactive pituitary gland, asthma, chronic bronchitis, or certain heart conditions.
Proprietary preparation: TRH-Cambridge.

Protium (Knoll) *See* PANTOPRAZOLE.

proton pump inhibitors Drugs that inhibit gastric (stomach) acid secretion and are used for the treatment of gastric and duodenal ulcers, reflux oesophagitis, and other types of *acid-peptic disease. They act by inhibiting the movements of hydrogen and potassium ions in the stomach – the so-called proton pump, which causes acid secretion. Proton pump inhibitors produce a more rapid response and promote ulcer healing at a faster rate than *H$_2$-receptor antagonists. In combination with antibiotics, they are used to eradicate *Helicobacter pylori*, a common cause of ulcers. *See* LANSOPRAZOLE; OMEPRAZOLE; PANTOPRAZOLE; RABEPRAZOLE SODIUM.

Side effects: diarrhoea, rash, and headache are among the most common side effects. More details are provided in entries for individual drugs.

Precautions: proton pump inhibitors should be used with caution in women who are pregnant or breastfeeding and in people with liver disease. They should not be used in patients in whom stomach cancer is a possibility without further investigation.

Interactions with other drugs: see entries for individual drugs.

protriptyline hydrochloride A *tricyclic antidepressant drug used for the treatment of depressive illness, particularly in patients who are apathetic and withdrawn. It is available as tablets on *prescription only.

Side effects: similar to those of *amitriptyline, but protriptyline is less sedating and can cause more agitation and anxiety, it can increase the heart rate and cause a fall in blood pressure, and is more likely to cause rashes (exposure to direct sunlight should be avoided).

Precautions and interactions with other drugs: see TRICYCLIC ANTIDEPRESSANTS.

Proprietary preparation: Concordin.

Provera (Pharmacia & Upjohn) *See* MEDROXYPROGESTERONE.

Provigil (Cephalon Europe) *See* MODAFINIL.

Pro-Viron (Schering Health Care) *See* MESTEROLONE.

proxymetacaine *See* LOCAL ANAESTHETICS.

Prozac (Dista) *See* FLUOXETINE.

Prozière (Ashbourne Pharmaceuticals) *See* PROCHLORPERAZINE.

pseudoephedrine A *sympathomimetic drug that constricts blood vessels. It is used mainly as a *decongestant and is included in many oral proprietary preparations for treating colds and coughs. It is similar in action to *ephedrine. Most preparations containing pseudoephedrine can be bought from pharmacies without a prescription.

Side effects, precautions, and interactions with other drugs: see DECONGESTANTS; EPHEDRINE HYDROCHLORIDE.

Proprietary preparations: Boots Decongestant Tablets; Galpseud (tablets and liquid); Sudafed (tablets and liquid); ACTIFED (combined with triprolidine; ACTIFED COMPOUND LINCTUS (combined with dextromethorphan and triprolidine); ACTIFED EXPECTORANT (combined with guaiphenesin <guaifenesin> and triprolidine); ADULT MELTUS EXPECTORANT WITH DECONGESTANT (combined with guaiphenesin <guaifenesin> and menthol); BENYLIN COUGH & CONGESTION (combined with dextromethorphan, diphenhydramine, and menthol); BENYLIN 4 FLU (combined with diphenhydramine and paracetamol); BOOTS CATARRH SYRUP FOR CHILDREN (combined with diphenhydramine); BOOTS NIGHT COLD COMFORT (combined with diphenhydramine, paracetamol, and pholcodine); BRONALIN DRY COUGH (combined with dextromethorphan); CATARRH-EX (combined with paracetamol); DIMOTANE CO (combined with brompheniramine and codeine); DIMOTANE EXPECTORANT (combined with brompheniramine and guaiphenesin <guaifenesin>); DIMOTANE PLUS (combined with brompheniramine); EXPULIN (combined with chlorpheniramine <chlorphenamine>, menthol, and pholcodine); GALPSEUD PLUS (combined with chlorpheniramine <chlorphenamine>); JUNIOR MELTUS DRY COUGH AND CATARRH (combined with dextromethorphan); LEMSIP PHARMACY POWERCAPS (combined with ibuprofen); LEMSIP PHARMACY POWER + PARACETAMOL (combined with paracetamol); MELTUS DRY COUGH (combined with dextromethorphan); NIROLEX FOR DRY COUGHS WITH DECONGESTANT (combined with dextromethorphan); NUROFEN COLDS & FLU (combined with ibuprofen); ROBITUSSIN CHESTY COUGH WITH CONGESTION (combined with guaiphenesin <guaifenesin>); ROBITUSSIN NIGHT-TIME (combined with codeine and brompheniramine); SUDAFED-CO (combined with paracetamol); SUDAFED EXPECTORANT (combined with guaiphenesin <guaifenesin>); SUDAFED LINCTUS (combined with dextromethorphan); SUDAFED PLUS (combined with triprolidine; TIXYLIX COUGH & COLD (combined with chlorpheniramine <chlorphenamine> and pholcodine); VICKS ACTION (combined with ibuprofen).

psoriasis A chronic skin disease in which scaly pink patches form on the elbows, knees, scalp, and other parts of the body, often causing itching. Its cause is not known, but the disorder often runs in families: it most commonly starts in adolescence. Psoriasis sometimes occurs in association with arthritis (psoriatic arthropathy). Occasionally the disease may be very severe, affecting much of the skin and causing considerable disability. While psychological stress may cause an exacerbation of psoriasis, the only significant event that precipitates the disease is a preceding streptococcal infection. Drugs, such as lithium or beta blockers, may occasionally be responsible.

Although there is as yet no cure, treatment of psoriasis has improved greatly in recent years. *Emollients provide relief of symptoms and may be the only treatment required for mild psoriasis. For mild to moderate psoriasis, *dithranol, *coal tar, and *salicylic acid, are often effective; *topical steroids may also be used. The *vitamin D analogues *calcipotriol and *tacalcitol and the *retinoid *tazarotene are newer *topical treatments for moderately severe disease. *Systemic therapy, with drugs such as *methotrexate, *acitretin, or *cyclosporin, is reserved for the worst cases.

Psoriderm (Dermal Laboratories) *See* COAL TAR.

PsoriGel (Galderma) *See* COAL TAR.

Psorin (Cortecs Healthcare) A proprietary combination of *coal tar and *salicylic acid (keratolytics) and *dithranol, used for the treatment of chronic *psoriasis. It is available as a ointment and can be obtained without a prescription, but only from pharmacies.
Precautions: Psorin should not come into contact with the eyes and should not be used with topical steroids. Exposure of treated skin to direct sunlight should be avoided.

Psorin Scalp Gel (Cortecs Healthcare) A proprietary combination of *dithranol and *salicylic acid (a keratolytic), used for the treatment of chronic *psoriasis of the scalp. It can be obtained without a prescription, but only from pharmacies.
Precautions: the gel should not come into contact with the eyes and should not be used with topical steroids. Exposure of the treated scalp to direct sunlight should be avoided. The gel should be washed off after one hour.

Pulmicort Inhaler (AstraZeneca) *See* BUDESONIDE.

Pulmicort Respules (AstraZeneca) *See* BUDESONIDE.

Pulmicort Turbohaler (AstraZeneca) *See* BUDESONIDE.

Pulmo Bailly (Roche Products) A proprietary combination of *codeine (a cough suppressant) and guaiacol (an *expectorant), used to relieve the symptoms of coughs, colds, bronchial catarrh, and other infections of the upper airways, such as pharyngitis or laryngitis. It is available as a liquid without a prescription, but only from pharmacies.
Side effects, precautions, and interactions with other drugs: see CODEINE.

pulmonary embolism *See* THROMBOSIS.

Pulmozyme (Roche Products) *See* DORNASE ALFA.

pumactant A synthetic pulmonary *surfactant that is used to treat breathing difficulties in premature babies who are receiving mechanical ventilation (*see* VENTILATOR). It is also used to prevent breathing difficulties in premature babies. Pumactant is available, on *prescription only, as a suspension that is administered through a tube placed in the trachea (windpipe).
Side effects: pumactant may increase the secretion of mucus, which can obstruct the tube.

Precautions: constant monitoring of heart rate and blood gases is necessary during treatment as pumactant can cause a rapid improvement in the baby's condition and high concentrations of oxygen in the tissues have toxic effects.

Proprietary preparation: Alec.

pumilio pine oil An aromatic oil obtained by distillation of the leaves of a pine tree, *Pino murgo pumilio.* It is used in combination with other aromatic oils in inhalations to relieve coughs and nasal congestion. Pumilio pine oil is also used as a *rubefacient.

Proprietary preparation: KARVOL (combined with other aromatic substances and chlorbutol <chlorobutanol>).

Pump-Hep (Leo Pharmaceuticals) *See* HEPARIN.

Puregon (Organon Laboratories) *See* FOLLITROPIN.

purgatives *See* LAXATIVES.

Puri-Nethol (GlaxoWellcome) *See* MERCAPTOPURINE.

Pylorid (GlaxoWellcome) *See* RANITIDINE BISMUTH CITRATE.

Pyralvex (Norgine) A proprietary combination of anthraquinone glycosides (anti-inflammatory agents) and *salicylic acid (a keratolytic), used for the treatment of mouth ulcers and sores caused by ill-fitting dentures. It is available as a solution and can be obtained without a prescription, but only from pharmacies.

Precautions: Pyralvex is not recommended for children. *See also* SALICYLIC ACID.

pyrazinamide A bactericidal *antibiotic drug used in combination with other drugs for the treatment of *tuberculosis. It is effective only during the first two or three months but is particularly useful in treating tuberculous meningitis. It is available as tablets on *prescription only.

Side effects: pyrazinamide may have adverse effects on the liver, including fever, loss of appetite, liver enlargement, and jaundice; other possible side effects are nausea, vomiting, muscle aches, and itching.

Precautions: people taking pyrazinamide should report symptoms of liver toxicity, such as persistent nausea and vomiting, malaise, and jaundice, to their doctor.

Interactions with other drugs:

Probenecid and sulphinpyrazone <sulfinpyrazone>: the effects of these drugs in treating gout are reduced.

Proprietary preparations: Zinamide; RIFATER (combined with rifampicin and isoniazid).

pyridostigmine An *anticholinesterase drug used for the treatment of myasthenia gravis and, less commonly, to restore motility in the small intestine following surgery. It is less powerful but longer acting than *neostigmine and may be preferable as dosing is less frequent. Pyridostigmine is available as tablets on *prescription only.

Side effects: nausea and vomiting, increased salivation, diarrhoea, and abdominal cramps are the most common side effects.

Precautions: pyridostigmine should not be taken by people with intestinal or urinary obstruction and should be used with caution in those with asthma, low blood pressure, peptic ulcers, epilepsy, Parkinson's disease, or kidney disease.

Interactions with other drugs:

Anti-arrhythmic drugs: procainamide and quinidine antagonize the action of pyridostigmine.

Antibiotics: aminoglycosides, clindamycin, and colistin antagonize the action of pyridostigmine.

Beta blockers: the risk of abnormal heart rhythms (*see* ARRHYTHMIA) is increased; propranolol antagonizes the action of pyridostigmine.

Proprietary preparation: Mestinon.

pyridoxine (vitamin B$_6$) A vitamin of the B group (*see* VITAMIN B COMPLEX) used as a vitamin supplement and to prevent the nerve damage that can occur in those receiving *isoniazid therapy. It is also used to treat a certain type of *anaemia (sideroblastic anaemia) and premenstrual syndrome (although its value in treating this is dubious). In the form of **pyridoxine hydrochloride** it is freely available *over the counter as tablets or *modified-release tablets; these cannot be prescribed on the NHS.

Precautions: pyridoxine may be toxic in high dosages; prolonged use is not recommended.

Interactions with other drugs:

Altretamine: pyridoxine reduces its activity.

Levodopa: its effect is reduced by pyridoxine.

Proprietary preparations: Benadon; Orovite Complement B6 (modified-release tablets); VIGRANON B (combined with other B vitamins).

pyrimethamine A drug that prevents the replication of the parasite that causes *malaria. It is used in combination with *dapsone or sulfadoxine (a *sulphonamide) for the treatment or prevention of malaria, but is no longer used alone for prevention of the disease due to the spread of resistant parasites and is unsuitable for travellers. Pyrimethamine may also be used in the treatment of toxoplasmosis, but it does not have a *licence for this. It is available as tablets on *prescription only.

Side effects: include rashes and insomnia; because pyrimethamine interferes with folic acid metabolism (the antifolate effect) there is a risk of anaemia or other blood disorders.

Precautions: pyrimethamine should be used with caution in people with liver or kidney disease and in women who are breastfeeding. Pregnant women should take folate supplements.

Interactions with other drugs:

Antibiotics: co-trimoxazole and trimethoprim enhance the antifolate effect of pyrimethamine.

Methotrexate: enhances the antifolate effect of pyrimethamine.

Phenytoin: enhances the antifolate effect of pyrimethamine.

Proprietary preparations: Daraprim; FANSIDAR (combined with sulfadoxine); MALOPRIM (combined with dapsone).

Pyrogastrone (Sanofi Winthrop) A proprietary combination of *carbenoxolone sodium (a cytoprotectant agent), *magnesium trisilicate, dried *aluminium hydroxide, and *sodium bicarbonate (antacids), and *alginic acid, used for the treatment of oesophagitis and oesophageal ulcers (*see* ACID-PEPTIC DISEASES). It is available as chewable tablets or a liquid on *prescription only.

Side effects, precautions, and interactions with other drugs: see CARBENOXOLONE SODIUM; ANTACIDS.

Q

Q-Mazine (Seton Scholl Healthcare) *See* PROMETHAZINE HYDROCHLORIDE.

Quellada-M (Stafford-Miller) *See* MALATHION.

Questran, Questran Light (Bristol-Myers Squibb) *See* CHOLESTYRAMINE <COLESTYRAMINE>.

quetiapine An atypical *antipsychotic drug that is used for the treatment of schizophrenia. It reduces both the positive symptoms (e.g. delusions) and the negative symptoms (e.g. apathy) of the disease without causing *extrapyramidal reactions. Quetiapine is available as tablets on *prescription only.

Side effects: include weight gain, dizziness, low blood pressure on standing (which can cause fainting in some people), sleepiness, indigestion, constipation, dry mouth, a running nose, and a fast heart rate. Quetiapine may prolong a certain phase of the heartbeat (the QT interval), which can lead to *arrhythmias, and reduce the numbers of certain white blood cells.

Precautions: quetiapine should not be taken by women who are breastfeeding. It should be used with caution in pregnant women and in people with cardiovascular disease, a history of stroke or epilepsy, Parkinson's disease, or liver or kidney impairment. It should also be used with care in people taking other drugs that prolong the QT interval (such as some antimalarial drugs, tricyclic antidepressants, and antihistamines).

Interactions with other drugs:

Anaesthetics: their effect in lowering blood pressure is increased.

Antidepressants: there is an increased risk of antimuscarinic effects and arrhythmias if quetiapine is taken with tricyclic antidepressants.

Antiepileptic drugs: quetiapine antagonizes the effects of these drugs in controlling seizures; phenytoin increases the metabolism of quetiapine, whose dosage may therefore need to be increased.

Antihistamines: there is an increased risk of arrhythmias if quetiapine is taken with astemizole or terfenadine.

Halofantrine: there is an increased risk of arrhythmias if this drug is taken with quetiapine.

Ritonavir: may increase the effects of quetiapine.

Sedatives: the sedative effects of quetiapine are increased if it is taken with anxiolytic or hypnotic drugs, or any other drug that causes sedation.

Proprietary preparation: Seroquel.

quinagolide A *dopamine receptor agonist, very similar to

*bromocriptine, used to reduce elevated prolactin concentrations in certain types of infertility. It is available as tablets on *prescription only.

Side effects: include nausea, headache, dizziness, fatigue, loss of appetite, gastrointestinal disturbances, insomnia, oedema (swelling), flushing, nasal congestion, low blood pressure, and psychiatric disturbances.

Precautions: quinagolide should not be taken by people with kidney or liver impairment and should be used with caution in those who have a history of psychiatric disorders. Women should stop taking the drug if they become pregnant.

Interactions with other drugs:

  Dopamine antagonists: may reduce its effect.

Proprietary preparation: Norprolac.

quinalbarbitone <secobarbital> An intermediate-acting *barbiturate used for the short-term treatment of severe insomnia in people who are already taking barbiturates. A *controlled drug, it is available as capsules.

Side effects, precautions, and interactions with other drugs: see BARBITURATES.

Proprietary preparations: Seconal Sodium; TUINAL (combined with amylobarbitone <amobarbital>).

quinapril An *ACE inhibitor used as an adjunct to *diuretics for the treatment of *heart failure. It is also used to treat all grades of *hypertension. It is available as tablets on *prescription only.

Side effects, precautions, and interactions with other drugs: see ACE INHIBITORS.

Proprietary preparations: Accupro; ACCURETIC (combined with hydrochlorothiazide).

See also ANTIHYPERTENSIVE DRUGS.

quinidine bisulphate A class I *anti-arrhythmic drug used for treatment and prevention of certain disorders of heart rhythms, usually ventricular or supraventricular tachycardia (*see* ARRHYTHMIA). It is available as tablets on *prescription only.

Side effects: include nausea, diarrhoea, hypotension (low blood pressure), rashes, fever, and arrhythmias (the so called 'quinidine syncope').

Precautions: quinidine should not be given to patients with heart block. Low doses are given initially and increased as necessary. *See also* ANTI-ARRHYTHMIC DRUGS.

Interactions with other drugs: quinidine interacts with a number of other drugs to increase the risk of ventricular arrhythmias. These drugs should therefore not be taken with quinidine (see below).

  Other anti-arrhythmic drugs: amiodarone should not be taken with quinidine; the plasma concentration of propafenone is increased by quinidine. Depression of heart function is increased if quinidine is taken with any other anti-arrhythmic.

Antihistamines: quinidine should not be taken with astemizole, terfenadine, or mizolastine.

Antimalarial drugs: the risk of arrhythmias is increased if mefloquine or halofantrine are taken with quinidine.

Antipsychotic drugs: quinidine should not be taken with thioridazine, pimozide, or sertindole.

Antiviral drugs: quinidine should not be taken with nelfinavir or ritonavir.

Cimetidine: increases the plasma concentration of quinidine.

Digoxin: quinidine increases the plasma concentration (and toxicity) of digoxin, whose dosage should therefore be reduced.

Rifampicin: reduces the plasma concentration of quinidine.

Sotalol: should not be taken with quinidine.

Tricyclic antidepressants: the risk of arrhythmias is increased if these drugs are taken with quinidine.

Proprietary preparation: Kinidin Durules.

quinine A drug used to treat falciparum *malaria and malarias in which the causative species of *Plasmodium* is not known. Quinine is also used, at a much lower dosage, to prevent leg cramps at night. It is available, on *prescription only, as tablets (quinine sulphate) or an injection (quinine dihydrochloride).

Side effects: at dosages used to treat malaria, side effects include ringing in the ears, headache, hot flushed skin, nausea, abdominal pain, rashes, disturbed vision, confusion, allergic reactions, blood disorders, acute kidney failure, *arrhythmias and other cardiovascular effects, and (especially after injection) low blood sugar.

Precautions: quinine is extremely toxic in overdosage: immediate advice must be sought from a poisons centre. Quinine must not be taken by people with certain blood disorders or optic neuritis (inflammation of the optic nerve). It should be used with caution by women who are pregnant or breastfeeding and by people with atrial fibrillation (*see* ARRHYTHMIA) or certain other heart conditions.

Interactions with other drugs:

Amiodarone: should not be used with quinine because the risk of ventricular arrhythmias is increased.

Antihistamines: astemizole and terfenadine should not be used with quinine because the risk of ventricular arrhythmias is increased.

Cimetidine: increases the plasma concentration (and possibly side effects) of quinine.

Cisapride: should not be used with quinine because the risk of ventricular arrhythmias is increased.

Digoxin: quinine increases the plasma concentration of digoxin, whose dosage may therefore need to be reduced.

Flecainide: quinine increases the plasma concentration of flecainide.

Halofantrine: should not be taken with quinine because of the risk of possibly fatal arrhythmias.

Mefloquine: there is an increased risk of convulsions.

Pimozide: should not be taken with quinine because the risk of ventricular arrhythmias is increased.

Quinocort (Quinoderm) A proprietary combination of *potassium hydroxyquinoline (an antifungal agent) and *hydrocortisone (a corticosteroid), used for the treatment of a variety of skin conditions in which infection is present or suspected. It is available as a cream on *prescription only.

Side effects and precautions: see TOPICAL STEROIDS.

Quinoderm (Quinoderm) A proprietary combination of *benzoyl peroxide (a keratolytic) and *potassium hydroxyquinoline sulphate (an antibacterial and antifungal drug), used for the treatment of acne and infected hair follicles. It is available as a cream or a lotion and can be obtained without a prescription, but only from pharmacies.

Side effects and precautions: see BENZOYL PEROXIDE.

quinolones (4-quinolones) A group of bactericidal *antibiotic drugs that are used mainly to treat infections that are resistant to *penicillin. They act by inhibiting enzymes that maintain the structure of bacterial DNA and are active against a wide range of bacteria. *See* CIPROFLOXACIN; CINOXACIN; LEVOFLOXACIN; NALIDIXIC ACID; NORFLOXACIN; OFLOXACIN.

Side effects: include nausea, vomiting, abdominal pain, diarrhoea, indigestion, and flatulence. More rare side effects are antibiotic-associated inflammation of the bowel, headache, dizziness, sleep disorders, rash, itching, fever, skin sensitivity to light, joint and muscle aches, and blood disorders.

Precautions: quinolones are not recommended for children or growing adolescents or for pregnant women. They should be discontinued if mental disturbance or allergic reactions (such as rashes) occur after the first dose. Driving ability may be impaired and the effects of alcohol are enhanced in people taking these drugs.

Interactions with other drugs:

Antacids: reduce the absorption of ciprofloxacin, levofloxacin, norfloxacin, and ofloxacin.

Anticoagulants: the anticoagulant effects of warfarin and nicoumalone <acenocoumarol> are increased by ciprofloxacin, nalidixic acid, norfloxacin, and ofloxacin.

Cyclosporin: there is an increased risk of kidney toxicity.

NSAIDs: there is an increased risk of convulsions.

Sucralfate: reduces the absorption of ciprofloxacin, levofloxacin, norfloxacin, and ofloxacin.

Theophylline: plasma concentration of theophylline is enhanced by ciprofloxacin and norfloxacin.

Quinoped (Quinoderm) A proprietary combination of *benzoyl peroxide (a keratolytic) and *potassium hydroxyquinoline sulphate (an antifungal drug), used for the treatment of athlete's foot and similar fungal infections. It is available as a cream and can be obtained without a prescription, but only from pharmacies.

Side effects and precautions: see BENZOYL PEROXIDE.

Qvar, Qvar Autohaler (3M Health Care) *See* BECLOMETHASONE <BECLOMETASONE> DIPROPRIONATE.

R

rabeprazole sodium A *proton pump inhibitor used for the treatment of gastric or duodenal ulcers and gastro-oesophageal reflux disease (*see* ACID-PEPTIC DISEASES). It is available as *enteric-coated tablets on *prescription only.

Side effects: include headache, diarrhoea, rashes, itching, dizziness, nausea and vomiting, constipation, flatulence, muscle and joint pain, chest pain, inflammation of the mouth lining, cough, and a running nose.

Precautions: see PROTON PUMP INHIBITORS.

Proprietary preparation: Pariet.

Radian-B Heat Spray (Roche Products) *See* RADIAN-B MUSCLE LOTION.

Radian-B Muscle Lotion (Roche Products) A proprietary combination of *camphor, *menthol, ammonium *salicylate, and *salicylic acid, used as a *rubefacient for the relief of muscular and rheumatic aches, pains, and stiffness, including pulled muscles, tennis elbow, and golf shoulder. **Radian-B Heat Spray** is an aerosol formulation. Both preparations are freely available *over the counter.

Side effects and precautions: see RUBEFACIENTS; SALICYLATES.

Radian-B Muscle Rub (Roche Products) A proprietary combination of *camphor, *menthol, *methyl salicylate, and capsicin (*see* CAPSICUM OLEORESIN) in the form of a cream, used as a *rubefacient for the relief of muscular and rheumatic aches, pains, and stiffness. It is freely available *over the counter.

Side effects and precautions: see RUBEFACIENTS; SALICYLATES.

Ralgex Cream (Seton Scholl Healthcare) A proprietary combination of glycol monosalicylate (*see* GLYCOL SALICYLATE), *methyl nicotinate, and *capsicum oleoresin, used as a *rubefacient for the relief of muscular and rheumatic aches, pains and stiffness. It is freely available *over the counter.

Side effects and precautions: see RUBEFACIENTS; SALICYLATES.

Ralgex Freeze Spray (Seton Scholl Healthcare) A proprietary combination of glycol monosalicylate (*see* GLYCOL SALICYLATE) in a propellant of isopentane and dimethylether that provides a cooling action on the skin (*see* RUBEFACIENTS). It is used for the relief of muscular and rheumatic pain and sprains and stiffness, including backache, sciatica, and lumbago. It is freely available *over the counter.

Side effects and precautions: see RUBEFACIENTS; SALICYLATES.

Ralgex Heat Spray (Seton Scholl Healthcare) A proprietary combination of glycol monosalicylate (*see* GLYCOL SALICYLATE) and *methyl nicotinate, used as a *rubefacient for the relief of muscular and rheumatic aches, pains, and stiffness, including backache, sciatica, and lumbago. It is freely available *over the counter .
Side effects and precautions: see RUBEFACIENTS; SALICYLATES.

Ralgex Stick (Seton Scholl Healthcare) A proprietary combination of *glycol salicylate, *ethyl salicylate, *methyl salicylate, capsicin (*see* CAPSICUM OLEORESIN), and *menthol, used as a *rubefacient for the relief of muscular and rheumatic aches, pains, and stiffness, including backache, sciatica, and lumbago. It is freely available *over the counter.
Side effects and precautions: see RUBEFACIENTS; SALICYLATES.

raloxifene A drug that acts selectively on *oestrogen receptors in the body: it mimics the action of oestrogen in the bones, heart, and arteries, but does not have oestrogenic effects in the uterus and breast. As a result, raloxifene can increase bone density and therefore protect against osteoporosis, which often develops after the menopause, without increasing the risk of cancer of the uterus or breast. Raloxifene is used to prevent fractures of the bones in the spine caused by osteoporosis in postmenopausal women; it has also been shown to reduce the concentrations of cholesterol in the blood and may therefore protect against cardiovascular disease. However, it does not relieve hot flushes and other symptoms of the menopause. Raloxifene is available as tablets on *prescription only.
Side effects: include hot flushes, leg cramps, and swelling (oedema) of the ankles. There is a risk of blood clots forming in the veins (*see* THROMBOSIS).
Precautions: raloxifene should not be taken by women with a history of venous thrombosis or by those with liver disease, severe kidney disease, cancer of the breast or lining of the uterus, or undiagnosed vaginal bleeding.
Interactions with other drugs:
  Anticoagulants: raloxifene opposes the anticoagulant effects of warfarin and nicoumalone <acenocoumarol>.
  Cholestyramine <colestyramine>: reduces the absorption of raloxifene.
Proprietary preparation: Evista.

raltitrexed An *antimetabolite used for the palliative treatment of advanced *cancers of the colon and rectum. It is usually given when *fluorouracil has not been effective or well tolerated or is inappropriate. Raltitrexed is available as an injection on *prescription only.
Side effects: include nausea and vomiting, diarrhoea, blood disorders, weight loss, dehydration, rash, weakness, fever, pain, and headache. *See also* CYTOTOXIC DRUGS.
Precautions: raltitrexed should not be given to patients with severe liver

or kidney disease or to women who are pregnant or breastfeeding. *See also* CYTOTOXIC DRUGS.

Proprietary preparation: Tomudex.

ramipril An *ACE inhibitor used as an adjunct to *diuretics for the treatment of *heart failure. It is also used to treat mild to moderate *hypertension and after heart attacks to prevent disease progression in patients with heart failure. It is available as capsules on *prescription only.

Side effects, precautions, and interactions with other drugs: see ACE INHIBITORS.

Proprietary preparation: Tritace.

See also ANTIHYPERTENSIVE DRUGS.

Ramysis (ISIS Products) *See* DOXYCYCLINE.

ranitidine An *H_2-receptor antagonist used in the treatment of gastric and duodenal ulcers, reflux oesophagitis, and Zollinger-Ellison syndrome and in the treatment and prevention of ulcers caused by the use of *NSAIDs (*see* ACID-PEPTIC DISEASES). It is available, as tablets, effervescent tablets, a sugar-free syrup, or an injection, on *prescription only. Packs containing no more than two weeks' supply of tablets, for the relief of indigestion and heartburn in people over 16 years old, can be obtained from pharmacies without a prescription.

Side effects: include diarrhoea, dizziness, rash, tiredness, and reversible liver changes; rare side effects are reversible confusion, blood disorders, and muscle or joint pain. In high doses ranitidine can cause breast enlargement in men.

Precautions: ranitidine should be used with caution by people who have poor kidney function and by women who are pregnant or breastfeeding.

Proprietary preparations: Rantac; Zaedoc; Zantac; Zantac Effervescent.

ranitidine bismuth citrate An *H_2-receptor antagonist with *cytoprotectant action, used for the treatment of duodenal or gastric ulcers and as an *adjunct to antibiotics (clarithromycin and amoxycillin <amoxicillin> or metronidazole) for the eradication of *Helicobacter pylori* (*see* ACID-PEPTIC DISEASES). It is available as tablets on *prescription only.

Side effects: include darkening of the tongue and blackening of stools, diarrhoea or other gastrointestinal upsets, headache, anaemia, and (rarely) blood disorders, confusion, and (in men) breast enlargement.

Precautions: ranitidine bismuth citrate should not be taken by people with severe kidney disease or by women who are pregnant or breastfeeding.

Proprietary preparation: Pylorid.

Rantac (APS-Berk) *See* RANITIDINE.

Rap-Eze (Roche Products) *See* CALCIUM CARBONATE.

Rapilysin (Roche Products) *See* RETEPLASE.

Rapitil (Pantheon Healthcare) *See* NEDOCROMIL SODIUM.

razoxane A *cytotoxic drug that has been used for the treatment of leukaemia (*see* CANCER); it has now largely been replaced by more effective drugs. Razoxane is available as tablets on *prescription only.
Side effects, precautions, and interactions with other drugs: see CYTOTOXIC DRUGS.

Rebif (Serono Laboratories) *See* INTERFERON-BETA.

reboxetine A drug that inhibits the reuptake of the neurotransmitter *noradrenaline <norepinephrine> and thus prolongs its action in the brain. It is used for the treatment of depression (*see* ANTIDEPRESSANT DRUGS). Reboxetine is available as tablets on *prescription only.
Side effects: include insomnia, sweating, low blood pressure on standing up, dizziness, difficulties in passing urine, impotence, dry mouth, constipation, and a fast heart rate.
Precautions: reboxetine is not recommended for women who are pregnant or breastfeeding. It should be used with caution in people with severe kidney or liver impairment, a history of epilepsy, manic depressive illness, urinary retention, or glaucoma.
Interactions with other drugs: reboxetine should not be taken with the following drugs: anti-arrhythmics, antipsychotics, cyclosporin, fluvoxamine, imidazoles and triazoles (antifungal drugs), macrolide antibiotics, and tricyclic antidepressants.
  MAOIs: reboxetine should not be started until two weeks after stopping MAOIs; MAOIs should not be started until at least one week after reboxetine has been stopped.
Proprietary preparation: Edronax.

Recombinate (Baxter Hyland) *See* FACTOR VIII.

Redoxon (Roche Products) *See* VITAMIN C.

Refludan (Hoechst Marion Roussel) *See* LEPIRUDIN.

reflux oesophagitis *See* ACID-PEPTIC DISEASES.

Refolinon (Pharmacia & Upjohn) *See* FOLINIC ACID.

Refresh Ophthalmic Solution (Allergan) *See* POLYVINYL ALCOHOL.

Regaine (Pharmacia & Upjohn) *See* MINOXIDIL.

Regulan (Procter & Gamble) *See* ISPAGHULA HUSK.

Regulose (Novartis Pharmaceuticals) *See* LACTULOSE.

Rehidrat (Searle) A proprietary combination of *potassium chloride, *sodium bicarbonate, *citric acid, and the sugars glucose, sucrose, and fructose, used for the replacement of fluid and *electrolytes in cases of dehydration (*see* ORAL REHYDRATION THERAPY). It is available as a powder to be dissolved in water and can be obtained without a prescription, but only from pharmacies.
Precautions: Rehidrat should not be taken by people with impaired kidney function or intestinal obstruction.

Relaxit Micro-enema (Crawford Pharmaceuticals) A proprietary combination of *sodium citrate (an osmotic laxative) and *sodium lauryl sulphoacetate (a wetting agent), used for the treatment of constipation. It can be obtained without a prescription, but only from pharmacies.
Precautions: see SODIUM CITRATE.

Relaxyl (Seton Scholl Healthcare) *See* ALVERINE CITRATE.

Relcofen (Cox Pharmaceuticals) *See* IBUPROFEN.

Relefact LH-RH (Hoechst Marion Roussel) *See* GONADORELIN.

Relifex (SmithKline Beecham Consumer Healthcare) *See* NABUMETONE.

Remedeine (Napp Pharmaceuticals) A proprietary combination of *paracetamol (a non-opioid analgesic) and *dihydrocodeine tartrate (a weak opioid analgesic), used for the relief of mild to moderate pain. It is available as tablets or effervescent tablets; **Remedeine Forte** contains higher doses of dihydrocodeine. Both preparations are available on *prescription only.
Side effects and precautions: see PARACETAMOL; MORPHINE. Remedeine preparations are not recommended for children, and the dosage of Remedeine Forte should be reduced for elderly people.
Interactions with other drugs: see OPIOIDS.

Remegel (Seton Scholl Healthcare) *See* CALCIUM CARBONATE.

Remnos (DDSA Pharmaceuticals) *See* NITRAZEPAM.

Rennie (Roche Products) A proprietary combination of the antacids *calcium carbonate and *magnesium carbonate, used for the relief of indigestion, heartburn, flatulence, and stomach upset (*see* ACID-PEPTIC DISEASES). It is freely available *over the counter in the form of chewable tablets.
Side effects and interactions with other drugs: see ANTACIDS.
Precautions: Rennies are not recommended for children under six years old.

Rennie Deflatine (Roche Products) A proprietary combination of *magnesium carbonate and *calcium carbonate (antacids) and activated *dimethicone <dimeticone> (an antifoaming agent), used for the relief of indigestion, heartburn, stomach upset, uncomfortable bloating, flatulence, and painful trapped wind (*see* ACID-PEPTIC DISEASES). It is freely available *over the counter in the form of chewable tablets.
Side effects, precautions, and interactions with other drugs: see ANTACIDS.

Rennie Rap-Eze (Roche Products) *See* CALCIUM CARBONATE.

ReoPro (Eli Lilly & Co) *See* ABCIXIMAB.

repaglinide An oral antidiabetic drug that acts by stimulating the release of *insulin; it is taken shortly before meals. Repaglinide is used for the treatment of noninsulin-dependent *diabetes mellitus that has not responded to dieting; it can also be given with *metformin when the diabetes is inadequately controlled by metformin alone. Repaglinide is available as tablets on *prescription only.
Side effects: include abdominal pain, constipation, diarrhoea, nausea and vomiting, and allergic reactions (such as rashes).
Precautions: repaglinide should not be taken by people with severe liver or kidney disease or by women who are pregnant or breastfeeding.
Interactions with other drugs:
  Antifungal drugs: fluconazole, itraconazole, and ketoconazole may increase the plasma concentration (and therefore effects) of repaglinide.
  Erythromycin: may increase the plasma concentration (and therefore effects) of repaglinide.
  Rifampicin: may reduce the plasma concentration (and therefore effects) of repaglinide.
Proprietary preparation: NovoNorm.

Replenate (Bio Products Laboratory) *See* FACTOR VIII.

Replenine (Bio Products Laboratory) *See* FACTOR IX.

Replens (Ethical Research Marketing) A proprietary non-hormonal vaginal preparation consisting of purified water with other ingredients that increase its acidity. Providing a high moisture content in the vagina, it is used to relieve the vaginal dryness, itching, and discomfort that can occur at the menopause; its effects last for 2–3 days. Replens is freely available *over the counter as a liquid in prefilled applicators.

reproterol hydrochloride A *sympathomimetic drug that stimulates beta *adrenoceptors. It is used as a *bronchodilator in the treatment of asthma, bronchitis, and emphysema. Reproterol is available as a metered-dose aerosol *inhaler on *prescription only.

Side effects, precautions, and interactions with other drugs: see
SALBUTAMOL.
Proprietary preparation: Bronchodil.

Requip (SmithKline Beecham Pharmaceuticals) *See* ROPINIROLE.

Resiston One (Rhône-Poulenc Rorer) A proprietary combination of
*sodium cromoglycate <cromoglicate> (a chromone) and
*xylometazoline (a decongestant), used for the treatment and prevention
of hay fever. It is available as a nasal spray and can be obtained without a
prescription, but only from pharmacies.
Side effects: there may be nasal irritation.

Resolve (Seton Scholl Healthcare) *See* PARACETAMOL.

Resonium-A (Sanofi Winthrop) *See* SODIUM POLYSTYRENE SULPHONATE.

resorcinol A *keratolytic that is used, usually in combination with
*sulphur, in skin preparations for the treatment of acne and other greasy
skin conditions. It is available without a prescription, but only from
pharmacies.
Side effects: resorcinol may cause mild irritation of the skin.
Precautions: resorcinol should not be applied to large areas of skin, in
high concentrations, or for a prolonged period, especially in children, as
it can be absorbed and interfere with the production of thyroid
hormones. It may deepen the colour of dark skins or darken light hair.
Proprietary preparation: ESKAMEL (combined with sulphur).

Respacal (UCB Pharma) *See* TULOBUTEROL HYDROCHLORIDE.

Respontin (Allen & Hanburys) *See* IPRATROPIUM BROMIDE.

Restandol (Organon Laboratories) *See* TESTOSTERONE.

reteplase A *fibrinolytic drug used to dissolve blood clots in the
coronary arteries (which supply the heart) in people who have had a
heart attack; treatment should be started within 12 hours of the attack.
Reteplase is available in a form for intravenous injection on *prescription
only.
Side effects, precautions, and interactions with other drugs: see
FIBRINOLYTIC DRUGS.
Proprietary preparation: Rapilysin.

Retin-A (Janssen-Cilag) *See* TRETINOIN.

retinoids A group of drugs derived from vitamin A. On the skin they
act to cause drying, peeling, and a reduction in the production of sebum
(oil). These effects can be useful in the treatment of *acne, *psoriasis, and

other skin disorders. Severe conditions may be treated with retinoids given by mouth, but this must be under hospital supervision. Retinoids include *acitretin, *tretinoin, *isotretinoin, and *tazarotene. They are available as tablets or topical preparations on *prescription only. Retinoids can cause abnormalities in the fetus. They should therefore not be taken during pregnancy, and precautions should be taken to avoid becoming pregnant during (and for some retinoids up to two years after) treatment. Breastfeeding should also be avoided during treatment as retinoids can have adverse effects on the babies of breastfeeding mothers.

retinol *See* VITAMIN A.

Retinova (Janssen-Cilag) *See* TRETINOIN.

Retrovir (GlaxoWellcome) *See* ZIDOVUDINE.

Revanil (Roche Products) *See* LYSURIDE MALEATE <LISURIDE MALEATE>.

reverse transcriptase inhibitors *See* ANTIVIRAL DRUGS.

Rheumacin LA (Hillcross Pharmaceuticals) *See* INDOMETHACIN <INDOMETACIN>.

Rheumox (Wyeth Laboratories) *See* AZAPROPAZONE.

Rhinocort Aqua (AstraZeneca) *See* BUDESONIDE.

Rhinolast (ASTA Medica) *See* AZELASTINE HYDROCHLORIDE.

Rhuaka (Anglian Pharma) A proprietary combination of the stimulant laxatives *cascara, *senna, and rhubarb, used for the relief of occasional constipation. It is freely available *over the counter as a syrup.
Side effects: see STIMULANT LAXATIVES.
Precautions: Rhuaka should not be given to children under seven years old. *See also* STIMULANT LAXATIVES.

Rhumalgan CR (Lagap Pharmaceuticals) *See* DICLOFENAC SODIUM.

ribavirin *See* TRIBAVIRIN.

riboflavine (<riboflavin>; **vitamin B$_2$**) A vitamin of the B group (*see* VITAMIN B COMPLEX). It is an ingredient of vitamin B and multivitamin preparations to treat vitamin deficiency.
Proprietary preparations: PABRINEX (combined with other B vitamins and vitamin C); VIGRANON B (combined with other B vitamins).

Ridaura (Yamanouchi Pharma) *See* AURANOFIN.

Rideril (DDSA Pharmaceuticals) *See* THIORIDAZINE.

rifabutin An *antibiotic used for the prevention of infection in immunocompromised patients and also for the treatment of *tuberculosis. It is available as capsules on *prescription only.

Side effects: include gastrointestinal upset, blood disorders, and discoloration of skin and urine.

Precautions: rifabutin should be used with caution in people with liver or kidney impairment and in women who are pregnant or breastfeeding.

Interactions with other drugs:

Anti-arrhythmic drugs: plasma concentrations of disopyramide, mexiletine, propafenone, and quinidine are reduced.

Anticoagulants: the effects of warfarin and nicoumalone <acenocoumarol> are reduced.

Antiepileptic drugs: the effects of carbamazepine and phenytoin are reduced.

Antifungal drugs: fluconazole and possibly other triazoles increase the effects of rifabutin, whose dosage should therefore be reduced.

Antiviral drugs: rifabutin should not be taken with ritonavir or saquinavir. When rifabutin is taken with indinavir its effects are increased and those of indinavir are reduced; their dosages should therefore be adjusted. Nelfinavir increases the effects of rifabutin, whose dosage should therefore be reduced.

Clarithromycin: increases the risk of the toxic effects of rifabutin, whose dosage should therefore be reduced.

Corticosteroids: the effects of these drugs are reduced.

Cyclosporin: plasma concentrations of cyclosporin are reduced.

Oral contraceptives: their contraceptive effect is reduced.

Sulphonylureas: the effects of these oral antidiabetic drugs are reduced.

Proprietary preparation: Mycobutin.

Rifadin (Hoechst Marion Roussel) *See* RIFAMPICIN.

rifampicin An *antibiotic that is especially useful in the treatment of *tuberculosis, when it is usually used in combination with other antituberculosis drugs, such as *isoniazid and *pyrazinamide. It is also used in the treatment of leprosy, brucellosis, legionnaires' disease, and serious staphylococcal infections. Rifampicin is used to prevent meningitis in carriers of the infecting organisms. It is available, on *prescription only, as tablets, capsules, or a syrup for oral use and as a solution for intravenous injection.

Side effects: transient disturbances of liver function may occur, but these do not normally require the treatment to be stopped. Other possible side effects are gastrointestinal disturbances, including nausea, vomiting, and diarrhoea. Intermittent therapy may cause influenza-like symptoms (fever, chills, dizziness, bone pain), wheezing and breathlessness, anaemia, kidney failure, flushing, urticaria and rashes, oedema, muscular weakness, blood disorders, and menstrual disturbances. Urine, saliva, and other body fluids may become coloured orange-red, but this is harmless; discoloration of contact lenses may occur.

Precautions: rifampicin should not be taken by patients with jaundice or porphyria and must be used with caution in those with impairment of liver or kidney function and in women who are pregnant or breastfeeding.

Interactions with other drugs:

Anti-arrhythmic drugs: plasma concentrations of disopyramide, mexiletine, propafenone, and quinidine are reduced.

Anticoagulant drugs: the effects of warfarin and nicoumalone <acenocoumarol> are reduced.

Antidiabetic drugs: the effects of sulphonylureas and repaglinide are reduced.

Antiepileptic drugs: the effects of carbamazepine and phenytoin are reduced.

Antifungal drugs: their effects are reduced.

Antiviral drugs: rifampicin should not be taken with indinavir, nelfinaquir, or saquinavir.

Atovaquone: its effects are reduced by rifampicin.

Calcium antagonists: the effects of diltiazem, nifedipine, and nisoldipine are reduced by rifampicin.

Chloramphenicol: plasma concentrations of chloramphenicol are reduced.

Corticosteroids: the effects of these drugs are reduced.

Cyclosporin: plasma concentrations of cyclosporin are reduced.

Oral contraceptives: their contraceptive effect is reduced; extra contraception is required by women who take them.

Proprietary preparations: Rifadin; Rimactane; RIFATER (combined with isoniazid and pyrazinamide); RIFINAH (combined with isoniazid); RIMACTAZID (combined with isoniazid).

Rifater (Hoechst Marion Roussel) A proprietary combination of *isoniazid, *pyrazinamide, and *rifampicin, used for the treatment of *tuberculosis. It is available as tablets on *prescription only.
Side effects, precautions, and interactions with other drugs: *see* ISONIAZID; PYRAZINAMIDE; RIFAMPICIN.

Rifinah (Hoechst Marion Roussel) A proprietary combination of *isoniazid and *rifampicin, used for the treatment of tuberculosis. It is available as tablets on *prescription only.
Side effects, precautions, and interactions with other drugs: *see* ISONIAZID; RIFAMPICIN.

Rilutek (Rhône-Poulenc Rorer) *See* RILUZOLE.

riluzole A drug used in the treatment of motor neurone disease. It can only be used under specialist supervision. Riluzole is available as tablets on *prescription only.

Side effects: include weakness, nausea, vomiting, a fast heart rate, abdominal pain, dizziness, somnolence, tingling.

Precautions: riluzole should not be taken by people with severe liver disease.

Proprietary preparation: Rilutek.

Rimacid (Norton Healthcare; Ranbaxy) *See* INDOMETHACIN <INDOMETACIN>.

Rimacillin (Ranbaxy) *See* AMPICILLIN.

Rimactane (Novartis Pharmaceuticals) *See* RIFAMPICIN.

Rimactazid (Novartis Pharmaceuticals) A proprietary combination of *isoniazid and *rifampicin, used for the treatment of tuberculosis. It is available as tablets on *prescription only.

Side effects, precautions, and interactions with other drugs: see ISONIAZID; RIFAMPICIN.

Rimafen (Ranbaxy) *See* IBUPROFEN.

Rimapam (Ranbaxy) *See* DIAZEPAM.

Rimapurinol (Ranbaxy) *See* ALLOPURINOL.

Rimoxallin (Ranbaxy) *See* AMOXYCILLIN <AMOXICILLIN>.

Rimso-50 (Britannia Pharmaceuticals) *See* DIMETHYL SULPHOXIDE.

Rinatec (Boehringer Ingelheim) *See* IPRATROPIUM BROMIDE.

ringworm *See* ANTIFUNGAL DRUGS.

Rinstead Adult Gel (Schering-Plough) A proprietary combination of *benzocaine (a local anaesthetic) and *chloroxylenol (an antiseptic), used for the treatment of mouth ulcers, sores caused by dentures, and general soreness of the mouth. It can be obtained without a prescription, but only from pharmacies.

Precautions: this medicine is not recommended for children under 12 years old.

Rinstead Sugar Free Pastilles (Schering-Plough) A proprietary combination of *chloroxylenol (an antiseptic) and *menthol (a soothing agent), used for the relief of mouth ulcers, sore spots caused by dentures, and soreness in the mouth. It is freely available *over the counter.

Precautions: these pastilles are not recommended for children.

Rinstead Teething Gel (Schering-Plough) A proprietary combination of *cetylpyridinium chloride (an antiseptic) and *lignocaine <lidocaine> hydrochloride (a local anaesthetic), used for the relief of teething pain and pain caused by mouth ulcers. It is freely available *over the counter.
Precautions: the gel is not recommended for children under three months old.

Risperdal (Janssen-Cilag; Organon Laboratories) *See* RISPERIDONE.

risperidone An atypical *antipsychotic drug used for the treatment of acute and chronic psychoses, including schizophrenia: it controls both the positive symptoms (e.g. delusions) and the negative symptoms (e.g. apathy) of the disease. Risperidone is available as tablets or a liquid on *prescription only.
Side effects: include weight gain, dizziness, low blood pressure on standing (which can cause fainting in some people), insomnia, agitation, anxiety, headache, drowsiness, lack of concentration, constipation, indigestion, nausea and vomiting, blurred vision, menstrual irregularities, and sexual dysfunction.
Precautions: risperidone should not be taken by women who are breastfeeding. It should be used with caution in elderly patients, pregnant women, and in people with liver, heart, or kidney disease, epilepsy, or Parkinson's disease. Drowsiness can affect skilled tasks.
Interactions with other drugs:
  Anaesthetics: their effect in lowering blood pressure is enhanced.
  Antidepressants: there is an increased risk of antimuscarinic effects and arrhythmias if risperidone is taken with tricyclic antidepressants.
  Antiepileptic drugs: their anticonvulsant effects are antagonized by risperidone; carbamazepine reduces the effects of risperidone.
  Antihistamines: there is an increased risk of arrhythmias if risperidone is taken with astemizole or terfenadine.
  Halofantrine: there is an increased risk of arrhythmias if this drug is taken with risperidone.
  Ritonavir: may increase the effects of risperidone.
  Sedatives: the sedative effects of risperidone are increased if it is taken with anxiolytic or hypnotic drugs, or any other drug that causes sedation.
Proprietary preparation: Risperdal.

Ritalin (Novartis Pharmaceuticals) *See* METHYLPHENIDATE HYDROCHLORIDE.

ritodrine A *sympathomimetic drug that acts on the beta *adrenoceptors to cause relaxation of the muscles of the uterus. It is used to prevent premature labour in women who are 24–33 weeks pregnant. Ritodrine is given by intravenous injection followed by tablets to prevent further episodes during the pregnancy; it is available on *prescription only.

Side effects: include a fast heart rate in the mother and the fetus, anxiety, tremor, flushing, sweating, nausea, vomiting, chest pain, a rise in blood glucose, low blood pressure, and a fall in blood *potassium concentrations. Ritodrine may cause accumulation of fluid in the lungs, in which case it should be discontinued immediately. Long-term therapy may produce a large baby.

Precautions: ritodrine should not be given to women who have eclampsia, pre-eclampsia, infection of the uterus or heart disease or to those who have lost a baby during a previous pregnancy. It must be used with caution in multiple pregnancies and in women with diabetes, suspected heart disease, or hyperthyroidism.

Interactions with other drugs:

Corticosteroids: increase the risk of low concentrations of potassium in the blood.

Diuretics: increase the risk of low concentrations of potassium in the blood.

Theophylline: increases the risk of low concentrations of potassium in the blood and of *arrhythmias.

Proprietary preparation: Yutopar.

ritonavir A protease inhibitor (*see* ANTIVIRAL DRUGS), similar to *indinavir, used in combination with other antivirals (usually nucleoside analogues) for the treatment of *HIV disease. It is available as capsules or a solution on *prescription only.

Side effects: include stomach and bowel upsets, disturbances of taste, tingling around the mouth or in the fingers and toes, and headache.

Precautions: ritonavir should not be taken by women who are breastfeeding. It should be used with caution in people with liver or kidney disease, diabetes, diarrhoea, and haemophilia and in pregnant women.

Interactions with other drugs: ritonavir is a potent inhibitor of several enzyme systems in the liver that are involved in metabolizing drugs; it therefore has the potential to interact with many drugs. A doctor should be consulted before ritonavir is taken with any other drug.

Proprietary preparation: Norvir.

rituximab A *monoclonal antibody that specifically destroys B-lymphocytes (a type of white blood cell). Rituximab is used to treat a type of non-Hodgkin's lymphoma (*see* CANCER) that affects B-lymphocytes and is resistant to standard *cytotoxic drugs. Since the drug acts relatively selectively against the cancerous B-lymphocytes, the widespread adverse effects associated with other cytotoxic drugs do not occur. The side effects of rituximab occur during infusion, mostly during the first course of treatment (see below); an analgesic and an antihistamine should be given before each infusion to reduce the severity of the side effects. Rituximab is available as a form for infusion on *prescription only.

Side effects: fever, chills, nausea, vomiting, allergic reactions (such as rash, itching, constriction of the airways, breathlessness, and a transient fall in blood pressure), flushing, and tumour pain commonly occur during infusion. The infusion may need to be stopped temporarily in order to treat these effects.

Precautions: rituximab should not be used in women who are breastfeeding and should be used with caution in pregnant women and in people with a history of heart disease. Treatment should be carefully monitored under the supervision of a specialist.

Proprietary preparation: Mabthera.

rivastigmine An *acetylcholinesterase inhibitor that increases the amounts of acetylcholine in the brain. It is used to treat the symptoms of mild to moderate dementia (including short-term memory loss) that occur in people with Alzheimer's disease. It is available as tablets on *prescription only, and treatment should be supervised by a specialist.

Side effects: include loss of appetite, nausea, vomiting, indigestion, abdominal pain, diarrhoea, weight loss, dizziness, sleepiness, agitation, confusion, and depression.

Precautions: rivastigmine should not be taken by women who are breastfeeding and it should be used with caution in pregnant women, people with liver or kidney disease, certain heart diseases, or peptic ulcers, and in people with a history of asthma or other obstructive lung diseases.

Interactions with other drugs:

  Muscle relaxants: rivastigmine either increases or reduces the effects of muscle relaxants used in surgery to paralyse muscles.

Proprietary preparation: Exelon.

Rivotril (Roche Products) *See* CLONAZEPAM.

rizatriptan A *5HT$_1$ agonist used to treat acute attacks of *migraine. A single dose can relieve a migraine headache at any stage of the attack. Rizatriptan is available as tablets or wafers on *prescription only.

Side effects: include sensations of tingling, heat, heaviness, pressure, or tightness; if tightness in the chest or throat is severe, treatment should be discontinued. Other side effects include flushing, dizziness, drowsiness, weakness, indigestion, diarrhoea, palpitations, a fast heart rate, breathlessness, headache, blurred vision, itching, and rash.

Precautions: rizatriptan should not be taken by people with certain heart conditions, uncontrolled high blood pressure, or disease of the peripheral blood vessels, or by those who have previously had a stroke. It should be used with caution by women who are pregnant or breastfeeding and by people with impaired liver or kidney function.

Interactions with other drugs:

Ergotamine: the risk of spasm of the blood vessels, which can have serious consequences, is increased if ergotamine is taken with rizatriptan. Ergotamine should not be taken for 6 hours after taking rizatriptan, and rizatriptan should not be taken for 24 hours after taking ergotamine.

MAOIs: cause restlessness and other signs of overactivity of the central nervous system if taken with rizatriptan, which should therefore not be started for two weeks after stopping MAOIs.

Propranolol: may increase the plasma concentration of rizatriptan, whose dosage should therefore be reduced.

Proprietary preparations: Maxalt; Maxalt Melt (wafers).

Roaccutane (Roche Products) *See* ISOTRETINOIN.

Robaxin (Shire Pharmaceuticals) *See* METHOCARBAMOL.

Robinul (Antigen Pharmaceuticals) *See* GLYCOPYRRONIUM BROMIDE.

Robinul-Neostigmine (Antigen Pharmaceuticals) A proprietary combination of *glycopyrronium bromide (an antimuscarinic drug) and *neostigmine (an anticholinesterase), used by anaesthetists after surgery to reverse the effects of muscle relaxants that have been used during surgery. Glycopyrronium prevents slowing of the heart rate, excessive salivation, and other unwanted effects of neostigmine. Robinul-Neostigmine is available as an injection on *prescription only.

Robitussin Chesty Cough (Whitehall Laboratories) *See* GUAIPHENESIN <GUAIFENESIN>.

Robitussin Chesty Cough with Congestion (Whitehall Laboratories) A proprietary combination of *pseudoephedrine (a decongestant) and *guaiphenesin <guaifenesin> (an expectorant), used to relieve the symptoms of productive coughs and nasal congestion. It is available as a liquid without a prescription, but only from pharmacies. It cannot be prescribed on the NHS.

Side effects and interactions with other drugs: *see* GUAIPHENESIN <GUAIFENESIN>; EPHEDRINE HYDROCHLORIDE; DECONGESTANTS.

Precautions: this medicine is not recommended for children under two years old. *See also* GUAIPHENESIN <GUAIFENESIN>; EPHEDRINE HYDROCHLORIDE; DECONGESTANTS.

Robitussin Dry Cough (Whitehall Laboratories) *See* DEXTROMETHORPHAN.

Robitussin Junior Persistent Cough (Whitehall Laboratories) *See* DEXTROMETHORPHAN.

Robitussin Night-Time (Whitehall Laboratories) A proprietary combination of *brompheniramine (a sedative antihistamine), *codeine (a cough suppressant), and *pseudoephedrine (a decongestant), used to relieve dry coughs and nasal congestion that interfere with sleep. It is available as a liquid without a prescription, but only from pharmacies.

Side effects and interactions with other drugs: see CODEINE; ANTIHISTAMINES; OPIOIDS; EPHEDRINE HYDROCHLORIDE; DECONGESTANTS.

Precautions: this medicine is not recommended for children under four years old, except on medical advice. *See also* ANTIHISTAMINES; OPIOIDS; EPHEDRINE HYDROCHLORIDE; DECONGESTANTS.

RoC (Johnson & Johnson) A proprietary *sunscreen preparation consisting of a cream containing avobenzone and ethylhexyl p-methoxycinnamate. It protects against both UVA and UVB (SPF 25) and can be prescribed on the NHS or obtained without a prescription.

Rocaltrol (Roche Products) *See* CALCITRIOL.

Rocephin (Roche Products) *See* CEFTRIAXONE.

Roferon-A (Roche Products) *See* INTERFERON-ALFA.

Rogitine (Novartis Pharmaceuticals) *See* PHENTOLAMINE.

Rohypnol (Roche Products) *See* FLUNITRAZEPAM.

Rommix (Ashbourne Pharmaceuticals) *See* ERYTHROMYCIN.

Ronicol (Tillomed Laboratories) *See* NICOTINYL ALCOHOL.

ropinirole A *dopamine receptor agonist, similar to *bromocriptine, used for the treatment of Parkinson's disease. It is available as tablets on *prescription only.

Side effects: include nausea, somnolence, oedema (swelling), abdominal pain, vomiting, and fainting. Occasionally slow heart rate and low blood pressure may occur.

Precautions: ropinirole should be used with caution in people who have liver or kidney disease and in women who are pregnant or breastfeeding.

Proprietary preparation: Requip.

rose bengal A red dye that is applied to the eye for diagnostic purposes: to highlight damaged areas of the cornea and locate foreign bodies. As it causes intense stinging, *local anaesthetic eye drops are applied first. Rose bengal is available as eye drops and can be obtained without a prescription, but only from pharmacies.

Proprietary preparation: Minims Rose Bengal.

Rowachol (Rowa Pharmaceuticals) A proprietary combination of essential oils (menthol, pinene, menthone, camphene, borneol, and

cineole) that has been used as an *adjunct to *bile acids for the dispersal
of gallstones. Its value has been questioned. Rowachol is available as
capsules on *prescription only.

Interactions with other drugs:

Anticoagulants: the effects of warfarin and nicoumalone
<acenocoumarol> may be reduced.

Rowatinex (Rowa Pharmaceuticals) A proprietary combination of
terpenes (volatile oils), including pinene, camphene, and borneol, that is
claimed to be of benefit in helping to dissolve and pass kidney stones. It
is available as capsules on *prescription only.

Rozex (Stafford-Miller) *See* METRONIDAZOLE.

rubefacients (counterirritants) Substances that, when rubbed into the
skin, cause the blood vessels to dilate, producing redness and a feeling of
warmth. This sensation competes with, and to some extent blocks, pain
in underlying muscles and joints, since both feelings are conveyed by the
same nerves. This action is called **counterirritation**. Rubefacients are
used for the relief of muscular aches and pains, rheumatism, and the
pain associated with sprains and strains. Common rubefacients include
*methyl salicylate, *ethyl salicylate, *glycol salicylate, *capsaicin,
*capsicum oleoresin, *methyl nicotinate, and **benzyl nicotinate**.
*Menthol and *camphor are also counterirritants, but act by cooling,
rather than warming, the skin.

Side effects: when used in large amounts or constantly, rubefacients may
irritate the skin.

Precautions: rubefacients are usually not recommended for children.
They should not be covered with dressings and should not come into
contact with the eyes, lips, or other mucous membranes, or broken or
inflamed skin, where they can cause stinging or burning. Hands should
be washed after use to avoid transmission to sensitive areas.

Rusyde (Cox Pharmaceuticals; CP Pharmaceuticals) *See* FRUSEMIDE
<FUROSEMIDE>.

Rynacrom (Pantheon Healthcare) *See* SODIUM CROMOGLYCATE
<CROMOGLICATE>.

Rynacrom Compound (Rhône-Poulenc Rorer) A proprietary
combination of *sodium cromoglycate (a chromone) and
*xylometazoline (a decongestant), used for the prevention and treatment
of hay fever. It is available as a nasal spray and can be obtained from
pharmacies without a prescription.

Side effects: there may be nasal irritation.

Rythmodan, **Rythmodan Retard** (Hoechst Marion Roussel) *See*
DISOPYRAMIDE.

S

Sabril (Hoechst Marion Roussel) *See* VIGABATRIN.

Saizen (Serono Laboratories) *See* SOMATROPIN.

Salactol (Dermal Laboratories) A proprietary combination of *salicylic acid and *lactic acid (both keratolytics), used for the treatment of warts, verrucas, corns, and calluses. It is available as a paint and can be obtained without a prescription, but only from pharmacies.
Side effects and precautions: see SALICYLIC ACID.

Salagen (Chiron) *See* PILOCARPINE.

Salamol Steri-Neb (Norton Healthcare) *See* SALBUTAMOL.

Salatac (Dermal Laboratories) A proprietary combination of *salicylic acid and *lactic acid (both keratolytics), used for the treatment of warts, verrucas, corns, and calluses. It is available as a gel and can be obtained without a prescription, but only from pharmacies.
Side effects and precautions: see SALICYLIC ACID.

Salazopyrin, Salazopyrin EN-Tabs (Pharmacia & Upjohn) *See* SULPHASALAZINE <SULFASALAZINE>.

salbutamol A *sympathomimetic drug that stimulates beta *adrenoceptors in the airways. It is used mainly as a *bronchodilator, to relieve constriction in the airways during attacks of asthma and to alleviate the symptoms of chronic bronchitis and emphysema. Salbutamol has its maximum effect 30–60 minutes after use; its duration of action is 3–6 hours. It also relaxes the muscles of the uterus and may be used intravenously to prevent premature labour. Salbutamol is available, on *prescription only, as tablets, *modified-release tablets, or a liquid for oral use, as an aerosol or powder for inhalation, as a solution for use in a *nebulizer or a ventilator, and as a solution for injection.
Side effects: fine tremor (particularly of the hands), restlessness, anxiety, and headache are the most common side effects; less likely are palpitation, dilatation of blood vessels in the extremities, increased heart rate, and muscle cramps. If salbutamol is injected, there may be pain at the injection site.
Precautions: salbutamol should be used with caution by people with an overactive thyroid gland, high blood pressure, certain heart conditions, or diabetes mellitus (particularly if the drug is given intravenously) and by women who are pregnant (unless salbutamol is used to delay labour) or breastfeeding. It is important not to exceed the stated dose; if a

previously effective dose does not provide at least three hours relief, a doctor's advice should be sought.

Interactions with other drugs:

Beta blockers: oppose the action of salbutamol.

Corticosteroids: there is an increased risk of low *potassium concentrations in the blood.

Diuretics: there is an increased risk of low potassium concentrations in the blood.

Theophylline: there is an increased risk of low potassium concentrations in the blood.

Proprietary preparations: Aerolin Autoinhaler (breath-activated metered-dose aerosol inhaler); Airomir (inhaler); Asmasal Clickhaler (breath-activated metered-dose powder inhaler); Asmaven (aerosol inhaler); Maxivent (aerosol inhaler); Salamol Steri-Neb (nebulizer solution); Salbutamol Spacehaler (metered-dose aerosol inhaler with spacer device); Ventodisks (discs containing powder blisters for use in an inhaler); Ventolin (syrup, injection, solution for infusion, aerosol inhalation, solution for respirator); Ventolin Accuhaler (breath-activated aerosol inhaler); Ventolin Easi-Breathe (aerosol inhalation); Ventolin Evohaler (aerosol inhalation); Ventolin Nebules (ampoules for use in a nebulizer); Ventolin Rotacaps (capsules containing powder for inhalation); Volmax (modified-release tablets); AEROCROM (combined with sodium cromoglycate <cromoglicate>); COMBIVENT (combined with ipratropium bromide); VENTIDE (combined with beclomethasone <beclometasone> dipropionate).

Salbutamol Spacehaler (Medeva) *See* SALBUTAMOL.

salcatonin <calcitonin (salmon)> A synthetic form of the hormone *calcitonin, which is identical in structure to the hormone produced by salmon. It is used to reduce abnormally high blood concentrations of calcium and to treat Paget's disease (in which the bones become deformed and fracture easily). Salcatonin is less likely to produce allergic reactions than calcitonin. It is available as an injection on *prescription only.

Side effects: include nausea, vomiting, and flushing (which diminish with use); less commonly tingling of hands, an unpleasant taste, and a rash may occur.

Precautions: some people are allergic to salcatonin and a scratch test may be necessary before taking the drug. It should be used with caution in women who are pregnant or breastfeeding.

Proprietary preparations: Calsynar; Miacalcic.

salicylates A group of drugs that are chemically related to *salicylic acid; they are *analgesics that also reduce fever and inflammation. *Aspirin (acetylsalicylic acid) and *diflunisal are salicylates that are taken by mouth to relieve pain, fever, and inflammation. Several salicylates are applied to the skin in the form of creams, ointments, sprays, or other *topical formulations to relieve pain and stiffness in muscles, joints, and ligaments. These salicylates, which are common ingredients of *rubefacient preparations, include *methyl salicylate (oil of wintergreen), *glycol salicylate, *ethyl salicylate, **ammonium salicylate**, **salicylamide**, and **tetrahydrofurfuryl salicylate**. *Choline salicylate is used as a gel to treat teething problems in babies.

Side effects and precautions: salicylates taken by mouth can irritate the stomach lining and may cause gastric ulceration and bleeding (*see* ASPIRIN). As a result of their wide use and ready availability, salicylates (mainly aspirin) are sometimes a cause of poisoning. Symptoms of mild chronic poisoning (**salicylism**) include headache, dizziness, ringing in the ears, and difficulty in hearing, which can be resolved by reducing the dosage. Topical preparations may cause skin irritation (*see also* RUBEFACIENTS). Excessive or prolonged use of topical preparations containing salicylates should be avoided as these drugs can be absorbed into the body and may cause adverse *systemic effects.

salicylic acid A *salicylate that has *keratolytic properties and is used topically, often in combination with *coal tar or other keratolytics, to remove surface skin in such conditions as dandruff, seborrhoeic *eczema, scaling of the skin, *psoriasis, and acne. It is also used to remove dead skin and promote healing of ulcers, sores, burns, or traumatic injuries and is included in some *rubefacient preparations. Higher concentrations can be used for the removal of hard skin associated with corns and calluses, warts, and verrucas. Salicylic acid is available, alone or in combination with other ingredients, as a liquid, cream, ointment, or shampoo. It can be obtained without a prescription but usually only from pharmacies (depending on the other ingredients).

Side effects: it may cause irritation and drying of the skin.

Precautions: salicylic acid should not be used on facial or genital warts or warts around the anus. It should not be applied to large areas of healthy skin or to broken skin and contact with the eyes should be avoided. High concentrations of salicylic acid should not be used by people with diabetes. *See also* SALICYLATES.

Proprietary preparations: Acnisal (liquid for acne); Carnation Corn Caps; Carnation Verruca Treatment; Corn Removal Pads; Corn Removal Plasters; Occlusal (liquid for warts); Polymer Gel Corn Removers; Soft Corn Remover Pads; Verruca Removal System; Verrugon (ointment for verrucas); ASERBINE (combined with benzoic acid and propylene glycol); CAPASAL (combined with coal tar; COCOIS (combined with coal tar and sulphur); CORN AND CALLUS REMOVAL LIQUID (combined with camphor); CUPLEX (combined with lactic acid and copper acetate); DIPROSALIC (combined with betamethasone); DUOFILM (combined with lactic acid); GELCOSAL (combined with coal tar); IONIL T (combined with benzalkonium chloride and coal tar); METED (combined with sulphur); MONPHYTOL (combined with chlorbutol <chlorobutanol>, methyl undecenoate, methyl salicylate, propyl salicylate, and propyl undecenoate); MOVELAT (combined with mucopolysaccharide polysulphate); PHYTEX (combined with borotannic complex, methyl salicylate, and acetic acid); POSALFILIN (combined with podophyllum resin); PRAGMATAR (combined with coal tar distillate and dithranol); PYRALVEX (combined with anthroquinone glycosides); RADIAN-B MUSCLE LOTION (combined with camphor, ammonium salicylate, and menthol); SALACTOL (combined with lactic acid); SEAL AND HEAL VERRUCA REMOVAL GEL (combined with camphor); STIEDEX LOTION (combined with desoxymethasone <desoximetasone>).

Saline Steri-Neb (Norton Healthcare) *See* SODIUM CHLORIDE.

Salivace (Penn Pharmaceuticals) A proprietary combination of salts of calcium, potassium, and sodium (*see* ELECTROLYTE), *xylitol (a sugar), and carboxymethylcellulose (a protective agent; *see* CARMELLOSE), used as an artificial saliva for the relief of dry mouth (which occurs, for example, after radiotherapy). It is freely available *over the counter in the form of a mouth spray.

Saliva Orthana (Nycomed Amersham) A proprietary combination of mucin (a constituent of mucus) obtained from the stomach of pigs and *xylitol (a sugar), used as an artificial saliva for the relief of dry mouth (which occurs, for example, after radiotherapy). It is freely available *over the counter in the form of a mouth spray or lozenges.

Saliveze (Wyvern Medical) A proprietary combination of carboxymethylcellulose (a protective agent; *see* CARMELLOSE) and salts of calcium, potassium magnesium and sodium (*see* ELECTROLYTE), used as an artificial saliva for the relief of dry mouth (which occurs, for example, after radiotherapy). It is freely available *over the counter in the form of a mouth spray.

Salivix (Cortecs Healthcare) A proprietary combination of *malic acid, acacia, and other ingredients, used as an artificial saliva for the relief of dry mouth (caused, for example, by radiotherapy). It is freely available *over the counter in the form of sugar-free pastilles.

salmeterol A *sympathomimetic drug that stimulates beta *adrenoceptors. It is used as a *bronchodilator in the treatment of asthma, bronchitis, and emphysema. Salmeterol has a longer duration of action than *salbutamol and is therefore taken less frequently. It is used to prevent asthma attacks during the night or induced by exercise; it is not suitable for the relief of acute attacks of asthma since it has a slower onset of action than salbutamol. Salmeterol is used mostly in conjunction with long-term prophylactic therapy, such as *corticosteroids or *chromones. It is available, on *prescription only, as an aerosol or powder for inhalation.

Side effects, precautions, and interactions with other drugs: see SALBUTAMOL.

Proprietary preparations: Serevent (metered-dose aerosol inhalation);

Serevent Accuhaler (breath-activated inhaler for powder); Serevent Diskhaler (inhaler for discs containing powder blisters).

Salofalk (Cortecs Healthcare) *See* MESALAZINE.

Salonair (Salonpas) A proprietary combination of *glycol salicylate, *menthol, *camphor, benzyl nicotinate, *methyl salicylate, and *squalane in the form of a spray, used as a *rubefacient for the relief of muscular and rheumatic pain. It is freely available *over the counter.
Side effects and precautions: see RUBEFACIENTS; SALICYLATES.

Salonpas Plasters (Salonpas) A proprietary combination of *methyl salicylate, *glycol salicylate, *menthol, and *camphor, used as a *rubefacient for the relief of minor aches and pains. It is freely available *over the counter.
Side effects: see RUBEFACIENTS; SALICYLATES.
Precautions: Salonpas should not be used by people who are allergic to aspirin. *See also* RUBEFACIENTS; SALICYLATES.

Saluric (Merck Sharp & Dohme) *See* CHLOROTHIAZIDE.

Salzone (Wallace Manufacturing) *See* PARACETAMOL.

Sandimmun (Novartis Pharmaceuticals) *See* CYCLOSPORIN.

Sandocal 400 (Novartis Pharmaceuticals) A proprietary combination of *calcium lactate gluconate and *calcium carbonate, used as a *calcium supplement. **Sandocal 1000** is a stronger formulation. Both preparations are available as effervescent tablets and can be obtained without a prescription, but only from pharmacies.
Side effects, precautions, and interactions with other drugs: see CALCIUM.

Sandoglobulin (Novartis Pharmaceuticals) *See* IMMUNOGLOBULINS.

Sando-K (HK Pharma) A proprietary combination of *potassium chloride and *potassium bicarbonate used as a *potassium supplement. It is available as tablets that dissolve in water to produce an effervescent drink and can be obtained without a prescription, but only from pharmacies.
Side effects, precautions, and interactions with other drugs: see POTASSIUM.

Sandostatin (Novartis Pharmaceuticals) *See* OCTREOTIDE.

Sandrena (Organon Laboratories) *See* OESTRADIOL <ESTRADIOL>; HORMONE REPLACEMENT THERAPY.

Sanomigran (Novartis Pharmaceuticals) *See* PIZOTIFEN.

saquinavir A protease inhibitor (*see* ANTIVIRAL DRUGS), similar to
*indinavir, used in combination with other antivirals (usually nucleoside
analogues) for the treatment of *HIV disease. It is available as capsules on
*prescription only.

Side effects: include diarrhoea, ulceration of the mouth, abdominal
discomfort, nausea, headache, peripheral neuropathy (causing tingling
and numbness in the limbs), and rashes.

Precautions: saquinavir should be used with caution by people with
impaired kidney or liver function or haemophilia and by pregnant
women. It should not be used during breastfeeding.

Interactions with other drugs: saquinavir interacts with a number of
drugs, including those listed below, and it is therefore important to
inform a doctor before taking any other medicines with saquinavir.

  Antiepileptic drugs: phenobarbitone <phenobarbital>, phenytoin, and
    carbamazepine can reduce the plasma concentration (and therefore
    effectiveness) of saquinavir.

  Antihistamines: saquinavir can increase the plasma concentrations (and
    therefore side effects) of astemizole and terfenadine.

  Cisapride: its plasma concentration (and therefore side effects) can be
    increased by saquinavir.

  Rifampicin and rifabutin: can reduce the plasma concentration (and
    therefore effectiveness) of saquinavir.

Proprietary preparation: Invirase.

Saventrine IV (Pharmax) *See* ISOPRENALINE HYDROCHLORIDE.

Savlon Antiseptic Cream, **Savlon Concentrated Antiseptic**
(Novartis Consumer Health) Proprietary combinations of the antiseptics
*chlorhexidine gluconate and *cetrimide, used for cleansing and
disinfecting all types of minor skin disorders and wounds. They are freely
available *over the counter.

Side effects: see CETRIMIDE.

Savlon Antiseptic Wound Wash (Novartis Consumer Health) *See*
CHLORHEXIDINE.

Savlon Dry Powder (Novartis Consumer Health) *See*
POVIDONE–IODINE.

scabicides *See* SCABIES.

scabies A skin disease caused by infestation with the mite *Sarcoptes
scabei*. A scabies infestation causes severe itching (particularly at night);
commonly infected areas are the nipples, penis, and the skin between
the fingers. Scratching to relieve the itch may lead to secondary
infection. Treatment is by application of a **scabicide** (a drug that kills the
mite), usually *permethrin or *malathion; it should be applied to all
parts of the skin from the neck down. *Benzyl benzoate can also be used

but it causes irritation. *Calamine or *crotamiton may be used to relieve itching that persists after the mites have been destroyed. All members of a family need to treated but clothing and bedding do not need to be disinfested.

Schering PC4 (Schering Health Care) A proprietary combination of *ethinyloestradiol <ethinylestradiol> and *norgestrel used as a postcoital *oral contraceptive ('morning-after pill'). To be effective it should be taken in spaced doses: two tablets within 72 hours of unprotected intercourse, followed by two tablets exactly 12 hours later. It is available on *prescription only.

Side effects: include nausea and vomiting, which may impair contraceptive action if the tablets have not been absorbed before vomiting occurs.

Precautions: women who become pregnant may be at risk of an ectopic pregnancy.

Interactions with other drugs: see ORAL CONTRACEPTIVES.

Scheriproct (Schering Health Care) A proprietary combination of *prednisolone hexanoate (a corticosteroid) and *cinchocaine hydrochloride (a local anaesthetic), used for the short-term relief of the discomfort and pain of *haemorrhoids and itching of the anus. It is available as an ointment or suppositories on *prescription only.

Side effects: see CORTICOSTEROIDS.

Precautions: Scheriproct should not be used when viral or fungal infection is present; prolonged use should be avoided.

sclerotherapy The injection of an irritant substance into a vein, which causes scarring and hardening so that the vein eventually closes up. Sclerotherapy using *ethanolamine oleate or *sodium tetradecyl sulphate is used in the treatment of varicose veins; *phenol is used as a sclerosant to treat *haemorrhoids.

Scopoderm TTS (Novartis Pharmaceuticals) *See* HYOSCINE HYDROBROMIDE.

scopolamine *See* HYOSCINE BUTYLBROMIDE; HYOSCINE HYDROBROMIDE.

Seal and Heal Verruca Removal Gel (Seton Scholl Healthcare) A proprietary combination of *salicylic acid (a keratolytic) and *camphor, used for the treatment of warts and verrucas. It is freely available *over the counter.

Precautions: this preparation is not recommended for children.

Sea-Legs (Seton Scholl Healthcare) *See* MECLOZINE HYDROCHLORIDE.

Secadrex (Rhône-Poulenc Rorer) A proprietary combination of *acebutolol (a beta blocker) and *hydrochlorothiazide (a thiazide diuretic), used in the treatment of mild to moderate *hypertension. It is available as tablets on *prescription only.

Side effects, precautions, and interactions with other drugs: see BETA BLOCKERS; THIAZIDE DIURETICS.

See also ANTIHYPERTENSIVE DRUGS; DIURETICS.

secobarbital *See* QUINALBARBITONE.

Seconal Sodium (Flynn Pharma) *See* QUINALBARBITONE <SECOBARBITAL>.

Sectral (Rhône-Poulenc Rorer) *See* ACEBUTOLOL.

Securon (Knoll) *See* VERAPAMIL HYDROCHLORIDE.

Securopen (Bayer) *See* AZLOCILLIN.

sedatives *See* ANXIOLYTIC DRUGS.

Select-a-Jet Dopamine (International Medication Systems) *See* DOPAMINE HYDROCHLORIDE.

selective serotonin reuptake inhibitors *See* SSRIS.

selegiline An inhibitor of monoamine oxidase type B, an enzyme that breaks down *dopamine and therefore increases dopamine concentrations in the brain (*compare* MONOAMINE OXIDASE INHIBITORS). It is used for the treatment of Parkinson's disease (*see* ANTIPARKINSONIAN DRUGS), either alone or in combination with *levodopa. It is available as tablets or a liquid on *prescription only.

Side effects: include low blood pressure, nausea and vomiting, confusion, and agitation.

Precautions: the side effects of levodopa may be increased when a combination of selegiline and levodopa is used; the dose of levodopa may need to be reduced.

Interactions with other drugs:

  Fluoxetine: there is a risk of high blood pressure and overstimulation of the central nervous system.

  MAOIs: there is a risk of a dangerous rise in blood pressure.

  Pethidine: there is a risk of toxic effects on the central nervous system.

Proprietary preparations: Centrapryl; Eldepryl (tablets or liquid); Stilline; Vivapryl; Zelapar (freeze-dried tablets).

selenium sulphide A drug with *antifungal properties that is applied to the scalp for the treatment of dandruff and seborrhoeic *eczema. It is available as a shampoo and can be obtained without a prescription, but only from pharmacies.

Precautions: selenium sulphide should not come into contact with the

eyes or broken skin. It should not be used within 48 hours of using perming or hair-colouring lotions.
Proprietary preparations: Lenium; Selsun.

Selsun (Abbott Laboratories) *See* SELENIUM SULPHIDE.

Semi-Daonil (Hoechst Marion Roussel) *See* GLIBENCLAMIDE.

Semprex (GlaxoWellcome) *See* ACRIVASTINE.

Senlax (Novartis Consumer Health) *See* SENNA.

senna A *stimulant laxative, isolated from the fruit of the senna plant, used for the treatment of constipation; the active ingredients are chemicals called **sennosides**. It is available as tablets, granules, or a syrup and can be obtained without a prescription, but some preparations are available only from pharmacies.
Side effects and precautions: see STIMULANT LAXATIVES.
Proprietary preparations: Boots Senna Tablets; Ex-Lax Senna (chocolate tablets); Nylax with Senna (tablets); Senlax (chocolate tablets); Senokot (tablets, granules, or syrup); BOOTS COMPOUND LAXATIVE (combined with figs); CALIFIG CALIFORNIA SYRUP OF FIGS (combined with figs); MANEVAC (combined with ispaghula husk); POTTER'S CLEANSING HERB (combined with aloes and cascara); PRIPSEN (combined with piperazine); RHUAKA (combined with cascara and rhubarb).

sennosides *See* SENNA.

Senokot (Reckitt & Colman) *See* SENNA.

Senselle (LRC Products) A proprietary non-hormonal water-based preparation used as a vaginal lubricant to relieve dryness of the vagina, which can occur at the menopause. Its effects last for up to 24 hours. Senselle is freely available *over the counter in the form of a liquid.

Septrin (GlaxoWellcome) *See* CO-TRIMOXAZOLE.

Serc (Solvay Healthcare) *See* BETAHISTINE.

Serdolect (Lundbeck) *See* SERTINDOLE.

Serenace (Norton Healthcare) *See* HALOPERIDOL.

Serevent (Allen & Hanburys) *See* SALMETEROL.

sermorelin An *analogue of *growth hormone releasing hormone (somatorelin), used to test the function of the pituitary gland in secreting growth hormone. It is available as a form for injection on *prescription only.

Side effects: sermorelin may cause flushing and there may be pain at the injection site.

Precautions: sermorelin should not be used in women who are pregnant or breastfeeding. It should be used with caution in people with epilepsy or hypothyroidism (underproduction of thyroid hormones), obese people, and people who are taking antithyroid drugs, insulin, corticosteroids, aspirin, or any other drugs that affect the production of growth hormone.

Proprietary preparation: Geref 50.

Seroquel (AstraZeneca) *See* QUETIAPINE.

serotonin (5-hydroxytryptamine; 5HT) A compound widely distributed in the tissues, particularly the brain and other parts of the nervous system, the blood platelets, and the intestinal wall. Serotonin is a transmitter of nerve impulses and also acts like a hormone. It causes contraction of smooth muscles (e.g. in the intestine) and constriction of blood vessels and may have a role in inflammation. Serotonin is thought to be involved in the development of a *migraine headache; drugs that act like serotonin (*see* 5HT$_1$ AGONISTS) are used to treat migraine, while drugs that antagonize its effects (such as *pizotifen) are used to prevent migraine attacks. In the brain, concentrations of serotonin are believed to have important effects on mood. Drugs that act to prolong the effects of serotonin in the brain, such as the selective serotonin reuptake inhibitors (*see* SSRIS), are used in the treatment of depression.

Seroxat (SmithKline Beecham Pharmaceuticals) *See* PAROXETINE.

sertindole An atypical *antipsychotic drug used for the treatment of schizophrenia. Because it can cause serious abnormalities in heart rhythm (*arrhythmias), sertindole is now used only for treating patients who are already taking it and who cannot be treated with other antipsychotic drugs. It is available for named patients as tablets on *prescription only.

Side effects: include arrhythmias, swelling of the ankles, weight gain, dizziness, low blood pressure on standing (which can cause fainting in some people), dry mouth, a running nose, nasal congestion, breathlessness, tingling in the fingers or toes, and (rarely) convulsions.

Precautions: sertindole should only be used for treating patients already taking it. It should not be taken by women who are pregnant or breastfeeding or by people with severe liver disease or arrhythmias. It should be used with caution in people with diabetes or mild or moderate liver disease. Heart activity should be monitored during treatment.

Interactions with other drugs:

Anaesthetics: their effect in lowering blood pressure is enhanced.

Anti-arrhythmic drugs: amiodarone, disopyramide, procainamide, and quinidine should not be taken with sertindole as this combination increases the risk of arrhythmias.

Antidepressants: tricyclic antidepressants should not be taken with sertindole as this combination increases the risk of arrhythmias. Fluoxetine and paroxetine increase the effects of sertindole.

Antiepileptic drugs: their anticonvulsant effects are antagonized by sertindole; carbamazepine and phenytoin reduce the effects of sertindole.

Antifungal drugs: itraconazole and ketoconazole increase the adverse effects of sertindole.

Antihistamines: astemizole and terfenadine should not be taken with sertindole as this combination increases the risk of arrhythmias.

Cisapride: should not be taken with sertindole as this combination increases the risk of arrhythmias.

Erythromycin: may increase the effects of sertindole.

Halofantrine: there is an increased risk of arrhythmias if this drug is taken with sertindole.

Ritonavir: may increase the effects of sertindole.

Sedatives: the sedative effects of sertindole are increased if it is taken with anxiolytic or hypnotic drugs, or any other drug that causes sedation.

Proprietary preparation: Serdolect.

sertraline An *antidepressant drug of the *SSRI group that is used for the treatment of depressive illness. It is available as tablets on *prescription only.

Side effects: *see* SSRIS.

Precautions: *see* SSRIS. In addition, at the end of treatment dosage of this drug should be reduced gradually (not suddenly).

Interactions with other drugs:

Selegiline: there is an increased risk of hypertension and adverse effects on the central nervous system.

See also SSRIS.

Proprietary preparation: Lustral.

Settlers Antacid Peppermint Tablets (Stafford-Miller) *See* CALCIUM CARBONATE.

Settlers Wind-Eze (Stafford-Miller) *See* DIMETHICONE <DIMETICONE>.

Sevredol (Napp Pharmaceuticals) *See* MORPHINE.

sildenafil A drug that is taken by mouth in the treatment of impotence. It enhances the erectile response to sexual stimulation and is used for the treatment of men who have difficulty in obtaining or maintaining an erection. During sexual stimulation, it acts as a selective enzyme inhibitor, causing relaxation of smooth muscle and increasing blood flow to the erectile tissue of the penis. Sildenafil has been shown to be effective in a broad range of men, including the elderly and those with high blood pressure, diabetes, coronary artery disease, depression, spinal-cord injury, or prostate problems. Sildenafil has also been reported to increase the sensation of orgasm in women, but it is not licensed for use in women or in males under 18 years old. It is available as tablets on *prescription only, and there are restrictions to its prescription on the NHS.

Side effects: include headache, flushing, dizziness, indigestion, nasal congestion, and visual disturbances (including effects on colour vision).

Precautions: sildenafil should not be used by men who are taking *nitrates (such as glyceryl trinitrate or isosorbide), or by those who have recently had a heart attack or a stroke, or who have cardiovascular conditions that make sexual activity inadvisable, severely impaired liver function, low blood pressure, or hereditary conditions that affect vision. It should be used with caution by men with abnormal anatomy of the penis, sickle-cell anaemia, multiple myeloma, leukaemia, active peptic ulcer, bleeding disorders, or impaired kidney function.

Interactions with other drugs:

  Cimetidine: increases the effect of sildenafil, whose dosage may therefore need to be reduced.

  Erythromycin: increases the effect of sildenafil, whose dosage may therefore need to be reduced.

  Ketoconazole: increases the effect of sildenafil, whose dosage may therefore need to be reduced.

  Nicorandil: sildenafil significantly enhances the effects of nicorandil in reducing blood pressure and should not be taken with this drug.

  Nitrates: sildenafil significantly enhances the effects of these drugs in reducing blood pressure and it should not be taken with nitrates.

Proprietary preparation: Viagra.

silver nitrate A *keratolytic used for the removal of warts and verrucas. It is available as a caustic pencil and can be obtained without a prescription, but only from pharmacies.

Side effects: silver nitrate stains skin and fabrics.

Precautions: silver nitrate should not be applied to facial or genital warts or to warts around the anus. Care should be taken to protect healthy skin and avoid broken skin during application.

Proprietary preparation: Avoca.

silver sulphadiazine <sulfadiazine> An *antibiotic that is active against a variety of bacteria; it has limited activity against viruses. It is used to prevent and treat infection in cases of severe burns and to disinfect skin graft sites, wounds, infected leg ulcers, and pressure sores. Silver sulphadiazine is available as a cream on *prescription only.

Side effects: discoloration of the skin has been reported; otherwise side effects are rare. However, if large areas of skin are treated enough sulphadiazine can be absorbed to cause the side effects of *sulphonamides.

Precautions: silver sulphadiazine should not be used during pregnancy or on newborn babies. It should be used with caution by people with impaired kidney or liver function.

Interactions with other drugs: if large areas of skin are treated enough sulphadiazine can be absorbed to cause interactions (*see* SULPHONAMIDES).

Proprietary preparation: Flamazine.

Simeco (Wyeth Laboratories) A proprietary combination of *aluminium hydroxide, *magnesium carbonate, and *magnesium hydroxide (antacids) and activated *dimethicone <dimeticone> (an antifoaming agent), used for the relief of indigestion (*see* ACID-PEPTIC DISEASES). It is available as tablets that can be obtained without a prescription, but only from pharmacies.

Side effects, precautions, and interactions with other drugs: see ANTACIDS.

simethicone *See* DIMETHICONE <DIMETICONE>.

Simplene (Chauvin Pharmaceuticals) *See* ADRENALINE <EPINEPHRINE>.

simvastatin A *statin used for the treatment of primary hypercholesterolaemia (*see* HYPERLIPIDAEMIA) that has not responded to dietary intervention. It is also used to prevent the progression of *atherosclerosis in patients with coronary artery disease and to reduce the incidence of coronary events in susceptible individuals. It is available as tablets on *prescription only.

Side effects and precautions: see STATINS.

Interactions with other drugs:

 Anticoagulants: the effects of warfarin and nicoumalone <acenocoumarol> are increased.

 Antifungal drugs: the risk of muscle damage is increased if simvastatin is taken with itraconazole, ketoconazole, and possibly other imidazole and triazole antifungals.

  See also STATINS.

Proprietary preparation: Zocor.

Sinemet, Sinemet CR, Sinemet LS, Sinemet Plus (Du Pont Pharmaceuticals) *See* CO-CARELDOPA.

Sinequan (Pfizer) *See* DOXEPIN.

Singulair (Merck Sharp & Dohme) *See* MONTELUKAST.

Sinthrome (Alliance Pharmaceuticals) *See* NICOUMALONE <ACENOCOUMAROL>.

Sinutab (Warner-Lambert Consumer Healthcare) A proprietary combination of *paracetamol (an analgesic and antipyretic) and *phenylpropanolamine (a decongestant), used for the treatment of nasal and sinus congestion, pain, and fever associated with colds and influenza. It is available as tablets and can be obtained without a prescription, but only from pharmacies.

Side effects: see EPHEDRINE HYDROCHLORIDE.

Precautions: Sinutab should not be given to children under six years old. *See also* PARACETAMOL; EPHEDRINE HYDROCHLORIDE.

Interactions with other drugs: see PHENYLPROPANOLAMINE; EPHEDRINE HYDROCHLORIDE.

Sinutab Night-time (Warner-Lambert Consumer Healthcare) A proprietary combination of *phenylpropanolamine (a decongestant), *paracetamol (an analgesic and antipyretic), and phenyltoloxamine (a sedative *antihistamine), taken at night for the relief of nasal and sinus congestion, pain, and fever associated with colds and influenza. It is available as tablets and can be obtained without a prescription, but only from pharmacies.

Side effects: see EPHEDRINE HYDROCHLORIDE; ANTIHISTAMINES.

Precautions: these tablets are not recommended for children. *See also* EPHEDRINE HYDROCHLORIDE; PARACETAMOL; ANTIHISTAMINES.

Interactions with other drugs: see EPHEDRINE HYDROCHLORIDE; PHENYLPROPANOLAMINE; ANTIHISTAMINES.

Siopel (AstraZeneca) A proprietary combination of *dimethicone <dimeticone> (a water repellent) and *cetrimide (an antiseptic), used as a barrier cream (*see* BARRIER PREPARATIONS). It is freely available *over the counter.

Skelid (Sanofi Winthrop) *See* TILUDRONIC ACID.

Skinoren (Schering Health Care) *See* AZELAIC ACID.

Slofedipine XL (Sanofi Winthrop) *See* NIFEDIPINE.

Slofenac SR (Sanofi Winthrop) *See* DICLOFENAC SODIUM.

Slo-Indo (Generics) *See* INDOMETHACIN <INDOMETACIN>.

Slo-Phyllin (Merck Pharmaceuticals) *See* THEOPHYLLINE.

Slow-Fe (Novartis Pharmaceuticals) *See* FERROUS SULPHATE.

Slow-Fe Folic (Novartis Pharmaceuticals) A proprietary combination of *ferrous sulphate and *folic acid, used to prevent deficiencies of iron and folic acid during pregnancy. It is available as *modified-release tablets and can be obtained without a prescription, but only from pharmacies.

Side effects, precautions, and interactions with other drugs: see IRON.

Slow-K (Alliance Pharmaceuticals) *See* POTASSIUM CHLORIDE.

Slow Sodium (HK Pharma) *See* SODIUM CHLORIDE.

Slow-Trasicor (Novartis Pharmaceuticals) *See* OXPRENOLOL HYDROCHLORIDE.

Slozem (Merck Pharmaceuticals) *See* DILTIAZEM HYDROCHLORIDE.

Sno Phenicol (Chauvin Pharmaceuticals) *See* CHLORAMPHENICOL.

Sno Tears (Chauvin Pharmaceuticals) *See* POLYVINYL ALCOHOL.

sodium A mineral element that is an important constituent of the human body. Sodium ions (*see* ELECTROLYTE) control the volume of extracellular fluid in the body (i.e. the body fluids surrounding cells) and are also necessary for the functioning of nerves and muscles. The amount of sodium in the body is controlled by the kidneys. Sodium is contained in most foods, most commonly in the form of *sodium chloride (common salt). An excessive intake of sodium can lead to fluid retention (*see* OEDEMA) and may also be implicated in *hypertension (high blood pressure).
  Sodium depletion is treated by means of oral or intravenous administration of sodium chloride or other sodium salts.

sodium acid phosphate A salt that is used as a *phosphate supplement. It also acts as an *osmotic laxative, being administered rectally for the treatment of constipation and to clear the bowel before examination or surgery. It is available from pharmacies without a prescription in the form of tablets, enemas, or suppositories.
Side effects and precautions: see PHOSPHATE SUPPLEMENTS; PHOSPHATE LAXATIVES.
Proprietary preparations: CARBALAX (combined with sodium bicarbonate); FLEET READY-TO-USE ENEMA (combined with sodium phosphate); FLETCHERS' PHOSPHATE ENEMA (combined with sodium phosphate); PHOSPHATE-SANDOZ (combined with sodium bicarbonate and potassium bicarbonate).

sodium alginate *See* ALGINIC ACID.

Sodium Amytal (Flynn Pharma) *See* AMYLOBARBITONE <AMOBARBITAL>.

sodium aurothiomalate A salt of gold that is used for the treatment of active progressive rheumatoid arthritis and juvenile arthritis. Unlike *NSAIDs, sodium aurothiomalate does not have an immediate therapeutic effect and it may take 4–6 months to obtain a full response. It is available as a solution for intramuscular injection on *prescription only.
Side effects: gold salts can cause blood disorders and affect the kidneys; severe reactions occur in up to 5% of patients. The following symptoms should be reported to a doctor: rash or itching, a metallic taste, fever,

sore throat or tongue, mouth ulcers, bleeding gums, bruising, heavy periods, and diarrhoea.

Precautions: blood counts and urine tests should be carried out regularly during treatment. Gold should not be given to those with kidney or liver disease, blood disorders, or exfoliative dermatitis or to women who are pregnant or breastfeeding; pregnancy should be avoided during its use. It should be used with caution in the elderly and in people with a history of urticaria, eczema, or colitis.

Interactions with other drugs: there is an increased risk of kidney damage if gold salts are given to patients who are taking other drugs that adversely affect the kidneys.

Proprietary preparation: Myocrisin.

sodium bicarbonate An *antacid used as an ingredient in many preparations for the relief of indigestion, heartburn, and the symptoms of ulcers; **sodium carbonate** has the same antacid action. Sodium bicarbonate is also used to treat metabolic acidosis (in which the acidity of the body fluids is abnormally high), such as occurs in kidney failure. For this it is given orally (as tablets or capsules) or, in severe cases, by intravenous injection or infusion. Solutions used to replace lost fluids or *electrolytes sometimes contain sodium bicarbonate. It is also taken orally to reduce the acidity of the urine in the treatment of mild infections of the urinary tract, such as cystitis. Sodium bicarbonate is also added to some preparations to make them effervescent, since it produces bubbles of carbon dioxide when dissolved in water. Oral preparations of sodium bicarbonate can be obtained without a prescription; infusions are available on *prescription only.

Side effects: antacid preparations cause belching. High doses of sodium bicarbonate may cause systemic alkalosis (in which the alkalinity of the body fluids is abnormally high).

Precautions: sodium bicarbonate should not be taken by people with kidney disease or by those who are on a low-sodium diet.

Proprietary preparations: Min-I-Jet Sodium Bicarbonate (injection); Nurse Harvey's Gripe Mixture; BISMAG TABLETS (combined with magnesium carbonate); BISODOL ANTACID POWDER (combined with magnesium carbonate); BISODOL ANTACID TABLETS (combined with calcium carbonate and magnesium carbonate); BISODOL EXTRA TABLETS (combined with calcium carbonate, magnesium carbonate, and simethicone); CARBALAX (combined with sodium acid phosphate); DE WITT'S ANTACID POWDER (combined with calcium carbonate, magnesium carbonate, magnesium trisilicate, kaolin, and peppermint oil); DIORALYTE TABLETS (combined with citric acid, glucose, sodium chloride, and potassium chloride); ENO (combined with sodium carbonate and citric acid); GASTROCOTE (combined with alginic acid, aluminium hydroxide, and magnesium trisilicate); GAVISCON LIQUID (combined with sodium alginate and calcium chloride); GAVISCON TABLETS (combined with alginic acid, aluminium hydroxide, and magnesium trisilicate); JAPP'S HEALTH SALTS (combined with sodium potassium tartrate and tartaric acid); KLEAN-PREP (combined with polyethylene glycol, sodium sulphate, sodium chloride, and potassium chloride); ELECTROLADE (combined with sodium chloride, potassium chloride, and glucose); MICTRAL (combined with nalidixic acid, sodium citrate, and citric acid); NEO GRIPE MIXTURE (combined with dill seed oil and ginger tincture); ORIGINAL ANDREWS SALTS (combined with magnesium sulphate and citric acid); PEPTAC (combined with alginic acid and calcium carbonate); PHOSPHATE-SANDOZ (combined with sodium acid phosphate and potassium bicarbonate); PYROGASTRONE (combined with carbenoloxone sodium, magnesium trisilicate, aluminium hydroxide, and alginic acid); URIFLEX G (combined with citric acid, magnesium oxide, and disodium edetate); WOODWARD'S GRIPE WATER (combined with dill seed oil).

sodium calcium edetate A drug used for the treatment of poisoning by lead and other heavy metals (*dimercaprol may be used as an adjunct in lead poisoning). Sodium calcium edetate is available as a form for intravenous infusion on *prescription only.
Side effects: include nausea and cramps; overdosage can cause kidney damage.
Precautions: sodium calcium edetate should be used with caution in people with kidney disease.
Proprietary preparation: Ledclair.

sodium carbonate *See* SODIUM BICARBONATE.

sodium cellulose phosphate A drug that binds to *calcium in the gut and is used to prevent too much calcium being absorbed in people with high plasma concentrations of calcium. However, it is not regarded as a very successful treatment and may also produce a harmful rise in serum phosphate concentrations. Sodium cellulose phosphate is available as granules that are sprinkled onto food; it can be obtained without a prescription, but only from pharmacies.
Side effects: this medicine may cause diarrhoea.
Precautions: sodium cellulose phosphate should not be taken by people with severe kidney disease or congestive heart failure. It should be used with caution in growing children and women who are pregnant or breastfeeding.
Proprietary preparation: Calcisorb.

sodium chloride (common salt) A salt of *sodium that is present in all tissues and is important in maintaining the balance of *electrolytes in the body. Intravenous infusions of sodium chloride are the basis of fluid replacement therapy and treatment for conditions associated with sodium depletion of electrolyte imbalance. Saline solutions of the correct concentration are similar to the body fluids and are therefore less disruptive to normal tissue structure and functioning than water. Sodium chloride can be combined with other ingredients (such as glucose, other sodium salts, and salts of potassium and calcium) in infusions. Sodium chloride can also be taken by mouth and is a basic ingredient of *oral rehydration therapy. Saline solutions are used widely to cleanse wounds and skin, irrigate the bladder, irrigate and lubricate the eyes (*see also* BALANCED SALT SOLUTION), flush out tubes and catheters, and as a mouthwash. They are also used for diluting drugs given by means of some *nebulizers. Sodium chloride is freely available *over the counter in the form of solutions, drops, or sprays; infusions are available on *prescription only.

Proprietary preparations: Irriclens; Minims Sodium Chloride (single-dose eye drops); Normasol; Saline Steri-Neb; Slow Sodium (tablets); Sterac Saline; Steripod Blue; Uriflex S; Uriflex SP; Uro-Tainer Saline; DIARREST (combined with codeine phosphate, dicyclomine <dicycloverine> hydrochloride, potassium chloride, and sodium citrate); DIOCALM REPLENISH (combined with glucose, sodium citrate, and potassium chloride); DIORALYTE NATURAL (combined with glucose, potassium chloride, and disodium hydrogen citrate); DIORALYTE RELIEF (combined with potassium chloride, sodium citrate, and precooked rice powder); DIORALYTE TABLETS (combined with sodium bicarbonate, citric acid, glucose, sodium chloride, and potassium chloride); ELECTROLADE (combined with potassium chloride, sodium bicarbonate, and glucose); MINIMS ARTIFICIAL TEARS (combined with hydroxyethylcellulose); MOVICOL (combined with polyethylene glycol, sodium sulphate, sodium bicarbonate, and potassium chloride).

sodium citrate A salt of sodium that is taken by mouth to make the urine alkaline in the treatment of cystitis and is instilled into the bladder to dissolve blood clots. It is also an *osmotic laxative used rectally to treat constipation. Sodium citrate is also an ingredient of electrolyte-replacement preparations used for the treatment of diarrhoea (*see* ORAL REHYDRATION THERAPY) and of *balanced salt solution for washing out the eyes. It can be obtained without a prescription in the form of granules to be dissolved in water or tablets (for cystitis) and as an enema.

Precautions: citrate tablets should be used with caution by elderly people, pregnant women, and by people with kidney or heart disease. Enemas should be used with caution in the elderly and should not be used by people with acute gastrointestinal conditions or inflammatory bowel disease.

Proprietary preparations: Boots Cystitis Relief (granules and tablets); Cymalon (granules); Cystemme (granules); Cystoleve (granules); DIARREST (combined with codeine phosphate, potassium chloride, and sodium chloride); DIOCALM REPLENISH (combined with glucose, sodium chloride, and potassium chloride); DIORALYTE RELIEF (combined with sodium chloride, potassium chloride, and precooked rice powder); FLEET MICRO-ENEMA (combined with sodium lauryl sulphoacetate); MICOLETTE MICRO-ENEMA (combined with sodium lauryl sulphoacetate); MICRALAX MICRO-ENEMA (combined with sodium alkylsulphoacetate); MICTRAL (combined with nalidixic acid, citric acid, and sodium bicarbonate); RELAXIT MICRO-ENEMA (combined with sodium lauryl sulphate).

sodium clodronate A *bisphosphonate used for the treatment of high blood concentrations of calcium and bone pain associated with primary or secondary bone cancers. It is available, on *prescription only, as tablets, capsules, or a solution for injection.

Side effects: include nausea, diarrhoea, and (rarely) allergic skin reactions.

Precautions: sodium clodronate should not be taken by women who are pregnant or breastfeeding. It should be used with caution in people with impaired kidney function.

Interactions with other drugs:

Aminoglycosides: in combination with sodium clodronate, they may cause abnormally low concentrations of calcium in the plasma.

Antacids: reduce the absorption of oral clodronate.

Calcium supplements: reduce the absorption of oral clodronate.

Iron supplements: reduce the absorption of oral clodronate.

NSAIDs: kidney damage may occur if these drugs are taken with clodronate.

Proprietary preparations: Bonefos; Loron.

sodium cromoglycate <sodium cromoglicate> A *chromone drug used to prevent attacks in the treatment of *asthma and a variety of other allergic conditions. It is available as liquid or powder aerosols for inhalation, sprays or drops for the nose, and drops or ointment for the eyes. For food allergy sodium cromoglycate is given as capsules. It is available on *prescription and some preparations can be bought from pharmacies without a prescription.

Side effects: inhalation, especially of powder, may cause local irritation of the throat, coughing, and transient wheezing and breathlessness. Taking capsules occasionally causes nausea, rashes, and joint pain. Local irritation may occur with preparations for the nose and eyes.

Proprietary preparations: Clariteyes (eye drops); Cromogen Easi-Breathe (breath-activated metered-dose aerosol inhalation); Cromogen Inhaler; Cromogen Steri-Neb (nebulizer solution); Hay-Crom (eye drops); Intal (metered-dose aerosol inhalation); Intal Fisonair (with spacer inhaler); Intal Spincaps (powder capsules for use with breath-activated Spinhaler device); Intal Syncroner (aerosol with spacer device); Nalcrom (capsules); Opticrom (eye drops and ointment); Optrex Hayfever Allergy Eye Drops; Rynacrom (nasal drops and spray); Vividrin (nasal spray); AEROCROM (combined with salbutamol); RESISTON ONE (combined with xylometazoline); RYNACROM COMPOUND (combined with xylometazoline).

sodium dihydrogen phosphate dihydrate See PHOSPHATE LAXATIVES.

sodium fluoride See FLUORIDE.

sodium iron edetate An *iron supplement used for the treatment of iron-deficiency anaemia. It is available as tablets without a prescription, but only from pharmacies.

Side effects, precautions, and interactions with other drugs: see IRON.

Proprietary preparation: Sytron.

sodium lauryl sulphoacetate A detergent and wetting agent (*see* SURFACTANT). It is used as an ingredient of shampoos, skin cleansers, and in toothpastes. It is also included in some *osmotic laxative preparations.

Side effects: sodium lauryl sulphoacetate can be irritating when applied directly to the skin.

Proprietary preparations: FLEET MICRO-ENEMA (combined with sodium citrate); MICOLETTE MICRO-ENEMA (combined with sodium citrate); RELAXIT MICRO-ENEMA (combined with sodium citrate).

sodium nitroprusside A cyanide-containing *vasodilator drug that is used in the emergency treatment of a sudden and severe rise in blood pressure (hypertensive crisis) and acute or chronic heart failure. It is also used by anaesthetists to control blood pressure during surgery. Nitroprusside is available as a solution for infusion on *prescription only.

Side effects: headache, dizziness, nausea, retching, abdominal pain, sweating, palpitations, and discomfort behind the breastbone are associated with rapid reduction of blood pressure induced by nitroprusside.

Precautions and interactions with other drugs: nitroprusside should not be used in people with severe liver disease or severe vitamin B_{12} deficiency. It should be used with caution in women who are pregnant or breastfeeding, in people with an overactive thyroid gland or certain heart conditions, and in the elderly. The blood-pressure-lowering effect of nitroprusside is increased by a large number of drugs (including anaesthetics).

sodium perborate A mild *antiseptic and disinfectant with deodorizing properties. It readily releases oxygen when dissolved in water and has an action similar to that of *hydrogen peroxide. Sodium perborate is used, in the form of a freshly prepared solution, as a mouthwash and, combined with *calcium carbonate, as a tooth powder.

Proprietary preparation: BOCASAN (combined with sodium hydrogen tartrate).

sodium phosphate *See* PHOSPHATE LAXATIVES.

sodium picosulphate <sodium picosulfate> A *stimulant laxative used for the treatment of constipation and for bowel evacuation before radiological examination, exploratory procedures, or surgery. It is available as an elixir (for constipation) and as a *bowel-cleansing solution (with magnesium citrate) and can be obtained without a prescription, but only from pharmacies.

Side effects and precautions: see STIMULANT LAXATIVES.

Proprietary preparations: Dulco-Lax Liquid; Laxoberal; PICOLAX (combined with magnesium citrate).

sodium polystyrene sulphonate   A resin that exchanges potassium ions for sodium ions in the intestine when it is taken by mouth or by enema. It is used to reduce high concentrations of potassium in blood associated with failure of the kidneys to produce adequate quantities of urine or in patients on dialysis. It is available as a powder and can be obtained without a prescription, but only from pharmacies.

Side effects: include high plasma sodium concentrations, low plasma potassium concentrations, loss of appetite, nausea and vomiting, constipation, and diarrhoea. If constipation occurs, treatment should be stopped and magnesium-containing laxatives avoided.

Precautions: sodium polystyrene sulphonate should not be taken by people with obstructive bowel disease and should be used with caution in women who are pregnant or breastfeeding. Plasma electrolytes may need to be monitored.

Interactions with other drugs:

  Lithium: sodium polystyrene sulphonate reduces the absorption of lithium.

Proprietary preparation: Resonium-A.

sodium potassium tartrate   *See* TARTARIC ACID.

sodium pyrrolidone carboxylate   A humectant (*see* EMOLLIENTS) used for the treatment of dry skin conditions. It is available as a cream and can be obtained without a prescription, but only from pharmacies. Some combined preparations are freely available *over the counter.

Proprietary preparations: Humiderm; HYDROMOL CREAM (combined with arachis oil, liquid paraffin, and sodium lactate); LACTICARE (combined with lactic acid).

sodium sulphate   An *osmotic laxative that is combined with other laxatives in a *bowel-cleansing solution for rapid evacuation of the bowel before investigation or surgery. It is also used alone for the treatment of constipation. Sodium sulphate is freely available *over the counter as a powder to be taken in water.

Precautions: sodium sulphate is not recommended for children.

Proprietary preparations: Fynnon Salts; KLEAN-PREP (combined with polyethylene glycol, sodium bicarbonate, sodium chloride, and potassium chloride).

sodium tetradecyl sulphate   An irritant substance that is used in *sclerotherapy to treat varicose veins. It is available, on *prescription only, as a solution for slow injection into the vein.

Side effects and precautions: see ETHANOLAMINE OLEATE.

Proprietary preparation: Fibro-Vein.

sodium valproate An *anticonvulsant drug used in the treatment of all forms of epilepsy: it is a drug of choice in major, absence, and partial seizures. It is suitable for long-term use, does not cause sedation, and can be taken with oral contraceptives. Sodium valproate is available, on *prescription only, as tablets, crushable tablets, a syrup, or a liquid for oral use and as an intravenous injection.

Side effects: include gastric irritation, nausea, unsteadiness, and weight gain. Transient hair loss, oedema, and blood disorders may occur; rare side effects are liver failure and bleeding disorders.

Precautions: patients who are planning on becoming pregnant, or who are already pregnant, should seek specialist advice.

Interactions with other drugs:

  Anticonvulsants: taking two or more anticonvulsants together may increase their adverse effects. Valproate often raises (but may lower) the plasma concentration of phenytoin; phenytoin often lowers the plasma concentration of valproate.

  Antidepressants: reduce the anticonvulsant effect of sodium valproate.

  Antimalarials: antagonize the anticonvulsant effect of sodium valproate.

  Antipsychotics: reduce the anticonvulsant effect of sodium valproate.

  Aspirin: enhances the effect of sodium valproate.

  Cimetidine: increases plasma concentrations of sodium valproate.

Proprietary preparations: Epilim; Orlept; Sondate 200 EC; EPILIM CHRONO (combined with valproic acid).

Sofradex (Hoechst Marion Roussel) A proprietary combination of *dexamethasone (a corticosteroid), *framycetin sulphate (an aminoglycoside antibiotic), and *gramicidin (an antibiotic), used for the treatment of inflammatory conditions of the eyes when infection is present or is likely to occur. It is also used to treat infections of the outer ear. Sofradex is available, on *prescription only, as eye drops or ointment or ear drops.

Side effects: see TOPICAL STEROIDS; FRAMYCETIN SULPHATE.

Precautions: long-term use of Sofradex should be avoided in infants. *See also* TOPICAL STEROIDS.

Soframycin (Hoechst Marion Roussel) A proprietary combination of the antibiotics *framycetin sulphate and *gramicidin in the form of an ointment, used for treating bacterial skin infections. Soframycin drops and ointment for treating eye infections contain framycetin as the sole ingredient. Soframycin preparations are available on *prescription only.

Side effects and precautions: see FRAMYCETIN SULPHATE.

Soft Corn Remover Pads (Seton Scholl Healthcare) *See* SALICYLIC ACID.

Solarcaine (Schering-Plough) A proprietary combination of *benzocaine (a local anaesthetic) and *triclosan (an antiseptic), used for the treatment of minor skin injuries and burns, including sunburn. It is available as a cream, lotion, or aerosol spray and can be obtained without a prescription, but only from pharmacies.

Precautions: Solarcaine is not recommended for children under three years old. It should not be used for longer than three days without medical advice.

Solian (Lorex Synthélabo) *See* AMISULPRIDE.

Solpadeine (SmithKline Beecham Consumer Healthcare) A proprietary combination of *paracetamol (an analgesic and antipyretic), *codeine (an opioid analgesic), and *caffeine (a stimulant), used for the relief of migraine, headache, rheumatic pains, period pains, toothache, and the fever and pain associated with colds and influenza. It is available as capsules, tablets, or effervescent tablets and can be obtained without a prescription, but only from pharmacies.

Side effects: *see* CODEINE.

Precautions: Solpadeine is not recommended for children. *See also* PARACETAMOL; OPIOIDS; CAFFEINE.

Interactions with other drugs: *see* OPIOIDS.

Solpadol (Sanofi Winthrop) *See* CO-CODAMOL.

Solpaflex (SmithKline Beecham Consumer Healthcare) A proprietary combination of *ibuprofen (an NSAID) and *codeine (an opioid analgesic), used to relieve the symptoms of colds and influenza, rheumatic and muscular pain, backache, migraine, headache, toothache, and period pains. It is available as tablets and can be obtained without a prescription, but only from pharmacies.

Side effects and interactions with other drugs: *see* NSAIDS; CODEINE; OPIOIDS.

Precautions: Solpaflex is not recommended for children. *See also* NSAIDS; CODEINE; OPIOIDS.

Solpaflex Gel (SmithKline Beecham Consumer Healthcare) *See* KETOPROFEN.

Solu-Cortef (Pharmacia & Upjohn) *See* HYDROCORTISONE.

Solu-Medrone (Pharmacia & Upjohn) *See* METHYLPREDNISOLONE.

Solvazinc (Cortecs Healthcare) *See* ZINC SULPHATE.

somatorelin *See* GROWTH HORMONE.

somatostatin *See* GROWTH HORMONE; LANREOTIDE; OCTREOTIDE.

somatropin A genetically engineered form of *growth hormone used for the treatment of children whose own secretion of growth hormone is insufficient to achieve normal stature. It is also used to treat underdevelopment of the ovaries or testes, Turner's syndrome (a genetic abnormality causing short stature and infertility in females), and the poor growth seen in children with kidney insufficiency. A *prescription only medicine, it is given by *subcutaneous injection; pens for self-injection are available.

Side effects: include fluid retention, inhibition of the functioning of the thyroid gland (causing tiredness, lethargy, and weight gain), and reactions at the injection site.

Precautions: somatropin should not be taken by people who have had a kidney transplant or by those with cancer; it should not be used to promote growth in children who have completed puberty. It should be used with caution in people with diabetes, poor thyroid function, or a history of malignant disease and by pregnant women.

Proprietary preparations: Genotropin; Humatrope; Norditropin; Saizen; Zomacton.

Somatuline LA (Ipsen) *See* LANREOTIDE.

Sominex (Seton Scholl Healthcare) *See* PROMETHAZINE HYDROCHLORIDE.

Somnite (Norgine) *See* NITRAZEPAM.

Sondate 200 EC (APS-Berk) *See* SODIUM VALPROATE.

Soneryl (Concord Pharmaceuticals) *See* BUTOBARBITONE <BUTOBARBITAL>.

Soothelip (Bayer) *See* ACICLOVIR.

Sorbichew (AstraZeneca) *See* ISOSORBIDE DINITRATE.

Sorbid SA (AstraZeneca) *See* ISOSORBIDE DINITRATE.

Sorbitrate (AstraZeneca) *See* ISOSORBIDE DINITRATE.

Sotacor (Bristol-Myers Squibb) *See* SOTALOL HYDROCHLORIDE.

sotalol hydrochloride A non-cardioselective *beta blocker that is also a class III *anti-arrhythmic drug; it is used for the treatment and prevention of heart *arrhythmias. It is available as tablets or solution for injection on *prescription only.

Side effects and precautions: see BETA BLOCKERS.

Interactions with other drugs: the risk of ventricular arrhythmias is increased if sotalol is taken with certain drugs. Sotalol should therefore not be taken with the following drugs: amiodarone, disopyramide, procainamide, and quinidine (all anti-arrhythmic drugs); astemizole,

terfenadine, and mizolastine (antihistamines); and cisapride. It should be used with caution with tricyclic antidepressants, phenothiazines, and halofantrine. *See also* BETA BLOCKERS.
Proprietary preparations: Beta-Cardone; Sotacor.

soya oil An oil expressed from soya beans. It is used as an *emollient for the relief of dry skin conditions.
Proprietary preparations: Balneum (bath oil); BALNEUM PLUS OIL (combined with lauromacrogols).

spansule A capsule. The term is usually restricted to *modified-release capsules.

Spasmonal, Spasmonal Forte (Norgine) *See* ALVERINE CITRATE.

SP Cold Relief Capsules (Sussex Pharmaceutical) A proprietary combination of *paracetamol (an analgesic and antipyretic), *phenylephrine (a decongestant), and *caffeine (a stimulant), used to treat the symptoms of colds and influenza. It is freely available *over the counter.
Side effects and interactions with other drugs: see PHENYLEPHRINE.
Precautions: see PARACETAMOL; PHENYLEPHRINE; CAFFEINE.

spectinomycin A narrow-spectrum *antibiotic used for the treatment of gonorrhoea caused by *penicillin-resistant organisms or gonorrhoea in patients who are allergic to penicillin. It is related in structure and in the way it functions to the *aminoglycosides. Spectinomycin is administered by deep *intramuscular injection and is available on *prescription only.
Side effects: include nausea, dizziness, urticaria, and fever.
Precautions: this drug should be used with caution in women who are pregnant or breastfeeding.
Interactions with other drugs:
  Botulinum toxin: spectinomycin enhances the toxic effects of botulinum toxin and the two drugs should not be used together.
  Lithium: the effects of lithium are enhanced and therefore there is an increased risk of toxicity.
Proprietary preparation: Trobocin.

Spectraban (Stiefel Laboratories) A proprietary *sunscreen preparation consisting of a lotion containing *aminobenzoic acid and padimate-O. It provides protection against UVB only (SPF 25). **Spectraban Ultra Lotion** also contains oxybenzone and *titanium dioxide but no aminobenzoic acid. It protects against both UVA and UVB (SPF 28). Both lotions can be prescribed on the NHS or obtained without a prescription.

spermicidal contraceptives Preparations in which the active ingredient is a **spermicide** (an agent that kills sperm). These contraceptives are applied locally and should be used in conjunction with barrier forms of contraception (condoms or diaphragms) as an additional safeguard against pregnancy: they are not very effective as the sole means of contraception. However, some preparations may be used alone in the year following the final menstrual period, when protection is still advisable. Spermicidal contraceptives are available, without a prescription, in the form of creams, gels, foams, or pessaries (*see* NONOXINOL-9).

Side effects: there may be local sensitivity to the active ingredient or to the perfume in the preparation.

Spiroctan (Roche Products) *See* SPIRONOLACTONE.

Spiroctan-M (Roche Products) *See* POTASSIUM CANRENOATE.

Spirolone (APS-Berk) *See* SPIRONOLACTONE.

spironolactone A *potassium-sparing diuretic that acts by inhibiting the activity of aldosterone, a hormone secreted by the adrenal gland that promotes potassium excretion and sodium retention by the kidneys. Spironolactone is used in the treatment of *oedema associated with cirrhosis of the liver, congestive *heart failure, kidney disorders, and primary hyperaldosteronism (a condition called Conn's syndrome, in which high concentrations of aldosterone occur as a result of increased activity of the adrenal gland). Its effects are slow and may only be seen after a few days' use. It may be given alone or in combination with *thiazide diuretics or *loop diuretics. Spironolactone is available as tablets or capsules on *prescription only. It is sometimes used to treat hirsutism (excess body hair) in women and acne vulgaris but it does not have a *licence for these uses. *See also* CO-FLUMACTONE.

Side effects: nausea and vomiting are more common with spironolactone than with other potassium-sparing diuretics (affecting 10% of individuals). Potassium retention may occur, causing muscle weakness and numbness. Men may experience breast enlargement and reversible impotence. Less commonly menstrual irregularities, diarrhoea, headache, confusion, and rash can occur.

Precautions: see POTASSIUM-SPARING DIURETICS.

Interactions with other drugs:

ACE inhibitors: see POTASSIUM-SPARING DIURETICS.

Carbenoxolone: its activity may be reduced by spironolactone.

Digoxin: concentrations may be increased, causing adverse effects.

Proprietary preparations: Aldactone; Laractone; Spiroctan; Spirolone; Spirospare; Aldactide 25 and Aldactide 50 (*see* CO-FLUMACTONE); LASILACTONE (combined with frusemide <furosemide>).

See also DIURETICS.

Spirospare (Ashbourne Pharmaceuticals) *See* SPIRONOLACTONE.

Sporanox (Janssen-Cilag) *See* ITRACONAZOLE.

Sprilon (Smith & Nephew Healthcare) A proprietary combination of *dimethicone <dimeticone> (a water repellent) and *zinc oxide (an astringent protective agent) in the form of a spray, used as a *barrier preparation to protect the skin around a *stoma after ileostomy or colostomy and for the treatment of eczema, leg ulcers, fissures (breaks in the skin), and pressure sores. It is freely available *over the counter.

squalane An oil that is included in some topical preparations to increase the absorption of the active ingredients. It is also a skin lubricant.
Proprietary preparations: DERMALEX (combined with hexachlorophane <hexachlorophene> and allantoin); SALONAIR (combined with glycol salicylate, menthol, camphor, benzyl nicotinate, and methyl salicylate).

squill An extract from the bulb of a species of lily (*Urginea maritima*) that is used as an *expectorant in cough remedies. It is available as a liquid, syrup, medicated sweets, and throat lozenges that are freely available *over the counter.
Side effects: squill may cause nausea and vomiting.
Proprietary preparations: Buttercup Honey and Lemon; Buttercup Syrup Traditional; ES BRONCHIAL MIXTURE (combined with ammonium bicarbonate, ipecacuanha, and senna); GALLOWAYS COUGH SYRUP (combined with ipecacuanha).

SSRIs (selective serotonin reuptake inhibitors) A class of *antidepressant drugs that act by inhibiting the reuptake of *serotonin (and possibly also of noradrenaline <norepinephrine>) and thus prolonging its action in the brain. They are less sedative than *tricyclic antidepressants (TCAs), with fewer *antimuscarinic side effects (dry mouth, blurred vision, constipation, and urinary retention), and fewer toxic effects on the heart. They do not cause weight gain. However, they have more gastrointestinal side effects (including nausea and vomiting) than the TCAs. The SSRIs are *citalopram, *fluoxetine, *fluvoxamine maleate, *paroxetine, and *sertraline. *Nefazodone hydrochloride and *venlafaxine are related to the SSRIs.
Side effects: include dose-related gastrointestinal effects (diarrhoea, nausea and vomiting, dyspepsia, abdominal pain, constipation, and loss of appetite) and weight loss; headache, restlessness, nervousness, and anxiety may also occur. Other possible side effects are dry mouth, palpitation, tremor, confusion, dizziness, low blood pressure, mania, convulsions, interference with sexual function, sweating, and movement disorders. Allergic reactions (rash, itching, swelling of the face) should be reported to a doctor.
Precautions: SSRIs should be used with caution in people who have liver, kidney, or heart disease or epilepsy, in women who are pregnant or breastfeeding, and in patients who are undergoing electroconvulsive therapy.
Interactions with other drugs:

Anticoagulants: the effects of warfarin and nicoumalone <acenocoumarol> are increased.

Antiepileptics: SSRIs increase the risk of convulsions recurring.

Astemizole: increases the risk of *arrhythmias and should not be taken with SSRIs.

Lithium: can increase the toxic effects of SSRIs.

MAOIs: the effects of MAOIs are increased. SSRIs should not be started until two weeks after stopping MAOIs; MAOIs should not be started until at least a week after SSRIs have been stopped (at least five weeks for fluoxetine, two weeks for paroxetine and sertraline).

Ritonavir: may increase plasma concentrations of SSRIs.

Sumatriptan: there is an increased risk of toxic effects on the central nervous system.

Other interactions are given in the entries for individual SSRIs.

stanozolol An *anabolic steroid used for the treatment of Behçet's disease (ulceration or inflammation affecting many parts of the body) and a hereditary form of angioedema (*see* ANAPHYLAXIS). It should not be used for promoting weight or appetite. Stanozolol is available as tablets on *prescription only.

Side effects: masculinizing effects (including acne, increased growth of body hair, and lack of periods) are usually reversible when treatment stops. Other side effects include irregular periods, headache, muscle cramps, indigestion, rash, hair loss, depression, and jaundice.

Precautions: stanozolol should not be taken by women who are pregnant or breastfeeding or by people with established liver disease, prostate cancer, or insulin-dependent diabetes. It should be used with caution in children (since it may affect stature) and in people with heart or kidney disease, high blood pressure, epilepsy, or migraine.

Interactions with other drugs: see ANABOLIC STEROIDS.

Proprietary preparation: Stromba.

Staril (Bristol-Myers Squibb) *See* FOSINOPRIL.

statins A group of *lipid-lowering drugs that act by inhibiting the enzyme HMG Co-A (hydroxy-3-methylglutaryl coenzyme A, which is involved in the synthesis of *cholesterol. They lower total cholesterol (typically LDL-cholesterol is reduced by 40%) and, to a lesser extent, plasma *triglycerides, and also increase plasma HDL (*see* LIPOPROTEINS). They are more effective than *bile-acid sequestrants in lowering LDL-cholesterol, but less effective than *fibrates in reducing triglycerides and raising HDL-cholesterol. Statins are used to treat *hyperlipidaemias in which high cholesterol concentrations are the main feature and which have not responded to dietary measures. They are also used to prevent the progression of *atherosclerosis and to reduce the incidence of untoward events in patients who have high cholesterol levels or known coronary artery disease. *See* ATORVASTATIN; CERIVASTATIN; FLUVASTATIN; PRAVASTATIN; SIMVASTATIN.

Side effects: reversible muscle inflammation and rhabdomyolysis (a serious condition involving muscle breakdown) can occur, but this is rare. Other side effects include headache, abdominal pain, nausea, and vomiting.

Precautions and interactions with other drugs: rhabdomyolysis is more likely to occur in people who are also taking *cyclosporin, *nicotinic acid, or *fibrates. Any muscle pain, tenderness, or weakness should be reported to a doctor promptly. Statins should not be taken by people with active liver disease and should be used with caution in those with a history of liver disease or alcoholism. Women should avoid pregnancy during and for one month after treatment.

status epilepticus *See* ANTICONVULSANT DRUGS.

stavudine An *antiviral drug that prevents retrovirus replication: it is a nucleoside analogue that inhibits the action of reverse transcriptase. Stavudine is used for the treatment of *HIV infection; it is available, on *prescription only, as capsules or an oral solution.

Side effects: include headache, fever, malaise, nausea, vomiting, diarrhoea, damage to peripheral nerves (causing weakness or numbness in the feet and hands), pancreatitis, chest pain, skin irritation and rash, and influenza-like symptoms.

Precautions: stavudine should be used with caution in people with a history of pancreatitis or disease of the peripheral nerves. It should not be taken by women who are pregnant or breastfeeding.

Interactions with other drugs:

Cytotoxic drugs: stavudine enhances the adverse effects of cyclophosphamide, doxorubicin, and etoposide. Doxorubicin may inhibit the effect of stavudine.

Proprietary preparation: Zerit.

Stelazine (Goldshield Pharmaceuticals) *See* TRIFLUOPERAZINE.

Stemetil (Rhône-Poulenc Rorer) *See* PROCHLORPERAZINE.

Sterac Saline (Galen) *See* SODIUM CHLORIDE.

sterculia A vegetable gum used as a *bulk-forming laxative for treating constipation. It is freely available *over the counter in the form of granules.

Side effects and precautions: see ISPAGHULA HUSK.

Proprietary preparations: Normacol; ALVERCOL (combined with alverine citrate); NORMACOL PLUS (combined with frangula).

Sterexidine (Galen) *See* CHLORHEXIDINE.

Steri-Neb Ipratropium (Norton Healthcare) *See* IPRATROPIUM BROMIDE.

Steripod Blue (Seton Scholl Healthcare) *See* SODIUM CHLORIDE.

Steripod Pink (Seton Scholl Healthcare) *See* CHLORHEXIDINE.

Steripod Yellow (Seton Scholl Healthcare) A proprietary combination of the antiseptics *chlorhexidine gluconate and *cetrimide, used for cleansing and disinfecting wounds and burns. It is available as a solution without a prescription, but only from pharmacies.
Side effects: see CETRIMIDE.
Precautions: the solution should not come into contact with the eyes.

steroids A group of chemically related compounds that includes the *corticosteroids, the *androgens (male sex hormones) and *anabolic steroids, the *oestrogens and *progestogens (female sex hormones), and the bile acids. When used without qualification, the term 'steroid' usually refers to a corticosteroid.

Ster-Zac Bath Concentrate (Seton Scholl Healthcare) *See* TRICLOSAN.

Ster-Zac DC, **Ster-Zac Powder** (Seton Scholl Healthcare) *See* HEXACHLOROPHANE <HEXACHLOROPHENE>.

Stesolid (Cox Pharmaceuticals) *See* DIAZEPAM.

Stiedex Lotion (Stiefel Laboratories) A proprietary combination of *desoxymethasone <desoximetasone> (a moderately potent topical steroid) and *salicylic acid (a keratolytic), used for the treatment of *psoriasis (particularly of the scalp), *eczema, lichen planus (an extremely itchy skin condition), and other disorders of the skin in which irritation is a predominant feature. It is available on *prescription only.
Side effects and precautions: see TOPICAL STEROIDS.

Stiedex LP (Stiefel Laboratories) *See* DESOXYMETHASONE <DESOXIMETASONE>.

Stiemycin (Stiefel Laboratories) *See* ERYTHROMYCIN.

stilboestrol <diethylstilbestrol> A synthetic *oestrogen used in the form of pessaries in *hormone replacement therapy for local relief of postmenopausal inflammation of the vagina. It is also taken as tablets for the treatment of breast cancer in postmenopausal women. Stilboestrol is available on *prescription only.
Side effects: see ETHINYLOESTRADIOL <ETHINYLESTRADIOL>; OESTROGENS.
Precautions and interactions with other drugs: see ETHINYLOESTRADIOL <ETHINYLESTRADIOL>.
Proprietary preparations: Apstil (tablets); Tampovagan (pessaries).

Stilline (APS-Berk) *See* SELEGILINE.

Stilnoct (Lorex Synthélabo) *See* ZOLPIDEM TARTRATE.

stimulant laxatives *Laxatives that stimulate motility of the intestines. They are used for the treatment of constipation and to clear the bowel before X-ray examination or surgery. Stimulant laxatives include *bisacodyl, *docusate sodium, *senna, and *sodium picosulphate. *See also* ALOIN; CASCARA; DANTHRON <DANTRON>; GLYCERIN; OXYPHENISATIN <OXYPHENISATINE>.
Side effects and precautions: stimulant laxatives may cause colicky pains. They should not be taken by people with gastrointestinal obstruction and are best avoided in children. Long-term use can cause low plasma *potassium concentrations and colonic atony (a nonfunctioning large intestine), with black staining of the colon.

stimulants Drugs that promote the activity of a body system or function. The term usually refers to **central nervous system stimulants**, which increase activity in the brain and spinal cord, producing feelings of alertness. Central nervous system stimulants include *dexamphetamine <dexamfetamine> sulphate, *methylphenidate hydrochloride, *modafinil, and *caffeine. **Respiratory stimulants** (also called **analeptic drugs**), mainly *doxapram hydrochloride, are occasionally used to stimulate breathing in comatose patients when mechanical ventilation cannot be used. They act on the central nervous system to stimulate the muscles involved in breathing, but since they also increase the activity of other muscles they may be harmful.

stoma The artificial opening created when part of the ileum or colon (small or large intestine, respectively) is brought to the surface of the body. The operation to create such an opening is an ileostomy or a colostomy. Various pouches and other appliances are designed to be used with stomas, and there is a variety of preparations, including *barrier preparations, for protecting the skin around a stoma.

Strepsils (Crookes Healthcare) A proprietary combination of the antiseptics *dichlorobenzyl alcohol and *amylmetacresol, used to relieve the symptoms of minor infections of the mouth and throat. It is freely available *over the counter in the form of lozenges (**Strepsils Original**, **Strepsils with Vitamin C**, and a variety of flavoured formulations).

Strepsils Dual Action Lozenges (Crookes Healthcare) A proprietary combination of *dichlorobenzyl alcohol and *amylmetacresol (antiseptics) and *lignocaine <lidocaine> (a local anaesthetic), used to relieve the pain and other symptoms of minor infections of the mouth and throat. It can be obtained without a prescription, but only from pharmacies.
Precautions: these lozenges should not be taken by children under 12 years old. *See also* LOCAL ANAESTHETICS.

Strepsils Pain Relief Spray (Crookes Healthcare) *See* LIGNOCAINE <LIDOCAINE>.

Streptase (Hoechst Marion Roussel) *See* STREPTOKINASE.

streptodornase An enzyme produced by *Streptococcus* bacteria. It liquefies pus and dead tissue and is combined with *streptokinase in a topical preparation for cleaning ulcers.
Proprietary preparation: VARIDASE TOPICAL (combined with streptokinase).

streptokinase A *fibrinolytic drug used for the treatment of deep-vein *thrombosis, pulmonary embolism, and an acute heart attack; treatment should be started rapidly (in the case of a heart attack, within 12 hours). Streptokinase is also used to dissolve blood clots in the shunts used to connect patients to kidney dialysis equipment. It is available in a form for intravenous injection or infusion on *prescription only. Because antibodies are formed against streptokinase, it is not usually used on more than one occasion.
Side effects: see FIBRINOLYTIC DRUGS. In addition, streptokinase may cause allergic reactions (such as rashes).
Precautions and interactions with other drugs: see FIBRINOLYTIC DRUGS.
Proprietary preparations: Kabikinase; Streptase; VARIDASE TOPICAL (combined with streptodornase).

streptomycin An *aminoglycoside antibiotic used for the treatment of *tuberculosis that has failed to respond to standard therapy; it is given in combination with other antituberculosis drugs. Streptomycin is also used in conjunction with *doxycycline to treat brucellosis. It is available as a form for intramuscular injection on *prescription only; its use is restricted to specialists.
Side effects, precautions, and interactions with other drugs: see GENTAMICIN.

Stromba (Sanofi Winthrop) *See* STANOZOLOL.

Stugeron, **Stugeron Forte** (Janssen-Cilag) *See* CINNARIZINE.

styrax The balsam obtained from the bark of the liquidambar tree, which has mild *antiseptic properties. It is used in *topical preparations for treatment of mouth ulcers and is a component of *benzoin tincture.
Proprietary preparation: FRADOR (combined with chlorbutol <chlorobutanol> and menthol).

subcutaneous injection The *injection of a drug under the skin, using a small volume of liquid (1–2 mL) and a narrow-gauge injection needle that is usually pushed through the skin at an angle of 45°. It is difficult and painful to inject larger volumes. A common site is the upper arm.

Sublimaze (Janssen-Cilag) *See* FENTANYL.

sublingual Beneath the tongue: refers to a route of administration of tablets or capsules of certain drugs (such as nitrates) that are placed under the tongue and allowed to dissolve there.

sucralfate A substance that can coat and stick to mucous membranes. It has a *cytoprotectant action, forming a barrier between peptic ulcers and the stomach acid, which allows the ulcers to heal (*see* ACID-PEPTIC DISEASES). It is also used for the prevention of gastric bleeding due to stress ulceration in seriously ill patients, and can be used as mouthwash to coat sore patches or mouth ulcers, especially in people who have mouth problems due to radiotherapy or chemotherapy. Sucralfate is available, on *prescription only, as tablets or a suspension.
Side effects: include constipation, diarrhoea, nausea, indigestion, dry mouth, and rash.
Precautions: sucralfate should not be used in people with impaired kidney function.
Interactions with other drugs:
  Digoxin: its absorption may be reduced by sucralfate: an interval of two hours should be left between taking digoxin and sucralfate.
  Phenytoin: its absorption is reduced by sucralfate: an interval of two hours should be left between taking phenytoin and sucralfate.
  Tetracyclines: their absorption is reduced by sucralfate: an interval of two hours should be left between taking tetracyclines and sucralfate.
  Warfarin: its absorption may be reduced by sucralfate.
Proprietary preparation: Antepsin.

Sudafed (Warner-Lambert Consumer Healthcare) *See* PSEUDOEPHEDRINE.

Sudafed-Co (Warner-Lambert Consumer Healthcare) A proprietary combination of *pseudoephedrine (a decongestant) and *paracetamol (an analgesic and antipyretic), used for the relief of nasal and sinus congestion, pain, and other symptoms associated with colds, influenza, and sinusitis. It is available as tablets and can be obtained without a prescription, but only from pharmacies.
Side effects and interactions with other drugs: see DECONGESTANTS; EPHEDRINE HYDROCHLORIDE.
Precautions: Sudafed-Co is not recommended for children under six years old. *See also* DECONGESTANTS; PARACETAMOL.

Sudafed Expectorant (Warner-Lambert Consumer Healthcare) A proprietary combination of *pseudoephedrine (a decongestant) and *guaiphenesin <guaifenesin> (an expectorant), used to relieve the symptoms of infections of the upper airways that are accompanied by a productive cough. It is available as a syrup without a prescription, but only from pharmacies.

Side effects and interactions with other drugs: see EPHEDRINE HYDROCHLORIDE; DECONGESTANTS; GUAIPHENESIN <GUAIFENESIN>.

Precautions: this medicine is not recommended for children under two years old. *See also* EPHEDRINE HYDROCHLORIDE; DECONGESTANTS; GUAIPHENESIN <GUAIFENESIN>.

Sudafed Linctus (Warner-Lambert Consumer Healthcare) A proprietary combination of *dextromethorphan (a cough suppressant) and *pseudoephedrine (a decongestant), used to relieve dry coughs and congestion associated with infections of the upper airways. It is available as a liquid without a prescription, but only from pharmacies.

Side effects and interactions with other drugs: see DEXTROMETHORPHAN; EPHEDRINE HYDROCHLORIDE; DECONGESTANTS.

Precautions: this medicine is not recommended for children under two years old. *See also* OPIOIDS; EPHEDRINE HYDROCHLORIDE; DECONGESTANTS.

Sudafed Nasal Spray (Warner-Lambert Consumer Healthcare) *See* OXYMETAZOLINE.

Sudafed Plus (Warner-Lambert Consumer Healthcare) A proprietary combination of *triprolidine hydrochloride (an antihistamine) and *pseudoephedrine (a decongestant), used for the treatment of hay fever. It is available as tablets without a prescription, but only from pharmacies.

Side effects: include drowsiness, rash, sleep disturbances, and (rarely) hallucinations.

Precautions: alcohol increases its sedative effects. Sudafed Plus should not be taken by people with severe high blood pressure or coronary artery disease. It should be used with caution by people with an enlarged prostate, an overactive thyroid gland, or diabetes.

Interactions with other drugs:

MAOIs: may cause a dangerous rise in blood pressure.

Sudocrem (Tosara Products) A proprietary combination of *zinc oxide (an astringent protective agent) anhydrous *lanolin (an emollient), benzyl alcohol (an antiseptic), benzyl benzoate (which improves its spreading properties), and benzyl cinnamate (a preservative), used for the prevention and treatment of bed sores and napkin rash and for the relief of burns and *eczema. It is freely available *over the counter in the form of a cream.

Sulazine EC (Cox Pharmaceuticals) *See* SULPHASALAZINE <SULFASALAZINE>.

sulconazole An imidazole *antifungal drug that is active against a wide range of fungi. It is used for the treatment of fungal skin infections, especially tinea (ringworm), candidiasis (thrush), and pityriasis versicolor (a chronic fungal infection of the skin). Sulconazole is available as a cream on *prescription only.

Side effects: sulconazole may cause irritation and reddening of the skin; if irritation occurs, treatment should be stopped.

Precautions: the cream should not come into contact with the eyes.

Proprietary preparation: Exelderm.

Suleo-M (Seton Scholl Healthcare) *See* MALATHION.

sulfadiazine *See* SULPHADIAZINE.

sulfadimidine *See* SULPHADIMIDINE.

sulfadoxine A long-acting *sulphonamide antibiotic used in combination with *pyrimethamine for the treatment of malaria.

Side effects, precautions, and interactions with other drugs: see CO-TRIMOXAZOLE.

Proprietary preparation: FANSIDAR (combined with pyrimethamine).

sulfamethoxazole *See* SULPHAMETHOXAZOLE.

sulfametopyrazine A *sulphonamide antibiotic used for the treatment of urinary-tract infections and chronic bronchitis. It is available as tablets on *prescription only.

Side effects, precautions, and interactions with other drugs: see CO-TRIMOXAZOLE.

Proprietary preparation: Kelfizine W.

sulfasalazine *See* SULPHASALAZINE.

sulfinpyrazone *See* SULPHINPYRAZONE.

sulindac An *NSAID used for the treatment of pain and inflammation in rheumatoid arthritis and other disorders of the joints or muscles and to relieve the pain of acute gout. It is available as tablets on *prescription only.

Side effects: see NSAIDS. In addition, sulindac may occasionally cause discoloration of the urine.

Precautions: see NSAIDS. In addition, sulindac should be used with caution in people with a history of kidney stones, who should be advised to drink plenty of fluids.

Interactions with other drugs: see NSAIDS.

Proprietary preparation: Clinoril.

Sulparex (Bristol-Myers Squibb) *See* SULPIRIDE.

sulphadiazine <sulfadiazine> A *sulphonamide antibiotic used to prevent the recurrence of rheumatic fever; it is also used for the treatment of toxoplasmosis (a protozoal infection that can cause blindness and mental retardation in a fetus), although it does not have a *licence in the UK for this. Sulphadiazine is available as tablets or an injection on *prescription only.
Side effects, precautions, and interactions with other drugs: see CO-TRIMOXAZOLE.

sulphadimidine <sulfadimidine> A *sulphonamide antibiotic used for the treatment of urinary-tract infections. It is available as tablets on *prescription only.
Side effects, precautions, and interactions with other drugs: see CO-TRIMOXAZOLE; SULPHONAMIDES.

sulphamethoxazole <sulfamethoxazole> A *sulphonamide antibiotic used in combination with the antibacterial drug trimethoprim (*see* CO-TRIMOXAZOLE) to treat a variety of serious infections.
Side effects, precautions, and interactions with other drugs: see CO-TRIMOXAZOLE.

sulphasalazine <sulfasalazine> A drug that is a combination of aminosalicylic acid and the sulphonamide sulphapyridine <sulfapyridene> (*see* AMINOSALICYLATES). It is used for the treatment of the inflammatory bowel diseases ulcerative colitis and Crohn's disease. Sulphasalazine is also used for the treatment of active rheumatoid arthritis that has not responded to *NSAIDs alone; unlike NSAIDs, it does not have an immediate therapeutic effect and it may take 4–6 months to obtain a full response. Sulphasalazine is available, on *prescription only, as tablets, *enteric-coated tablets, a suspension, suppositories, or an enema.
Side effects: include nausea, diarrhoea, headache, rashes and more severe allergic reactions, fever, loss of appetite, blood disorders (see below), and damage to the kidneys and liver.
Precautions: blood counts and liver-function tests should be carried out at the start of treatment and may be necessary during treatment. Sulphasalazine should not be taken by people who are allergic to aminosalicylates or sulphonamides and should be used with caution in those with a history of allergy or impaired liver or kidney function. Unexplained bleeding, bruising, sore throat, fever, or malaise should be reported to a doctor immediately as this may indicate a blood disorder. *See* AMINOSALICYLATES.
Proprietary preparations: Salazopyrin, Salazopyrin EN-Tabs; Sulazine EC.

sulphinpyrazone <sulfinpyrazone> A drug used for the long-term treatment of gout and recurrent gouty arthritis; it acts by increasing the amount of uric acid excreted in the urine. It is not used to control acute attacks, and may in fact exacerbate symptoms if started during an attack.

Sulphinpyrazone may be used in conjunction with *allopurinol. It is available as tablets on *prescription only.

Side effects: include gastrointestinal disturbances and occasionally rashes and salt and water retention. Rarely, blood disorders and gastrointestinal ulcers and bleeding may occur.

Precautions: people taking sulphinpyrazone must maintain an adequate fluid intake (at least 2 litres a day) to prevent crystals of uric acid being passed in the urine (which can cause pain and bleeding). Sulphinpyrazone should not be taken by people with peptic ulcers or kidney disease.

Interactions with other drugs:

Anticoagulants: sulphinpyrazone enhances the anticoagulant effects of warfarin and nicoumalone <acenocoumarol>.

Aspirin: antagonizes the effect of sulphinpyrazone.

Phenytoin: the plasma concentration of phenytoin is increased.

Sulphonylureas: their effects are enhanced by sulphinpyrazone.

Theophylline: the plasma concentration of theophylline is reduced.

Proprietary preparation: Anturan.

sulphonamides A group of *antibiotics, derived from sulphanilamide (a red dye), that prevent the growth of bacteria (i.e. they are bacteriostatic). They act by inhibiting the production of an essential bacterial growth factor, folic acid. Most sulphonamides are taken orally and are short-acting, therefore they may need to be taken several times day. Because they are rapidly excreted and are very soluble in the urine, some of them may be used for treating urinary-tract infections. Topical sulphonamides are used in the treatment of infected burns.

A variety of side effects may occur with sulphonamide treatment, including nausea, vomiting, headache, and loss of appetite; more severe effects include blood disorders, skin rashes, and fever. Because of increasing bacterial resistance to sulphonamides and their adverse effects, and with the development of more effective less toxic antibiotics, the clinical use of these drugs has declined. Those still used include sulphamethoxazole <sulfamethoxazole> (combined with trimethoprim as *co-trimoxazole), *sulphadimidine <sulfadimidine>, *sulphadiazine <sulfadiazine>, *silver sulphadiazine <sulfadiazine>, *sulfametopyrazine, sulfadoxine (combined with pyrimethamine as *Fansidar), and sulphathiazole <sulfathiazole>, sulphacetamide <sulfacetamide>, and sulphabenzamide <sulfabenzamide> (combined in *Sultrin).

sulphonylureas A group of *oral hypoglycaemic drugs derived from sulphonamide. They act by stimulating *insulin secretion from functioning beta cells of the pancreas and are therefore used to treat people with noninsulin-dependent *diabetes mellitus, who are still producing some natural insulin. Sulphonylureas cause weight gain and should be used in conjunction with a carefully controlled diet; they should only be taken if strict dietary measures have failed to control blood-sugar levels. The main sulphonylureas are *chlorpropamide, *glibenclamide, *gliclazide, *glimepiride, *glipizide, *gliquidone, *tolazamide, and *tolbutamide. They are available as tablets on *prescription only.

Side effects: these are usually mild and include stomach and bowel upsets (nausea, vomiting, diarrhoea, etc.) and headache. Allergic reactions (including transient rashes) may rarely occur.

Precautions: sulphonylureas should be used with caution in the elderly and people with impaired liver or kidney function; they should not be taken by women who are breastfeeding.

Interactions with other drugs:

Antibiotics: chloramphenicol, co-trimoxazole, quinolones, sulphonamides, and trimethoprim enhance the effects of sulphonylureas.

Antifungal drugs: fluconazole and miconazole increase the plasma concentrations of sulphonylureas.

Corticosteroids: reduce the effects of sulphonylureas.

NSAIDs: enhance the effects of sulphonylureas.

Oral contraceptives: antagonize the effects of sulphonylureas.

Phenothiazines: enhance the effects of sulphonylureas.

Sulphinpyrazone <sulfinpyrazone>: enhances the effects of sulphonylureas.

sulphur An element with *keratolytic and mild *antiseptic properties that also has some activity against fungi and kills parasites. It was formerly widely used in creams, lotions, and ointments to treat a variety of skin conditions, including acne, dandruff, scabies, and fungal infections. Sulphur has been replaced by more effective drugs for many purposes, although it is still used as an ingredient in some skin preparations.

Precautions: preparations containing sulphur should not be applied near the eyes or mouth.

Proprietary preparations: ACTINAC (combined with chloramphenicol, hydrocortisone acetate, butoxyethyl nicotinate, and allantoin); CLEARASIL TREATMENT CREAM REGULAR (combined with triclosan); COCOIS (combined with coal tar and salicylic acid); METED (combined with salicylic acid); PRAGMATAR (combined with coal tar distillate and salicylic acid).

sulpiride An *antipsychotic drug used for the treatment of schizophrenia; it controls both the positive symptoms (e.g. delusions) and the negative symptoms (e.g. apathy) of the disease. Sulpiride is available as tablets on *prescription only.

Side effects: as for *chlorpromazine, but sulpiride is less sedating and does not cause jaundice or skin reactions.

Precautions: see CHLORPROMAZINE HYDROCHLORIDE.

Interactions with other drugs:

Anaesthetics: their effect in lowering blood pressure is enhanced.

Antidepressants: there is an increased risk of antimuscarinic effects and arrhythmias if sulpiride is taken with tricyclic antidepressants.

Antiepileptic drugs: their anticonvulsant effects are antagonized by sulpiride.

Antihistamines: there is an increased risk of arrhythmias if sulpiride is taken with astemizole or terfenadine.

Halofantrine: there is an increased risk of arrhythmias if this drug is taken with sulpiride.

Ritonavir: may increase the effects of sulpiride.

Sedatives: the sedative effects of sulpiride are increased if it is taken with anxiolytic or hypnotic drugs, or any other drug that causes sedation.

Proprietary preparations: Dolmatil; Sulparex; Sulpitil.

Sulpitil (Pharmacia & Upjohn) *See* SULPIRIDE.

Sultrin (Janssen-Cilag) A proprietary combination of three *sulphonamides (sulphathiazole <sulfathiazole>, sulphacetamide <sulfacetamide>, and sulphabenzamide <sulfabenzamide>), used for the treatment of vaginal infections caused by the bacterium *Haemophilus vaginalis*. It is available as a cream on *prescription only.

Side effects: Sultrin may cause allergic reactions, and if absorbed it may produce *systemic effects (*see* SULPHONAMIDES).

Precautions: Sultrin should not be used by pregnant women or by people who are allergic to peanuts. It may damage latex condoms and diaphragms.

sumatriptan A *$5HT_1$ agonist used for treating acute attacks of *migraine. A single dose can relieve a migraine headache at any stage of the attack. Sumatriptan is available, on *prescription only, as tablets, an injection, or a nasal spray.

Side effects: include sensations of heaviness, pressure, heat, tingling, or tightness; if tightness in the chest or throat is severe, treatment should be stopped. Other side effects include flushing, fatigue, dizziness, and in increase in blood pressure (which does not last).

Precautions: sumatriptan should not be taken by people who have previously had a heart attack or who have uncontrolled high blood pressure. It should be used with caution in people with kidney or liver disease, heart conditions, or epilepsy, and in women who are pregnant or breastfeeding.

Interactions with other drugs:

Antidepressants: if MAOIs are taken with sumatriptan the risk of adverse effects on the central nervous system (CNS) is increased; sumatriptan should therefore not be started until two weeks after MAOIs have been stopped. SSRIs should not be taken with sumatriptan as this combination also has adverse effects on the CNS.

Ergotamine: the risk of spasm of the blood vessels, which can have serious consequences, is increased if ergotamine is taken with sumatriptan. Ergotamine should not be taken for 6 hours after taking sumatriptan, and sumatriptan should not be taken for 24 hours after taking ergotamine.

Lithium: should not be taken with sumatriptan as the risk of adverse effects on the CNS is increased.

Proprietary preparation: Imigran.

Sun E45 (Crookes Healthcare) A proprietary combination of *zinc oxide and *titanium dioxide used as a *sunscreen preparation; it reflects and thus protects against both UVA and UVB radiation. Sun E45 is available as a lotion (SPF 15 or 25) and a sunblock lotion (SPF 50); all these lotions can be prescribed on the NHS and can also be obtained without a prescription.

sunscreen preparations Preparations that protect the skin against the harmful effects of the sun's ultraviolet (UV) radiation. The two ranges of solar UV wavelengths that cause skin damage are UVB (long wavelengths in the range 280–310 nanometres) and UVA (long wavelengths in the range 310–400 nm). UVB causes sunburn and contributes to the development of skin cancer but its strength varies during daylight depending on the extent to which it is filtered out by clouds and the atmosphere. UVA is not filtered by the atmosphere, does not cause sunburn, and penetrates more deeply into the skin, causing the wrinkles, yellowing, and blotching associated with ageing. It also causes some photosensitive reactions in patients taking such drugs as *amiodarone and *phenothiazines; it can also contribute to skin cancer.

Sunscreen preparations contain absorbent substances, such as *aminobenzoic acid, which absorb UVB only, or reflective substances, such as *zinc oxide and *titanium dioxide, which reflect both UVA and UVB radiation. The amount of protection to be expected from a sunscreen preparation effective against UVB is indicated by its sun protection factor (SPF). For example, a preparation with an SPF of 8 should enable a person to remain in the sun without burning eight times longer than an unprotected person. These preparations do not, however, protect against the long-term damage associated with UVA. Some manufacturers indicate the extent to which their product does offer UVA protection by means of an arbitrary star rating system. A four-star product can be expected to provide roughly equal UVA and UVB protection, while three, two, and one stars indicate greater protection against UVB than UVA roughly in proportion to the number of stars. Thus a three-star product will provide about 33% less protection to UVA than a four-star product.

The following proprietary preparations provide protection against both UVA and UVB: *Ambre Solaire, *Coppertone, *Piz Buin, *RoC, *Spectraban, *Sun E45, and *Uvistat.

suppository A bullet-shaped plug containing a drug that is administered by insertion into the rectum. It is used when the drug needs to be delivered to the lining of the rectum or when an individual cannot take a drug by mouth, for example because he or she is unable to swallow or is vomiting. Since the lining of the rectum is well supplied with blood vessels, the absorption of a drug from a suppository is quite rapid. *Compare* PESSARY (vaginal suppository).

supraventricular tachycardia *See* ARRHYTHMIA.

Suprax (Rhône-Poulenc Rorer) *See* CEFIXIME.

Suprecur (Shire Pharmaceuticals) *See* BUSERELIN.

Suprefact (Shire Pharmaceuticals) *See* BUSERELIN.

surfactant A substance that is added to a cream or ointment to reduce its surface tension and thus increase its spreading or wetting properties. **Pulmonary** (or **lung**) **surfactant** is a complex mixture of proteins, fats, and carbohydrates that is made by cells in the lungs and prevents the lungs from collapsing by reducing surface tension. Premature babies often have difficulties in breathing because their lungs have not yet made enough surfactant. They are treated with synthetic pulmonary surfactants (*see* BERACTANT; COLFOSCERIL PALMITATE; PORACTANT ALFA; PUMACTANT).

Surgam, **Surgam SA** (Florizel) *See* TIAPROFENIC ACID.

Surmontil (Rhône-Poulenc Rorer) *See* TRIMIPRAMINE.

Survanta (Abbott Laboratories) *See* BERACTANT.

Suscard (Pharmax) *See* GLYCERYL TRINITRATE.

Sustac (Pharmax) *See* GLYCERYL TRINITRATE.

sustained-release preparation *See* MODIFIED-RELEASE PREPARATION.

Sustanon 100, **Sustanon 250** (Organon Laboratories) *See* TESTOSTERONE.

Symmetrel (Novartis Pharmaceuticals) *See* AMANTADINE HYDROCHLORIDE.

sympathetic nervous system A part of the nervous system that works in conjunction with another series of nerves (the parasympathetic system) to control the diameter of blood vessels and certain functions of the heart, lungs, intestines and pancreas, sweat glands, salivary glands, bladder, and genitalia. Both the sympathetic and parasympathetic nervous systems function automatically – we are not aware of their actions and have no voluntary control over them. The substances that relay information in the sympathetic nervous system are predominantly *noradrenaline <norepinephrine> and, to a lesser extent, *adrenaline

<epinephrine>. They act on very small specialized areas of the cells of the target tissues called *adrenoceptors. Many drugs act on the sympathetic nervous system, either by stimulating or by blocking these receptors or by increasing or preventing the release of noradrenaline from sympathetic nerve endings. *See* ALPHA BLOCKERS; BETA BLOCKERS; SYMPATHOMIMETIC DRUGS.

sympathomimetic drugs Drugs that mimic the effects of stimulating the *sympathetic nervous system. They act on the blood vessels, airways, and heart. There are two main types (although several drugs belong to both types). The **alpha-adrenoceptor stimulants** (also called **alpha stimulants** or **alpha agonists**) stimulate the alpha *adrenoceptors; they are *vasoconstrictors and are used as nasal *decongestants (e.g. *ephedrine, *xylometazoline, *phenylephrine). Centrally acting alpha stimulants (e.g. *clonidine, *methyldopa) act on alpha receptors in the brain that control blood pressure, decreasing the sympathetic stimulation of arteries and thus causing them to relax. These drugs are used in treating *hypertension. **Beta-adrenoceptor stimulants** (also called **beta stimulants** or **beta agonists**) stimulate beta adrenoceptors. They are *bronchodilators (e.g. *salbutamol), used to treat asthma; heart stimulants (e.g. *dobutamine hydrochloride, *dopamine); or relaxants of uterine muscle (e.g. *ritodrine). Some drugs act by directly stimulating the release of noradrenaline <norepinephrine>. *See also* ADRENALINE <EPINEPHRINE>; NORADRENALINE <NOREPINEPHRINE>.

Synacthen (Alliance Pharmaceuticals) *See* TETRACOSACTRIN <TETRACOSACTIDE> ACETATE.

Synalar (AstraZeneca) *See* FLUOCINOLONE ACETONIDE.

Synalar C (AstraZeneca) A proprietary combination of *fluocinolone acetonide (a potent topical steroid) and *clioquinol (an antifungal agent), used for the treatment of infected conditions of the skin. It is available as a cream or an ointment on *prescription only.
Side effects and precautions: see TOPICAL STEROIDS; CLIOQUINOL.

Synalar N (AstraZeneca) A proprietary combination of *fluocinolone acetonide (a potent topical steroid) and *neomycin sulphate (an antibiotic), used for the treatment of infected conditions of the skin. It is available as a cream or an ointment on *prescription only.
Side effects and precautions: see TOPICAL STEROIDS.

Synarel (Searle). *See* NAFARELIN.

Syndol (Seton Scholl Healthcare) A proprietary combination of *paracetamol and *codeine phosphate (analgesics), *doxylamine (an antihistamine), and *caffeine (a stimulant), used for the relief of headache, migraine, neuralgia, toothache, sore throat, period pains, and rheumatic aches and pains. It is available as tablets and can be obtained without a prescription, but only from pharmacies.

Side effects: see CODEINE; ANTIHISTAMINES; CAFFEINE.

Precautions: Syndol is not recommended for children. *See also* PARACETAMOL; ANTIHISTAMINES; CAFFEINE.

Interactions with other drugs: see ANTIHISTAMINES; OPIOIDS.

Synflex (Roche Products) *See* NAPROXEN.

Synphase (Searle) A proprietary combination of *ethinyloestradiol <ethinylestradiol> and *norethisterone used as an *oral contraceptive of the triphasic type. These tablets are packaged in three phases, which differ in the amounts of the active ingredients they contain. Synphase is available on *prescription only.

Side effects, precautions, and interactions with other drugs: see ORAL CONTRACEPTIVES.

Syntaris (Roche Products) *See* FLUNISOLIDE.

Syntocinon (Alliance Pharmaceuticals) *See* OXYTOCIN.

Syntometrine (Alliance Pharmaceuticals) A proprietary combination of *ergometrine maleate and *oxytocin, which causes contraction of the uterus and is used to stop the bleeding of an incomplete abortion or to assist delivery of the placenta in childbirth. It is available, on *prescription only, as a solution for intramuscular injection.

Side effects, precautions, and interactions with other drugs: see OXYTOCIN; ERGOMETRINE.

Syscor MR (Bayer) *See* NISOLDIPINE.

systemic Throughout the body. A drug that is given systemically, e.g. by *injection or by mouth, is absorbed into the bloodstream and reaches most parts of the body; it therefore has effects on the body as a whole, rather than on individual tissues or organs. Drugs that are inhaled have systemic effects, as do those administered *transdermally or as *enemas, *suppositories, or *pessaries. Some drugs given by a *topical route of administration may have systemic effects.

Sytron (Link Pharmaceuticals) *See* SODIUM IRON EDETATE.

tablet A small disc or other shape containing one or more drugs, made by compressing a powdered form of the drug(s). It is usually taken by mouth but may be inserted into a body cavity *see* PESSARY; SUPPOSITORY).

tacalcitol An *analogue of *vitamin D that is used in the treatment of *psoriasis. It acts by slowing down the division of skin cells whose overgrowth causes the formation of scaly patches seen in this disease. Tacalcitol is available as an ointment on *prescription only.
Side effects: tacalcitol may irritate the skin, causing itching, reddening, or a burning sensation.
Precautions: tacalcitol should not be used by people with disorders of calcium metabolism. It should be used with caution by people with peeling psoriasis or impaired kidney function and by pregnant women. Tacalcitol should not be used on the face.
Proprietary preparation: Curatoderm.

tacrolimus An *immunosuppressant, similar to *cyclosporin, used for the prevention of rejection in transplant patients. It is available as tablets on *prescription only.
Side effects: include tremor, headache, tingling in the fingers and toes, kidney impairment, fatigue, gum swelling, gastrointestinal disturbances, and visual disturbances. There may be an increased susceptibility to infection.
Precautions: tacrolimus should not be taken by women who are pregnant or breastfeeding. It may affect the performance of such skilled tasks as driving or operating machinery.
Interactions with other drugs:
  Cyclosporin: should not be used in conjunction with tacrolimus.
  Hormonal contraceptives: tacrolimus may affect their contraceptive action; non-hormonal contraception should be used during treatment.
Proprietary preparation: Prograf.

Tagamet (SmithKline Beecham Pharmaceuticals) *See* CIMETIDINE.

Tambocor (3M Health Care) *See* FLECAINIDE ACETATE.

Tamofen (Pharmacia & Upjohn) *See* TAMOXIFEN.

tamoxifen An *oestrogen antagonist used to treat women with breast cancer, both before and after the menopause, in which oestrogen stimulates growth of the tumour. It is also used to prevent a recurrence of breast cancer, and for women at particularly high risk of developing the disease it may be a primary preventive treatment. Tamoxifen is also used, sometimes in conjunction with *human chorionic gonadotrophin, to treat infertility in women caused by failure of the ovaries to produce egg cells. As a side benefit, tamoxifen also reduces the risk of a heart attack. It is available as tablets on *prescription only.

Side effects: the most common are hot flushes, vaginal bleeding, and nausea or other stomach and bowel upsets; there may also be loss of periods, vaginal discharge or itching, light-headedness, loss of hair, rashes, and visual disturbances (in which case treatment should be stopped). Any abnormal vaginal bleeding or discharge or pelvic pain should be reported to a doctor promptly to exclude the possibility of cancer of the endometrium (womb lining).

Precautions: tamoxifen should not be used by women who are pregnant or breastfeeding. In women taking this drug there is a small increase in the risks of developing endometrial cancer and venous thrombosis.

Interactions with other drugs:

Aminoglutethimide: reduces plasma concentrations of tamoxifen.

Anticoagulants: tamoxifen increases the effects of warfarin and nicoumalone <acenocoumarol>.

Proprietary preparations: Emblon; Fentamox; Nolvadex-D; Nolvadex Forte (a stronger preparation); Oestrifen; Tamofen.

Tampovagan (Co-Pharma) *See* STILBOESTROL <DIETHYLSTILBESTROL>.

tamsulosin hydrochloride An *alpha blocker used to relieve urinary retention in men with an enlarged prostate gland. It is available as *modified-release tablets on *prescription only.

Side effects and interactions with other drugs: *see* ALPHA BLOCKERS.

Precautions: tamsulosin should not be taken by men with severe liver disease. *See also* ALPHA BLOCKERS.

Proprietary preparation: Flomax MR.

tar A substance obtained from the distillation of the wood of various trees of the pine family. A *keratolytic that relieves itching, it is used in combination with other drugs in various preparations for the treatment or relief of a variety of skin disorders, including *eczema, *psoriasis, and dandruff.

Side effects and precautions: *see* COAL TAR.

Proprietary preparations: GELCOSAL (combined with coal tar and salicylic acid); GELCOTAR (combined with coal tar); POLYTAR (combined with cade oil, coal tar, arachis oil, and oleyl alcohol).

Tarcortin (Stafford-Miller) A proprietary combination of *hydrocortisone (a corticosteroid) and *coal tar extract (a keratolytic), used for the treatment of eczema, psoriasis, and other skin conditions. It is available as a cream on *prescription only.

Side effects and precautions: *see* TOPICAL STEROIDS; COAL TAR.

Targocid (Hoechst Marion Roussel) *See* TEICOPLANIN.

Tarka (Knoll) A proprietary combination of *verapamil hydrochloride (a calcium antagonist), in a modified-release form, and *trandolapril (an ACE inhibitor). It is used for the treatment of *hypertension in people who have been stabilized on the individual drugs at the same dosages and is available as capsules on *prescription only.
Side effects, precautions, and interactions with other drugs: see CALCIUM ANTAGONISTS; ACE INHIBITORS.

tartaric acid A weak acid with laxative properties used in the preparation of effervescent powders, granules, and tablets. Tartaric acid or its salt **sodium potassium tartrate** are ingredients of *antacid preparations used to relieve indigestion and heartburn and of mild *laxatives, which are freely available *over the counter.
Side effects: strong solutions are irritant and when swallowed can cause vomiting, diarrhoea, abdominal pains, and thirst.
Proprietary preparation: JAPP'S HEALTH SALTS (combined with sodium bicarbonate).

Tarvid (Hoechst Marion Roussel) *See* OFLOXACIN.

Tavanic (Hoechst Marion Roussel) *See* LEVOFLOXACIN.

Tavegil (Novartis Pharmaceuticals) *See* CLEMASTINE.

taxanes A group of drugs originally isolated from the bark of the Pacific yew (*Taxus brevifolia*). They are used for the treatment of advanced ovarian *cancer and advanced breast cancer, especially when standard treatment has failed. The common taxanes are *paclitaxel and *docetaxel.

Taxol (Bristol-Myers Squibb) *See* PACLITAXEL.

Taxotere (Rhône-Poulenc Rorer) *See* DOCETAXEL.

tazarotene A *retinoid used for the treatment of mild to moderate *psoriasis affecting up to 10% of the skin area. It is available as a gel on *prescription only.
Side effects: include local irritation, burning, redness, peeling of the skin, rash, dermatitis, and (rarely) skin pain.
Precautions: tazarotene should not be used by women who are pregnant or breastfeeding, and contraception must be used during treatment (*see* RETINOIDS). It should not be applied to skin folds, the face or scalp, normal or inflamed skin, or the eyes. Prolonged exposure to ultraviolet light (including sunlight) should be avoided.
Proprietary preparation: Zorac.

tazobactam An agent that inhibits the activity of of beta-lactamases, enzymes that are produced by bacteria and destroy *penicillins. It is given in combination with *piperacillin to prevent the destruction of this antibiotic (*see* TAZOCIN).

Tazocin (Wyeth Laboratories) A proprietary combination of *piperacillin (a penicillin) and *tazobactam (a beta-lactamase inhibitor), used for the treatment of infections of the lower respiratory tract, urinary tract, and skin. It is available as an injection on *prescription only.
Side effects, precautions, and interactions with other drugs: see BENZYLPENICILLIN.

TCAs *See* TRICYCLIC ANTIDEPRESSANTS.

TCP First Aid Antiseptic Cream (Pfizer Consumer Healthcare) A proprietary combination of *triclosan, *chloroxylenol, and *TCP Liquid Antiseptic, used for the treatment of minor cuts, grazes, scratches, insect bites, stings, spots, and blisters. It is freely available *over the counter.

TCP Liquid Antiseptic (Pfizer Consumer Healthcare) A proprietary preparation of halogenated *phenols used an an *antiseptic for treating cuts, grazes, insect bites and stings, spots, mouth ulcers, and as a gargle for sore throats. It is freely available *over the counter.

TCP Sore Throat Lozenges (Pfizer Consumer Healthcare) *See* HEXYLRESORCINOL.

Tears Naturale (Alcon Laboratories) A proprietary combination of *dextran and *hypromellose, used as a substitute for natural tears when the production of these is deficient. It is available as eye drops and can be obtained without a prescription, but only from pharmacies.
Precautions: the drops should not be used with soft contact lenses.

Tegretol (Novartis Pharmaceuticals) *See* CARBAMAZEPINE.

teicoplanin An *antibiotic, similar to *vancomycin, used for the treatment of serious infections, including endocarditis (infection of the heart membranes or valves) and peritonitis in dialysis patients, and to prevent infection after orthopaedic surgery. It is available, on *prescription only, as a solution for *intramuscular or *intravenous injection.
Side effects: include nausea, vomiting, diarrhoea, rash, fever, bronchospasm, anaphylactic reactions, dizziness, headache, blood disorders, and mild hearing loss.
Precautions: blood counts and liver and kidney function tests should be carried out during treatment; hearing tests are required for patients on long-term treatment. Teicoplanin should not be given to patients who are

allergic to vancomycin, and it should be used with caution in people with kidney disease and in women who are pregnant or breastfeeding.
Proprietary preparation: Targocid.

Telfast (Hoechst Marion Roussel) *See* FEXOFENADINE HYDROCHLORIDE.

temazepam A short-acting *benzodiazepine used for the short-term treatment of insomnia and anxiety. It is also used to relax patients before operations. Temazepam is available as tablets, gel-filled capsules, or an oral solution. Since it has been used as a drug of abuse, temazepam is now a *controlled drug and the capsules are no longer available on the NHS.
Side effects and precautions: see BENZODIAZEPINES; DIAZEPAM.
Interactions with other drugs: see BENZODIAZEPINES.

Temgesic (Schering-Plough) *See* BUPRENORPHINE.

Tenben (Galen) A proprietary combination of *atenolol (a cardioselective beta blocker) and *bendrofluazide <bendroflumethiazide> (a thiazide diuretic), used for the treatment of *hypertension. It is available as capsules on *prescription only.
Side effects, precautions, and interactions with other drugs: see BETA BLOCKERS; THIAZIDE DIURETICS.
See also ANTIHYPERTENSIVE DRUGS; DIURETICS.

Tenchlor (APS-Berk) *See* CO-TENIDONE.

Tenif (AstraZeneca) A proprietary combination of *atenolol (a beta blocker) and *nifedipine (a calcium antagonist), used for the treatment of *angina or *hypertension, usually when a single drug has been inadequate. It is available as capsules on *prescription only.
Side effects, precautions, and interactions with other drugs: see BETA BLOCKERS; CALCIUM ANTAGONISTS.
See also ANTIHYPERTENSIVE DRUGS.

Tenkicin (Kent Pharmaceuticals) *See* PHENOXYMETHYLPENICILLIN.

Tenkorex (Kent Pharmaceuticals) *See* CEPHALEXIN <CEFALEXIN>.

Tenoret 50 (AstraZeneca) *See* CO-TENIDONE.

Tenoretic (AstraZeneca) *See* CO-TENIDONE.

Tenormin (AstraZeneca) *See* ATENOLOL.

tenoxicam An *NSAID used for the treatment of pain and inflammation in rheumatoid arthritis and other disorders of the joints or muscles. It is available as tablets or an injection on *prescription only.

Side effects, precautions, and interactions with other drugs: see NSAIDS.
Proprietary preparation: Mobiflex.

Tensipine MR (Ethical Generics) *See* NIFEDIPINE.

Tensium (DDSA Pharmaceuticals) *See* DIAZEPAM.

Teoptic (CIBA Vision Ophthalmics) *See* CARTEOLOL HYDROCHLORIDE.

terazosin An *alpha blocker used to treat mild to moderate
*hypertension and to relieve the obstruction of urine flow that can occur
in men with an enlarged prostate gland. It is available as tablets on
*prescription only.
Side effects, precautions, and interactions with other drugs: see ALPHA
BLOCKERS.
Proprietary preparation: Hytrin.
See also ANTIHYPERTENSIVE DRUGS; VASODILATORS.

terbinafine An *antifungal drug used for the treatment of fungal
infections of the skin, scalp, or nails. It is available as a cream or tablets
on *prescription only.
Side effects: the tablets may cause stomach and bowel upsets, changes in
taste, headache, and aches or pains in the muscles and joints. If either
preparation causes a rash a doctor should be consulted, as treatment may
need to be discontinued if the rash worsens.
Precautions: terbinafine should be used with caution by people with
chronic liver disease or impaired kidney function and by women who are
pregnant or breastfeeding.
Interactions with other drugs:
  Cimetidine: increases the plasma concentration of terbinafine.
  Rifampicin: reduces the plasma concentration of terbinafine.
Proprietary preparations: Lamisil; Lamisil Cream.

terbutaline sulphate A *sympathomimetic drug that stimulates beta
*adrenoceptors in the airways. It is used mainly as a *bronchodilator to
relieve constriction of the airways in attacks of *asthma and to alleviate
wheezing and breathlessness in bronchitis and emphysema. It also
relaxes the uterus and can be used in obstetrics to prevent or delay
premature labour. Terbutaline is available, on *prescription only, as a
metered-dose aerosol or as a powder for inhalation, as tablets, *modified-
release tablets, or a syrup for oral use, as a solution for use in a
*nebulizer or a ventilator, and as a solution for injection.
Side effects, precautions, and interactions with other drugs: see
SALBUTAMOL.
Proprietary preparations: Bricanyl; Bricanyl SA (modified-release tablets);
Monovent (syrup).

terfenadine One of the newer (non-sedating) *antihistamines, used for the relief of the symptoms of allergic rhinitis (particularly hay fever), urticaria, and other itching skin conditions. It is available as tablets or a suspension on *prescription only.

Side effects: see ANTIHISTAMINES. The most likely side effects are indigestion, stomach ache, and headache; the risk of sedation is low. At high doses terfenadine may cause palpitation or irregular heart rhythms (*see* ARRHYTHMIA); a doctor should be informed if these occur.

Precautions: grapefruit juice can increase the plasma concentration of terfenadine, increasing risk of arrhythmias. The stated dose should not be exceeded. Terfenadine should not be taken by people with liver disease.

Interactions with other drugs: the following drugs should not be given with terfenadine as this increases the risk of arrhythmias: anti-arrhythmic drugs; antipsychotic drugs; clarithromycin; diuretics; erythromycin; imidazole antifungals (e.g. itraconazole, ketoconazole); monoamine oxidase inhibitors; sotalol; tricyclic antidepressants.

Proprietary preparations: Histafen; Terfenor; Terfinax; Triludan (tablets or suspension); Triludan Forte (twice the strength of Triludan tablets).

Terfenor (Norton Healthcare) *See* TERFENADINE.

Terfinax (Ashbourne Pharmaceuticals) *See* TERFENADINE.

Teril CR (Lagap Pharmaceuticals) *See* CARBAMAZEPINE.

terlipressin An analogue of *vasopressin that used for the treatment of bleeding varicose veins in the oesophagus. It is available in a form for injection on *prescription only.

Side effects: similar to those of *vasopressin, but milder.
Precautions and interactions with other drugs: see VASOPRESSIN.
Proprietary preparation: Glypressin.

terpineol A constituent of various aromatic oils that has mild disinfectant properties. It is used in combination with other volatile agents in inhalations to relieve the congestion associated with colds and catarrh.

Proprietary preparations: CHYMOL EMOLLIENT BALM (combined with eucalyptus oil, methyl salicylate, and phenol); KARVOL (combined with other aromatic substances and chlorbutol <chlorobutanol>).

Terra-Cortril (Pfizer) A proprietary combination of *oxytetracycline (an antibiotic) and *hydrocortisone (a corticosteroid), used for the treatment of infected eczema, insect bites, and inflammation (and sometimes infection) of skin surfaces that rub together (e.g. in the groin or armpits). It is available as an ointment on *prescription only.

Side effects and precautions: see TOPICAL STEROIDS.

Terra-Cortril Nystatin (Pfizer) A proprietary combination of *oxytetracycline (an antibiotic), *hydrocortisone (a corticosteroid), and *nystatin (an antifungal agent), used for the treatment of infected skin conditions. It is available as an ointment on *prescription only.

Side effects and precautions: see TOPICAL STEROIDS.

Terramycin (Pfizer) *See* OXYTETRACYCLINE.

Tertroxin (Goldshield Pharmaceuticals) *See* LIOTHYRONINE SODIUM.

testosterone The main *androgen (male sex hormone). It is available as a variety of esters (**testosterone enanthate <enantate>, propionate**, and **undecanoate**) for the treatment of underdevelopment of the testes or as replacement therapy in castrated men. It can also be used to prevent osteoporosis caused by lack of androgens. Testosterone is available, on *prescription only, as capsules, an injection, a *depot implant, or *transdermal (skin) patches.

Side effects: include excessive frequency and duration of penile erections, sodium and fluid retention, increased bone growth, enlargement of the prostate, reduced production of sperm, headache, depression, anxiety, generalized tingling sensations, gastrointestinal bleeding, nausea, jaundice, changes in libido, abnormal hair growth in women, male pattern baldness, and acne.

Precautions: testosterone should not be taken by men with cancer of the breast or prostate or by women who are pregnant or breastfeeding. It should be used with caution in people who have heart, liver, or kidney disease, in elderly men and prepubertal boys, and in people who suffer from high blood pressure, epilepsy, or migraine.

Interactions with other drugs:

Anticoagulants: testosterone enhances the effects of warfarin, nicoumalone <acenocoumarol>, and phenindione.

Antidiabetic drugs: testosterone may increase their effects in lowering blood-sugar concentrations.

Proprietary preparations: Andropatch (transdermal patches); Restandol (capsules); Primoteston Depot; Sustanon 100 and Sustanon 250 (depot formulation); Virormone (injection).

tetrabenazine A drug that acts by reducing the amount of available *dopamine in the brain. It is used to control the jerky involuntary movements that occur in Huntington's disease and related disorders. Tetrabenazine is available as tablets on *prescription only.

Side effects: depression can develop (which may restrict the use of tetrabenazine); other side effects include drowsiness, nausea, vomiting, *extrapyramidal reactions, and low blood pressure.

Precautions: tetrabenazine should be used with caution in women who are pregnant and should not be taken by women who are breastfeeding. It may affect driving ability.

Interactions with other drugs:

MAOIs: stimulation of the central nervous system and increased blood pressure can occur if these antidepressants are taken with tetrabenazine.

tetracaine *See* AMETHOCAINE.

Tetrachel (APS-Berk) *See* TETRACYCLINE HYDROCHLORIDE.

tetracosactrin acetate <tetracosactide acetate> A drug that stimulates the adrenal glands to produce *corticosteroids; it is a synthetic form of the pituitary hormone corticotrophin. Tetracosactrin is used to test whether or not the adrenal glands are functioning normally to produce corticosteroids. It is available as a *depot injection on *prescription only.
Side effects: allergic reactions may occur.
Precautions: tetracosactrin should not be given to people who are allergic to it.
Proprietary preparation: Synacthen.

tetracycline hydrochloride A broad-spectrum antibiotic that gave its name to the *tetracyclines. It is used for the treatment of chronic bronchitis, brucellosis, chlamydial infections, and infections due to mycoplasmas and rickettsias. It is also used to treat mouth ulcers and *acne. Tetracycline is available, on *prescription only, as tablets, capsules, or a solution for topical application.
Side effects, precautions, and interactions with other drugs: see TETRACYCLINES.
Proprietary preparations: Achromycin; Tetrachel; Topicycline (topical solution); DETECLO (combined with chlortetracycline and demeclocycline hydrochloride).

tetracyclines A group of broad-spectrum antibiotics whose value has decreased since many infective organisms have developed resistance to them. However, they are still the treatment of choice against *Chlamydia* bacteria (which cause a variety of diseases, notably sexually transmitted infections, parrot disease, and eye infections), rickettsias (which cause Q fever and typhus), and mycoplasmas (bacteria that cause respiratory and genital infections). They are also used to treat brucellosis, Lyme disease, acne, gum disease, and exacerbations of chronic bronchitis. Tetracyclines act by inhibiting protein synthesis in sensitive organisms. *See* CHLORTETRACYCLINE; DEMECLOCYCLINE HYDROCHLORIDE; DOXYCYCLINE; LYMECYCLINE; MINOCYCLINE; OXYTETRACYCLINE; TETRACYCLINE HYDROCHLORIDE.
Side effects: include nausea and vomiting, diarrhoea, headache, and visual disturbances. If a rash occurs, treatment should be discontinued. A rash on exposure to sunlight may occur in rare cases.
Precautions: the tetracyclines are deposited in growing bones and teeth, causing discoloration. For this reason they should not be taken by

children under 12 years old or by women who are pregnant or breastfeeding. Absorption of most tetracyclines (except doxycycline and minocycline) from the stomach is reduced in the presence of milk and other dairy products. Most tetracyclines (except doxycycline and minocycline) can exacerbate kidney failure and should not be taken by people with kidney disease.

Interactions with other drugs:

Antacids: reduce the absorption of tetracyclines.

Calcium salts: reduce the absorption of tetracyclines.

Iron salts: reduce the absorption of tetracyclines.

Oral contraceptives: there is a small risk that tetracyclines may reduce the effectiveness of oral contraceptives.

Sucralfate: reduces the absorption of tetracyclines.

Zinc salts: reduce the absorption of tetracyclines.

tetrahydrofurfuryl salicylate *See* SALICYLATES.

Tetralysal 300 (Galderma) *See* LYMECYCLINE.

T/Gel (Johnson & Johnson) *See* COAL TAR.

Theo-Dur (AstraZeneca) *See* THEOPHYLLINE.

theophylline A *xanthine used for the treatment of *asthma and in some cases of emphysema and chronic bronchitis (*see* BRONCHODILATORS). It is available as tablets or capsules, in both usual or *modified-release formulations, and as a liquid and can be obtained from pharmacies without a prescription.

Side effects: include nausea, headache, gastrointestinal disturbances, palpitation, and insomnia. *See also* XANTHINES.

Precautions: theophylline should be used with caution by people with some types of heart disease, liver disease, or peptic ulcer, and by women who are in late pregnancy or breastfeeding. Fluvoxamine seriously increases the plasma concentration of theophylline, and these two drugs should not be taken together. There may be a need to monitor concentrations of plasma potassium.

Interactions with other drugs: see XANTHINES.

Proprietary preparations: Lasma (modified-release tablets); Nuelin; Nuelin SA (modified-release tablets); Slo-Phyllin (modified-release capsules); Theo-Dur (modified-release tablets); Uniphyllin Continus (modified-release tablets); DO-DO CHESTEZE (combined with ephedrine and caffeine); FRANOL (combined with ephedrine).

Thephorin (Sinclair Pharmaceuticals) *See* PHENINDAMINE TARTRATE.

thiabendazole <tiabendazole> An *anthelmintic used for the treatment of infestations by worms, especially species of the roundworm *Strongyloides*, which live in the intestines but may migrate to other tissues. It is also used in conjunction with other drugs for treating mixed infestations that do not involve roundworms. Thiabendazole is available as chewable tablets on *prescription only.

Side effects: include loss of appetite, nausea, vomiting, dizziness, diarrhoea, headache, itching, drowsiness, and allergic reactions, including fever, chills, and rashes.

Precautions: thiabendazole should not be taken by women who are pregnant or breastfeeding and should be used with caution in people with liver or kidney disease. It may impair the performance of such tasks as driving and operating machinery.

Interactions with other drugs:

　Theophylline: its plasma concentration (and therefore side effects) may be increased.

Proprietary preparation: Mintezol.

thiamine (vitamin B₁) A vitamin of the B group *see* VITAMIN B COMPLEX) that is taken orally (as **thiamine hydrochloride**) to treat vitamin B_1 deficiency. In combination with other B vitamins and vitamin C (ascorbic acid), it is given by injection to relieve severe deficiency states, such as those caused by alcoholism or occurring after acute infections, surgery, or in some psychiatric conditions; injections may also be needed by people undergoing kidney dialysis. Thiamine tablets are freely available *over the counter; the injection is a *prescription only medicine.

Side effects: rarely, an allergic reaction and anaphylactic shock (*see* ANAPHYLAXIS) can occur after injection.

Proprietary preparations: Benerva (tablets); PABRINEX (combined with other B vitamins and ascorbic acid).

thiazide diuretics A class of *diuretics that bring about a moderate loss of fluid as urine. They are used for long-term treatment of such conditions as *hypertension or *oedema associated with congestive *heart failure. Thiazides and thiazide-like diuretics may be used for extended periods in the treatment of hypertension; in this situation their diuretic activity decreases but their *antihypertensive activity continues. *Potassium supplements may be required with the thiazide diuretics; alternatively, they may be used in combination with *potassium-sparing diuretics. Thiazide diuretics start to act within 1–2 hours of oral administration and have a duration of action of 12–24 hours. They are therefore usually given early during the day.

See BENDROFLUAZIDE <BENDROFLUMETHIAZIDE>; BENZTHIAZIDE; CHLOROTHIAZIDE; CHLORTHALIDONE <CHLORTALIDONE>; CYCLOPENTHIAZIDE; HYDROCHLOROTHIAZIDE; HYDROFLUMETHIAZIDE; INDAPAMIDE HEMIHYDRATE; MEFRUSIDE; METOLAZONE; POLYTHIAZIDE; XIPAMIDE.

Side effects: if the loss of potassium, sodium, and water is too great, thiazide diuretics can cause weakness, lethargy, and cramps; dizziness may occur as a result of postural hypotension (low blood pressure on standing up from a sitting or lying posture); less commonly mild gastrointestinal upsets, rashes, photosensitivity (skin sensitivity to light), anorexia, reversible impotence, blood disorders, and pancreatitis may occur.

Precautions: thiazide diuretics should not be taken by people with certain liver or kidney disorders, and they can aggravate gout or diabetes. They should be used with caution by men with an enlarged prostate gland, women who are breastfeeding, and by elderly people. They should not be taken by women who are pregnant, as they can cause jaundice in the newborn baby and because they also cause a reduction in the total volume of the blood.

Interactions with other drugs:

Anti-arrhythmic drugs: if potassium loss occurs, amiodarone, disopyramide, flecainide, and quinidine are more likely to have adverse effects on the heart and the action of lignocaine <lidocaine> and mexiletine are antagonized.

Antihistamines: the risk of *arrhythmias with astemizole and terfenadine is increased if potassium concentrations are low.

Antihypertensive drugs: their effects in lowering blood pressure are increased.

Corticosteroids: may further increase the loss of potassium when taken with thiazide diuretics.

Digitalis drugs: the adverse effects of these drugs may be increased if potassium concentrations are low.

Lithium: concentrations of lithium may be increased, leading to the risk of serious side effects.

NSAIDs: may reduce the diuretic effect of thiazides, requiring dosage modification.

Pimozide: if potassium loss occurs, pimozide is more likely to cause arrhythmias.

thioguanine <tioguanine> An *antimetabolite used for the treatment of acute myeloid and lymphocytic leukaemia (*see* CANCER), particularly in children. It is available as tablets on *prescription only.

Side effects and precautions: *see* MERCAPTOPURINE; CYTOTOXIC DRUGS.

Proprietary preparation: Lanvis.

thiopentone <thiopental> *See* BARBITURATES.

thioridazine A phenothiazine *antipsychotic drug used for the treatment of schizophrenia and other psychoses and mania, and as an *adjunct to the short-term treatment of severe anxiety, agitation, and violent or otherwise dangerous behaviour. It is also used to treat agitation and restlessness in elderly patients and severe mental or behavioural disorders in children. Thioridazine is available, on *prescription only, as tablets, a syrup, or a suspension.

Side effects: as for *chlorpromazine, but thioridazine is less sedating and *extrapyramidal reactions rarely occur; however, it has marked antimuscarinic effects (e.g. dry mouth, constipation, difficulty in passing urine, blurred vision) and it is more likely to cause low blood pressure and possibly disturbances in heart rhythm (*arrhythmias).

Precautions: see CHLORPROMAZINE HYDROCHLORIDE.

Interactions with other drugs:

Anaesthetics: their effect in lowering blood pressure is enhanced.

Anti-arrhythmic drugs: amiodarone, disopyramide, procainamide, and quinidine should not be taken with thioridazine as this combination increases the risk of arrhythmias.

Antidepressants: there is an increased risk of antimuscarinic effects and arrhythmias if thioridazine is taken with tricyclic antidepressants.

Antiepileptic drugs: their anticonvulsant effects are antagonized by thioridazine.

Antihistamines: astemizole and terfenadine should not be taken with thioridazine as this combination increases the risk of arrhythmias.

Beta blockers: the risk of arrhythmias is increased if sotalol is taken with thioridazine.

Cisapride: should not be taken with thioridazine as this combination increases the risk of arrhythmias.

Halofantrine: there is an increased risk of arrhythmias if this drug is taken with thioridazine.

Ritonavir: may increase the effects of thioridazine.

Sedatives: the sedative effects of thioridazine are increased if it is taken with anxiolytic or hypnotic drugs, or any other drug that causes sedation.

Proprietary preparations: Melleril; Rideril.

thiotepa An *alkylating drug that is administered directly into the chest or abdomen to treat metastases in accumulations of fluid that are caused by certain *cancers. It is also instilled into the bladder to treat bladder cancer and is occasionally used to treat breast cancer. Thiotepa is available as an injection on *prescription only.

Side effects and precautions: see CYTOTOXIC DRUGS.

Throaties Family Cough Linctus (Ernest Jackson) *See* IPECACUANHA.

thromboembolism *See* THROMBOSIS.

thrombolytic drugs *See* FIBRINOLYTIC DRUGS.

thrombosis Blockage of a blood vessel by a blood clot (thrombus). Blood clots can form in arteries or veins. Thrombosis in an artery obstructs the blood flow to the tissue it supplies: obstruction of an artery to the brain is one of the causes of a stroke, and thrombosis in an artery supplying the heart (**coronary thrombosis**) results in a heart attack. Obstruction of a vein by a blood clot is most common in the deep veins of the calf of the leg (**deep-vein thrombosis; DVT**). A blood clot may form in one place, break off, and be carried in the blood to block another vessel some distance away; this is known as **thromboembolism**. For example, a blood clot that breaks off from a larger clot in a leg vein often lodges in the pulmonary artery, which brings blood to the lungs, resulting in **pulmonary embolism**.

Drugs used in the prevention and treatment of thrombosis and thromboembolism include *anticoagulants, *antiplatelet drugs, and *fibrinolytic drugs.

thrush   *See* ANTIFUNGAL DRUGS.

thymol   An aromatic liquid extracted from thyme oil. An antiseptic with antibacterial and antifungal activity, it is used in combination with *glycerin (**compound thymol glycerin**) as a mouthwash to relieve the pain of mouth ulcers and for general oral hygiene. It is also included, with other volatile substances, in inhalations for the relief of coughs, colds, and nasal congestion. Preparations containing thymol are freely available *over the counter.

Side effects: if swallowed, thymol may irritate the stomach.

Proprietary preparation: KARVOL (combined with other aromatic substances and chlorbutol <chlorobutanol>).

thymoxamine <moxisylyte>   An *alpha blocker taken by mouth for the short-term treatment of Raynaud's syndrome (poor circulation of the hands and feet). It can also be injected directly into the penis to produce an erection in men with erectile impotence. Thymoxamine is available, on *prescription only, as tablets or an injection.

Side effects: see ALPHA BLOCKERS. Injections may cause local pain or swelling and prolonged erection.

Precautions: thymoxamine should be used with caution in people with diabetes or angina and in those who have had a recent heart attack (*see also* ALPHA BLOCKERS). Injections should not be given to men with a predisposition to prolonged erection (as in sickle-cell anaemia or leukaemia) or anatomical deformity of the penis. Thymoxamine should not be used in conjunction with other drugs for treating impotence.

Interactions with other drugs:

Alpha blockers and beta blockers: may cause a severe fall in blood pressure on standing.

Proprietary preparations: Erecnos (injection); Opilon (tablets).

See also VASODILATORS.

thyroid hormones   Two iodine-containing hormones, **thyroxine (T_4)** and **triiodothyronine (T_3)**, that are secreted by the thyroid gland. They are essential for normal metabolic processes and mental and physical development. Lack of these hormones, resulting from underactivity of the thyroid gland (**hypothyroidism**), causes mental and physical slowing, undue sensitivity to cold, slowing of the pulse, weight gain, and coarsening of the skin (**myxoedema**). Hypothyroidism may develop in those who have received treatment for an overactive thyroid gland. If present at birth, lack of thyroid hormones causes mental retardation and stunted growth (the condition of **cretinism**). Treatment of hypothyroidism is with *thyroxine sodium <levothyroxine sodium> or *liothyronine; affected babies must be treated promptly for normal development to occur.

Excessive amounts of thyroid hormones in the bloodstream causes **thyrotoxicosis**, producing a rapid heartbeat, sweating, tremor, anxiety, increased appetite, loss of weight, and intolerance of heat. Causes include simple overactivity of the thyroid gland (**hyperthyroidism**), a hormone-secreting tumour of the gland, and **Graves' disease**, in which there are additional symptoms, including swelling of the neck (**goitre**), due to enlargement of the gland, and protrusion of the eyes (**exophthalmos**). Treatment may be by the use of antithyroid drugs (*see* CARBIMAZOLE; PROPYLTHIOURACIL; IODINE), which interfere with the production of thyroid hormones. Alternatively, radioactive iodine is given by mouth to destroy some thyroid tissue, or part of the thyroid gland is surgically removed.

thyrotoxicosis *See* THYROID HORMONES.

thyroxine sodium <levothyroxine sodium> A preparation of the *thyroid hormone thyroxine that is given to replace a lack of the natural hormone. It is also used for the treatment of goitre and thyroid cancer. Thyroxine sodium is available as tablets on *prescription only.

Side effects: these are usually the result of overdosage at the start of treatment and diminish as the dosage is adjusted according to the level of thyroid hormones measured in the blood. They include irregular heart rhythms, anginal pain, muscle cramps, headache, restlessness, excitability, insomnia, flushing, sweating, diarrhoea, excessive weight loss, and muscular weakness.

Precautions: thyroxine sodium should be used with caution by people with poorly functioning adrenal glands, cardiovascular disorders, diabetes mellitus, or diabetes insipidus and by women who are pregnant or breastfeeding.

Interactions with other drugs:

   Antiepileptic drugs: carbamazepine, phenobarbitone <phenobarbital>, phenytoin, and primidone increase the requirement for thyroxine sodium.

   Cholestyramine <colestyramine>: reduces the absorption of thyroxine sodium.

   Oral anticoagulants: their anticoagulant effects are enhanced.

   Propranolol: reduces the effect of thyroxine sodium.

   Rifampicin: increases the requirement for thyroxine sodium.

   Sucralfate: reduces the absorption of thyroxine sodium.

Proprietary preparation: Eltroxin.

tiabendazole *See* THIABENDAZOLE.

tiagabine An *anticonvulsant drug used as an *adjunct in the treatment of partial epileptic seizures. It is available as tablets on *prescription only.
Side effects: include diarrhoea, dizziness, tiredness, difficulty in concentrating, tremor, mood changes, and impaired speech.
Precautions: tiagabine may impair driving ability and the performance of other skilled tasks. It should be used with caution in patients with liver disease.
Proprietary preparation: Gabitril.

tiaprofenic acid An *NSAID used for the treatment of pain and inflammation in rheumatoid arthritis and other disorders of the joints or muscles. It is available as tablets or *modified-release capsules on *prescription only.
Side effects and precautions: see NSAIDS. Tiaprofenic acid may cause severe cystitis and should not be taken by people with urinary disorders. If symptoms of cystitis develop (such as frequency or pain in passing urine or blood in the urine) treatment should be stopped and a doctor informed.
Interactions with other drugs: see NSAIDS.
Proprietary preparations: Surgam; Surgam SA (modified-release capsules).

tibolone A synthetic steroid that mimics the effects of *oestrogens and *progestogens (it also has weak androgenic effects). It is used for the relief of hot flushes and other physical symptoms of the menopause and helps to relieve depression and decreased libido. It is also used to prevent osteoporosis in postmenopausal women. If natural periods have been absent for a year or more before taking tibolone, the lining of the uterus will not be stimulated and bleeding will not occur; otherwise there may be some irregular vaginal bleeding (*see* HORMONE REPLACEMENT THERAPY). Tibolone is available as tablets on *prescription only.
Side effects: include changes in body weight, dizziness, headache, migraine, visual disturbances, dermatitis, skin rashes and itching, vaginal bleeding, stomach upsets, and growth of facial hair.
Precautions: tibolone should not be taken during pregnancy or breastfeeding or by women with hormone-dependent tumours, undiagnosed vaginal bleeding, a history of cardiovascular disorders, or severe liver disorders. It should be taken with caution by women with epilepsy, migraine, or diabetes.
Interactions with other drugs:
  Antiepileptic drugs: carbamazepine, phenobarbitone <phenobarbital>, phenytoin, and primidone reduce the effect of tibolone.
  Rifampicin: reduces the effect of tibolone.
Proprietary preparation: Livial.

ticarcillin A broad-spectrum *penicillin that is active against *Pseudomonas* and *Proteus* bacteria. It is used in combination with *clavulanic acid for the treatment of systemic (generalized) and local infections (such as infected wounds or burns) and respiratory and urinary-tract infections. Given by injection or infusion, it is available on *prescription only. It is sometimes used in conjunction with an *aminoglycoside antibiotic.

Side effects, precautions, and interactions with other drugs: see BENZYLPENICILLIN.

Proprietary preparation: TIMENTIN (combined with clavulanic acid).

Tiger Balm (LRC Products) A proprietary combination of *camphor, *clove oil, *menthol, *peppermint oil, and *cajuput oil, used as a *rubefacient for the relief of minor muscular aches and pains. It is freely available *over the counter.

Side effects and precautions: see RUBEFACIENTS.

Tiger Balm Red Extra Strength (LRC Products) A proprietary combination of *camphor, *menthol, *cajuput oil, *clove oil, cinnamon oil, and *peppermint oil, used as a *rubefacient for the relief of minor muscular aches and pains. It is freely available *over the counter.

Side effects and precautions: see RUBEFACIENTS.

Tilade (Pantheon Healthcare) *See* NEDOCROMIL SODIUM.

Tilarin (Pantheon Healthcare) *See* NEDOCROMIL SODIUM.

Tildiem LA, **Tildiem Retard** (Lorex Synthélabo) *See* DILTIAZEM HYDROCHLORIDE.

Tiloryth (Tillomed Laboratories) *See* ERYTHROMYCIN.

tiludronic acid A *bisphosphonate used for the treatment of Paget's disease, in which the bones are deformed and fracture easily. It is available as tablets on *prescription only.

Side effects: include stomach pain, nausea, diarrhoea, and (rarely) weakness of the muscles, dizziness, headache, and rashes.

Precautions: tiludronic acid should not be taken by women who are pregnant or breastfeeding. It should be used with caution in people with kidney disease.

Interactions with other drugs:

Aminoglycosides: in combination with tiludronic acid, they may cause abnormally low concentrations of calcium in the plasma.

Antacids: reduce the absorption of tiludronic acid.

Calcium supplements: reduce the absorption of tiludronic acid.

Iron supplements: reduce the absorption of tiludronic acid.

Proprietary preparation: Skelid.

Timecef (Hoechst Marion Roussel) *See* CEFODIZIME.

Timentin (SmithKline Beecham Pharmaceuticals) A proprietary combination of *ticarcillin (a penicillin) and *clavulanic acid (a penicillinase inhibitor), used for the treatment of severe infections in hospitalized patients with suppressed or impaired immune systems (*see* TICARCILLIN). It is available, on *prescription only, in a form for injection or infusion.
Side effects, precautions, and interactions with other drugs: see BENZYLPENICILLIN.

Timodine (Reckitt & Colman) A proprietary combination of *nystatin (an antifungal agent), *hydrocortisone (a corticosteroid), *benzalkonium chloride (an antiseptic), and *dimethicone <dimeticone> (a water repellent), used for the treatment of a variety of skin conditions and napkin rash infected with *Candida*. It is available as a cream on *prescription only and should be stored in a refrigerator.
Side effects and precautions: see TOPICAL STEROIDS.

timolol maleate A *beta blocker used for the treatment and prevention of cardiac *arrhythmias, *angina, and after heart attacks to prevent recurrence. It is also used to prevent the occurrence of *migraine and as eye drops for the treatment of *glaucoma. Timodol is available, on *prescription only, as tablets or as a solution for ophthalmic use.
Side effects, precautions, and interactions with other drugs: see BETA BLOCKERS.
Proprietary preparations: Betim; Blocadren; Timoptol (eye drops); Timoptol LA (long-acting eye drops); COSOPT (combined with dorzolamide); MODUCREN (combined with amiloride hydrochloride and hydrochlorothiazide); PRESTIM (combined with bendrofluazide <bendroflumethiazide>).
See also ANTI-ARRHYTHMIC DRUGS.

Timonil Retard (CP Pharmaceuticals) *See* CARBAMAZEPINE.

Timoptol, **Timoptol-LA** (Merck Sharp & Dohme) *See* TIMOLOL MALEATE.

Timpron (APS-Berk) *See* NAPROXEN.

Tinaderm-M (Schering-Plough) A proprietary combination of *tolnaftate and *nystatin (both antifungal drugs), used for the treatment of fungal infections of the skin and nails. It is available as a cream on *prescription only.
Side effects and precautions: see NYSTATIN.

tincture A medicinal preparation consisting of an extract of a drug derived from a plant in a solution of alcohol. Many plants contain active ingredients that are used as drugs and are extracted in this way.

tinea *See* ANTIVIRAL DRUGS.

tinidazole An *antibiotic that is active against protozoa (including amoebae) and some bacteria. It is similar to *metronidazole and has similar uses, including the treatment or prevention of intestinal amoebic infections (such as amoebic dysentery), giardiasis (a protozoal infection of the intestines), bacterial infections of the vagina or urethra, and ulceration of the gums and gingivitis. Tinidazole is longer acting than metronidazole and therefore needs to be taken only once daily. It is available as tablets on *prescription only.
Side effects: include nausea, vomiting, stomach upset, furred tongue, an unpleasant taste in the mouth, itching, swelling of the face, and darkening of the urine. Long-term therapy can decrease the numbers of white blood cells.
Precautions: the combination of alcohol and tinidazole may lead to vomiting, therefore alcohol should be avoided during treatment. Tinidazole should not be taken by women during the first three months of pregnancy and should be used with caution during the remainder of the pregnancy.
Proprietary preparation: Fasigyn.

tinzaparin sodium A *low molecular weight heparin used for the prevention and treatment of deep-vein *thrombosis and in the treatment of pulmonary embolism. It is also used in patients undergoing kidney dialysis, in order to prevent the formation of blood clots. Tinzaparin is available as a solution for subcutaneous injection on *prescription only.
Side effects, precautions, and interactions with other drugs: see HEPARIN.
Proprietary preparation: Innohep.

tioconazole An imidazole *antifungal drug that is active against a wide range of fungi. It is used for the treatment of fungal infections of the nail bed and is available, on *prescription only, as a solution for painting on the nails.
Side effects: there may be mild local irritation.
Precautions: tioconazole should not be used during pregnancy.
Proprietary preparation: Trosyl.

tioguanine *See* THIOGUANINE.

Tisept, **Tisept Concentrate** (Seton Scholl Healthcare) Proprietary combinations of the antiseptics *chlorhexidine gluconate and *cetrimide, used for cleansing and disinfecting wounds and burns, changing dressings, and in obstetrical procedures. They are available as solutions without a prescription, but only from pharmacies.

Side effects: see CETRIMIDE.
Precautions: the solution should not come into contact with the eyes.

titanium dioxide A white compound that protects the skin and reflects sunlight. It is an ingredient of many *sunscreen preparations, since it protects the skin against the damaging effects of ultraviolet light (both UVA and UVB). It is also included in *barrier preparations for the prevention of napkin rash. Preparations containing titanium dioxide are freely available *over the counter.

Proprietary preparations: AMBRE SOLAIRE (combined with UVB-absorbing agents); METANIUM (combined with a water-repellent emollient base); PIZ BUIN (combined with UVB-absorbing agents); SPECTRABAN (ULTRA LOTION) (combined with UVB-absorbing agents); SUN E45 (combined with zinc oxide); UVISTAT (combined with UVB-absorbing agents).

Titralac (3M Health Care) A proprietary combination of *calcium carbonate and glycine (an amino acid), used as a *calcium supplement or as a *phosphate-binding agent in people with kidney failure. It is freely available *over the counter in the form of tablets.

Precautions: Titralac should not be taken by people with low concentrations of phosphate in the blood or high concentrations of calcium in the blood or urine. Plasma *electrolytes and albumin may therefore need to be monitored.
Interactions with other drugs: see CALCIUM.

Tixylix Catarrh Syrup (Novartis Consumer Health) A proprietary combination of *diphenhydramine (a sedative antihistamine) and *menthol, used for the relief of productive coughs, catarrh, and nasal congestion in children. It is available without a prescription, but only from pharmacies.
Side effects and interactions with other drugs: see ANTIHISTAMINES.
Precautions: this medicine is not recommended for children under one or over ten. *See also* ANTIHISTAMINES.

Tixylix Chesty Cough (Novartis Consumer Health) *See* GUAIPHENESIN <GUAIFENESIN>.

Tixylix Cough & Cold (Novartis Consumer Health) A proprietary combination of *chlorpheniramine <chlorphenamine> (an antihistamine), *pholcodine (a cough suppressant), and *pseudoephedrine (a decongestant), used for the relief of dry irritating coughs and the running nose, congestion, and other symptoms associated with colds. It is available as a linctus without a prescription, but only from pharmacies.
Side effects and interactions with other drugs: see ANTIHISTAMINES; EPHEDRINE HYDROCHLORIDE; DECONGESTANTS; PHOLCODINE.
Precautions: this medicine is not recommended for children under one

year old. *See also* ANTIHISTAMINES; EPHEDRINE HYDROCHLORIDE; DECONGESTANTS; OPIOIDS.

Tixylix Daytime (Novartis Consumer Health) *See* PHOLCODINE.

Tixylix Inhalant (Novartis Consumer Health) A proprietary combination of *turpentine oil, *eucalyptus oil, *camphor, and *menthol in the form of capsules. The contents are placed on a handkerchief or in hot water and the vapour is inhaled to relieve nasal congestion and catarrh. It is freely available *over the counter.

Tixylix Night-time (Novartis Consumer Health) A proprietary combination of *pholcodine (a cough suppressant) and *promethazine hydrochloride (a sedative antihistamine), used to relieve the symptoms of coughs and colds, especially irritating dry coughs that interfere with sleep. It is available as a linctus without a prescription, but only from pharmacies. It cannot be prescribed on the NHS.
Side effects and interactions with other drugs: see PHOLCODINE; ANTIHISTAMINES.
Precautions: this medicine is not recommended for children under one year old. *See also* OPIOIDS; ANTIHISTAMINES.

tizanidine A *muscle relaxant that is used for the relief of spasticity associated with multiple sclerosis or injury or disease of the spinal cord. It is available as tablets on *prescription only.
Side effects: include drowsiness, fatigue, dizziness, dry mouth, nausea, stomach upset, and low blood pressure.
Precautions: tizanidine should not be taken by people with severe liver disease, and should be used with caution in women who are pregnant or breastfeeding and in elderly people. Tizanidine enhances the sedative effects of alcohol.
Interactions with other drugs:
  Antihypertensive drugs: tizanidine increases their effects in lowering blood pressure.
  Anxiolytics and hypnotic drugs: tizanidine enhances their sedative effects.
  Digoxin: heart rate may be slowed if digoxin is given with tizanidine.
  Diuretics: tizanidine enhances their effects in lowering blood pressure.
Proprietary preparation: Zanaflex.

tobramycin An *aminoglycoside antibiotic used for the treatment of serious infections that are resistant to *gentamicin. It is also used to treat eye infections. It is given as an *intramuscular or *intravenous injection and is available on *prescription only.
Side effects, precautions, and interactions with other drugs: see GENTAMICIN.
Proprietary preparation: Nebcin.

tocopherols *See* VITAMIN E.

Tofranil (Novartis Pharmaceuticals) *See* IMIPRAMINE HYDROCHLORIDE.

Tolanase (Pharmacia & Upjohn) *See* TOLAZAMIDE.

tolazamide A *sulphonylurea used for the treatment of noninsulin-dependent (type II) *diabetes mellitus. It is available as tablets on *prescription only.
Side effects, precautions, and interactions with other drugs: see SULPHONYLUREAS.
Proprietary preparation: Tolanase.

tolbutamide A *sulphonylurea used for the treatment of noninsulin-dependent (type II) *diabetes mellitus. It is available as tablets on *prescription only.
Side effects, precautions, and interactions with other drugs: see SULPHONYLUREAS.

tolerance The reduction or loss of the normal response to a drug or other substance that usually provokes a reaction in the body. Tolerance may develop after taking a particular drug over a long period of time. In such cases the dosage of the drug may need to be increased in order to produce the desired effect. Examples of drugs that bring about tolerance are *ephedrine (used in nasal decongestants), *glyceryl trinitrate (for treating angina), and *opioids (used for pain relief). Tolerance does not imply *dependence, although some drugs that cause tolerance also cause dependence.

tolfenamic acid An *NSAID used to relieve the pain of *migraine attacks. It is available as rapid tablets on *prescription only.
Side effects: see NSAIDS. Additional side effects may include difficulty or pain in passing urine (especially in men) and tremor.
Precautions and interactions with other drugs: see NSAIDS.
Proprietary preparation: Clotam.

tolnaftate An *antifungal drug that is active against a wide range of fungi, but not *Candida* (causing thrush). It is used for the treatment and prevention of various forms of tinea (ringworm) and pityriasis versicolor, a chronic fungal infection of the skin; it is not suitable for deep-seated infections of the nail bed. Tolnaftate is available, alone or in combination with other drugs, as a foot spray, ointment, powder, or cream; most preparations can be obtained without a prescription.
Proprietary preparations: Mycil Foot Spray; MYCIL OINTMENT (combined with benzalkonium chloride); MYCIL POWDER (combined with chlorhexidine); TINADERM-M (combined with nystatin).

tolterodine tartrate An *antimuscarinic drug used to treat urinary incontinence and abnormal frequency or urgency in passing urine. It is available as tablets on *prescription only.

Side effects: include dry mouth, constipation, indigestion, nausea, abdominal discomfort, flatulence, vomiting, headache, dry skin, dry eyes, drowsiness, nervousness, tingling in the fingers, and (more rarely) blurred vision, chest pain, and difficulty in passing urine.

Precautions: tolterodine should not be taken by people with urinary retention, uncontrolled acute glaucoma, myasthenia gravis, or severe ulcerative colitis. It should be used with caution in people in whom the outlet of the bladder is obstructed (for example by an enlarged prostate) and in those with a hiatus hernia, disease of peripheral nerves, or impaired liver or kidney function.

Interactions with other drugs: see ANTIMUSCARINIC DRUGS.

Proprietary preparation: Detrusitol.

Tomudex (AstraZeneca) *See* RALTITREXED.

tonic A medicinal preparation purporting to increase vigour and liveliness and produce a feeling of wellbeing. Ingredients of tonics include bitters (such as *gentian mixtures), which are supposed to increase the appetite; minerals, such as iron; and vitamins. Any beneficial effects of tonics, however, are likely to be due to their *placebo effect.

Topal (Novex Pharma) A proprietary combination of *alginic acid, *aluminium hydroxide, and *magnesium carbonate, used as an *antacid for the treatment of indigestion, heartburn and oesophagitis due to reflux, and gastritis (*see* ACID-PEPTIC DISEASES). It is freely available *over the counter in the form of tablets.

Side effects and interactions with other drugs: see ANTACIDS.

Precautions: Topal has a high sugar content and should therefore be used with caution by people with diabetes.

Topamax (Janssen-Cilag) *See* TOPIRAMATE.

topical Describing the route of administration of a drug that is applied directly to the surface of the body, where its effects are required. The term usually refers to application of a drug, in the form of a cream, ointment, or gel, to a region of skin, but is also used for application to the eyes, ears, nasal passages, and mouth cavity. Since a drug administered topically is intended to exert its effects only locally, any *systemic effects would be unwanted. Most drugs applied to the skin and other surfaces are not absorbed into the circulation and therefore do not reach other parts of the body. However, potent drugs (notably corticosteroids), for example in ointments and eye drops, can be absorbed and have systemic effects.

topical steroids *Corticosteroids formulated for use on the skin. They reduce inflammation and are effective for treating such conditions as

*eczema, dermatitis, and *psoriasis. Steroids may also be used to reduce keloid scars and granulomas (growths of tissue that form over wounds or healing ulcers). Topical steroids may also be used in the nose, eyes, and ears; nasal preparations may be used for the treatment of hay fever. The side effects of topical steroids are less severe than those of systemic steroids, but care must still be taken; the number and degree of side effects will depend on the strength of the steroid, the duration of treatment, and the area of the body being treated. Topical steroids are classified in four groups: mild, moderately potent, potent, and very potent. More steroid is absorbed from the face, the genitals, and areas where skin surfaces rub together (as in the groin); there is little absorption from nose, ear, or eye preparations. Potent topical steroids are not usually used in children. Some compound preparations for topical use combine corticosteroids with antibiotics or antifungal agents; these must also be used with care, as the steroid will be absorbed.

See ALCLOMETASONE DIPROPIONATE; BECLOMETHASONE <BECLOMETASONE> DIPROPIONATE; BETAMETHASONE; CLOBETASOL PROPIONATE; CLOBETASONE BUTYRATE; DESOXYMETHASONE <DESOXIMETASONE>; DIFLUCORTOLONE VALERATE; FLUMETHASONE <FLUMETASONE> PIVALATE; FLUOCINOLONE ACETONIDE; FLUOCINONIDE; FLUOCORTOLONE; FLURANDRENOLONE <FLUDROXYCORTIDE>; HALCINONIDE; HYDROCORTISONE; HYDROCORTISONE BUTYRATE; MOMETASONE FUROATE.

Side effects: there may be local irritation and allergic reactions at the site of application; disturbances in taste or smell may occur with nasal sprays. With long-term use of potent topical steroids, the most common side effect is atrophy (thinning) of the skin, with the development of stretch marks (striae) and possibly localized collections of fine blood vessels, which appear as red – sometimes spidery – spots. There may be increased growth of hair. Very potent preparations may be absorbed through the skin and produce effects throughout the body (*see* CORTICOSTEROIDS).

Precautions: topical steroids should not be used to treat acne or rosacea (since they will exacerbate these conditions), dermatitis around the mouth, scabies, leg ulcers, ringworm, or viral skin diseases. They should not be used for bacterial or fungal infections unless antimicrobials are used as well. Topical steroids should not be used for ear or eye infections if viral, tuberculous, or purulent infections are present. Extensive use during pregnancy should be avoided. Use of steroids on the face and in children should be limited to five days unless a specialist has advised longer treatment; steroids should not be used for prolonged periods to treat nappy rash. Topical steroids should be withdrawn gradually after prolonged use.

Topicycline (Monmouth Pharmaceuticals) *See* TETRACYCLINE HYDROCHLORIDE.

topiramate A drug used as an *adjunct in the treatment of partial seizures of epilepsy that are inadequately controlled by other *anticonvulsants. It is available as tablets on *prescription only.

Side effects: include shaky movements, impaired concentration, confusion, dizziness, fatigue, tingling, agitation, and depression.

Precautions: topiramate should not be taken by women who are breastfeeding. Dosage should be reduced gradually at the end of treatment.

Interactions with other drugs:

Anticonvulsants: carbamazepine and phenytoin often lower the plasma concentration of topiramate; topiramate sometimes increases the plasma concentration of phenytoin.

Oral contraceptives: the contraceptive effect of these drugs is reduced by topiramate.

Proprietary preparation: Topamax.

topoisomerase inhibitors A class of *cytotoxic drugs that block the action of topoisomerase, an enzyme that is required for DNA replication and hence cell division. Topoisomerase inhibitors are therefore used to treat *cancer, in which rapid cell division must be prevented. The drugs of this class are *irinotecan and *topotecan.

topotecan A *topoisomerase inhibitor used for the treatment of *cancer of the ovaries that has spread to other parts of the body and has not responded to other treatments. It may also be used to treat a certain form of lung cancer (small cell lung cancer) that has not responded to other therapy. Topotecan is available as a form for intravenous infusion on *prescription only.

Side effects: include *bone marrow suppression, hair loss, nausea, abdominal pain, loss of appetite, sore mouth, fatigue, and weakness.

Precautions: topotecan should not be given to patients with severe liver or kidney disease or bone marrow suppression, or to women who are pregnant or breastfeeding. *See also* CYTOTOXIC DRUGS.

Proprietary preparation: Hycamtin.

Toptabs (Sussex Pharmaceutical) A proprietary combination of *aspirin (an analgesic) and *caffeine (a stimulant), used for the relief of mild to moderate pain. It is available as tablets and can be obtained without a prescription, but only from pharmacies.

Side effects, precautions, and interactions with other drugs: see ASPIRIN; CAFFEINE.

Toradol (Roche Products) *See* KETOROLAC TROMETAMOL.

torasemide A *loop diuretic used for the treatment of congestive *heart failure and *oedema associated with liver or kidney disease and for pulmonary oedema (fluid in the spaces of the lungs causing breathing difficulties). It is available as tablets or an injection on *prescription only.

Side effects, precautions, and interactions with other drugs: see LOOP DIURETICS.

Proprietary preparation: Torem.
See also DIURETICS.

Torem (Roche Products) *See* TORASEMIDE.

toremifene An *oestrogen antagonist used for the treatment of advanced breast cancer in postmenopausal women in which oestrogens stimulate growth of the tumour (*see* CANCER). It is available as tablets on *prescription only.
Side effects: include hot flushes, vaginal bleeding or discharge, sweating, nausea, vomiting, dizziness, fluid retention, and chest or back pain. Vaginal bleeding or discharge or pelvic pain should be reported to a doctor promptly to exclude the possibility of cancer of the endometrium (womb lining).
Precautions: toremifene should not be taken by women who are pregnant or breastfeeding or by those who have severe liver disease, hyperplasia (overgrowth) of the endometrium, or a history of severe thromboembolic disease.
Interactions with other drugs:
  Anticoagulants: toremifene increases the effects of warfarin and nicoumalone <acenocoumarol>.
  Antiepileptic drugs: the effects of toremifene may be reduced by carbamazepine, phenobarbitone <phenobarbital>, and phenytoin.
  Thiazide diuretics: increase the risk of high concentrations of calcium in the blood, especially in women in whom the cancer has spread to the bones.
Proprietary preparation: Fareston.

Totamol (CP Pharmaceuticals) *See* ATENOLOL.

Totaretic (CP Pharmaceuticals) *See* CO-TENIDONE.

tramadol hydrochloride An *opioid analgesic used for the treatment of moderate to severe pain. It causes less depression of breathing and constipation than other opioids and is less likely to cause dependence. Tramadol is available, on *prescription only, as capsules, soluble tablets, an effervescent powder in sachets, *modified-release capsules and tablets, and an injection.
Side effects: include low blood pressure and (occasionally) high blood pressure, hallucinations, and confusion. *See also* MORPHINE.
Precautions: tramadol should be used with caution in people who have a history of epilepsy and in women who are pregnant or breastfeeding. *See also* MORPHINE.
Interactions with other drugs:
  Antidepressants: the risk of convulsions may be increased if tramadol is taken with tricyclic antidepressants or SSRIs. MAOIs should not be taken with tramadol.

Carbamazepine: reduces the effects of tramadol.

See also OPIOIDS.

Proprietary preparations: Tramake (capsules); Tramake Insts (sachets); Zamadol (capsules); Zamadol SR (modified-release capsules); Zydol; Zydol SR (modified-release tablets).

Tramake, Tramake Insts (Galen) *See* TRAMADOL HYDROCHLORIDE.

tramazoline hydrochloride A *sympathomimetic drug that constricts blood vessels. Tramazoline is used as a nasal *decongestant to relieve the symptoms of hay fever; it is included as an ingredient of a nasal spray that is available on *prescription only.

Side effects, precautions, and interactions with other drugs: *see* EPHEDRINE HYDROCHLORIDE; DECONGESTANTS.

Proprietary preparation: DEXA-RHINASPRAY DUO (combined with dexamethasone).

Tramil 500 (Whitehall Laboratories) *See* PARACETAMOL.

Trandate (Medeva) *See* LABETALOL HYDROCHLORIDE.

trandolapril An *ACE inhibitor used as an adjunct to *diuretics for the treatment of *heart failure. It is also used after a heart attack to prevent deterioration of left ventricular function and to treat mild to moderate *hypertension. It is available as capsules on *prescription only.

Side effects, precautions, and interactions with other drugs: *see* ACE INHIBITORS.

Proprietary preparations: Odrik; Gopten; TARKA (combined with verapamil).

See also ANTIHYPERTENSIVE DRUGS.

tranexamic acid A drug that prevents the breakdown of blood clots in the circulation (fibrinolysis). It acts by preventing the activation of the enzyme that digests fibrin, the protein in blood clots, i.e. it is an antifibrinolytic drug (*see* HAEMOSTATIC DRUGS). Tranexamic acid is used to reduce excessive menstrual bleeding, especially when this is caused by an intrauterine contraceptive device (IUCD) and the woman does not wish to change to another form of contraception. It is also used to control excessive bleeding after surgery or tooth extraction. Tranexamic acid is available, on *prescription only, as tablets, syrup, or a solution for intravenous injection.

Side effects: include nausea, vomiting, diarrhoea, and giddiness if the drug is injected rapidly.

Precautions: tranexamic acid should not be taken by people with thromboembolic disease (*see* THROMBOSIS) and should be used with caution in people with kidney disease or haematuria (blood in the urine).

Proprietary preparation: Cyklokapron.

Tranquax (APS-Berk) *See* CLOMIPRAMINE HYDROCHLORIDE.

tranquillizers *See* ANTIPSYCHOTIC DRUGS; ANXIOLYTIC DRUGS.

transdermal Across the skin: describing a route of administration of drugs that enables them to be absorbed slowly and steadily into the circulation. Such drugs are usually incorporated into adhesive patches; examples are nicotine (for treating smoking dependence), female sex hormones for (*hormone replacement therapy), and nitrates (for angina).

Transiderm-Nitro (Novartis Pharmaceuticals) *See* GLYCERYL TRINITRATE.

Transvasin Heat Rub (Seton Scholl Healthcare) A proprietary combination of *ethyl nicotinate, *hexyl nicotinate, and tetrahydrofurfuryl salicylate (*see* SALICYLATES), used as a *rubefacient for the relief of muscular aches and pains, sprains, and strains. It is freely available *over the counter in the form of a cream.
Side effects and precautions: see RUBEFACIENTS.

Transvasin Heat Spray (Seton Scholl Healthcare) A proprietary combination of *2-hydroxyethyl salicylate, *diethylamine salicylate, and *methyl nicotinate, used as a *rubefacient for the relief of muscular aches and pains. It is freely available *over the counter.
Side effects and precautions: see RUBEFACIENTS.

Tranxene (Boehringer Ingelheim) *See* CLORAZEPATE DIPOTASSIUM.

tranylcypromine A *monoamine oxidase inhibitor used for the treatment of depressive illness. It is available as tablets on *prescription only.
Side effects and precautions: see MONOAMINE OXIDASE INHIBITORS. Tranylcypromine causes insomnia if taken in the evening; it should therefore not be taken later than 3 pm.
Interactions with other drugs: see MONOAMINE OXIDASE INHIBITORS.
Proprietary preparations: Parnate; PARSTELIN (combined with trifluoperazine).

Trasicor (Novartis Pharmaceuticals) *See* OXPRENOLOL HYDROCHLORIDE.

Trasidrex (Novartis Pharmaceuticals) A proprietary combination of *oxprenolol hydrochloride (a beta blocker), and *cyclopenthiazide (a thiazide diuretic), used in the treatment of mild to moderate *hypertension. It is available as tablets on *prescription only.
Side effects, precautions, and interactions with other drugs: see BETA BLOCKERS; THIAZIDE DIURETICS.
See also ANTIHYPERTENSIVE DRUGS; DIURETICS.

Trasylol (Bayer) *See* APROTININ.

Travasept 100 (Baxter Healthcare) A proprietary combination of the antiseptics *chlorhexidine gluconate and *cetrimide, used for cleansing and disinfecting wounds and burns. It is available as a solution without a prescription, but only from pharmacies.
Side effects: see CETRIMIDE.
Precautions: the solution should not come into contact with the eyes.

Travogyn (Schering Health Care) *See* ISOCONAZOLE NITRATE.

Traxam, **Traxam Pain Relief** (Wyeth Laboratories) *See* FELBINAC.

trazodone An *antidepressant drug, related to the *tricyclic antidepressants, used for the treatment of depressive illness, particularly when sedation is desirable. It is available, on *prescription only, as capsules, *modified-release tablets, or a liquid.
Side effects: similar to those of *amitriptyline hydrochloride, but trazodone has fewer effects on the heart. Rarely, it can cause priapism (painful and persistent erection of the penis), in which case treatment should be stopped immediately.
Precautions and interactions with other drugs: see TRICYCLIC ANTIDEPRESSANTS.
Proprietary preparations: Molipaxin; Molipaxin CR (modified-release tablets).

Trental (Hoechst Marion Roussel) *See* OXPENTIFYLLINE <PENTOXIFYLLINE>.

treosulfan An *alkylating drug used for the treatment of ovarian *cancer. It is available, on *prescription only, as capsules or an injection.
Side effects: include pigmentation of the skin and (rarely) irritation and bleeding in the bladder. *See also* CYTOTOXIC DRUGS.
Precautions: see CYTOTOXIC DRUGS.

tretinoin A *retinoid used topically for the treatment of *acne and to reduce the wrinkling and other damage to the skin caused by overexposure to the sun. Tretinoin is also administered orally to treat certain types of leukaemia (*see* CANCER). A *prescription only medicine, it is available as a lotion, cream, gel, or (for chemotherapy) as capsules.
Side effects: skin preparations may cause redness, local irritation, and peeling at the start of treatment, but this should not last; they may cause changes in skin pigmentation and make the skin more sensitive to light. Side effects caused by the capsules include stomach upsets, irregular heart rhythms, flushing, headache, dry skin and mucous membranes, rash, visual impairment, hearing disturbances, confusion, dizziness, bone pain, and chest pain; the retinoic acid syndrome (including fever, breathlessness, and *oedema) requires immediate treatment.
Precautions: skin preparations should not be used on damaged or sunburnt skin, by people with eczema or a personal or family history of skin cancer, or by pregnant women. These preparations should not come

into contact with the eyes, nostrils, or mouth, and exposure of treated skin to ultraviolet light (including excessive sunlight) should be avoided. Skin preparations should not be used with other topical agents (e.g. *keratolytics) that may cause irritation. Capsules should not be taken by women who are pregnant or breastfeeding, and contraception must be used for one month before and during treatment and for at least one month after stopping treatment (*see* RETINOIDS). They should be used with caution in people with liver or kidney disease. Blood tests to monitor concentrations of fats should be carried out during treatment; there is a risk of thrombosis during the first month of treatment.

Interactions with other drugs:
  Keratolytics: see precautions above.
  Oral contraceptives: tretinoin reduces the contraceptive effects of progestogen-only pills and possibly also of combined pills.
Proprietary preparations: Retin-A (for acne); Retinova (for sun-damaged skin); Vesanoid (capsules).

TRH-Cambridge (Cambridge Laboratories) *See* PROTIRELIN.

Tri-Adcortyl (Bristol-Myers Squibb) A proprietary combination of *triamcinolone acetonide (a potent steroid), *nystatin (an antifungal drug), and the antibiotics *neomycin and *gramicidin, used for the treatment of inflammatory skin conditions when bacterial or *Candida* (thrush) infection may be present. It is available as a cream or ointment on *prescription only.
Side effects, precautions, and interactions with other drugs: *see* TOPICAL STEROIDS.

Tri-Adcortyl Otic (Bristol-Myers Squibb) A proprietary combination of *triamcinolone acetonide (a potent steroid), *nystatin (an antifungal drug), and the antibiotics *neomycin and *gramicidin, used for the treatment of bacterial infections of the outer ear. It is available as an ear ointment on *prescription only.
Side effects: this medicine may impair hearing and kidney function.
Precautions: the ointment should not be used for treating tuberculous or viral infections and should not be applied when the eardrum is perforated. It should be used with caution by people with hearing loss and by pregnant women. Long-term use in infants should be avoided.

Triadene (Schering Health Care) A proprietary combination of *ethinyloestradiol <ethinylestradiol> and *gestodene used as an *oral contraceptive of the triphasic type. These tablets are packaged in three phases, which differ in the amounts of the active ingredients they contain. Triadene is available on *prescription only.
Side effects and interactions with other drugs: *see* ORAL CONTRACEPTIVES.
Precautions: Triadene should not be used by women who are at risk of developing thromboembolism, for example because they are very overweight or have varicose veins or a history of thrombosis. It should

therefore only be taken by women who cannot tolerate other brands and who are prepared to accept the increased risk. *See also* ORAL CONTRACEPTIVES.

triamcinolone acetonide A potent glucocorticoid (*see* CORTICOSTEROIDS), similar to *prednisolone, used for the treatment of inflammatory disorders, including the swelling, pain, and stiffness associated with rheumatoid arthritis, osteoarthritis, bursitis, or tenosynovitis (inflammation of the tendon); skin diseases, such as *eczema, *psoriasis, and dermatitis; eczematous inflammation of the outer ear; and mouth sores and ulcers. It is also used for the prevention and treatment of allergic rhinitis (including hay fever). Triamcinolone is available, on *prescription only, as tablets, a solution for injection into joints or muscles, a skin cream or ointment, ear drops or ointment, a paste, and a metered-dose nasal spray.

Side effects, precautions, and interactions with other drugs: see CORTICOSTEROIDS; TOPICAL STEROIDS.

Proprietary preparations: Adcortyl; Kenalog (injection); Lederspan (injection); Nasacort (nasal spray); ADCORTYL WITH GRANEODIN (combined with neomycin and gramicidin); ADCORTYL IN ORABASE (combined with carmellose); AUDICORT (combined with neomycin); AUREOCORT (combined with chlortetracycline); NYSTADERMAL (combined with nystatin); PEVARYL TC (combined with econazole nitrate); TRI-ADCORTYL (combined with nystatin, neomycin, and gramicidin); TRI-ADCORTYL OTIC (combined with nystatin, neomycin, and gramicidin).

Triam-Co (Norton Healthcare) A proprietary combination of *triamterene (a potassium-sparing diuretic) and *hydrochlorothiazide (a thiazide diuretic), used for the treatment of *hypertension and *oedema associated with heart failure, liver disease, or kidney disease. It is available as tablets on *prescription only.

Side effects, precautions, and interactions with other drugs: see THIAZIDE DIURETICS; POTASSIUM-SPARING DIURETICS.

See also ANTIHYPERTENSIVE DRUGS; DIURETICS.

triamterene A *potassium-sparing diuretic used for the treatment of *oedema associated with heart failure, liver disease, or kidney disease. It is available as capsules on *prescription only.

Side effects, precautions, and interactions with other drugs: see POTASSIUM-SPARING DIURETICS.

Proprietary preparations: Dytac; DYAZIDE (combined with hydrochlorothiazide); DYTIDE (combined with benzthiazide); FRUSENE (combined with frusemide <furosemide>); KALSPARE (combined with chlorthalidone <chlortalidone>); TRIAM-CO (combined with hydrochlorothiazide).

See also DIURETICS.

tribavirin (ribavirin) An *antiviral drug that is used in the treatment of severe infection caused by the respiratory syncytial virus in infants and children. Available on *prescription only, it is given by inhalation.

Side effects: include worsening of the respiratory condition, bacterial pneumonia, and anaemia.

Precautions: women who are pregnant or attempting to become pregnant should avoid exposure to this aerosol.

Proprietary preparation: Virazid.

triclofos sodium A *hypnotic drug used for the short-term treatment of insomnia. It is taken by mouth and is available as a solution on *prescription only.

Side effects: similar to those of *chloral hydrate, but triclofos causes less stomach irritation and fewer other gastrointestinal side effects.

Precautions and interactions with other drugs: see CHLORAL HYDRATE.

triclosan An *antiseptic that is active against a wide range of bacteria and fungi. As a soap or liquid it is used as a preoperative hand wash for surgeons and for cleansing and disinfecting the skin of patients before surgery, injections, or taking blood samples. It is also included in various skin preparations to prevent infection of minor wounds and for treating such conditions as eczema and acne. Triclosan is freely available *over the counter.

Precautions: triclosan should not come into contact with the eyes.

Proprietary preparations: Aquasept; Manusept; Ster-Zac Bath Concentrate; CLEARASIL TREATMENT CREAM REGULAR (combined with sulphur); DETTOL ANTISEPTIC CREAM (combined with chloroxylenol and edetic acid); OILATUM PLUS (combined with liquid paraffin and benzalkonium chloride; OILATUM JUNIOR FLARE UP (combined with benzalkonium chloride and liquid paraffin); SOLARCAINE (combined with benzocaine); TCP FIRST AID ANTISEPTIC CREAM (combined with chloroxylenol and TCP Liquid Antiseptic).

tricyclic antidepressants (TCAs) A class of *antidepressant drugs that block the reuptake of noradrenaline <norepinephrine> and serotonin into nerve endings, thus prolonging their action in the brain. TCAs can be divided roughly into two groups: those with sedative properties (*amitriptyline hydrochloride, *dothiepin <dosulepin> hydrochloride, *doxepin, and *trimipramine), which tend to be of greater benefit to patients who are anxious and agitated; and those with only weakly sedative action (*clomipramine hydrochloride, *imipramine, *lofepramine, *nortriptyline, and *protriptyline hydrochloride), which are more useful for treating lethargic and withdrawn patients. Related to the TCAs are the antidepressants *maprotiline hydrochloride, *mianserin hydrochloride, *trazodone, and *viloxazine hydrochloride. Some TCAs are used to treat bedwetting in children and as an *adjunct for pain relief (*see also* MIGRAINE).

Side effects: all tricyclic antidepressants can have significant *antimuscarinic effects (dry mouth, blurred vision, drowsiness, constipation, and urinary retention), but *tolerance to these effects develops with continued use. Abnormal heart rhythms (*see* ARRHYTHMIA) and heart block can occasionally follow the use of TCAs, particularly amitriptyline. TCAs are sometimes associated with convulsions.

Precautions: TCAs and related antidepressants should not be taken by people who have recently suffered a heart attack, who have severe liver disease, or who are manic. They should be used with caution in people with heart disease, a history of epilepsy, thyroid disease, acute glaucoma, or a history of urinary retention, and in women who are pregnant or breastfeeding. Alcohol should be avoided, as it enhances the sedative effects of these drugs.

Interactions with other drugs:

Anti-arrhythmics: TCAs increase the risk of recurrence of ventricular arrhythmias.

Antiepileptics: TCAs increase the risk of convulsions recurring; plasma concentrations of some tricyclics are reduced.

Antihistamines: increase the sedative effects of TCAs; astemizole and terfenadine increase the risk of ventricular arrhythmias and should not be taken with TCAs.

Cimetidine: increases plasma concentrations of TCAs and therefore dosages of these may need to be reduced.

Halofantrine: increases the risk of ventricular arrhythmias.

MAOIs: cause restlessness and other signs of overactivity of the central nervous system and should not be taken until at least a week after stopping a course of TCAs. TCAs should not be taken until two weeks after stopping an MAOI.

Sotalol: increases the risk of ventricular arrhythmias.

Sympathomimetics: cause raised blood pressure.

Tridestra (Orion Pharma) A proprietary preparation of *oestradiol <estradiol> tablets and combined oestradiol/*medroxyprogesterone tablets used as sequential combined *hormone replacement therapy for the relief of menopausal symptoms and prevention of osteoporosis in women who have not had a hysterectomy. The tablets, which are available on *prescription only, must be taken in the prescribed order.

Side effects, precautions, and interactions with other drugs: *see* HORMONE REPLACEMENT THERAPY.

trientine dihydrochloride A drug used to treat Wilson's disease (a condition in which copper accumulates in the body) in people who cannot tolerate treatment with *penicillamine. It is available as capsules on *prescription only.

Side effects: include nausea.

Precautions: trientine should be used with caution during pregnancy.

Interactions with other drugs:

Iron: the absorption of iron supplements given by mouth is reduced by trientine.

trifluoperazine An *antipsychotic drug used for the treatment of schizophrenia and other psychoses and for the short-term treatment of severe anxiety, agitation, and violent or dangerous behaviour. It is also used to treat severe nausea and vomiting. Trifluoperazine is available, on *prescription only, as tablets, *modified-release capsules, or a syrup.

Side effects: as for *chlorpromazine, but trifluoperazine is less sedating, has fewer antimuscarinic effects, and *extrapyramidal reactions are more frequent.

Precautions and interactions with other drugs: see CHLORPROMAZINE HYDROCHLORIDE.

Proprietary preparations: Stelazine; Stelazine Spansules (modified-release capsules); PARSTELIN (combined with tranylcypromine).

Trifyba (Sanofi Winthrop) *See* BRAN.

triglycerides A class of important lipids consisting of glycerol combined with three fatty acids. Increased concentrations of triglycerides in the blood (**hypertriglyceridaemia**: *see* HYPERLIPIDAEMIA) are a risk factor for coronary heart disease, and very high levels can cause life-threatening pancreatitis (inflammation of the pancreas). Triglycerides are transported in the blood by *lipoproteins, and high circulating concentrations can be reduced by dietary modification, which is the usual first-line treatment. When triglyceride concentrations are particularly high, *lipid-lowering drugs may be used.

trihexyphenidyl hydrochloride *See* BENZHEXOL HYDROCHLORIDE.

trilostane A drug that inhibits the production of both mineralocorticoids and glucocorticoids (*see* CORTICOSTEROIDS). It is therefore used to treat conditions that arise from overproduction of these hormones (such as Cushing's syndrome). It can also be used to treat postmenopausal breast cancer. Trilostane is available as capsules on *prescription only.

Side effects: include flushing, nausea, a running nose, and diarrhoea.

Precautions: trilostane should not be taken by pregnant women or by those with severe kidney or liver disease. It should be used with caution by people with impaired kidney or liver function. Nonhormonal contraception should be used (if appropriate) during treatment.

Interactions with other drugs:

Potassium-sparing diuretics: there is an increased risk of high concentrations of potassium in the blood.

Proprietary preparation: Modrenal.

Triludan (Hoechst Marion Roussel) *See* TERFENADINE.

trimeprazine tartrate <alimemazine tartrate> One of the original (sedating) *antihistamines, used to relieve the symptoms of such allergic conditions as urticaria and other itching skin conditions. It is available as tablets or a syrup on *prescription only.

Side effects: *see* ANTIHISTAMINES. Trimeprazine may also cause *antimuscarinic effects, abnormal heart rhythms, low blood pressure, breathing difficulties, *extrapyramidal reactions, and (in high doses) convulsions.

Precautions and interactions with other drugs: *see* ANTIHISTAMINES.

Proprietary preparations: Vallergan; Vallergan Syrup; Vallergan Forte Syrup.

trimetaphan camsylate <trimetaphan camsilate>

A drug that is used during surgery to maintain a low blood pressure; it acts by reducing the tension of the blood vessels. Trimetaphan is available as an injection on *prescription only.

Side effects: include an increase in heart rate and depression of breathing, constipation, increased pressure in the eye, and dilation of the pupils.

Precautions: trimetaphan should not be used in pregnant women or in people with severe atherosclerosis, severe heart disease, or pyloric stenosis (narrowing of the outlet of the stomach). It should be used with caution in people with liver or kidney disease, diabetes, disease of the coronary or cerebral arteries, Addison's disease, or degenerative diseases of the brain.

trimethoprim

An antibacterial drug whose action is similar to that of the *sulphonamides. It is used for the treatment of many bacterial infections, especially infections of the urinary and respiratory tracts. It is sometimes given as a combination with sulphamethoxazole <sulfamethoxazole> (*see* CO-TRIMOXAZOLE); however, it is currently recommended that trimethoprim alone is sufficient for the treatment of most infections and has fewer side effects. It is available, on *prescription only, as tablets or as a solution for *intramuscular or *intravenous injection.

Side effects: gastrointestinal disturbances, including nausea and vomiting, may occur; other possible side effects are itching and rashes. Blood disorders may very rarely occur with long-term treatment – such symptoms as fever, sore throat, bruising, and rashes should be reported to a doctor immediately.

Precautions: trimethoprim should not be taken by patients with severe kidney disease, by pregnant women, or by newborn babies. It should be used with caution in people who have kidney disease and in women who are breastfeeding. Blood counts are required for those on long-term therapy.

Proprietary preparations: Monotrim; Trimogal; Trimopan; Triprimix; Bactrim (*see* CO-TRIMOXAZOLE); Chemotrim Paediatric (*see* CO-TRIMOXAZOLE); POLYTRIM (combined with polymyxin B sulphate and bacitracin); Septrin (*see* CO-TRIMOXAZOLE).

trimetrexate A drug used for the treatment of moderate to severe *Pneumocystis carinii* pneumonia in AIDS patients who are resistant to, or cannot tolerate, standard therapy. It destroys the parasites that cause the disease by inhibiting an enzyme involved in folate metabolism. To protect the body's cells from these antifolate effects (which include *bone marrow suppression, ulceration of the mouth, stomach, and intestines, and liver or kidney disease), trimetrexate is given with calcium folinate (*see* FOLINIC ACID). It is used only under specialist supervision and is available as a form for intravenous infusion on *prescription only.

Side effects: include blood disorders, vomiting, diarrhoea, ulceration of the mouth or stomach, fever, and confusion.

Precautions: trimetrexate should not be given to women who are pregnant or breastfeeding; people receiving trimetrexate should avoid conception for at least six months following treatment. It should be used with caution in people with liver or kidney disease. Blood tests and monitoring of liver and kidney function should be done regularly during treatment.

Interactions with other drugs: drugs (such as zidovudine) that suppress the bone marrow should not be used during treatment with trimetrexate.

Proprietary preparation: Neutrexin.

Tri-Minulet (Wyeth Laboratories) A proprietary combination of *ethinyloestradiol <ethinylestradiol> and *gestodene used as an *oral contraceptive of the triphasic type. These tablets are packaged in three phases, which differ in the amounts of the active ingredients they contain. Tri-Minulet is available on *prescription only.

Side effects and interactions with other drugs: see ORAL CONTRACEPTIVES.

Precautions: Tri-Minulet should not be used by women who are at risk of developing thromboembolism, for example because they are very overweight or have varicose veins or a history of thrombosis. It should therefore only be taken by women who cannot tolerate other brands and who are prepared to accept the increased risk. *See also* ORAL CONTRACEPTIVES.

trimipramine A *tricyclic antidepressant drug used for the treatment of depressive illness, especially when sedation is required. It is available as tablets or capsules on *prescription only.

Side effects, precautions, and interactions with other drugs: see AMITRIPTYLINE HYDROCHLORIDE; TRICYCLIC ANTIDEPRESSANTS.

Proprietary preparation: Surmontil.

Trimogal (Lagap Pharmaceuticals) *See* TRIMETHOPRIM.

Trimopan (APS-Berk) *See* TRIMETHOPRIM.

Trimovate (GlaxoWellcome) A proprietary combination of *clobetasone butyrate (a moderately potent topical steroid), *nystatin (an antifungal agent), and *oxytetracycline (an antibiotic), used for the treatment of infected conditions of the skin in moist or covered areas. It is available as a cream on *prescription only.

Side effects and precautions: see TOPICAL STEROIDS.

Trinordiol (Wyeth Laboratories) A proprietary combination of *ethinyloestradiol <ethinylestradiol> and *levonorgestrel used as an *oral contraceptive of the triphasic type. These tablets are packaged in three phases, which differ in the amounts of the active ingredients they contain. Trinordiol is available on *prescription only.

Side effects, precautions, and interactions with other drugs: see ORAL CONTRACEPTIVES.

TriNovum (Janssen-Cilag) A proprietary combination of *ethinyloestradiol <ethinylestradiol> and *norethisterone used as an *oral contraceptive of the triphasic type. These tablets are packaged in three phases, which differ in the amounts of the active ingredients they contain. TriNovum is available on *prescription only.

Side effects, precautions, and interactions with other drugs: see ORAL CONTRACEPTIVES.

Triogesic (Novartis Consumer Health) A proprietary combination of *paracetamol (an analgesic) and *phenylpropanolamine (a decongestant), used for the relief of nasal and sinus congestion and associated headache and sinus pain. It is available as tablets and can be obtained without a prescription, but only from pharmacies.

Side effects: see EPHEDRINE HYDROCHLORIDE.

Precautions: Triogesic is not recommended for children under six years old. *See also* PARACETAMOL; EPHEDRINE HYDROCHLORIDE.

Interactions with other drugs: see PHENYLPROPANOLAMINE; EPHEDRINE HYDROCHLORIDE.

Triominic (Novartis Consumer Health) A proprietary combination of pheniramine (an antihistamine) and *phenylpropanolamine (a decongestant), used for the relief of nasal congestion associated with allergic and infectious disorders of the upper airways. It is available as tablets without a prescription, but only from pharmacies.

Side effects and interactions with other drugs: see ANTIHISTAMINES; EPHEDRINE HYDROCHLORIDE.

Precautions: this medicine is not recommended for children under six years old. *See also* ANTIHISTAMINES; EPHEDRINE HYDROCHLORIDE.

tripotassium dicitratobismuthate A bismuth-containing drug with *cytoprotectant action, used for the treatment of gastric and duodenal ulcers (*see* ACID-PEPTIC DISEASES). It is available as a liquid or tablets and can be obtained without a prescription, but only from pharmacies.

Side effects: tripotassium dicitratobismuthate may cause blackening of the tongue and stools.

Precautions: this medicine should not be taken by people with kidney disease or by pregnant women.

Proprietary preparations: De-Nol (liquid); De-Noltab (tablets).

Triprimix (Ashbourne Pharmaceuticals) *See* TRIMETHOPRIM.

triprolidine hydrochloride One of the original (sedating) *antihistamines. It is available in combination with *pseudoephedrine for the treatment of hay fever and is also an ingredient in some cough medicines and decongestant preparations. Preparations containing triprolidine can be bought from pharmacies without a prescription.

Side effects, precautions, and interactions with other drugs: see ANTIHISTAMINES.

Proprietary preparations: ACTIFED (combined with pseudoephedrine); ACTIFED COMPOUND LINCTUS (combined with dextromethorphan and pseudoephedrine); ACTIFED EXPECTORANT (combined with guaiphenesin <guaifenesin> and pseudoephedrine); ACTIFED JUNIOR COUGH RELIEF (combined with dextromethorphan); SUDAFED PLUS (combined with pseudoephedrine).

Triptafen (Forley) A proprietary combination of *amitriptyline hydrochloride (a *tricyclic antidepressant) and *perphenazine (an antipsychotic drug), used for the treatment of depression with anxiety. It is available as tablets on *prescription only. **Triptafen-M** is a similar preparation but contains a lower proportion of amitriptyline.

Side effects, precautions, and interactions with other drugs: see TRICYCLIC ANTIDEPRESSANTS; AMITRIPTYLINE HYDROCHLORIDE; PERPHENAZINE; CHLORPROMAZINE HYDROCHLORIDE.

triptorelin An analogue of *gonadorelin that is used for the treatment of *endometriosis. It is also used to treat advanced prostate cancer, having an action similar to that of *leuprorelin. Triptorelin is given by *intramuscular injection and is available on *prescription only.

Side effects: see GOSERELIN. Other side effects include dry mouth, excessive salivation, and difficulty in urinating.

Precautions: for women, *see* GOSERELIN. In cancer treatment, triptorelin should not be used by men in whom there is compression of the spinal cord or secondary tumours in the spinal cord.

Proprietary preparation: De-capeptyl sr.

Trisequens (Novo Nordisk Pharmaceutical) A proprietary preparation of combined *oestradiol/*oestriol <estradiol>/<estriol> tablets and combined oestradiol/oestriol/*norethisterone tablets used as sequential combined *hormone replacement therapy for the relief of menopausal symptoms in women who have not had a hysterectomy. **Trisequens Forte** contains a higher dose of oestrogens. The tablets, which are available on *prescription only, must be taken in the prescribed order.

Side effects, precautions, and interactions with other drugs: *see* HORMONE REPLACEMENT THERAPY.

trisodium edetate A chelating agent that binds free *calcium. It is used rarely as an infusion to lower high plasma calcium concentrations due to overproduction of *parathyroid hormone by the parathyroid gland. It is also applied to the eyes to remove deposits of calcium in the cornea in the treatment of lime burns of the eyes. A *prescription only medicine, trisodium edetate is available as a solution for injection or for use as eye drops.

Precautions: infusions should not be used in people with kidney disease or tuberculosis.

Proprietary preparation: Limclair.

Tritace (Hoechst Marion Roussel) *See* RAMIPRIL.

Trobocin (Pharmacia & Upjohn) *See* SPECTINOMYCIN.

Tropergen (Norgine) *See* CO-PHENOTROPE.

tropicamide An *antimuscarinic drug that is applied to the eye to dilate the pupil before examination of the interior of the eye. It is shorter acting than *atropine sulphate and *cyclopentolate hydrochloride. Tropicamide is available as eye drops on *prescription only.

Side effects: tropicamide may cause transient stinging and an increase in pressure in the eye; with prolonged use local irritation and conjunctivitis can occur.

Precautions and interactions with other drugs: *see* ANTIMUSCARINIC DRUGS.

Proprietary preparations: Mydriacyl; Minims Tropicamide (single-dose eye drops).

tropisetron An *antiemetic used for the prevention or treatment of nausea and vomiting associated with *cytotoxic chemotherapy or occurring after surgery. It acts by opposing the action of the neurotransmitter 5-hydroxytryptamine (*serotonin) at receptors in the central nervous system and in the gut. It is available, on *prescription only, as capsules or an intravenous injection.

Side effects: include headache, constipation, diarrhoea, and abdominal pain.

Precautions: tropisetron should be used with caution in people with uncontrolled high blood pressure (*hypertension) and in women who are pregnant or breastfeeding.

Proprietary preparation: Navoban.

Tropium (DDSA Pharmaceuticals) *See* CHLORDIAZEPOXIDE.

Trosyl (Pfizer) *See* TIOCONAZOLE.

Trusopt (Merck Sharp & Dohme) *See* DORZOLAMIDE.

Tryptizol (Merck Sharp & Dohme) *See* AMITRIPTYLINE HYDROCHLORIDE.

tryptophan An amino acid that appears to benefit some people with resistant depression (*see* ANTIDEPRESSANT DRUGS). It is available as tablets on *prescription only, and under hospital supervision, for those who are unsuited to alternative treatments. Patients and prescribers must be registered with the Optimax Information and Clinical Support Unit.
Side effects: include drowsiness, nausea, headache, and light-headedness. The risk of eosinophilia-myalgia syndrome (a blood disorder associated with muscle pain) has been reduced since nonprescription preparations containing tryptophan were withdrawn.
Precautions: dosage should be reduced gradually at the end of treatment to avoid withdrawal reactions.
Interactions with other drugs:
 Antidepressants: there is a risk of confusion, agitation, and nausea.
Proprietary preparation: Optimax.

tuberculosis An infectious disease caused by the bacillus *Mycobacterium tuberculosis* and characterized by the formation of nodular lesions (tubercles) in the tissues. In **pulmonary tuberculosis** the bacillus is inhaled into the lungs, where it sets up a primary tubercle and spreads to the nearest lymph nodes. Natural immune defences may heal it at this stage; alternatively the disease may smoulder for months or years and fluctuate with the patient's resistance. Many people become infected but show no symptoms. Others develop a chronic infection and can transmit the bacillus by coughing and sneezing. In some cases the bacilli spread from the lungs to the bloodstream, setting up millions of tiny tubercles throughout the body **miliary tuberculosis**, or migrate to the brain to cause **tuberculous meningitis**.
 Tuberculosis is treated with a combination of antibiotics that should be continued for six months in order to prevent the development of drug-resistant strains of the bacillus. The recommended treatment is divided into two phases. In the first phase a combination of at least three of the following drugs – *isoniazid, *rifampicin, *pyrazinamide, and *ethambutol hydrochloride – is taken for two months. This is followed by a combination of isoniazid and rifampicin, which is continued for four months. *See also* CAPREOMYCIN; CYCLOSERINE; RIFABUTIN; STREPTOMYCIN.

Tuinal (Flynn Pharma) A proprietary combination of the barbiturates *amylobarbitone <amobarbital> and *quinalbarbitone <secobarbital> used for the short-term treatment of severe insomnia in patients who are already taking barbiturates. Tuinal is available as capsules; it is a *controlled drug.
Side effects, precautions, and interactions with other drugs: see BARBITURATES.

tulobuterol hydrochloride A *sympathomimetic drug that stimulates beta *adrenoceptors in the airways. It is used as a *bronchodilator in the treatment of asthma, bronchitis, and emphysema. Tulobuterol is available as tablets or a syrup on *prescription only.

Side effects: see SALBUTAMOL.

Precautions: see SALBUTAMOL. In addition it should not be used by people with impaired kidney function or by pregnant women.

Interactions with other drugs: see SALBUTAMOL.

Proprietary preparation: Respacal.

Tums (SmithKline Beecham Consumer Healthcare) *See* CALCIUM CARBONATE.

turpentine oil An aromatic oil that is an ingredient of *rubefacient liniments, embrocations, and creams for relief of aches, pains, and stiffness in muscles, tendons, and joints. It is also included in inhalant preparations to relieve the congestion caused by colds, catarrh, influenza, and hay fever. Preparations containing turpentine oil are freely available *over the counter.

Side effects and precautions: see RUBEFACIENTS.

Proprietary preparations: BN LINIMENT (combined with ammonia solution and ammonium chloride); ELLIMAN'S UNIVERSAL EMBROCATION (combined with acetic acid); GODDARD'S WHITE OIL EMBROCATION (combined with dilute ammonia solution and acetic acid); DEEP HEAT RUB (combined with eucalyptus oil, menthol, and methyl salicylate); TIXYLIX INHALANT (combined with camphor, eucalyptus oil, and menthol); VICKS VAPORUB (combined with camphor, eucalyptus oil, and menthol); WOODWARD'S BABY CHEST RUB (combined with eucalyptus oil and menthol).

Tylex (Schwartz Pharma) *See* CO-CODAMOL.

tyrothricin An antibiotic that is too toxic to be taken systemically (into the body) but is used topically in low doses as an ingredient of lozenges for local treatment of infections of the skin and mouth.

Side effects: there may be blackening or soreness of the tongue.

Precautions: tyrothricin should not be used in the nose.

Proprietary preparation: TYROZETS (combined with benzocaine).

Tyrozets (Johnson & Johnson) A proprietary combination of *tyrothricin (an antibiotic) and *benzocaine (a local anaesthetic), used for the relief of sore throat and mild irritations of the mouth. It is available as lozenges and can be obtained without a prescription, but only from pharmacies.

Precautions: Tyrozets are not recommended for children under three years old.

Ubretid (Rhône-Poulenc Rorer) *See* DISTIGMINE BROMIDE.

Ucerax (UCB Pharma) *See* HYDROXYZINE HYDROCHLORIDE.

Ukidan (Serono Laboratories) *See* UROKINASE.

Ultec (APS-Berk) *See* CIMETIDINE.

Ultrabase (Schering Health Care) A proprietary combination of *liquid paraffin and *white soft paraffin (both emollients) in the form of a cream, used for the treatment of dry skin conditions. It is freely available *over the counter.

Ultralanum (Schering Health Care) *See* FLUOCORTOLONE.

Ultraproct (Schering Health Care) A proprietary combination of *fluocortolone (a corticosteroid) and *cinchocaine hydrochloride (a local anaesthetic), used to relieve the discomfort and pain of *haemorrhoids and itching of the anus. It is available as an ointment or suppositories on *prescription only.
Side effects: see CORTICOSTEROIDS.
Precautions: Ultraproct should not be used when viral or fungal infection is present; prolonged use should be avoided.

undecenoic acid An *antifungal drug. Undecenoic acid and its salts (mainly **zinc undecenoate**) are used to treat tinea (ringworm) infections of the skin, especially athlete's foot. Undecenoic acid and undecenoates are available in creams, dusting powders, sprays, paints, and shampoos, which can be obtained from pharmacies without a prescription.
Proprietary preparations: Mycota (cream, dusting powder, or spray); CEANEL CONCENTRATE (combined with cetrimide and phenylethyl alcohol); MONPHYTOL (combined with methyl salicylate, salicylic acid, and chlorbutol).

Unguentum M (Crookes Healthcare) A proprietary combination of *liquid paraffin, *white soft paraffin, and other *emollients and silicic acid (an anti-caking agent), used for the treatment of dry skin conditions and napkin rash. It is freely available *over the counter in the form of a cream.

Uniflu with Gregovite C (Unigreg) A proprietary combination of *codeine (an analgesic and cough suppressant), *diphenhydramine (an antihistamine), *paracetamol (an analgesic and antipyretic), and *phenylephrine (a decongestant), used to relieve the symptoms of coughs and colds. It is available as tablets without a prescription, but only from pharmacies. It cannot be prescribed on the NHS.

Side effects, precautions, and interactions with other drugs: see CODEINE; ANTIHISTAMINES; PARACETAMOL; PHENYLEPHRINE; DECONGESTANTS.

Unihep (Leo Pharmaceuticals) *See* HEPARIN.

Uniparin Calcium, **Uniparin Forte** (CP Pharmaceuticals) *See* HEPARIN.

Uniphyllin Continus (Napp Pharmaceuticals) *See* THEOPHYLLINE.

Unipine XL (Ethical Generics) *See* NIFEDIPINE.

Uniroid-HC (Unigreg) A proprietary combination of *hydrocortisone (a corticosteroid) and *cinchocaine hydrochloride (a local anaesthetic), used to relieve the discomfort and pain of *haemorrhoids and itching of the anus. It is available as an ointment or suppositories on *prescription only.
Side effects: see CORTICOSTEROIDS.
Precautions: Uniroid should not be used when viral or fungal infection is present and should be used for longer than seven days. It is not recommended for children under 12 years old.

Unisept (Seton Scholl Healthcare) *See* CHLORHEXIDINE.

Univer (Rhône-Poulenc Rorer) *See* VERAPAMIL HYDROCHLORIDE.

Urdox (CP Pharmaceuticals) *See* URSODEOXYCHOLIC ACID.

urea A compound used alone or in combination with other drugs as a hydrating (moisturizing) agent in *emollient creams and lotions for treating dry skin conditions. It is also included in ear-drop preparations used for dissolving and washing out earwax (*see* UREA HYDROGEN PEROXIDE). Urea-containing preparations can be obtained without a prescription, but only from pharmacies.
Precautions: some people find the smell unpleasant. Urea may irritate sensitive skin.
Proprietary preparations: Aquadrate (cream); Eucerin (cream); Nutraplus (cream); ALPHADERM (combined with hydrocortisone); BALNEUM PLUS CREAM (combined with lauromacrogols); CALMURID (combined with lactic acid); CALMURID HC (combined with hydrocortisone and lactic acid).

urea hydrogen peroxide A combination of *urea and *hydrogen peroxide in equal amounts, which releases hydrogen peroxide locally on application. Its foaming action softens and facilitates the removal of earwax: it is therefore included in ear drops for this purpose. Urea hydrogen peroxide can be obtained without a prescription, but only from pharmacies.

Precautions: urea hydrogen peroxide may cause irritation; it should not be used on perforated eardrums.

Proprietary preparations: Otex; EXTEROL (combined with glycerin).

Uriben (Rosemont Pharmaceuticals) *See* NALIDIXIC ACID.

Uriflex (Seton Scholl Healthcare) *See* SODIUM CHLORIDE.

Uriflex C (Seton Scholl Healthcare) *See* CHLORHEXIDINE.

Uriflex G (Seton Scholl Healthcare) A proprietary combination of *citric acid, *magnesium oxide, *sodium bicarbonate, and *disodium edetate in the form of a solution, used for flushing catheters. It is available from pharmacies without a prescription.

Uriflex R (Seton Scholl Healthcare) A proprietary combination of *citric acid, *magnesium carbonate, *gluconolactone, and *disodium edetate in the form of a solution, used for flushing catheters. It is available from pharmacies without a prescription.

Urispas 200 (Shire Pharmaceuticals) *See* FLAVOXATE HYDROCHLORIDE.

urofollitrophin <urofollitropin> A preparation of follicle-stimulating hormone (a *gonadotrophin) used for the treatment of infertility in men and women that is due to underactivity of the pituitary gland (resulting in insufficient production of gonadotrophins). It is extracted from natural sources; a synthetic preparation (*see* FOLLITROPIN) is also available. Urofollitrophin is also used to induce superovulation (production of a large number of eggs) in women undergoing fertility treatment, such as *in vitro* fertilization. It is available as an injection on *prescription only.

Side effects: include ovarian hyperstimulation (the uncontrolled production of large numbers of follicles in the ovaries) and multiple pregnancy; allergic reactions may occur in both sexes.

Precautions: urofollitrophin should be used with caution in women with ovarian cysts and in people with thyroid or adrenal disorders or pituitary tumours.

Proprietary preparations: Metrodin High Purity; Orgafol.

urokinase A *fibrinolytic drug used for the treatment of *thrombosis in the blood vessels of the eye and to dissolve blood clots in the shunts used to connect patients to kidney dialysis equipment. It is also used to treat deep-vein thrombosis and pulmonary embolism. Urokinase is available in a form for injection on *prescription only.

Side effects, precautions, and interactions with other drugs: *see* FIBRINOLYTIC DRUGS.

Proprietary preparation: Ukidan.

Uromitexan (ASTA Medica) *See* MESNA.

Uro-Tainer Chlorhexidine (B. Braun (Medical)) *See* CHLORHEXIDINE.

Uro-Tainer Saline (B. Braun (Medical)) *See* SODIUM CHLORIDE.

Uro-Tainer Suby G (B. Braun (Medical)) A proprietary combination of *citric acid, magnesium oxide, sodium bicarbonate, and *disodium edetate in the form of a solution, used for flushing catheters in the bladder to keep them unblocked. It is available from pharmacies without a prescription.

ursodeoxycholic acid A *bile acid used in the treatment of gallstones or to prevent recurrence after they have dissolved. Ursodeoxycholic acid is suitable for people with mild symptoms who cannot be treated by other means. It is also used, with limited effect, to treat primary biliary cirrhosis (a disease affecting the liver and bile ducts). It is available as tablets or capsules on *prescription only.

Side effects: diarrhoea may occur, but this is rare.

Precautions: ursodeoxycholic acid should not be taken by women who are pregnant or planning to become pregnant, or by people with inflammatory bowel disease.

Interactions with other drugs:

Clofibrate: reduces the beneficial effect of ursodeoxycholic acid.

Oral contraceptives: oestrogens reduce the effect of ursodeoxycholic acid; women should use nonhormonal methods of contraception while undergoing treatment.

Proprietary preparations: Destolit; Urdox; Ursofalk; Ursogal.

Ursofalk (Cortecs Healthcare) *See* URSODEOXYCHOLIC ACID.

Ursogal (Galen) *See* URSODEOXYCHOLIC ACID.

Utinor (Merck Sharp & Dohme) *See* NORFLOXACIN.

Utovlan (Searle) *See* NORETHISTERONE.

Uvistat (Boehringen Ingelheim) A proprietary *sunscreen preparation that is available in a variety of forms. Uvistat cream, which contains ethylhexyl *p*-methoxycinnamate, avobenzone, and *titanium dioxide, offers protection against both UVA and UVB (SPF 22). Uvistat Ultrablock cream contains a higher proportion of *titanium dioxide and has an SPF of 30. A lotion, in which the cinnamate is replaced by methylbenzylidene camphor, has an SPF of 25. All these products can be prescribed on the NHS or obtained without a prescription.

Vagifem (Novo Nordisk Pharmaceutical) *See* OESTRADIOL <ESTRADIOL>; HORMONE REPLACEMENT THERAPY.

Vaginyl (DDSA Pharmaceuticals) *See* METRONIDAZOLE.

Vagisil Medicated Creme (Combe International) *See* LIGNOCAINE <LIDOCAINE>.

valaciclovir An *antiviral drug that is converted to *aciclovir in the body. It is used for the treatment of herpesvirus infections of the skin and mucous membranes, including shingles and genital herpes. Valaciclovir is available as tablets on *prescription only.
Side effects, precautions, and interactions with other drugs: see ACICLOVIR.
Proprietary preparation: Valtrex.

Valclair (Sinclair Pharmaceuticals) *See* DIAZEPAM.

Valium (Roche Products) *See* DIAZEPAM.

Vallergan (Rhône-Poulenc Rorer) *See* TRIMEPRAZINE <ALIMEMAZINE> TARTRATE.

Valoid (GlaxoWellcome) *See* CYCLIZINE.

valproic acid An *anticonvulsant drug used for the treatment of epilepsy. It is available as *enteric-coated capsules on *prescription only.
Side effects, precautions, and interactions with other drugs: see SODIUM VALPROATE.
Proprietary preparations: Convulex; EPILIM CHRONO (combined with sodium valproate).

valsartan An *angiotensin II inhibitor used in the treatment of *hypertension. It is available as tablets on *prescription only.
Side effects and precautions: see ANGIOTENSIN II INHIBITORS.
Interactions with other drugs: see ACE INHIBITORS.
Proprietary preparation: Diovan.
See also ANTIHYPERTENSIVE DRUGS.

Valtrex (GlaxoWellcome) *See* VALACICLOVIR.

Vancocin (Eli Lilly & Co) *See* VANCOMYCIN.

vancomycin An *antibiotic used for the prevention and treatment of endocarditis (infection of the heart membranes and valves) and for the treatment of other serious infections, including staphylococcal infections resistant to other antibiotics. It is not absorbed after oral administration and must therefore be given intravenously for systemic infections. Vancomycin is also used for the treatment of pseudomembranous colitis, an inflammation of the large bowel associated with severe diarrhoea that is caused by broad-spectrum antibiotics. For this it can be given orally, as capsules (as it does not need to be absorbed). Vancomycin is available on *prescription only.

Side effects: high concentrations of vancomycin in the blood can cause kidney damage and tinnitus (ringing in the ears; if this occurs treatment should be discontinued). Other side effects include blood disorders, nausea, chills, and fever; rashes and low blood pressure may occur if the drug is infused rapidly.

Precautions: rapid infusions should be avoided. Vancomycin should be used with caution in people who have impaired kidney function or who are deaf and in women who are pregnant or breastfeeding. Blood and urine tests are required to monitor kidney function.

Interactions with other drugs:

   Antibiotics: aminoglycosides and capreomycin increase the risk of ear and kidney damage.

   Loop diuretics: increase the risk of ear damage.

Proprietary preparation: Vancocin.

Varidase Topical (Wyeth Laboratories) A proprietary combination of *streptokinase and *streptodornase, which is applied to ulcers in order to liquefy blood clots and dead tissue so that these can be easily removed. It is also used to dissolve blood clots in the bladder and in urinary catheters. Varidase Topical is available, on *prescription only, as a powder to be dissolved in saline solution.

Side effects: allergic reactions and a burning sensation may occur, but this is rare.

Precautions: Varidase Topical should not be applied to bleeding ulcers.

Vascace (Roche Products) *See* CILAZAPRIL.

Vaseline Dermacare (Elida Gibbs) A proprietary combination of *dimethicone <dimeticone> and *white soft paraffin (both emollients), used to relieve the symptoms of *eczema and itching conditions associated with dry skin. It is freely available *over the counter in the form of a cream or lotion.

vasoconstriction Narrowing of the blood vessels, especially arteries and arterioles (small arteries). Constricted blood vessels can cause insufficient blood supply to the tissues and can contribute to high blood pressure (*hypertension).

vasoconstrictor drugs (vasoconstrictors) Drugs that cause narrowing of blood vessels, reduction in blood flow, and an increase in blood pressure. They are used to increase blood pressure in disorders of the circulation, in cases of shock, or when blood pressure has fallen in lengthy surgical procedures. Some vasoconstrictors are *sympathomimetic drugs and are used to relieve nasal congestion.

vasodilatation An increase in the diameter of blood vessels, especially the arteries and arterioles (small arteries), brought about by relaxation of the muscle forming the vessel wall.

vasodilators Drugs that cause widening of blood vessels (mainly small arteries) and therefore an increase in blood flow. Because blood pressure depends partly on the diameter of blood vessels, vasodilators are used to lower blood pressure in *hypertension. **Coronary vasodilators** increase the blood flow through the heart and are used to relieve or prevent *angina. **Peripheral vasodilators** affect the blood flow to the limbs and are used to treat conditions of poor circulation, such as acrocyanosis (purple-bluish discoloration of hands and feet due to slow circulation of blood in the skin), chilblains, and Raynaud's syndrome (poor circulation in hands and feet). Poor peripheral blood flow can also cause claudication (a cramp-like pain felt in the legs on walking or exercise). The main classes of vasodilator drugs are *alpha blockers, *nicotinic acid derivatives, *nitrates, class II *calcium antagonists, *potassium channel activators, and *ACE inhibitors. Potent vasodilators used in the treatment of severe hypertension include *diazoxide, *sodium nitroprusside, *minoxidil, and *hydralazine. The blood vessels are widened either by affecting the action of the muscles of the vessel walls (nitrates and calcium antagonists) or by interfering with nerve signals that govern the tone of the blood vessels (alpha blockers).
Side effects: flushing and headaches are common at the start of treatment. Dizziness and fainting can also occur as a result of lowered blood pressure. See also entries for individual classes of drugs.
Precautions: the major risk is that blood pressure may sometimes fall too low. See also entries for individual classes of drugs. *See also* ANTIHYPERTENSIVE DRUGS.

Vasogen Cream (Pharmax) A proprietary combination of *zinc oxide (an astringent protective agent), *calamine (a mild astringent), and *dimethicone <dimeticone> (a water repellent), used as a *barrier preparation for the prevention and treatment of bedsores and napkin rash and for the protection of the skin around a *stoma after an ileostomy or colostomy. It is freely available *over the counter.

vasopressin (antidiuretic hormone) A hormone, secreted by the pituitary gland, that decreases the excretion of water from the kidneys and also constricts blood vessels. A lack of vasopressin results in **diabetes insipidus**, a condition in which the patient passes large amounts of urine and is always thirsty. Vasopressin is used to treat diabetes insipidus and to stop the bleeding from varicose veins in the oesophagus, which can in serious cases be life-threatening. It is given by subcutaneous or intramuscular injection and is available on *prescription only.

Synthetic analogues of vasopressin include *terlipressin and *desmopressin.

Side effects: include pallor, nausea, belching, abdominal cramps, an urge to defecate, and headache; allergic reactions (such as rash) may rarely occur, and vasopressin may cause constriction of coronary vessels, resulting in angina.

Precautions: vasopressin should not be given to people with vascular disease or chronic kidney disease; it should be used with caution in those with asthma, epilepsy, migraine, or poor kidney function and in pregnant women.

Interactions with other drugs:

Carbamazepine: may increase the effect of vasopressin.

Chlorpropamide: may increase the effect of vasopressin.

Clofibrate: may increase the effect of vasopressin.

Proprietary preparation: Pitressin.

Vasoxine (GlaxoWellcome) *See* METHOXAMINE HYDROCHLORIDE.

Vectavir (SmithKline Beecham Pharmaceuticals) *See* PENCICLOVIR.

Veganin (Warner-Lambert Consumer Healthcare) A proprietary combination of *aspirin and *paracetamol (analgesics and antipyretics) and *codeine (an opioid analgesic), used to treat the symptoms of influenza and to relieve mild to moderate pain, such as headache, period pains, rheumatic pains, and toothache. It is available as tablets and can be obtained without a prescription, but only from pharmacies.

Side effects and precautions: *see* ASPIRIN; PARACETAMOL; CODEINE.

Interactions with other drugs: *see* ASPIRIN; OPIOIDS.

vehicle Any substance that acts as the medium in which a drug is administered. Examples are sterile water, isotonic sodium chloride, and dextrose solutions.

Velbe (Eli Lilly & Co) *See* VINBLASTINE SULPHATE.

Velosef (Bristol-Myers Squibb) *See* CEPHRADINE <CEFRADINE>.

venlafaxine An *antidepressant drug that is related to the *SSRI group; it inhibits the reuptake of *serotonin and *noradrenaline <norepinephrine>. It is used for the treatment of depressive illness and may be more effective for treating resistant depression than the SSRIs. Venlafaxine is available as tablets or modified-release capsules on *prescription only.

Side effects: include nausea, constipation, headache, insomnia, drowsiness, dizziness, weakness, sweating, and nervousness; if convulsions occur, treatment should be stopped. At the end of treatment, dosage should be reduced gradually.

Precautions: venlafaxine should not be taken by people with a history of heart disease, by those with severely impaired liver or kidney function, or by women who are pregnant or breastfeeding. Driving ability may be impaired. If an allergic rash develops, a doctor should be informed.

Interactions with other drugs:

  MAOIs: venlafaxine should not be taken with MAOIs and should not be started until two weeks after stopping MAOIs; MAOIs should not be started until at least a week after stopping venlafaxine.

Proprietary preparations: Efexor (tablets); Efexor XL (capsules).

Venofer (Syner-Med) *See* FERRIC HYDROXIDE SUCROSE.

Ventide (Allen & Hanburys) A proprietary combination of *salbutamol (a bronchodilator) and *beclomethasone <beclometasone> dipropionate (a corticosteroid) used for the long-term management of asthma and to treat chronic bronchitis. It is available, on *prescription only, as a metered-dose aerosol or as a powder for inhalation.

Side effects, precautions, and interactions with other drugs: see SALBUTAMOL; BECLOMETHASONE <BECLOMETASONE> DIPROPIONATE.

ventilator A piece of equipment that is mechanically operated to maintain a flow of air into and out of the lungs of a patient who is unable to breathe normally.

Ventodisks (Allen & Hanburys) *See* SALBUTAMOL.

Ventolin, Ventolin Accuhaler, Ventolin Easi-Breathe, Ventolin Evohaler, Ventolin Nebules, Ventolin Rotacaps (Allen & Hanburys) *See* SALBUTAMOL.

ventricular tachycardia *See* ARRHYTHMIA.

Vepesid (Bristol-Myers Squibb) *See* ETOPOSIDE.

Veracur (Typharm) *See* FORMALDEHYDE.

verapamil hydrochloride A class I *calcium antagonist used for the treatment of mild to moderate *hypertension, *angina, and supraventricular tachycardia (*see* ARRHYTHMIA). It is available as short-acting or *modified-release tablets on *prescription only.

Side effects: constipation is the most common side effect. *See also* CALCIUM ANTAGONISTS.

Precautions: verapamil should not be taken by people with low blood pressure, a slow heart rate, a history of heart failure, or certain other heart conditions. *See also* CALCIUM ANTAGONISTS; ANTIHYPERTENSIVE DRUGS.

Interactions with other drugs:

Anaesthetics: verapamil increases the effect of general anaesthetics in lowering blood pressure.

Anti-arrhythmic drugs: verapamil increases the risk of amiodarone slowing the heart rate and having other adverse effects on the heart; the risk of the heart ceasing to beat is increased if verapamil is taken with disopyramide or flecainide; verapamil increases the plasma concentration of quinidine, which may result in a severe fall in blood pressure.

Antiepileptic drugs: verapamil enhances the effects of carbamazepine; the effects of verapamil are reduced by phenytoin and phenobarbitone <phenobarbital>.

Beta blockers: verapamil should not be taken with beta blockers as this combination increases the risk of a severe fall in blood pressure, leading to heart failure.

Cyclosporin: its plasma concentration is increased by verapamil.

Digoxin: its plasma concentration is increased by verapamil; bradycardia (slowing of heart rate) is increased.

Rifampicin: reduces the effects of verapamil.

Theophylline: its effects are enhanced by verapamil.

 See also CALCIUM ANTAGONISTS.

Proprietary preparations: Berkatens; Ethimil MR (modified-release tablets); Univer (modified-release capsules); Cordilox; Half Securon SR (modified-release tablets); Securon; Securon SR (modified-release tablets); Verapress MR (modified-release tablets); TARKA (combined with trandolapril).

Verapress MR (Dexcel Pharma) *See* VERAPAMIL HYDROCHLORIDE.

Veripaque (Sanofi Winthrop) *See* OXYPHENISATIN <OXYPHENISATINE>.

Vermox (Janssen-Cilag) *See* MEBENDAZOLE.

Verruca Removal Gel (Seton Scholl Healthcare) *See* SALICYLIC ACID.

Verrugon (J. Pickles & Sons) *See* SALICYLIC ACID.

Vesanoid (Roche Products) *See* TRETINOIN.

Viagra (Pfizer) *See* SILDENAFIL.

Viazem XL (Du Pont Pharmaceuticals) *See* DILTIAZEM HYDROCHLORIDE.

Vibramycin, **Vibramycin-D** (Pfizer) *See* DOXYCYCLINE.

Vicks Action (Procter & Gamble) A proprietary combination of *ibuprofen (an NSAID) and *pseudoephedrine (a decongestant), used to relieve the symptoms of colds and influenza, including nasal congestion, aches and pains, headache, fever, and sore throat. It is available as tablets and can be obtained without a prescription, but only from pharmacies.

Side effects and interactions with other drugs: see NSAIDS; DECONGESTANTS; EPHEDRINE HYDROCHLORIDE.

Precautions: this medicine should not be given to children. *See also* NSAIDS; EPHEDRINE HYDROCHLORIDE.

Vicks Coldcare (Procter & Gamble) A proprietary combination of *paracetamol (an analgesic and antipyretic), *phenylpropanolamine (a decongestant), and *dextromethorphan (a cough suppressant), used to relieve the symptoms of colds and influenza. It is freely available *over the counter in the form of capsules.

Side effects: see EPHEDRINE HYDROCHLORIDE; DEXTROMETHORPHAN.

Precautions: see PARACETAMOL; EPHEDRINE HYDROCHLORIDE; OPIOIDS.

Interactions with other drugs: see PHENYLPROPANOLAMINE; EPHEDRINE HYDROCHLORIDE; OPIOIDS.

Vicks Inhaler (Procter & Gamble) A proprietary combination of *menthol and *camphor, used to relieve nasal congestion. It is freely available *over the counter in the form of a stick; this is inserted into the nostril, and the vapour is inhaled.

Vicks Medinite (Procter & Gamble) A proprietary combination of *dextromethorphan (a cough suppressant), *pseudoephedrine (a decongestant), *doxylamine (an antihistamine), and *paracetamol (an analgesic and antipyretic), used to relieve the symptoms of colds and influenza, including nasal congestion, irritating coughs, headache, fever, and aches and pains. It is available as a syrup and can be obtained without a prescription, but only from pharmacies.

Side effects: see DEXTROMETHORPHAN; EPHEDRINE HYDROCHLORIDE; DECONGESTANTS; ANTIHISTAMINES.

Precautions: this syrup should not be taken by children under 10 years old. *See also* OPIOIDS; DECONGESTANTS; ANTIHISTAMINES; PARACETAMOL.

Interactions with other drugs: see OPIOIDS; EPHEDRINE HYDROCHLORIDE; ANTIHISTAMINES.

Vicks Sinex (Procter & Gamble) A proprietary combination of *oxymetazoline (a sympathomimetic drug), *menthol, and eucalyptol (*see* EUCALYPTUS OIL), used as a nasal *decongestant to relieve the congestion associated with colds, hay fever, and sinusitis. It is freely available freely *over the counter in the form of a nasal spray.

Side effects, precautions, and interactions with other drugs: see DECONGESTANTS.

Vicks Ultra Chloraseptic (Procter & Gamble) *See* BENZOCAINE.

Vicks Vaporub (Procter & Gamble) A proprietary combination of *menthol, *camphor, *eucalyptus oil, and *turpentine oil, used to relieve nasal and catarrhal congestion associated with colds. It can be rubbed on the chest or back or added to hot water and used as an inhalation. Vicks Vaporub is freely available *over the counter.

Side effects and precautions: see RUBEFACIENTS.

Vicks Vaposyrup Chesty Cough (Procter & Gamble) *See* GUAIPHENESIN <GUAIFENESIN>.

Vicks Vaposyrup Dry Cough, Vicks Vaposyrup Children's Dry Cough (Procter & Gamble) *See* DEXTROMETHORPHAN.

Vicks Vaposyrup for Tickly Coughs (Procter & Gamble) *See* MENTHOL.

Videx (Bristol-Myers Squibb) *See* DIDANOSINE.

Vidopen (APS-Berk) *See* AMPICILLIN.

vigabatrin An *anticonvulsant drug used for the treatment of epilepsy that has not been controlled by other anticonvulsants. It is available, on *prescription only, for oral use as tablets or a powder to be made into a solution.

Side effects: include drowsiness, fatigue, dizziness, nervousness, irritability, agitation, depression, headache, and impaired concentration. Less commonly, confusion, aggression, memory disturbance, and disturbances of vision (including loss of visual field) may occur.

Precautions: vigabatrin should be used with caution in people who have liver or kidney disease. Visual-field tests should be performed before and during treatment, and patients should report any new visual symptoms to a doctor. Women who are planning to become pregnant, or who are already pregnant, should seek specialist advice. Vigabritin is not recommended for women who are breastfeeding. Dosage should be reduced gradually at the end of treatment.

Interactions with other drugs:

  Anticonvulsants: taking two or more anticonvulsants together may increase their adverse effects.

Proprietary preparation: Sabril.

Vigam (Bio Products Laboratory) *See* IMMUNOGLOBULINS.

Vigranon B (Wallace Manufacturing) A proprietary combination of *nicotinamide (a B vitamin), *riboflavine (vitamin B_2), *pyridoxine hydrochloride (vitamin B_6), *thiamine hydrochloride (vitamin B_1), and pantothenol (a B vitamin), used to prevent vitamin B deficiency (*see* VITAMIN B COMPLEX). It is available as tablets and can be bought without a prescription, but only from pharmacies.

viloxazine hydrochloride An *antidepressant drug, related to the *tricyclic antidepressants, used for the treatment of depressive illness, especially when sedation is not desirable. It is available as tablets on *prescription only.

Side effects: similar to those of *amitriptyline hydrochloride, but viloxazine is less sedating, has fewer and milder antimuscarinic effects (dry mouth, blurred vision, problems in urinating), and is less likely to cause palpitation and a fast heart rate.

Precautions: see TRICYCLIC ANTIDEPRESSANTS.

Interactions with other drugs: see TRICYCLIC ANTIDEPRESSANTS. In addition, viloxazine can increase the plasma concentrations of carbamazepine, phenytoin, and theophylline.

Proprietary preparation: Vivalan.

vinblastine sulphate A *vinca alkaloid used for the treatment of acute leukaemias, lymphomas, and some solid tumours (see CANCER). It is available as an injection on *prescription only.

Side effects and precautions: see VINCA ALKALOIDS; CYTOTOXIC DRUGS.

Proprietary preparation: Velbe.

vinca alkaloids A class of *cytotoxic drugs originally extracted from the periwinkle plant (*Catharanthus roseus*; formerly called *Vinca rosea*). They are used to treat acute lymphomas, acute leukaemias, and some solid tumours, such as breast and lung cancer (see CANCER). The commonly used vinca alkaloids are *vinblastine sulphate, *vincristine sulphate, *vindesine sulphate, and *vinorelbine. They are usually given by intravenous injection or infusion and are available on *prescription only. *See also* ETOPOSIDE.

Side effects: vinca alkaloids commonly cause reversible peripheral neurological side effects, which include tingling of the fingers or toes, abdominal pain, constipation, and muscle weakness. Other side effects include *bone marrow suppression and reversible hair loss. There may also be pain and irritation at the injection site. *See also* CYTOTOXIC DRUGS.

Precautions: vinca alkaloids should not be given to women who are pregnant or breastfeeding. The dosage may need to be reduced for people with liver disease. Any signs of fever, sore throat, or infection should be reported to a doctor. *See also* CYTOTOXIC DRUGS.

vincristine sulphate A *vinca alkaloid used for the treatment of acute leukaemias, lymphomas, and some solid tumours (see CANCER). It is available as a solution for injection on *prescription only.

Side effects and precautions: see VINCA ALKALOIDS; CYTOTOXIC DRUGS.

Interactions with other drugs:

Itraconazole: may increase the risk of neurological side effects of vincristine.

Proprietary preparation: Oncovin.

vindesine sulphate A *vinca alkaloid used for the treatment of acute leukaemias, lymphomas, and some solid tumours (*see* CANCER). It is available as an injection on *prescription only.

Side effects and precautions: see VINCA ALKALOIDS; CYTOTOXIC DRUGS.
Proprietary preparation: Eldisine.

vinorelbine A semisynthetic *vinca alkaloid used for the treatment of some forms of lung cancer and also for advanced breast cancer when treatment with anthracyclines (*cytotoxic antibiotics) has failed. It is available as an injection on *prescription only.

Side effects and precautions: see VINCA ALKALOIDS; CYTOTOXIC DRUGS.
Proprietary preparation: Navelbine.

Vioform-Hydrocortisone (Novartis Consumer Health) A proprietary combination of *clioquinol (an antifungal drug) and *hydrocortisone (a corticosteroid), used for the treatment of infected inflammatory skin conditions and itching of the anal and genital regions. It is available as a cream or ointment on *prescription only.

Side effects and precautions: see TOPICAL STEROIDS; CLIOQUINOL.

Viracept (Roche Products) *See* NELFINAVIR.

Viraferon (Schering-Plough) *See* INTERFERON-ALFA.

Viramune (Boehringer Ingelheim) *See* NEVIRAPINE.

Virasorb (Seton Scholl Healthcare) *See* ACICLOVIR.

Virazid (ICN Pharmaceuticals) *See* TRIBAVIRIN.

Viridal (Schwartz Pharma) *See* ALPROSTADIL.

Virormone (Ferring Pharmaceuticals) *See* TESTOSTERONE.

Virovir (Opus) *See* ACICLOVIR.

Visclair (Sinclair Pharmaceuticals) *See* METHYLCYSTEINE HYDROCHLORIDE.

Viscotears (CIBA Vision Ophthalmics) *See* CARBOMER.

Viskaldix (Novartis Pharmaceuticals) A proprietary combination of *pindolol (a non-cardioselective beta blocker) and clopamide (a *thiazide diuretic), used in the treatment of mild to moderate *hypertension. It is available as tablets on *prescription only.

Side effects, precautions, and interactions with other drugs: see BETA BLOCKERS; THIAZIDE DIURETICS.
See also ANTIHYPERTENSIVE DRUGS; DIURETICS.

Visken (Novartis Pharmaceuticals) *See* PINDOLOL.

Vista-Methasone (Martindale Pharmaceuticals) *See* BETAMETHASONE.

Vista-Methasone N (Martindale Pharmaceuticals) A proprietary combination of *betamethasone (a corticosteroid) and *neomycin sulphate (an antibiotic), used for the treatment of infected inflammatory conditions of the eyes. It is available as eye drops on *prescription only.
Side effects: include increased pressure in the eye, thinning of the cornea, and cataracts.
Precautions: see TOPICAL STEROIDS; NEOMYCIN SULPHATE. In addition, soft contact lenses should not be worn during treatment.

Vistide (Pharmacia & Upjohn) *See* CIDOFOVIR.

vitamin Any of a group of substances that are required, in very small amounts, for healthy growth and development: they cannot be synthesized by the body and are therefore essential constituents of the diet. Vitamins are divided into two groups, according to whether they are soluble in water or fat. The water-soluble group includes the vitamin B complex and vitamin C; the fat-soluble vitamins are vitamins A, D, E, and K. Lack of sufficient quantities of any of the vitamins in the diet results in specific vitamin deficiency diseases.
   Vitamin supplements are readily available for treating and preventing vitamin deficiencies.

vitamin A (retinol) A fat-soluble vitamin that is necessary for healthy vision, particularly vision in dim light. It is also essential for growth and the integrity of mucous tissue (in the mouth, eyes, nose, and genitals). Vitamin A deficiency causes stunted growth, night blindness, and drying and thickening of the cornea, which can progress eventually to blindness. The vitamin occurs in foods of animal origin, especially milk products, egg yolk, and liver, and it can be formed in the body from beta-carotene, a pigment found in vegetables, especially carrots, cabbage, and lettuce. Deficiency is rare in the UK.
   Supplements of vitamin A are given usually in combination with *vitamin D as tablets or capsules of fish oils (*see* HALIBUT-LIVER OIL) for adults and children; these are freely available *over the counter. Vitamin A is also available as an injection (as **vitamin A palmitate**) on *prescription only for the treatment of acute deficiency states.
Side effects: none reported in low doses, but vitamin A is one of the few vitamins that can be toxic in overdose, causing rough dry skin, dry hair, and an enlarged liver.
Precautions: there is evidence suggesting that vitamin A may cause birth defects, therefore women who are pregnant or planning to become pregnant should not take vitamin A supplements (unless advised to by a doctor) or eat large amounts of liver products, such as paté.
Interactions with other drugs:
   Retinoids: the risk of vitamin A poisoning is increased if isotretinoin or acetretin are taken with vitamin A supplements.

Proprietary preparations: HALYCITROL (combined with vitamin D); MINADEX (combined with vitamins C and D); MOTHERS' AND CHILDREN'S VITAMIN DROPS (combined with vitamins C and D).

vitamin B₁ *See* THIAMINE; VITAMIN B COMPLEX.

vitamin B₂ *See* RIBOFLAVINE; VITAMIN B COMPLEX.

vitamin B₆ *See* PYRIDOXINE; VITAMIN B COMPLEX.

vitamin B₁₂ *See* VITAMIN B COMPLEX.

vitamin B complex A group of water-soluble vitamins that, although not chemically related, are often found together in the same kinds of food (including milk, liver, and cereals).

Vitamin B₁ (*see* THIAMINE) is required for carbohydrate metabolism; a deficiency leads to beriberi. **Vitamin B₂** (*see* RIBOFLAVINE) is important for oxygen exchange in the tissues. **Vitamin B₆** (*see* PYRIDOXINE) is involved in protein metabolism. **Vitamin B₁₂** (*see* CYANOCOBALAMIN; HYDROXOCOBALAMIN) is necessary for the synthesis of nucleic acids (DNA and RNA), the maintenance of myelin (an important component of certain nerve cells), and the proper functioning of *folic acid. B₁₂ can be absorbed only in the presence of **intrinsic factor**, a protein secreted in the stomach. A deficiency of vitamin B₁₂ affects nearly all the body tissues, particularly those containing rapidly dividing cells. The most serious effects of a deficiency are pernicious *anaemia (due to deficiency of intrinsic factor) and degeneration of the nervous system. Vitamin B₁₂ is contained only in foods of animal origin. Other members of the B complex include *nicotinamide, *aminobenzoic acid, **pantothenic acid**, **panthenol**, **inositol**, and **biotin**.

B group vitamins are used to treat specific diseases due to deficiencies of these vitamins and also to prevent deficiency in people considered to be at risk (e.g. pregnant women). They are available as specific vitamin supplements and are also included in numerous multivitamin preparations; many *iron supplements also contain B group vitamins.

Proprietary preparations: Vigranon B (syrup); ABIDEC (combined with vitamins A, C, and D); DALIVIT (combined with vitamins A, C, and D); PABRINEX (combined with vitamin C).

vitamin C (ascorbic acid) A water-soluble vitamin that is essential for maintaining healthy connective tissues and the integrity of cell membranes: it is necessary for the synthesis of collagen, which is required to produce connective tissue. Vitamin C has antioxidant properties, i.e. it neutralizes oxygen free radicals, which are produced by various disease processes and toxic substances and have damaging effects on the body. Vitamin C occurs in fruits and vegetables, especially citrus fruits. Elderly people may suffer mild vitamin C deficiency, which leads to an increased susceptibility to infection. Severe vitamin C deficiency causes scurvy. There have been claims that large doses of vitamin C help to prevent colds and influenza, and consequently vitamin C is often included in cold preparations, but these claims are unproven. Vitamin C is freely available *over the counter as tablets or effervescent tablets; these cannot be prescribed on the NHS. It is also included as an ingredient in numerous multivitamin preparations.

Proprietary preparations: Redoxon; PABRINEX (combined with B group vitamins); plus many other proprietory preparations.

vitamin D A fat-soluble *vitamin that promotes the absorption of *calcium and phosphorus from the intestine and their deposition in bone. It occurs in the form of a group of closely related steroid-based compounds, including **vitamin D₂** (*ergocalciferol), manufactured from ergosterol by plants when exposed to ultraviolet light, and **vitamin D₃** (*cholecalciferol <colecalciferol>), which is formed from a derivative of cholesterol by the action of sunlight on the skin. Deficiency of vitamin D interferes with the absorption of calcium from the intestine, causing rickets in children and osteomalacia (softening of the bones) in adults. Vitamin D supplements may be required by people who do not get enough sunlight (for example, the housebound elderly and members of certain ethnic groups or cultures who always keep their skin covered) and menopausal women. People who have kidney disease, especially those on dialysis, may also need vitamin D therapy to avoid bone disease.

Simple vitamin D deficiency is treated with oral supplements of ergocalciferol or cholecalciferol <colecalciferol>. Deficiency caused by poor absorption of calcium from the intestines or chronic liver disease is treated with *calciferol tablets. People with kidney disease or poorly functioning parathyroid glands (which produce *parathyroid hormone) are treated with *alfacalcidol, *calcitriol, or *dihydrotachysterol. Since vitamin D promotes absorption of calcium from food, care must be taken to ensure that not too much calcium is absorbed, which may cause adverse effects (see below); blood tests may be necessary. *See also* CALCIPOTRIOL.

Side effects: these are most commonly related to increased concentrations of calcium in the blood, caused by overdosage of vitamin D. Symptoms of overdosage include loss of appetite, tiredness, nausea, vomiting, stomach pains, thirst, headache, dizziness, and excessive urination.

Precautions: vitamin D preparations should not be taken by people with high plasma concentrations of calcium or calcification due to malignant disease. Plasma calcium may need to be monitored during treatment. Vitamin D should be used with caution during pregnancy and breastfeeding.

Interactions with other drugs:

  Antiepileptic drugs: carbamazepine, phenobarbitone <phenobarbital>, phenytoin, and primidone reduce the effects of vitamin D: increased dosage of vitamin D may be required.

  Thiazide diuretics: increase the risk of absorbing too much calcium.

Proprietary preparations: ABIDEC (combined with vitamins A, B, and C);

DALIVIT (combined with vitamins A, B, and C); HALYCITROL (combined with vitamin A).

vitamin E (tocopherols) A group of fat-soluble vitamins that stabilize cell membranes by protecting them from the damaging effects of oxygen free radicals, which are produced by various disease processes and toxic substances, i.e. they have antioxidant effects. The most important member of the vitamin E group is **alpha-tocopherol**, which is found in vegetable oils, eggs, butter, and wholemeal cereals. There is evidence to suggest that it may reduce the risk of a heart attack in susceptible individuals. It is available, as **alpha tocopheryl acetate**, in the form of a suspension or tablets that can be obtained without a prescription, but only from pharmacies.

Side effects: there may be diarrhoea and abdominal pain with higher dosages.

Proprietary preparations: Ephynal; FORCEVAL (combined with other vitamins); KETOVITE (combined with other vitamins).

vitamin K A fat-soluble vitamin that is necessary for the production of factors (including prothrombin) that are essential for blood clotting. Because vitamin K dissolves in fat, people who do not absorb fat properly also do not absorb vitamin K and become deficient in the vitamin. In such people vitamin K can be replaced orally by a soluble synthetic form, *menadiol sodium phosphate. An injectable form of the vitamin, *phytomenadione, is given to premature newborn babies to protect against haemorrhage and to people taking anticoagulant therapy to counteract the effects of an overdosage of *warfarin sodium.

Vitamin Tablets (with Calcium and Iodine) for Nursing Mothers (Sussex) A proprietary combination of ascorbic acid (*see* VITAMIN C), *vitamin A, *ergocalciferol (vitamin D_2), calcium hydrogen phosphate (a *calcium supplement), and potassium iodide (a source of *iodine), used as a vitamin and mineral supplement for women who are breastfeeding. It is available without a prescription.

Side effects and interactions with other drugs: see VITAMIN A.

Precautions: these tablets are not recommended for women who are pregnant or likely to become pregnant unless a doctor advises otherwise.

Vivalan (AstraZeneca) *See* VILOXAZINE HYDROCHLORIDE.

Vivapryl (ASTA Medica) *See* SELEGILINE.

Vividrin (Pharma-Global) *See* SODIUM CROMOGLYCATE <CROMOGLICATE>.

Volmax (Allen & Hanburys) *See* SALBUTAMOL.

Volraman (Eastern Pharmaceuticals) *See* DICLOFENAC SODIUM.

Volsaid Retard (Trinity Pharmaceuticals) *See* DICLOFENAC SODIUM.

Voltarol, **Voltarol Emulgel**, **Voltarol 75 mg SR**, **Voltarol Retard**
(Novartis Pharmaceuticals) *See* DICLOFENAC SODIUM.

Voltarol Ophtha (CIBA Vision Ophthalmics) *See* DICLOFENAC SODIUM.

warfarin sodium An oral *anticoagulant used for the prevention and treatment of deep-vein *thrombosis and pulmonary embolism and for the prevention of embolism in people with atrial fibrillation (*see* ARRHYTHMIA) and in those who have an artificial heart valve or a cardiac aneurysm (a weakness in the wall of a coronary artery). Warfarin is available as tablets on *prescription only.

Side effects: excessive bleeding is the most serious side effect (*see* ANTICOAGULANTS); if this occurs, immediate medical advice should be sought and *phytomenadione may need to be given. Other side effects include allergic reactions and rashes.

Precautions: patients are required to have regular blood tests to ensure that they are on a suitable dose of warfarin. Warfarin should not be used during the first three months or the last three months of pregnancy or by women who are trying to become pregnant, unless the patient's condition makes this unavoidable. It should also be avoided in people with peptic ulcer and used with caution in people with kidney or liver disease. Excessive consumption of alcohol increases the anticoagulant effects of warfarin, and radical changes in diet can affect the anticoagulant effect of warfarin.

Interactions with other drugs: warfarin interacts with many other drugs, the most important of which are listed below. If warfarin and the interacting drug are both taken regularly, the dosage of warfarin will need to be adjusted to take this into account. Short courses of interacting drugs may also affect the dose of warfarin needed.

Acitretin: may reduce the anticoagulant effect of warfarin.

Aminoglutethimide: reduces the anticoagulant effect of warfarin.

Anabolic steroids: enhance the anticoagulant effect of warfarin.

Analgesics: co-proxamol and paracetamol may enhance the anticoagulant effect of warfarin.

Anti-arrhythmic drugs: amiodarone and propafenone enhance the anticoagulant effect of warfarin.

Antibiotics: the anticoagulant effect of warfarin is enhanced by cephamandole <cefamandole>, chloramphenicol, ciprofloxacillin, co-trimoxazole, erythromycin, metronidazole, oxfloxacin, and possibly by certain other antibiotics. Rifampicin reduces the anticoagulant effect of warfarin.

Antiepileptic drugs: carbamazepine, phenobarbitone <phenobarbitol>, and primidone reduce the anticoagulant effect of warfarin; valproate enhances its anticoagulant effect. Phenytoin may either reduce or enhance the anticoagulant effect of warfarin.

Antifungal drugs: griseofulvin reduces the anticoagulant effect of warfarin; fluconazole, itraconazole, ketoconazole, and miconazole enhance its anticoagulant effect.

Aspirin: increases the risk of excessive bleeding.

Cholestyramine <colestyramine>: may enhance or reduce the anticoagulant effect of warfarin.

Corticosteroids: may alter the anticoagulant effect of warfarin.

Danazol: increases the anticoagulant effect of warfarin.

Disulfiram: enhances the anticoagulant effect of warfarin.

Flutamide: increases the anticoagulant effect of warfarin.

Ifosfamide: may enhance the anticoagulant effect of warfarin.

Lipid-lowering drugs: clofibrate and simvastatin enhance the anticoagulant effect of warfarin.

NSAIDs: the anticoagulant effect of warfarin is seriously enhanced by azapropazone and phenylbutazone. Diclofenac, difusinal, flurbiprofen, mefenamic acid, meloxicam, piroxicam, and sulindac can cause peptic ulcers, giving a site for possibly severe bleeding if these drugs are used with warfarin.

Oral contraceptives: reduce the anticoagulant effect of warfarin.

Proguanil: may enhance the anticoagulant effect of warfarin.

Ritonavir: may enhance the anticoagulant effect of warfarin.

SSRIs: these antidepressants may increase the anticoagulant effect of warfarin.

Sulphinpyrazone <sulfinpyrazone>: enhances the anticoagulant effect of warfarin.

Tamoxifen: increases the anticoagulant effect of warfarin.

Testosterone: enhances the anticoagulant effect of warfarin.

Thyroxine: enhances the anticoagulant effect of warfarin.

Ulcer-healing drugs: cimetidine and omeprazole enhance the anticoagulant effect of warfarin.

Vitamin K: reduces the anticoagulant effect of warfarin.

Proprietary preparation: Marevan.

Warticon (Perstorp Pharma) *See* PODOPHYLLOTOXIN.

Wasp-Eze Ointment (Seton Scholl Healthcare) *See* ANTAZOLINE.

Wasp-Eze Spray (Seton Scholl Healthcare) A proprietary combination of *mepyramine maleate (an antihistamine) and *benzocaine (a local anaesthetic), used for the relief of insect stings. It is available from pharmacies without a prescription.

Side effects: the spray may occasionally cause allergic reactions.

Precautions: the spray should not be applied to the eyes, mouth, or other mucous membranes or to broken skin.

Waxsol (Norgine) *See* DOCUSATE SODIUM.

Welldorm (Smith & Nephew Healthcare) *See* CHLORAL BETAINE <CLORAL BETAINE>.

Welldorm Elixir (Smith & Nephew Healthcare) *See* CHLORAL HYDRATE.

Wellferon (GlaxoWellcome) *See* INTERFERON-ALFA.

Wellvone (GlaxoWellcome) *See* ATOVAQUONE.

white soft paraffin (white petroleum jelly) A purified mixture of hydrocarbons obtained from petroleum. A bleached version of *yellow soft paraffin, it is used as an *emollient and as a base for ointments. It is odourless when rubbed into the skin and not readily absorbed.
Side effects: very rarely it may cause allergic reactions or acne.
Proprietary preparations: DIPROBASE (combined with liquid paraffin); E45 CREAM (combined with lanolin and liquid paraffin); GERMOLENE OINTMENT (combined with zinc oxide, octaphonium <octafonium> chloride, methyl salicylate, and other emollients); HEWLETTS CREAM (combined with zinc oxide); LACRI-LUBE (combined with liquid paraffin and wool fat); LIPOBASE (combined with liquid paraffin); LUBRI-TEARS (combined with liquid paraffin and wool fat); ULTRABASE (combined with liquid paraffin and stearyl alcohol); UNGUENTUM M (combined with silicic acid, liquid paraffin, and other emollients); VASELINE DERMACARE (combined with dimethicone <dimeticone>).

Windcheaters (Seton Scholl Healthcare) *See* DIMETHICONE <DIMETICONE>.

witch hazel *See* HAMAMELIS.

withdrawal symptoms *See* DEPENDENCE.

Woodward's Baby Chest Rub (Seton Scholl Healthcare) A proprietary combination of *turpentine oil, *eucalyptus oil, and *menthol in the form of an ointment that is rubbed onto the chests of infants for the relief of nasal catarrh and congestion due to colds. It is freely available *over the counter.

Woodward's Colic Drops (Seton Scholl Healthcare) *See* DIMETHICONE <DIMETICONE>.

Woodward's Gripe Water (Seton Scholl Healthcare) A proprietary combination of *sodium bicarbonate and *dill seed oil, used for the relief of wind pain in babies and children over one month old. It is freely available *over the counter.

Woodward's Teething Gel (Seton Scholl Healthcare) A proprietary combination of *cetylpyridinium chloride (an antiseptic) and *lignocaine <lidocaine> hydrochloride (a local anaesthetic), used for the relief of pain associated with teething problems. It is freely available *over the counter.

Precautions: this medicine is not recommended for babies under three months old.

wool fat *See* LANOLIN.

Xalatan (Pharmacia & Upjohn) *See* LATANOPROST.

xamoterol A beta-adrenoceptor stimulant (*see* SYMPATHOMIMETIC DRUGS) that was designed for the treatment of chronic mild heart failure. Its use has declined since it has been shown to worsen heart failure in some cases. It is available as tablets on *prescription only.

Side effects: include gastrointestinal upset, headache, dizziness, and cramps.

Precautions: xamoterol should not be taken by people who are taking high doses of *frusemide <furosemide> or *ACE inhibitors or by those with severe heart failure.

Proprietary preparation: Corwin.

Xanax (Pharmacia & Upjohn) *See* ALPRAZOLAM.

xanthines A group of nitrogen-containing compounds found widely in nature. Natural xanthines include caffeine and theobromine, which are consumed in tea and coffee. Xanthine drugs relax smooth muscle, especially in the airways (*see* BRONCHODILATORS), and are therefore used primarily in the treatment of *asthma (*see also* PHOSPHODIESTERASE INHIBITORS). *Modified-release formulations are particularly useful for the prevention of nocturnal asthma attacks. *See* AMINOPHYLLINE; THEOPHYLLINE; OXPENTIFYLLINE <PENTOXIFYLLINE>.

Side effects: up to one-third of children experience gastrointestinal disturbances, sleep disruption, and/or psychological changes. Adults experience gastrointestinal upset, nausea, headaches, vertigo, and flushes.

Precautions: smoking and alcohol shorten the duration of action of xanthines and higher doses may be necessary in smokers. The duration of action is increased in heart failure, cirrhosis of the liver, and viral infections and by certain drugs.

Interactions with other drugs:

Aminoglutethimide: reduces plasma concentration of xanthines.

Antibiotics: ciprofloxacin, clarithromycin, erythromycin, and norfloxacin increase plasma concentration of xanthines; rifampicin reduces plasma concentration of xanthines.

Anti-epileptics: carbamazepine, phenobarbitone <phenobarbital>, phenytoin, and primidone reduce plasma concentration of xanthines.

Calcium antagonists: diltiazem and verapamil increase plasma concentration of xanthines.

Cimetidine: increases plasma concentration of xanthines.

Disulfiram: increases plasma concentration of xanthines.

Fluvoxamine: increases plasma concentration of xanthines.

Oral contraceptives: increase plasma concentration of xanthines.

Sympathomimetics: salbutamol and terbutaline may reduce plasma concentration of potassium.

Xanthomax (Ashbourne Pharmaceuticals) *See* ALLOPURINOL.

Xatral, **Xatral SR** (Lorex Synthélabo) *See* ALFUZOSIN HYDROCHLORIDE.

Xenical (Roche Products) *See* ORLISTAT.

Xepin (Bioglan Laboratories) *See* DOXEPIN.

xipamide A thiazide-like diuretic (*see* THIAZIDE DIURETICS) used for the treatment of *hypertension and *oedema associated with heart failure, liver disease, or kidney disease. More potent than many of the thiazide diuretics, it is available as tablets on *prescription only.
Side effects, precautions, and interactions with other drugs: see THIAZIDE DIURETICS.
Proprietary preparation: Diurexan.
See also DIURETICS.

xylitol A sugar, obtained from birch and other trees, that increases the production of saliva and inhibits bacterial growth. It is used as a bulk sweetener in foods and a toothpaste and as a component of artificial salivas.
Proprietary preparations: ORALBALANCE (combined with oxidase enzymes); SALIVACE (combined with carboxymethylcellulose and electrolytes; SALIVA ORTHANA (combined with mucin).

Xylocaine (AstraZeneca) *See* LIGNOCAINE <LIDOCAINE>.

Xylocaine Antiseptic Gel (AstraZeneca) A proprietary combination of *lignocaine <lidocaine> (a local anaesthetic) and *chlorhexidine gluconate (an antiseptic), used for anaesthetizing and cleansing the urethra before examinations or minor surgical procedures are performed. It is available on *prescription only.
Side effects: see LIGNOCAINE <LIDOCAINE>.

Xylocard (AstraZeneca) *See* LIGNOCAINE <LIDOCAINE>.

xylometazoline A *sympathomimetic drug that stimulates alpha *adrenoceptors. It is used for the treatment of nasal congestion (*see* DECONGESTANTS) and is also used in combination with other drugs to treat allergic conjunctivitis. It is available from pharmacies without a *prescription in the form of a nasal spray or drops and eye drops.
Side effects: include nasal irritation, headache, and increased heart rate. Prolonged use may cause rebound congestion.

Precautions: xylometazoline should not be used during pregnancy. Prolonged use should be avoided.

Interactions with other drugs: *see* DECONGESTANTS.

Proprietary preparations: Nazo-Mist; Otrivine (adult nasal drops, children's nasal drops, and adult nasal spray); OTRIVINE-ANTISTIN (combined with antazoline sulphate); RESISTON ONE (combined with sodium cromoglycate <cromoglicate>); RYNACROM COMPOUND (combined with sodium cromoglycate <cromoglicate>).

Xyloproct (AstraZeneca) A proprietary combination of *zinc oxide and aluminium acetate (astringents), *lignocaine <lidocaine> (a local anaesthetic), and *hydrocortisone acetate (a corticosteroid), used to relieve the discomfort of *haemorrhoids, itching of the anus or vulva, and the pain of anal fissures. It is available as an ointment or suppositories on *prescription only.

Side effects: Xyloproct may cause dermatitis. *See also* CORTICOSTEROIDS.

Precautions: Xyloproct should not be used when viral or fungal infection is present; prolonged use should be avoided.

8Y (Bio Products Laboratory) *See* FACTOR VIII.

yellow soft paraffin (yellow petroleum jelly) A purified mixture of hydrocarbons obtained from petroleum. Semisolid, pale yellow to amber, and translucent, it is used as an *emollient and as a base for ointments. It is odourless when rubbed into the skin and not readily absorbed.
Side effects: very rarely it may cause allergic reactions or acne.
Proprietary preparations: EPADERM (combined with liquid paraffin and wax); GERMOLENE OINTMENT (combined with zinc oxide, octaphonium <octafonium> chloride, methyl salicylate, and other emollients).

Yomesan (Bayer) *See* NICLOSAMIDE.

Yutopar (Solvay Healthcare) *See* RITODRINE.

Z

Zacin (Bioglan Laboratories) *See* CAPSAICIN.

Zaditen (Novartis Pharmaceuticals) *See* KETOTIFEN.

Zaedoc (Ashbourne Pharmaceuticals) *See* RANITIDINE.

zafirlukast A *leukotriene receptor antagonist used for the treatment of mild to moderate asthma that is not adequately controlled by the usual combination of an inhaled *corticosteroid and a beta stimulant (such as *salbutamol). It should not be used to treat acute attacks. Zafirlukast is available as tablets on *prescription only.

Side effects: include abdominal pain, headache, allergic reactions (including rashes), and bronchial infections in the elderly.

Interactions with other drugs:
  Aspirin: increases the plasma concentration of zafirlukast.
  Erythromycin: reduces the plasma concentration of zafirlukast.
  Terfenadine: reduces the plasma concentration of zafirlukast.
  Theophylline: reduces the plasma concentration of zafirlukast; the plasma concentration of theophylline is increased by zafirlukast.
  Warfarin: its anticoagulant effect is increased by zafirlukast.

Proprietary preparation: Accolate.

zalcitabine An *antiviral drug that prevents retrovirus replication: it is a nucleoside analogue that inhibits reverse transcriptase. Zalcitabine is used to treat HIV infection in patients who cannot tolerate zidovudine or in whom zidovudine has failed. It is available as tablets on *prescription only.

Side effects: include damage to peripheral nerves (causing weakness and numbness in the limbs), pancreatitis, nausea, vomiting, diarrhoea, constipation, abdominal pain, mouth ulcers, pharyngitis, headache, dizziness, muscle and joint pains, rash, itching, weight loss, fatigue, fever, chest pain, and blood disorders.

Precautions: zalcitabine should not be taken by patients with disease of the peripheral nerves. It should be used with caution in people with kidney or liver disease, in those with a history of pancreatitis, alcohol abuse, or heart failure, and in women who are pregnant or breastfeeding.

Interactions with other drugs: zalcitabine should not be used with other drugs that have the potential to cause damage to peripheral nerves, specifically: chloramphenicol, cisplatin, dapsone, didanosine, disulfiram, ethionamide, glutethamide, gold salts, hydralazine, isoniazid, metronidazole, nitrofurantoin, phenytoin, ribavirin, and vincristine.

  Aminoglycosides: may increase the plasma concentration of zalcitabine.

Amphotericin: may increase the plasma concentration of zalcitabine.
Foscarnet: may increase the plasma concentration of zalcitabine.
Proprietary preparation: Hivid.

Zamadol, Zamadol SR (ASTA Medica) *See* TRAMADOL HYDROCHLORIDE.

Zanaflex (Elan Pharma) *See* TIZANIDINE.

Zanidip (Napp Pharmaceuticals) *See* LERCANIDIPINE.

Zantac (GlaxoWellcome) *See* RANITIDINE.

Zarontin (Parke-Davis Medical) *See* ETHOSUXIMIDE.

Zavedos (Pharmacia & Upjohn) *See* IDARUBICIN.

ZeaSORB (Stiefel Laboratories) A proprietary combination of aldioxa (aluminium dihydroxyallantoinate; an astringent), *chloroxylenol (an antiseptic), and powdered maize core. It is used as an antiperspirant dusting powder to prevent excessive sweating of the feet, hands, and armpits. ZeaSORB can be obtained without a prescription, but only from pharmacies.

Zelapar (Athena Neurosciences) *See* SELEGILINE.

Zemtard (Ashbourne Pharmaceuticals) *See* DILTIAZEM HYDROCHLORIDE.

Zenoxone (Biorex Laboratories) *See* HYDROCORTISONE.

Zerit (Bristol-Myers Squibb) *See* STAVUDINE.

Zestoretic (AstraZeneca) A proprietary combination of *lisinopril (an ACE inhibitor) and *hydrochlorothiazide (a thiazide diuretic), used in the treatment of mild to moderate *hypertension. A *prescription only medicine, it is available as tablets of two strengths: **Zestoretic 10** and **Zestoretic 20**.
Side effects, precautions, and interactions with other drugs: *see* ACE INHIBITORS; THIAZIDE DIURETICS.

Zestril (AstraZeneca) *See* LISINOPRIL.

Zida-Co (Opus) *See* CO-AMILOZIDE.

Zidoval (3M Health Care) *See* METRONIDAZOLE.

zidovudine (azidothymidine; AZT) An *antiviral drug that prevents retrovirus replication: it is a nucleoside analogue that inhibits reverse transcriptase. One of the oldest antiviral drugs, zidovudine is used, in combination with other antivirals, for the treatment of *HIV infection and to prevent transmission of HIV from mother to fetus. Zidovudine is available, on *prescription only, as capsules, a syrup, or a solution for injection.

Side effects: include anaemia, nausea and vomiting, loss of appetite, abdominal pain, indigestion, headache, rash, fever, aching muscles, pigmentation of the skin, nails, and mouth, and reduced production of white blood cells.

Precautions: zidovudine should not be given to people with severe anaemia or a very low white-blood-cell count; blood tests may be required during the first three months of treatment. It should be used with caution in those with kidney or liver disease and in pregnant women; breastfeeding is not recommended during treatment.

Interactions with other drugs:

Aciclovir: causes extreme lethargy.

Clarithromycin: reduces the absorption of zidovudine.

Ganciclovir: greatly reduces production of blood cells in the bone marrow.

Methadone: increases the plasma concentration (and therefore side effects) of zidovudine.

Phenytoin: the plasma concentration of phenytoin is altered.

Probenecid: increases the plasma concentration of zidovudine.

Proprietary preparations: Retrovir; COMBIVIR (combined with lamivudine).

Zileze (Opus) *See* ZOPICLONE.

Zimovane (Rhône-Poulenc Rorer) *See* ZOPICLONE.

Zinacef (GlaxoWellcome) *See* CEFUROXIME.

Zinamide (Merck Sharp & Dohme) *See* PYRAZINAMIDE.

zinc A metallic element required in minute amounts for the normal functioning of many enzymes in the body. Deficiency is rare with a balanced diet but it may occur in people with some forms of kidney disease or conditions in which absorption of food substances from the intestine is reduced or it may result from burns or trauma. Zinc deficiency can affect the skin, oesophagus (gullet), or eyes. It is treated with supplementary *zinc sulphate.

zinc oxide A soothing and protective agent that is mildly *astringent and used in the form of a cream, ointment, or dusting power to treat napkin rash, urine rashes, *eczema, *haemorrhoids, and mild skin abrasions. Creams and ointments often also contain *emollients, such as castor oil, arachis oil, and wool fat. Zinc oxide is also used as a paste in medicated bandages to treat leg ulcers. Combined with *coal tar or *ichthammol, it is used as a paste to treat *psoriasis or eczema. Zinc oxide reflects sunlight and is therefore included in some *sunscreen preparations. Zinc oxide can be obtained without a prescription but some compound preparations are *prescription only medicines.

Proprietary preparations: ANUGESIC-HC (combined with pramoxine <pramocaine> hydrochloride, hydrocortisone acetate, benzyl benzoate, Peru balsam, and bismuth oxide); ANUGESIC-HC SUPPOSITORIES (combined with pramoxine <pramocaine> hydrochloride, hydrocortisone acetate, benzyl benzoate, bismuth oxide, and bismuth subgallate); ANUSOL (combined with bismuth oxide, bismuth subgallate, and Peru balsam); ANUSOL-HC (combined with bismuth oxide, bismuth subgallate, Peru balsam, benzyl benzoate, and hydrocortisone acetate); BOOTS HAEMORRHOID OINTMENT (combined with lignocaine <lidocaine>); BOOTS SUPPOSITORIES FOR HAEMORRHOIDS (combined with benzyl alcohol, glycol monosalicylate, and methyl salicylate); E45 WASH CREAM (combined with light liquid paraffin); GERMOLENE OINTMENT (combined with methyl salicylate, octaphonium <octafonium> chloride, phenol, and emollients); GERMOLOIDS (combined with lignocaine <lidocaine>); HEMOCANE (combined with benzoic acid, cinnamic acid, and lignocaine <lidocaine>); HEWLETTS CREAM (combined with white soft paraffin); MORHULIN (combined with cod liver oil); SUDOCREM (combined with anhydrous lanolin, benzyl benzoate, benzyl cinnamate, and benzyl alcohol); SUN E45 (combined with titanium dioxide); VASOGEN CREAM (combined with calamine and dimethicone <dimeticone>); XYLOPROCT (combined with lignocaine <lidocaine>, aluminium acetate, and hydrocortisone).

zinc sulphate A salt of zinc used as an oral supplement for treating *zinc deficiency. It is also used as an *astringent for the treatment of excessive tear production or watery eyes. Zinc sulphate is available as effervescent tablets, *modified-release capsules, or eye drops and can be obtained without a prescription, but only from pharmacies.

Side effects: oral preparations may cause abdominal pain and indigestion.

Precautions: oral zinc sulphate should be used with caution by people with kidney disease.

Interactions with other drugs (oral preparations):

Iron supplements: reduce the absorption of zinc and their own absorption is reduced by zinc.

Penicillamine: its absorption is reduced.

Quinolone antibiotics: the absorption of ciprofloxacin and norfloxacin is reduced.

Tetracyclines: reduce the absorption of zinc and their own absorption is reduced by zinc.

Proprietary preparations: Solvazinc (tablets); Z Span Spansules (modified-release capsules); DENCYL (combined with ferrous sulphate and folic acid); DITEMIC (combined with ferrous sulphate and B vitamins); FESOVIT Z (combined with ferrous sulphate and vitamins B and C).

zinc undecenoate *See* UNDECENOIC ACID.

Zineryt (Yamanouchi Pharma) A proprietary combination of *erythromycin (a macrolide antibiotic) and zinc acetate (an *astringent), used for the treatment of *acne. It is available as a solution for topical application on *prescription only.

Side effects: local irritation may occur.

Precautions: when applying the solution, care should be taken to avoid the eyes and mucous membranes.

Interactions with other drugs: *see* ERYTHROMYCIN.

Zinga (Ashbourne Pharmaceuticals) *See* NIZATIDINE.

Zinnat (GlaxoWellcome) *See* CEFUROXIME.

Zirtek (UCB Pharma) *See* CETIRIZINE HYDROCHLORIDE.

Zispin (Organon Laboratories) *See* MIRTAZAPINE.

Zita (Eastern Pharmaceuticals) *See* CIMETIDINE.

Zithromax (Pfizer) *See* AZITHROMYCIN.

Zocor (Merck Sharp & Dohme) *See* SIMVASTATIN.

Zofran (GlaxoWellcome) *See* ONDANSETRON.

Zoladex (AstraZeneca) *See* GOSERELIN.

Zoleptil (Orion Pharma) *See* ZOTEPINE.

Zollinger-Ellison syndrome *See* ACID-PEPTIC DISEASES.

zolmitriptan A *5HT$_1$ agonist used for treating acute attacks of *migraine. A single dose can relieve a migraine headache at any stage of the attack. Zolmitriptan is available as tablets on *prescription only.

Side effects: include sensations of heat, heaviness, pressure, tingling or tightness; if tightness in the chest or throat is severe, treatment should be stopped. Other side effects may include drowsiness, an increase in blood pressure (which does not last), and (rarely) dry mouth and muscle weakness.

Precautions: zolmitriptan should not be taken for 12 hours before or after taking other 5HT$_1$ agonists. It should not be taken by people who have previously had a heart attack or who have uncontrolled high blood pressure or certain heart conditions. Zolmitriptan should be used with caution in people with liver disease and in women who are pregnant or breastfeeding.

Interactions with other drugs:

Ergotamine: the risk of spasm of the blood vessels, which can have serious consequences, is increased if ergotamine is taken with zolmitriptan. Ergotamine should not be taken for six hours after taking zolmitriptan, and zolmitriptan should not be taken for six hours after taking ergotamine.

Fluvoxamine: this antidepressant may enhance the effects of zolmitriptan, whose dosage should therefore be reduced.

Moclobemide: the dosage of zolmitriptan should be reduced if it is taken with this MAOI (an antidepressant) to avoid the risk of adverse effects on the central nervous system.

Proprietary preparation: Zomig.

zolpidem tartrate A short-acting drug that is used for the short-term treatment of insomnia (*see* HYPNOTIC DRUGS). It acts in the same way as *benzodiazepines, but takes a shorter time to act and has little or no hangover effect. Zolpidem is available as tablets on *prescription only.

Side effects: include diarrhoea, nausea, vomiting, vertigo, dizziness, headache, daytime drowsiness, memory disturbances, and nightmares. *Dependence can occur with prolonged use.

Precautions: zolpidem should not be taken by people with obstructive sleep apnoea (in which airflow from the nose to the lungs is obstructed during sleep), myasthenia gravis, or severe liver or lung disease, or by women who are pregnant or breastfeeding. It should be used with caution by people with a history of drug abuse or depression. *See also* HYPNOTIC DRUGS.

Interactions with other drugs: the sedative effects of zolpidem are increased by a number of drugs, including anaesthetics, opioid analgesics, antidepressants, antihistamines, antipsychotics, and most importantly by ritonavir, which increases the plasma concentration of zolpidem, causing profound sedation; these two drugs should therefore not be taken together.

Proprietary preparation: Stilnoct.

Zomacton (Ferring Pharmaceuticals) *See* SOMATROPIN.

Zomig (AstraZeneca) *See* ZOLMITRIPTAN.

Zomorph (Link Pharmaceuticals) *See* MORPHINE.

Zonivent (Ashbourne Pharmaceuticals) *See* BECLOMETHASONE <BECLOMETASONE> DIPROPIONATE.

zopiclone A short-acting drug that is used for the short-term treatment of insomnia (*see* HYPNOTIC DRUGS). It acts in the same way as *benzodiazepines, but takes a shorter time to act and has little or no hangover effect. Zopiclone is available as tablets on *prescription only.

Side effects: include a bitter or metallic taste, diarrhoea, nausea, vomiting, vertigo, dizziness, headache, irritability, confusion, daytime drowsiness, memory disturbances, and nightmares. *Dependence can occur with prolonged use.

Precautions: zopiclone should not be taken by people with depressed breathing, severe obstructive sleep apnoea (in which the airflow from mouth to lungs is obstructed during sleep), myasthenia gravis, or severe liver disease, or by women who are pregnant or breastfeeding. It should be used with caution by people with a history of drug abuse or depression. *See also* HYPNOTIC DRUGS.

Interactions with other drugs: the sedative effects of zopiclone are enhanced by a number of other drugs, including anaesthetics, opioid analgesics, antidepressants, antihistamines, and antipsychotic drugs, and importantly:

Erythromycin: inhibits the metabolism of zopiclone, which increases its sedative effects.

Ritonavir: may increase the plasma concentration of zopiclone, enhancing its sedative effects.

Proprietary preparations: Zileze; Zimovane.

Zorac (Allergan) *See* TAZAROTENE.

zotepine An atypical *antipsychotic drug used for the treatment of schizophrenia. It is available as tablets on *prescription only.

Side effects: include weight gain, dizziness, low blood pressure on standing (which can cause fainting in some people), constipation, indigestion, dry mouth, a fast heart rate, headache, insomnia, drowsiness, and fever. Zotepine may also prolong a certain phase of the heartbeat (the QT interval) and cause blood disorders.

Precautions: zotepine should not be given to those suffering from acute gout, to people who have had kidney stones, or to women who are breastfeeding. It should be used with caution in people with cardiovascular disease, a history of epilepsy or Parkinson's disease, liver or kidney disease, an enlarged prostate gland, or acute glaucoma, and in pregnant women. It should also be used with care in people taking other drugs that prolong the QT interval (since this may give rise to *arrhythmias; see below) or that cause loss of potassium (such as some diuretics).

Interactions with other drugs:

Anaesthetics: their effect in lowering blood pressure is increased.

Anti-arrhythmic drugs: there is an increased risk of arrhythmias if these drugs are taken with zotepine.

Antidepressant drugs: there is an increased risk of arrhythmias if zotepine is taken with tricyclic antidepressants; fluoxetine increases the plasma concentration of zotepine.

Antiepileptic drugs: zotepine antagonizes the effects of these drugs in controlling seizures.

Antihistamines: there is an increased risk of arrhythmias if zotepine is taken with astemizole or terfenadine.

Halofantrine: there is an increased risk of arrhythmias if this drug is taken with zotepine.

Ritonavir: may increase the effects of zotepine.

Sedatives: the sedative effects of zotepine are increased if it is taken with anxiolytic or hypnotic drugs; diazepam increases the plasma concentration of zotepine.

Proprietary preparation: Zoleptil.

Zoton (Wyeth Laboratories) *See* LANSOPRAZOLE.

Zovirax (GlaxoWellcome) *See* ACICLOVIR.

Zoxin (Opus) *See* FLUCLOXACILLIN.

Z Span Spansules (Goldshield Pharmaceuticals) *See* ZINC SULPHATE.

zuclopenthixol A thioxanthene *antipsychotic drug. **Zuclopenthixol dihydrochloride** is used for the treatment of schizophrenia and other psychoses, especially in patients who are agitated, hostile, or aggressive (it should not be given to patients who are apathetic or withdrawn); **zuclopenthixol decanoate** is given by <depot injection> for the maintenance treatment of such patients. **Zuclopenthixol acetate** is given by injection for the short-term treatment of acute psychosis, mania, or exacerbations of chronic psychosis; it is used to stabilize patients and treatment should not last longer than two weeks. Zuclopenthixol is available, on prescription only, as tablets or injections.

Side effects and precautions: *see* CHLORPROMAZINE HYDROCHLORIDE.

Interactions with other drugs:

Anaesthetics: their effect in lowering blood pressure is enhanced.

Antidepressants: there is an increased risk of antimuscarinic effects and arrhythmias if zuclopenthixol is taken with tricyclic antidepressants.

Antiepileptic drugs: their anticonvulsant effects are antagonized by zuclopenthixol.

Antihistamines: there is an increased risk of arrhythmias if zuclopenthixol is taken with astemizole or terfenadine.

Halofantrine: there is an increased risk of arrhythmias if this drug is taken with zuclopenthixol.

Ritonavir: may increase the effects of zuclopenthixol.

Sedatives: the sedative effects of zuclopenthixol are increased if it is taken with anxiolytic or hypnotic drugs, or any other sedating drug.

Proprietary preparations: Clopixol (tablets or depot injection); Clopixol Acuphase (injection); Clopixol Conc. (depot injection).

Zumenon (Solvay Healthcare) *See* OESTRADIOL <ESTRADIOL>; HORMONE REPLACEMENT THERAPY.

Zydol, Zydol SR (Searle) *See* TRAMADOL HYDROCHLORIDE.

Zyloric (GlaxoWellcome) *See* ALLOPURINOL.

Zyprexa (Eli Lilly & Co) *See* OLANZAPINE.

APPENDIX

Some proprietary preparations containing aspirin and/or paracetamol

Preparation	Active ingredients	Form
Alka-Seltzer	aspirin	effervescent tablets
Alka-Seltzer XS	aspirin, caffeine, paracetamol	effervescent tablets
Alvedon	paracetamol	suppositories
Anadin	aspirin, caffeine	tablets
Anadin Extra, Anadin Extra Soluble	aspirin, caffeine, paracetamol	tablets, soluble tablets
Anadin Maximum Strength	aspirin, caffeine	capsules
Anadin Paracetamol	paracetamol	tablets
Angettes 75	aspirin	tablets (75 mg antiplatelet)
Askit	aspirin, aloxiprin, caffeine	capsules, powders
*Aspav	aspirin, papaveretum	dispersible tablets
Aspro, Aspro Clear, Maximum Strength Aspro Clear	aspirin	tablets, soluble tablets
Bayer Aspirin	aspirin	tablets
Beechams All-in-One	paracetamol, guaiphenesin, phenylephrine	liquid
Beechams Flu-Plus Hot Lemon, Beechams Flu-Plus Hot Berry Fruits	paracetamol, phenylephrine	powders
Beechams Flu-Plus Caplets	paracetamol, caffeine, phenylephrine	tablets
Beechams Lemon Tablets	aspirin	tablets
Beechams Powders	aspirin, caffeine	powders
Beechams Powders Capsules	paracetamol, caffeine, phenylephrine	capsules
Beechams Warmers	paracetamol, phenylephrine	powders
Benoral	aspirin, paracetamol [benorylate]	tablets, granules, suspension
Benylin 4 Flu	paracetamol, diphenhydramine, pseudoephedrine	tablets, liquid
Boots Children's Pain Relief Syrup	paracetamol	liquid
Boots Pain Relief Extra Caplets, Boots Pain Relief Extra Soluble	paracetamol, caffeine	tablets, soluble tablets
Boots Infant Pain Relief	paracetamol	oral suspension

Preparation	Active ingredients	Form
Calpol Infant, Calpol 6 Plus, Calpol Paediatric	paracetamol	oral suspensions
Caprin	aspirin	enteric-coated tablets (75 mg antiplatelet; 300 mg standard)
Catarrh-Ex	paracetamol, caffeine, phenylephrine	capsules
Codis 500	aspirin, codeine	dispersible tablets
Coldrex Tablets	paracetamol, caffeine, phenylephrine	tablets
Day Nurse	paracetamol, dextromethorphan, phenylpropanolamine	capsules, liquid
De Witt's Analgesic Pills	paracetamol, caffeine	tablets
Disprin, Disprin Direct	aspirin	dispersible tablets
Disprin CV	aspirin	modified-release tablets (100 mg antiplatelet)
Disprin Extra	aspirin, paracetamol	soluble tablets
Disprol Paediatric Suspension	paracetamol	sugar-free suspension for children
Disprol Soluble Paracetamol Tablets	paracetamol	dispersible tablets for children
*Distalgesic	paracetamol, dextropropoxyphene [co-proxamol]	tablets
Dristan Decongestant Tablets	aspirin, caffeine, chlorpheniramine, phenylephrine	tablets
Fanalgic	paracetamol	tablets, capsules
Femigraine	aspirin, cyclizine	effervescent tablets
Feminax	paracetamol, caffeine, codeine, hyoscine	tablets
Fennings Children's Cooling Powders	paracetamol	powders
†Fortagesic	paracetamol, pentazocine	tablets
Fynnon Calcium Aspirin	aspirin	tablets
Hedex Caplets	paracetamol	tablets
Hedex Extra	paracetamol, caffeine	tablets
Infadrops	paracetamol	drops
Lemsip Cold + Flu Combined Relief Capsules	paracetamol, caffeine, phenylephrine	capsules
Lemsip Cold + Flu Original Lemon	paracetamol, phenylephrine, vitamin C	powders
Medinol Over 6	paracetamol	oral suspension for children

Preparation	Active ingredients	Form
Medinol Paediatric	paracetamol	sugar-free suspension for children
Medised	paracetamol, promethazine	liquid (standard or sugar-free)
Migraleve	paracetamol, codeine, buclizine,	tablets (pink)
	paracetamol, codeine	tablets (yellow)
Mu-Cron Tablets	paracetamol, phenylpropanolamine	tablets
Night Nurse	paracetamol, dextromethorphan, promethazine	capsules, liquid
Nurse Sykes Powders	aspirin, caffeine, paracetamol	powders
Nu-Seals Aspirin	aspirin	enteric-coated tablets (75 mg antiplatelet; 300 mg standard)
Paldesic	paracetamol	suspension for children
*Panadeine	paracetamol, codeine [co-codamol]	effervescent or dispersible tablets
Panadol, Panadol Soluble	paracetamol	capsules, tablets, soluble tablets
Panadol Baby and Infant	paracetamol	sugar-free suspension
Panadol Extra	paracetamol, caffeine	tablets, soluble tablets
Panadol Junior	paracetamol	powder
Panadol Ultra	paracetamol, codeine	tablets
Panaleve Junior	paracetamol	syrup
Panaleve 6+	paracetamol	suspension for children
Paracets	paracetamol	tablets, capsules
Paraclear	paracetamol	soluble tablets, plain tablets
Paraclear Extra Strength	paracetamol, caffeine	tablets
*Paracodol	paracetamol, codeine [co-codamol]	capsules
Paradote	paracetamol, co-methiamol	tablets
Paramin	paracetamol	capsules
Paramol	paracetamol, dihydrocodeine	tablets
Phensic	aspirin, caffeine	tablets
Placidex	paracetamol	syrup
PostMI 75EC	aspirin	enteric-coated tablets (75 mg antiplatelet)
Powerin	aspirin, caffeine, paracetamol	tablets
Propain	paracetamol, caffeine, codeine, diphenhydramine	tablets
Resolve	paracetamol	powder
*Remedeine	paracetamol, dihydrocodeine	tablets, effervescent tablets

Preparation	Active ingredients	Form
Salzone	paracetamol	suspension for children
Sinutab	paracetamol, phenylpropanolamine	tablets
Sinutab Night-time	paracetamol, phenylpropanolamine, phenyltoloxamine	tablets
Solpadeine	paracetamol, caffeine, codeine	tablets, souble tablets, capsules
*Solpadol	paracetamol, codeine [co-codamol]	tablets, effervescent tablets
Sudafed-Co	paracetamol, pseudoephedrine	tablets
Syndol	paracetamol, caffeine, codeine	tablets
Toptabs	aspirin, caffeine	tablets
Tramil 500	paracetamol	capsules
Triogesic	paracetamol, phenylpropanolamine	tablets
*Tylex	paracetamol, codeine [co-codamol]	capsules, effervescent tablets
Veganin	aspirin, paracetamol, codeine	tablets
Vick's Coldcare	paracetamol, dextromethorphan, phenylpropanolamine	capsules
Vick's Medinite	paracetamol, dextromethorphan, doxylamine, ephedrine	syrup

* prescription only medicine
† controlled drug